# THE TOBACCO BOOK

A Reference Guide of Facts, Figures, and Quotations about Tobacco

by

## David B. Moyer, M.D.

SUNSTONE
PRESS

SANTA FE

Sunstone books may be purchased for educational, business, or sales promotional use. For information please write: Special Markets Department, Sunstone Press, P.O. Box 2321, Santa Fe, New Mexico 87504-2321.

---

Library of Congress Cataloging-in-Publication Data:

Moyer, David B., 1946-
    The Tobacco book: a reference guide of facts, figures, and quotations about tobacco / by David B. Moyer.
        p.cm
"A new edition of the 2000 book The tobacco reference guide"—Pref.
Includes bibliographical references and index.
        ISBN: 0-86534-382-9 (pbk.)
1. Tobacco habit. 2. Tobacco habit—Statistics. 3. Tobacco habit—United States. 4. Tobacco industry—United States. 5. Smoking.
I. Moyer, David B., 1946-Tobacco reference guide. II. Title.
YV5735.M68 2004
362.29'6—dc22

                2004003575

---

**WWW.SUNSTONEPRESS.COM**
SUNSTONE PRESS / POST OFFICE BOX 2321 / SANTA FE, NM 87504-2321 /USA
(505) 988-4418 / *ORDERS ONLY* (800) 243-5644 / FAX (505) 988-1025

# Contents

## REFERENCE ABBREVATIONS

ANR        Americans for Nonsmokers' Right

ASH        Action on Smoking and Health

JAMA     Journal of the American Medical Association

NEJM     New England Journal of Medicine

SCARC...Smoking Control Advocacy Resource Center

# Preface

The data in this book has been compiled from medical and media sources, and are represented as reported, although I make no claim for their accuracy. This project was completed as a resource for the tobacco control community, and funding for publication was provided by the Luther Terry Foundation. I would like to express my appreciation to Kathy Jacobs for her excellent computer and desktop publishing skills in the production of the book.

"It is now proved beyond doubt that smoking is one of the leading causes of statistics."
—Fletcher Krebel, Reader's Digest, December 1961

# CHAPTER 1
# SCOPE OF THE PROBLEM AND OVERALL DEATH AND DISABILITY

1.  "Tobacco is the single, chief, avoidable cause of death in our society, and the most important public health issue of our time."          C. Everett Koop, M.D. Preface to the 1982 Surgeon General report
    *The Health Consequences of Smoking--Cancer*

2.  "Smoking represents the most extensively documented cause of disease ever investigated in the history of biomedical research."          Antonia Novello, preface to 1990 Surgeon General report

3.  There have been more than 60,000 studies in the medical literature linking tobacco use and disease.
    *Tobacco Use*, p. iii

4.  Tobacco accounted for 2.6% of the worldwide burden of disease in 1990; by 2020, that figure will grow to 9%.
    Washington Post National Weekly Edition, April 13, 1998 (World Health Organization data)

5.  10 million Americans have died from tobacco in the last 30 years.          Frontline, PBS television, May 1998

6.  Among current cigarette smokers, 52% of deaths from all causes in men and 43% in women are attributable to cigarette smoking.          *Changes in Cigarette-Related Disease Risks*, p. 405

7.  There are more deaths from tobacco every six weeks than there were Americans killed in the entire Vietnam war.

8.  Total AIDS cases in the US from 1981 through October 1995 were 494,493 adults and adolescents and 6817 children. Total AIDS deaths in this fourteen-year period were 311,381, equal to about nine months of deaths caused by tobacco.          US News and World Report, January 8, 1996, p. 16

9.  Deaths from AIDS in the United States peaked at 43,115 in 1995, and declined to 31,130 in 1996 and 16,685 in 1997.          New York Times, October 8, 1998

10. Deaths caused by smoking in developed countries from 1950 to 2000 will total an estimated 52 million men (20% of the total deaths) and 10.5 million women (4% of all deaths of women in this time period).
    *Tobacco or Health: A Global Status Report*, 1997, p. 44

11. Annual tobacco–attributable mortality is expected to increase from three million deaths in 1990 to 8.4 million in 2020, with almost all of this annual increase (4.7 million out of 5.4 million deaths) expected to occur in developing countries.          *The Global Burden of Disease*, Christopher Murray and Alan Lopez, Harvard University Press, 1996, p. 317

12. The 434,000 Americans who die from smoking each year exceed the combined total of deaths from car accidents, plane crashes, homicide, suicide, AIDS, alcohol, and drug abuse.          *Saving Lives and Raising Revenue*
    Coalition on Smoking or Health, February 1995

13. Tobacco kills more Americans every year and a half than have all the wars of this century.

14. Total war deaths for the US are: Vietnam, 58,167; Korea, 43,891; World War II, 405,399; World I, 116,516; and the Civil War, 624,511.          From *Gettysburg*, Mort Kunstler, Turner, 1992

15. Cigarette smoking accounts for 30% of all deaths in adults in the District of Columbia. Among black men, 40% of the deaths are attributable to smoking.          Journal of the National Medical Association 1989; 81:1125

16. Tobacco is responsible for 19.4% of all the deaths in the United States, or 1147 deaths each day.
    Tobacco Control, Fall 1994, p. 196

17. Tobacco control has had the dismal luxury of unimaginably "great" statistics to make its case. Globally, an estimated four million people die each year from tobacco related illness, compared to 2.7 million from malaria, and 2.8 million from AIDS. After deaths from malnutrition (5.9 million in 1990) and violence and injury (5.8 million), tobacco claims more deaths than any other single cause. Between 1950 and 2000, it was estimated that smoking caused about 62 million deaths in developed countries (12.5 % of all deaths: 20% of male deaths and 4% of female deaths). More than half of these deaths (38 million) will have occurred at ages 35-69 years. Currently, smoking is the cause of more than one in three (36%) male deaths in middle age, and about one in eight (13%) of female deaths. Each smoker who dies in this age group loses, on average, 22 years of life compared with average life expectancy. By 2020, the World Health Organization estimates that "the burden of disease attributable to tobacco will outweigh that caused by any single disease". One person dies every 8 seconds from smoking.

Tobacco Control, March 2002, p.1 (quote)

18. During 1995-1999, a total of 442,398 persons in the United States died prematurely each year as a result of smoking. This number reflects the inclusion of 35,053 secondhand smoking-attributable heart disease deaths. Deaths attributable to cigar smoking, pipe smoking, and smokeless tobacco use were not included.

JAMA, May 8, 2002, p. 2356

19. If present smoking patterns persist, there will be one billion deaths from tobacco in the 21$^{st}$ century, compared with 100 million in the past century. There are 1.1 billion smokers at present and by 2030, about another billion people will become smokers. If present trends hold, about 15% of all adult deaths worldwide in the second half of the 21$^{st}$ century will be due to tobacco.

Tobacco Control, March 2002

20. The 434,000 tobacco-related deaths in 1988 in the United States included 198,000 from cardiovascular disease (including 26,000 from stroke), 112,000 from lung cancer, 31,000 from other cancers, 83,000 from emphysema and related disease, and 1300 burn deaths from fires caused by smoking.

Morbidity and Mortality Weekly Report 1991; 40:62

21. 1991 tobacco deaths were 491,000, including 195,000 from heart disease, stroke, and vascular disease, 157,000 from cancer, 83,000 from pulmonary disease, 53,000 from passive smoking, and 3500 from burns and pediatric diseases.

Archives of Family Medicine, September 1992, p. 129

22. At present smoking rates, at least 5 million American children, none of whom yet smoke, will eventually die from tobacco-induced disease. Worldwide, 200 million children now alive will die from disease caused by tobacco.

World Health Organization and Antonia Novello, M.D.

23. The number of US tobacco-related deaths each year equals the number of American troops stationed in Saudi Arabia in February 1991 at the peak of the Desert Shield/Desert Storm buildup.

24. The number of deaths caused by tobacco in the decade of the 1990s in the United States will exceed the current combined populations of the cities of Washington, D.C., Boston, San Francisco, Denver, Minneapolis, Seattle, Miami, Atlanta, and Kansas City.

Preventive Medicine 1993, 22:514

25. The yearly death toll from tobacco in the United States is equal to the disappearance of a city the size of Denver, Seattle, or Miami.

26. The number of deaths that will be caused by tobacco in the decade of the 1990's in the United States, about 4.5 million, is greater than the current population of 35 of the 50 states.

San Francisco Chronicle, November 10, 1993

27. Annual deaths from avoidable causes: smokers from smoking, 434,000; alcohol (including drunk driving), 105,000; nonsmokers from second-hand smoke, 53,000; car accidents, 50,000; AIDS, 31,000; firearms, 35,000; homicide, 22,000; and illicit drugs, 20,000.

*Saving Lives and Raising Revenue*, Coalition on Smoking or Health, February 1995

28. "While Americans recognize smoking as hazardous to health, they greatly underestimate the dangers of smoking, both in absolute terms and relative to other health hazards."

    American Journal of Public Health, July 1991, p. 841 (Kenneth Warner)

29. Every ton of tobacco consumed results in approximately one death (it may be closer to 1.3). One in eight deaths in less developed countries is caused by tobacco, one in four in developed countries, and one in six for the world as a whole.

    Tobacco Control, Winter 1994, p. 359

30. Each ton of tobacco produces one million cigarettes, which eventually leads to one death.

    World Health Organization

31. The World Health Organization estimates that at least 750 million people worldwide will have their lives substantially shortened by the use of cigarettes.

    Western Journal of Medicine, June 1994, p. 552

32. Smoking kills 17 times more people each year than are victims of homicide, and 50 times more than die from illegal drugs.

    Mother Jones magazine, May-June 1996, p. 69

33. Nicotine dependence causes 70 times more deaths in the United States than all other types of drug dependence combined.

    JAMA, February 23, 1994, p. 585

34. Tobacco use, passive smoke exposure, and fires caused by cigarettes were responsible for the deaths of five million Americans in the decade of the 1980's.

    New York Times, October 25, 1996, p. A39

35. "To the most fearsome plagues devastating humanity during this millennium—the Black Death, smallpox, malaria, yellow fever, Asiatic cholera, and tuberculosis—is now added the manmade plague: tobaccosis, the foremost scourge of the twentieth century."Population and Development Review, June 1990, p. 213 (R.T. Ravenholt)

36. In 1997, Life magazine ranked the global spread of smoking as number 54 in the magazine's list of the 100 most important events of the last 1000 years of human history.

    *Nicotine and Public Health*, p. 10

37. In 2030, one third of deaths in adults worldwide will be from tobacco, compared to one in six in 2000, and 70% of these will be in developing countries.

    11th World Conference on Tobacco and Health, Chicago, 2000

38. There is one death from tobacco every 8 seconds, or 4 million deaths worldwide each year.

    CBS news, May 31, 2000

39. Smoking causes an average man to lose more than 13 years of life, and an average woman to lose 14.5 years.

    Morbidity and Mortality Weekly Report, April 12, 2002

40. A 2002 World Health Organization report ranks the major threats to health worldwide. In developed (high-income) countries, the top-ranked health risk is tobacco, accounting for 12.2% of "lost healthy years" in the population, followed by high blood pressure (10.9%), alcohol (9.2%), high cholesterol (7.6%), and obesity (7.4%). In developing countries with low mortality, tobacco (4.0%) ranks third behind alcohol and hypertension, and in developing countries with high mortality, it accounts for only 2.0% of lost healthy years (compared to 14.9% for underweight and 10.2% for unsafe sex).

    Associated Press, October 31, 2002

41. A 2002 World Health Organization report concluded that 47% of premature deaths in the world could be averted if 20 hazards to health, ranging from unsafe sex to zinc deficiency, could be eliminated. In developed countries, tobacco is the leading risk factor, 12.2%, in percentage of lost years of healthy life attributable to 10 leading selected risk factors. (This is followed by blood pressure, 10.9%, alcohol, 9.2%, cholesterol, 7.6%, overweight, 7.4%, and physical activity, 3.3%). In high-mortality developing countries, the leading risk factors are underweight, unsafe sex, unsafe water, and indoor smoke from cooking, with tobacco ninth at 2%. In low-mortality developing countries tobacco is third (4%) in percentage of lost years of healthy life, behind alcohol (6.2%) and blood pressure (5%).

    Washington Post National Weekly Edition, November 11-17, 2002, p. 35

42. Within 25 years, illnesses caused by tobacco are expected to surpass infectious diseases as the single leading threat to human health worldwide.                                          World Watch, July-August 1997, p. 19

43. "In the United States during this century alone, the smoking of 26 trillion cigarettes and 556 billion cigars and the consumption of 25 billion pounds of 'manufactured tobacco' (pipe tobacco, chewing tobacco, and snuff) have produced more than 2.7 million deaths from lung cancer; more than 7 million deaths from cardiovascular disease; and more than 14 million deaths from all forms of tobaccosis."
                                          Population and Development Review, June 1990, p. 237 (R.T. Ravenholt)

44. The global death toll from tobacco in the 20th century will be about 100 million, a number roughly equal to the global death toll from all the international wars over the same period.
                                          San Francisco Chronicle, September 1, 1996, p. 4

45. Every day in the United States, nearly 5000 people who smoke either quit or die.
                                          Journal of Pediatrics, April 1997, p. 518

46. An estimated 25 million Americans alive today will die prematurely from smoking-related illnesses.
                                          Morbidity and Mortality Weekly Report, May 23, 1997, p. 449

47. In the U.S., tobacco is the cause of one third of all deaths in people under age 70.        Reuters, September 7, 1998

48. Deaths in the Hiroshima bombing, 140,000, are less than one third of the yearly US tobacco-induced deaths.
                                          San Francisco Chronicle, August 6, 1994, p. A14

49. Worldwide, unless many adult smokers stop, there will be 100 million deaths from smoking in the next 20 years. In China alone, one third of all males now ages 2 to 29 will be killed by tobacco at present smoking rates. This is 100 million out of this group of 340 million males, or 3 million each year eventually.
                                          10Th World Conference on Tobacco or Health, Beijing 1997 (Richard Peto)

50. 40% of total mortality is related to lifestyle issues. Tobacco is responsible for 20%, poor diet and sedentary lifestyle accounts for 15%, and alcohol causes 5%.
                                          R. Taylor Hays, M.D., Mayo Clinic Nicotine Dependence Center conference, May 12, 1997

51. Causes of premature death in the United States include tobacco 38%; obesity, diet, and sedentary life style, 28% (300,000 deaths per year); alcohol, 10%; infections, 8%; toxins, 6%; firearms, 4%; sexually transmitted disease, 2%; motor vehicle accidents, 2%; and, illicit drugs, 2%. Overall, unhealthy lifestyles account for 48% of premature mortality.                              Centers for Disease Control data presented at Navy Healthy Lifestyle
                                          Symposium, Pensacola, Florida, September 17, 1997 (Rob Brawley)

52. The following conditions and outcomes in the United States could be avoided each year if pregnant women and their partners did not smoke:
    19,000 to 141,000 spontaneous abortions
    32,000 to 61,000 infants with low birth weight
    14,000 to 26,000 infants admitted to the neonatal intensive care unit
    1900 to 4800 infant deaths as a result of various perinatal disorders
    1200 to 2200 infant deaths from SIDS.            Journal of Family Practice, Vol. 40, 1995, pp. 1-10 (Joe DiFranza)

53. Smoking kills one in 10 adults worldwide. By the year 2030 the proportion will be one in six, or 10 million deaths per year, more than any other single cause.                                          *Curbing the Epidemic*, p. 1

54. At current smoking prevalence rates, it is estimated that by 2025, tobacco use will account for 9% of the world's total death and disability, triple the current share.                              JAMA, October 6, 1999, p. 1284

55. Tobacco is responsible for 24% of adult deaths in North America.
                                          Journal of the National Cancer Institute, January 2003, p. 12

56.  Tobacco accounts for 9% of the total global burden of disease, and is responsible for 4.9 million deaths a year.

Dean Edell, M.D., ABC radio, March 19, 2003 (rebroadcast)

57.  There will be 150 million tobacco deaths in the first quarter of this century.

Tobacco Control, December 2002, p. 289

58.  Each day, 80,000 to 100,000 young people around the world become addicted to tobacco.

British Medical Association (www.tobaccofactfile.org)

59.  On a global basis, tobacco accounts for 71% of all drug-related premature deaths. Alcohol is responsible for 26% of these deaths, and all illicit drugs combined cause only 3% of drug-related deaths.

Dean Edell, M.D. , ABC radio, March 19, 2003
rebroadcast, and Reuters, February 25, 2003

JAMA: Journal of the American Medical Association
NEJM: New England Journal of Medicine

# CHAPTER 2
# DEMOGRAPHICS OF TOBACCO USE

1.  The World Health Organization estimates that 500 million of the 5.3 billion people populating the earth in 1990 will die from disease caused by tobacco.                    British Medical Journal, September 28, 1991, p. 732

2.  The World Health Organization estimates that unless present trends change, 200 to 250 million of the world's children, none of whom yet smoke, will eventually die from smoking-induced disease. Two thirds of these are from developing countries, and each will lose an average of 20 years of life.

3.  About a third of the global population age 15 and older are smokers, 1.1 billion people in all. 800 million of these are in developing countries, and most of these smokers in developing countries are men (700 out of 800 million).                    *Tobacco or Health: A Global Status Report*, 1997, p. 12

4.  There are 1.1 billion smokers in the world, 300 million in developed or "rich" countries and 800 million in the developing world. Of the total, 900 million are males and 200 million are females.
                    9th World Conference on Tobacco or Health, Paris, 1994 (Alan Lopez)

5.  Globally, about 47% of men and 12% of women smoke. The figures are 42% for men and 24% for women in the developed countries, compared to 48% of men and 7% of women in the developing countries. The global per capita yearly cigarette consumption is 1640.                    *Tobacco or Health: A Global Status Report*, 1997, p. 12,
                    and 9th World Conference on Tobacco or Health, Paris, 1994 (Alan Lopez)

6.  Smoking has been declining by about one percent per year in the United States and the developed world. In developing and third world countries, however, smoking rates are increasing by about two per cent per year.
                    9th World Conference on Tobacco or Health, Paris, 1994

7.  In the United States, on average among 1000 20-year-olds who smoke cigarettes regularly, about 6 will die from homicide, about 12 will die in motor vehicle accidents, and about 500 will be killed by smoking (250 in middle age 35-69, and 250 more in old age). In the United Kingdom in this group, about one will die from homicide, 6 from motor vehicle accidents, and the same 500 from smoking.
                    *Mortality from Smoking in Developed Countries 1950-2000*, Richard Peto et al,
                    Oxford University, 1994, p. A97

8.  It is estimated that 34% of all deaths in men between 35 and 69 years of age in the European Union are attributable to smoking. In some parts of Eastern Europe, this proportion is as high as 40-45%.
                    9th World Conference on Tobacco or Health, Paris, 1994 (Richard Doll)

9.  Tobacco is the largest single cause of premature death in the developed world, responsible for about 30% of all deaths among persons 35 to 69 years of age.                    *Growing Up Tobacco Free*, p. vii

10. The death toll from smoking in the decade of the 1990's is expected to total 3 million for Eastern Europe and 5 million throughout the former Soviet Union.                    American Medical News, October 3, 1994, p. 14

11. Over the period from 1950 to 2000, 60 million people (50 million men and 10 million women) in developed countries alone have died or will die from smoking.                    New York Times, September 21, 1994, p. A16

12. One of the national health objectives for 2010 is to reduce the prevalence of cigarette smoking among adults to no more than 12%. In 1998, 24.1% of adults were current smokers, an estimated 47.2 million adults. Rates were higher among persons aged 19 to 24 years (27.9%) and 25 to 44 years (27.5%).
                    JAMA, November 1, 2000, p. 2180

13. Past and projected annual tobacco-related deaths:

| Year | Total | Developed countries | Developing countries |
|------|-------|---------------------|----------------------|
| 1950 | 300,000 | 300,000 | Negligible |
| 1965 | 1,000,000 | 900,000 | 100,000 |
| 1975 | 1,500,000 | 1,300,000 | 200,000 |
| 1995 | 3,000,000 | 2,000,000 | 1,000,000 |
| 2000 | 3,500,000 | 2,400,000 | 1,100,000 |
| 2025 | 10,000,000 | 3,000,000 | 7,000,000 |

*The Tobacco Epidemic*, p. 81

14. At present smoking rates, there will be 100 million deaths from tobacco in the next 20 years.

10th World Conference on Tobacco or Health, Beijing, 1997 (Richard Peto)

15. About half a billion of the 5.5 billion people now alive will eventually be killed by tobacco. Of the 800 million smokers alive today in developing countries, about 200 million will be killed by tobacco, half in middle age. "What we've seen so far is nothing compared to what you'll see in developing countries...We are expecting a tidal wave of mortality."

Dr. Alan Lopez, World Health Organization (New York Times, September 21, 1994, p. A16)

16. For young adults who smoke cigarettes regularly, just over half of those who die in middle age will have been killed by tobacco. Overall, regular cigarette smokers lose about 8 years of projected life expectancy (or 16 years, for the half who are killed by the habit: 20 to 25 years for those killed in middle age, plus 5 to 10 years for those killed at older ages). *Mortality from Smoking*, p. A1

17. The annual toll of premature deaths caused by tobacco will rise from 3 million worldwide in the 1990's to 10 million by the year 2025. Half a billion people alive today, including 200 million at present under the age of 20, will eventually die from tobacco-induced disease, half of them in middle age.

The Lancet, April 28, 1990, p. 1026

18. The global cigarette market in 1995 was worth $262.3 billion, an increase of 4.5% from 1994 and 33.8% compared to 1990. The Asian Pacific region accounted for 51.6% of global cigarette sales, and increased by 8% per year between 1990 and 1995; China alone accounted for 1.693 trillion cigarettes, or 32.3% of global sales. The United States had 9.4% of world cigarette sales. Asian Business Review, March 1998, pp. 31-32, from the World Tobacco File 1997

19. In 1995, 760 billion cigarettes were manufactured in the United States, of which 487 billion (64%) were consumed domestically. There were also 2.5 billion cigars smoked and 14.2 million pounds of pipe and roll-your-own tobacco consumed. Consumption of chewing tobacco was 63.3 million pounds, and snuff, 60 million pounds. 243 billion cigarettes were exported to 111 countries. U.S. domestic cigarette consumption was highest in 1981, at 640 billion. *The Tobacco Epidemic*, pp. 37 and 42

20. Smoking prevalence among US physicians dropped from 53% in 1955 to 3% in 1993. In Europe, 20 to 30% of doctors still smoked in the early 1990's.

Hospital Practice, August 15, 1994, p. 12, and American Medical News, June 6, 1994

21. The average smoking prevalence among medical students at the Johns Hopkins medical school was 65% for the years 1948-51. By the 1980's, the maximum prevalence in medical school surveys was less than 3 percent.

*Tobacco and the Clinician*, p. 16

22. 74% of all men born between the years of 1910 and 1940 were smokers at some point in their lives. In contrast, only 38% of men born in the 1960's are expected to be "ever-smokers."

Journal of the National Cancer Institute, September, 1983, p. 475, and Smoking and Health: A Report to Congress, 1987

23. Cigarette smoking in males peaked in the 1941-1945 birth cohort, with 84% having ever smoked. The peak in females was 70% in the 1956-1960 cohort.                    American Journal of Public Health, January 1998, pp. 27-33

24. In a 1980 survey of white males born between 1921 and 1930, only 24 percent had never smoked. 40 percent were current smokers, and 36 percent were ex-smokers.                    *Strategies to Control Tobacco Use*, p. 114

25. Smoking prevalence for men was highest in the 1940's and 1950's. For women, smoking prevalence peaked later, in the 1960's, at 44% for women born between 1931 and 1940.                    JAMA, December 1, 1993, p. 2542

26. Successive birth cohorts of males from 1870 to 1919 reached higher levels of smoking. Among males born before 1890, the cumulative percentage eventually becoming smokers was 26%. In the 1890-1899 birth cohort, it rose to 50%, and was 60% for the 1900-1909 cohort and 68% in the 1910-1919 group. For females, the prevalence was only 2% in the group born before 1890, 4% 1890-1899, 14% 1900-1909, and rose to a cumulative percentage of 30% in females born between 1910-1919.                    Health Psychology 1995; 14:502

27. Peak smoking prevalence for white women born in 1910 with less than a high school education was 28%. For the same group of women born in 1960, the peak prevalence had risen to 71%. For white men with less than a high school education, in the cohort born in 1910, the peak prevalence was 70%, and was 78% for the 1960 cohort (but only 32% for the 1960 group with a high school education).
American Journal of Public Health, February 1996, p. 233

28. In 1955, 60% of men and 28% of women smoked. By 1990, the male smoking rate had plunged to 28%, compared with a drop of only five percentage points to 23% for women.
USA Today, November 18, 1992, p. 6D

29. Smoking prevalence for Americans living below the poverty level in 1993 was 39% for men and 29% for women.                    Cancer Facts and Figures 1994 (American Cancer Society)

30. About 3500 Americans successfully stop smoking every day. This group, when added to the 1200 customers a day who die as a result of smoking, create an ongoing problem for the tobacco companies: they need to recruit almost 5000 new smokers every day simply to maintain the "status quo" and their current sales. Virtually all of these new smokers are children.                    *Tobacco Biology and Politics*, Stanton Glantz, p. 7

31. The decade of the 1980's began with 50 million American smokers. By 1990, 10 million had quit, but 10 million children had started to smoke, balancing each other out. The decade ended with about 45 million smokers, a decline of 5 million. The 5 million difference are the deaths.    Tobacco Control, Winter 1993, p. S51

32. Prevalence of smoking among adults peaked at 42.4% in 1965.
Morbidity and Mortality Weekly Report 1994; 43:925

33. Heavy smokers (more than 25 cigarettes per day) have lifetime medical care expenditures that are 47% higher (for males) and 41% higher (for females) than never-smokers.                    Milbank Quarterly, Vol. 70, No. 1, 1992

34. Each year, decisions by young people to begin smoking commit the health care system to extra medical care expenses of $9.4 billion, spread out over the lifetimes of each new crop of smokers.
Milbank Quarterly, Vol. 70, No. 1, 1992, p. 100

35. Since the 1960's, smoking prevalence among college graduates has dropped by more than half to 18%, but prevalence rates among high school dropouts are unchanged.                    Pediatrics, May 1994, p. 866

36. In China today, there are 50 million children alive who will eventually die from smoking-related illness. Of the 2.3 billion of the world's children who are under 20 years old, about 800 million are expected to become smokers. If current smoking patterns continue, about 250 million of these children will eventually die from tobacco-induced disease.                    JAMA, January 6, 1989

37. While smoking mortality is expected to increase by 50% in developed countries in the next 30 years, it is expected to increase by 700% during the same time period in the less developed parts of the world.

ASH Review, January 1994, p. 6

38. Global cigarette production is increasing by about 3% per year, compared to the world's annual 1.2% annual population growth rate. 5.3 trillion cigarettes were produced in 1989, with China accounting for a third of the total.

Social Science and Medicine 1993; 38:106

39. In most of the developed world, smoking rates tend to be inversely proportional to socioeconomic class, with more educated groups having lower rates.

40. The average US smoker consumes about 11,000 cigarettes (550 packs) a year.

*Nicotine Addiction*, p. 47

41. From 1973 to 1992, smoking rates for college graduates declined from 28% to 14%, but for those without a high school education decreased from 44% only to 37%. Smoking among men dropped from 43% to 28%, and in women from 33% to 24%.

Cancer Facts and Figures 1994, American Cancer Society, p. 22

42. From 1965 through 1985, smoking prevalence in the US declined at a rate of 0.5 percentage points per year, and from 1986 to 1990, the rate of decline accelerated to 1.1 percentage points per year. In 1990, 25.5% of adults smoked. However, in 1991, the smoking rate increased to 25.7%, or 46.3 million Americans. The Centers for Disease Control blamed cheap discount cigarettes and a 16% increase in tobacco advertising for the reversal. Tobacco industry advertising and promotion increased from $3.99 billion in 1990 to $4.6 billion in 1991.

Morbidity and Mortality Weekly Report, May 20,1994, p. 346

43. In 1991, 46.3 million adults (25.7%) were current smokers, and 43.5 million (or 48.5% of ever smokers) Americans were former smokers.

JAMA, April 21, 1993, p. 1931

44. The number of Americans dying from cigarette smoking dropped from 434,000 in 1988 to 419,000 in 1990. The drop was due primarily from a 10% drop in deaths from cardiovascular disease. However, lung cancer deaths rose by 4% and COPD deaths rose by 5% during the same period. Even so, smoking is still responsible for one of every five deaths in the US. The average smoker loses 5 years of life from the habit, or seven minutes for each cigarette smoked. The total years of life lost annually is 5 million.

Morbidity and Mortality Weekly Report, August 27, 1993

45. The decline in the overall prevalence of smoking in the US (from 42.3% in 1965 to 25.5% in 1990) is not reflected in a corresponding decline in the actual number of adult smokers. Because of increasing population, numbers of smokers declined only from 50 million in 1965 to 46 million in 1990.

American Journal of Public Health, September 1992, p. 1204

46. In 1993, 25% of adults, or 46 million Americans, were current smokers. The group with the highest prevalence of smoking was male high school dropouts, 42% of whom smoked. Other groups with high rates were 39% among American Indians and Alaskan Natives, and 32% among persons living below the poverty level.

JAMA, February 1, 1995, p. 369

47. In Nevada, 24% of all deaths in 1990 were attributable to tobacco use, the highest percentage of any state. Neighboring Utah, with Mormons accounting for 70 percent of the population, had the nation's lowest smoking-related death rate of 13.4%.

Associated Press, June 27, 1994

48. By 1989, 50% of all adults (and 60% of college graduates) who had ever smoked regularly had quit. Dr. C. Everett Koop wrote: "This achievement has few parallels in the history of public health."

*Nicotine Addiction*, p. 59

49. Among men alive today, there are more former smokers than current smokers.

JAMA, February 23, 1994, p. 628

50. Young adults who watch TV for four or more hours a day are more than twice as likely to be smokers as those who watch TV for a hour a day or less. San Francisco Chronicle, March 19, 1994, p. A1

51. White men ages 18 to 24 in the US had the same rates of smoking in 1993 as they did in 1980, the only group not showing a decline. San Francisco Chronicle, November 13, 1993

52. If youth initiation rates in the United States can be brought down to 20%, overall smoking prevalence will decline from 25% in 1995 to 19% in 2005, 15% in 2015, 13% in 2025, and just over 12% in 2035 at a "steady state." If youth initiation rates remain at 25%, then the steady state prevalence will be 15.5%.
10th World Conference on Tobacco or Health, Beijing, 1997 (Kenneth Warner)

53. Groups with high smoking prevalence are unemployed men (44%), divorced or separated men (48%), psychiatric outpatients (52%), psychiatric inpatients (72%), and alcoholics (83%).
*Nicotine Addiction*, pp. 73, 311, and 328

54. In 1994, 48 million adults, or 25.5% of the adult population were current smokers, no change from the previous year. This included 28.2% of men and 23.1% of women. Groups with the highest smoking prevalence were American Indians (42.2%), those with less than a high school education (38.2%), and persons living below the poverty level (34.7%). There were 46 million former smokers in 1994; 69.3% of current smokers indicated a desire to quit completely, and 46.4% had stopped smoking for at least one day during the preceding year. The plateau in prevalence and consumption corresponded with a 10.4% decrease in the real price per pack of cigarettes during 1992-1994, after annual increases averaging 4% since 1984. In addition, domestic cigarette marketing expenditures are increasing at more than four times the rate of inflation, with the largest increases in expenditures for coupons and other items that make cigarettes more affordable.
JAMA, August 28, 1996, p. 595

55. In 1996, the median prevalence of current smoking for adults was 23.6%, similar to the previous year and ranging from 15.9% in Utah to 31.5% in Kentucky. The estimated percentage of children exposed to environmental tobacco smoke in the home ranged from 11.7% in Utah to 34.2% in Kentucky. About one third to one half of adult smokers have children in their homes, and in most (more than 70%) of those homes, smoking was permitted in some or all indoor areas. Therefore, during 1996, approximately 15 million (21.9%) of all children and adolescents younger than age 18 were exposed to ETS in the home.
Morbidity and Mortality Weekly Report, November 7, 1997, pp. 1038-43

56. Smoking prevalence is 53.7% for Native American men in Alaska and 33.1% for women in this group, compared to nationwide rates of 28% among white men and 24.7% among white females.
American Lung Association Fact Sheet (1997)

57. About 24.7% of American adults smoked cigarettes in 1995, according to the Centers for Disease Control and Prevention, continuing the "no change" prevalence pattern of the 1990's. There were 47 million current and 44.3 million former smokers; of ever-smokers, 48.6% had quit the habit. Among active smokers, 68% reported wanting to quit, and 46% had stopped smoking for at least one day in the previous year. Smoking was most prevalent, 37.5%, among people with between 9 and 11 years of education (high school dropouts), but was only 14% for college graduates. 32.5% of people living below the federal poverty level were smokers, compared to 23.8% of the rest of the adult population. The smoking rates in different ethnic groups were as follows: American Indians and Alaska natives 36.2% (including 37.3% of men in this group); blacks, 25.8%; whites, 25.6%; Hispanics, 18.3%; and Asians and Pacific Islanders, 16.6% (but only 4.3% of women in this last group).
Washington Post, December 26, 1997 (from Morbidity and Mortality Report, CDC)

58. In California in 1991, 26% of adults with less than a high school education were smokers, compared with only 12.7% of college graduates. Tobacco Use in California, California Department of Health Services, 1992, p. 16

59. Cigarette smoking among military personnel was 31.9% in 1995, with the highest prevalence, 39.4%, in the 18 to 25 year old group. 18.2% of military personnel used smokeless tobacco, including 21.9% of men under age 25. 1995 DOD Survey of Health Related Behaviors Among Military Personnel

60. College graduates had a smoking prevalence of 14% in 1991. For high school graduates, the rate is 29%, and is 37% for the group with less than a high school education. Tobacco Control, Autumn 1995, p. 311

61. In the developed world, tobacco causes about a third of all deaths at ages 35 to 69 years old, and about 25 diseases are positively associated with smoking. JAMA, June 5, 1995, p. 1683

62. In 1992-93, current cigarette smoking among adults ranged from a low of 15% in Utah to as high as 28% in Alaska, 29% in Kentucky, and 30% in Nevada.
State Tobacco Control Highlights 1996, Centers for Disease Control

63. In the United States in 1900, 7.4 pounds of tobacco were consumed per person age 15 years and older: 2% as cigarettes, 48% as chewing tobacco, 27% as cigars, and 19% as smoking tobacco (pipe and hand-rolled). By 1952, 12.9 pounds were consumed per person: 81% cigarettes, 3% chewing tobacco, 10% cigars, and 4% as smoking tobacco. In 1991, the figure was 5.1 pounds, with 87% cigarettes, 9% smokeless tobacco, 4% cigars, and 1% smoking (mostly pipe) tobacco. Epidemiologic Reviews 1995; 17:48

64. College freshmen have smoking prevalence rates of less than 10%, whereas Job Corps applicants of the same age have rates exceeding 60%. Only 15% of college graduates are current smokers and 28% are former smokers; almost two-thirds of college graduates who ever smoked have successfully quit.
Clinics in Chest Medicine, December 1991, pp. 638-639

65. In 1993, the prevalence of current smoking was 37% for persons who had completed 9-11 years of education, but only 14% for persons who had completed at least 16 years of education.
Epidemiologic Reviews 1995; 17:52

66. Among mothers on Medicaid in Washington state, the maternal smoking prevalence was 44%, compared to 16.3% of mothers not on Medicaid. Among married Medicaid-funded mothers, the smoking prevalence was 2.6 times higher in whites, 1.4 times higher in blacks, and 1.8 times higher in American Indians than for married mothers not funded by Medicaid. American Journal of Preventive Medicine 1994; 10:91

67. In 1993, Kentucky had the nation's highest percentage of adults who smoked, more than 30%. Nearly 50% of sixth through 12th grade students at schools in Madison County (Lexington area) regularly use tobacco. The state has 60,000 tobacco growers who produce almost 500 million pounds of burley tobacco; tobacco is a $900 million annual business in Kentucky. San Francisco Chronicle, June 5, 1995, p. 1683

68. In a 1985 survey, twenty states reported smoking rates higher than 30%, led by Nevada (36.5%), Alaska (35.5%), and Kentucky (35.4%). By 1993, only two states, Kentucky (32.2%) and West Virginia (30.5%) reported smoking rates of 30% or greater. Journal of the National Cancer Institute, December 4, 1996, p. 1753

69. Las Vegas has the highest lung cancer death rate in the country, and Nevada the highest percentage of adult smokers (36%). Nevada also has very weak laws regulating smoking, consistent with the state's "frontier ethic" about personal behavior and government interference. Utah has the lowest state smoking prevalence of 14% for adults. Kentucky and Nevada have the highest rates of 36%. In 1990, 39.7% of adult males in Kentucky and 38.4% in Nevada were smokers. Morbidity and Mortality Weekly Report, June 10, 1994, p.5

70. The states with the lowest adult prevalence of cigarette smoking in 1995 were Utah, 13.2%, California, 15.5%, Hawaii, 17.8%, New Jersey, 19.2%, Idaho, 19.8%, Washington, 20.2%, Minnesota and Georgia, 20.5%, and Connecticut, 20.8%. The states with the highest prevalence were Kentucky, 27.8%, Indiana, 27.2%, Tennessee, 26.5%, Nevada, 26.3%, Ohio, 26%, and North Carolina, 25.8%. Three states, Nevada, Rhode Island, and West Virginia, have more women smokers than men. A disturbing fact was that rates of current smoking among young adults ages 18 to 30 years were much higher, led by Maine with 32% and Ohio with 31%; 13 additional states had prevalence rates of 27% to 31%.
Morbidity and Mortality Weekly Report, November 8, 1996, pp. 963 and 972

71. Smoking among California adults increased by 11% from 1995 to 1996, rising to 18.6% from 16.7% the previous year. This was the first increase in prevalence in the state since 1988.

San Francisco Chronicle, March 26, 1997, p. A15

72. About 13% of college graduates smoke, but 40% of people with only high school degrees do.

New York Times, July 29, 1997, p. C8

73. In a 1992 survey of the Harvard class of 1942, only 4% of the men (at the time about 71 years old) were current smokers. 57% were former smokers, and 39% had never smoked.　　Harvard College Gazette, October 1997

74. Domestic cigarette sales peaked at 640 billion in 1981, and declined to 511 billion cigarettes in 1991, 506 billion in 1992, and 485 billion in 1993. Sales have since leveled off at 487 billion cigarettes in 1995 and 483 billion in 1996.　　Tobacco Control, Fall 1994, p. 287, Wall Street Journal,

January 30, 1997, p. B10, and USA Today, June 23, 1997, p. 1B

75. Cigarette consumption in the United States increased at a rate of 5% to 15% per year in the first half of this century. Adult yearly per capita cigarette consumption rose from 53 in 1900 to 650 cigarettes per year in 1920, and peaked at 4345 (217 packs per capita) in 1963. There has been a gradual decline since to 4148 in 1973, 3488 in 1983, 2675 in 1992, and 2414 (121 packs) in 1993. The 1993 figure was the lowest level since 1942.

Medical Clinics of North America, March 1992, p. 290,

Time, November 28, 1994, p. 24, and Tobacco Control, Autumn 1995, p. 311

76. Adult per capita yearly cigarette consumption in the United States was 128 packs per year in 1997 (estimate), compared to 140 packs, or 2800 cigarettes, in 1990. This compares to an average of 70 packs per year in California, and 72 packs in Massachusetts.

10th National Conference on Nicotine Dependence, Minneapolis, 1997 (Greg Connolly)

77. Total world cigarette consumption in trillions increased from 2 in 1956 to 2.5 in 1964, 2.8 in 1967, 4.5 in 1980, 5.5 in 1988, and 6 trillion in 1996.

10th World Conference on Tobacco or Health, Beijing, 1997 (Garfield Mahood)

78. Worldwide cigarette consumption for adults age 15 and older in 1997 was 1650 cigarettes, or 82.5 packs, per capita each year, for a total of 6 trillion cigarettes smoked.

10th World Conference on Tobacco or Health, Beijing, 1997

79. The countries with the highest annual per capita smoking rates are Greece, 2774 cigarettes (139 packs), Japan, 2669 (133 packs), and Poland, 2365 (118 packs). The United States ranks number 11 at 1831 cigarettes per capita per year, or 92 packs.　　Wall Street Journal, June 1997

80. Judith Mackay, M.D., reviewed trends and future predictions for tobacco use in her closing address at the 10th World Conference on Tobacco or Health in Beijing on August 28, 1997. In the year 2025, the total number of smokers is expected to increase to 1.64 billion from the present 1.1 billion; only 15% of these will live in developed countries. Total yearly deaths will increase from 3.5 million to 10 million, accounting for 9% of total deaths compared to 3% in 1997. The smoking prevalence in developing countries will increase from 8% to 20% in women, and decline from 60% to 45% in men. (In developed countries, the prevalence rate for men is expected to drop from 35% to 25%.) Deaths from AIDS are expected to peak at 1.7 million in the year 2006. Asia and the Indian subcontinent, the home of half the world's population, have only ten full time workers in tobacco control.

81. The 1998 National Household Survey on Drug Abuse was released by the U.S. Department of Health and Human Services. Based on interviews with 25,500 people, it is one of the most carefully conducted surveys in the nation. 60 million Americans, or 27.7% of the population age 12 and older, were current cigarette smokers in 1998, a decrease from 29.6% a year earlier. This included 29.7% of men and 25.7% of women. The highest rates were in young adults ages 18 to 25, 41.6%, a significant increase from 34.6% in this age group in 1994. 18.2% of youth ages 12 to 17 (18.7% of boys and 17.7% of girls) were current smokers, a total of 4.1 million and a rate similar to the 18.9% in 1994. Levels of education were correlated with smoking rates; 50% of adults

ages 26 to 34 who had not completed high school smoked, while only 15% of college graduates in this group smoked.

82. The American Lung Association estimates that there are 47 million smokers and 46 million former smokers in the United States.
Contra Costa Times, January 4, 2000

83. In 1997, 48 million American adults (24.7%) were current smokers. Prevalence was highest in the age group 18 to 24 years (28.7%) and 25 to 44 years (28.6%). The prevalence was highest among persons with less than a higher school education (35.4%, and lowest among college graduates (11.6%). 33.3% of persons living below the poverty level were smokers. An estimated 44.3 million adults were former smokers.
Morbidity and Mortality Weekly Report, November 5, 1999, p. 994

84. Cigarettes manufactured in the United States increased from 4 billion in 1900 to 720 billion (estimated) in 2000.
US News and World Report, December 27, 1999, p. 44

85. Tobacco will be responsible for 100 million deaths worldwide in the first two decades of the new millennium.
The Lancet, March 13, 1999, p. 909

86. Tobacco's share of death and disability worldwide is expected to increase from 3% at present to 9% in 2025.
Public Health Reports, January 1998, p. 17

87. The number of smokers worldwide is expected to rise from 1.1 billion in 2000 to 1.6 billion in 2025. Every day, worldwide, between 82,000 and 99,000 young people start to smoke.      *Curbing the Epidemic*, pp. 2 and 19

88. The number of worldwide smokers will increase from 1.1 billion in 1998 to an estimated 1.64 billion in 2025, as tobacco deaths increase from 3 million a year to 10 million. By comparison, annual HIV deaths will peak at 1.7 million in the year 2006. By 2025, the prevalence of smoking among women worldwide is expected to rise from 8% to 20%, but for men, to fall to 25% in developed countries (as low as 15% in some), and to decrease from 60% to 45% in developing countries. "By 2025, the transfer of the tobacco epidemic from rich to poor countries will be well advanced, with only 15% of the world's smokers living in the rich countries."
Public Health Reports, January 199, pp. 14-17 (Judith Mackay)

89. Worldwatch Institute and U.S. Department of Agriculture figures for world cigarette production in trillions of cigarettes:

| 1950 | 1.68 | 1995 | 5.60 |
| 1960 | 2.15 | 1996 | 5.68 (peak) |
| 1970 | 3.11 | 1997 | 5.64 |
| 1980 | 4.39 | 1998 | 5.61 trillion |
| 1990 | 5.42 | | |

90. In a survey of medical students graduating in 1996, 2% were current smokers, and 13% were former smokers.
JAMA, October 7, 1998, p. 1192

91. 48% of gay men in a survey were current smokers, a rate much higher than the smoking prevalence of 28.6% of men in the general population.
American Journal of Public Health, December 1999, p. 1875

92. Worldwide, there were 2.6 million deaths from AIDS in 1999, and a total of 16.3 million deaths since the epidemic began. 33.6 million people are living with AIDS or are infected with HIV; more than two thirds are in sub-Saharan Africa. 5.6 million people were newly infected with HIV in 1999.
Report for World AIDS Day, December 1, 1999

93. Deaths from AIDS in the United States decreased from 49,357 in 1995 to 36,792 in 1996, 21,222 in 1997 and 17,047 in 1998. In the late 1990's there were about 40,000 new cases of AIDS each year, a decrease from a peak of 150,000 cases a year a decade earlier.
CDC Data

94. The median adult smoking rate in the United States was 23.2% in 1997. The highest prevalence rates were Kentucky, 30.8%, Missouri, 28.7%, Arkansas, 28.5%, Nevada, 27.7%, and West Virginia, 27.4%. The lowest rates were in Utah, 13.7%, California, 18.4%, Hawaii, 18.6%, the District of Columbia, 18.8%, and Idaho, 19.9%. The highest smoking prevalence for men was Kentucky (33.1%), and for women highest in Nevada (29.8%). The prevalence of adult smokeless tobacco use ranged from 1.4% in Arizona, the lowest, up to 8.8% in West Virginia.                                                            Morbidity and Mortality Weekly Report, November 6, 1998

95. In 1997, Kentucky had the highest smoking rate in the nation, 30.8%, up from 27.8% in 1995. 47% of Kentucky high school students were current smokers, and two thirds of farms in Kentucky grow tobacco.
                                                            Associated Press, August 25, 1999 (CDC Data)

96. Nearly 40% of American Indian and Alaska Native adults smoke cigarettes, and since 1983, very little progress has been made in reducing tobacco use among this group.
                                                            1998 Surgeon General report, Tobacco Use Among Minority Groups

97. Smoking rates among American Indians is highest in the northern plains (47% for men and 42% for women) and lowest in the southwest (25.4% for men and 17.8% for women) in surveys from 1993 through 1996. In Alaska, 41.8% of Alaska Native and American Indian women were smokers, the highest prevalence of any area.
                                                            JAMA, March 15, 2000, p. 1415

98. The number of Navajo high school students who smoke regularly increased from 29% in 1992 to 47.5% in 1997.                                                            Associated Press, August 11, 1999

99. Native American youth have the highest tobacco use rates of any other group in Oklahoma, with 50% of Native American high school and 26% of middle school children reporting current tobacco use.
                                                            2002 National Conference on Tobacco or Health Abstract D+ D- 187-57

100. In 2001, 23.1% of adult Americans were smokers. 32.8% of adults with less than a high school education were smokers, compared to 15.8% of those with more than a high school education.
                                                            Associated Press, December 25, 2002

101. In 2000, 36% of the 32 million low income Medicaid recipients, and 25% of pregnant Medicaid patients, were cigarette smokers, compared to 23% of the general population and 12% of all pregnant women.
                                                            American Journal of Public Health, December 2002, p. 1940

102. In a CDC survey released on November 2, 2000 (Associated Press), the states with the highest smoking rates were Nevada (31.5%) and Kentucky (29.7%). Ohio, Arkansas, Alaska, West Virginia, Missouri and Indiana were next highest, between 27% and 28%. The lowest rates were in Utah (13.9%), Hawaii (18.6%), California (18.7%), Massachusetts (19.4%), and Minnesota (19.5%). Arizona, Montana, Maryland and the District of Columbia were between 20.0% and 20.6%.

103. Nevada has the highest adult smoking rate and also the highest death rate from smoking. The state also has a strict "pre-emption" law which prohibits localities from enacting any antismoking regulations that are stricter than the lenient state standards. Casinos, hotels and restaurants are permeated with secondhand smoke, and businesses are not required to provide no-smoking areas.                New York Times, May 20, 2001

104. The portion of adults in California who smoke decreased from 22.8% in 1988 to 18% in 1999, and California lung cancer rates dropped 14% between 1988 and 1997, while the estimated drop nationwide was 2.7%.
                                                            Washington Post National Weekend Edition, December 11, 2000, p. 30

105. In 1999, an estimated 46.5 million adults (23.5%) were current smokers. Overall, 19.2% of adults were everyday smokers and 4.3% were some day smokers. The prevalence of smoking was higher among men (25.7%) than women (21.5%). Among racial/ethnic groups, Hispanics (18.1%) and Asians/Pacific Islanders (15.1%) had the lowest prevalence of cigarette use; American Indians/Alaska Natives had the highest prevalence (40.8%). Adults who had earned a General Education Development diploma had the highest smoking prevalence (44.4%); persons with masters, professional and doctoral degrees had the lowest prevalence

(8.5%). Prevalence was highest among persons aged 18-24 years (27.9%) and 25-44 years (27.3%) and lowest among those aged ≥65 years (10.6%). The prevalence of smoking was highest among adults living below the poverty level (33.1%). In 1999, an estimated 45.7 million adults (23.1%) were former smokers; 25.8 million were men and 19.9 million were women. Former smokers constituted 49.5% of persons who had ever smoked ≥100 cigarettes. Some occupations showed a disproportionate number of smokers. Nearly half of waiters, construction workers, mechanics, and movers smoked, while less than one fifth of teachers and sales representatives smoked. 43% of unemployed people smoked, compared with 30% of employed people and 23% of those not in the labor force.                         2002 AMA Annual Tobacco Report

106. An estimated 65.5 million Americans reported current use of a tobacco product in 2000, a prevalence rate of 29.3% for the population aged 12 and older. Among this group, 55.7 million (24.9%) smoked cigarettes, 10.7 million (4.8%) smoked cigars, 7.6 million (3.4%) used smokeless tobacco and 2.1 million (1.0%) smoked tobacco in pipes. Although the rate of cigarette use was lower in 2000 than in 1999, the difference between 25.8% to 24.9% is not statistically significant. However, the rate of past year use of cigarettes decreased significantly between 1999 and 2000, from 30.1% to 29.1%                2002 AMA Annual Tobacco Report

107. Among Hispanic smokers, 30% are not daily smokers. Almost 20% of California smokers do not smoke daily.
                                                                *Nicotine and Public Health*, p. 303

108. 24.1% of Americans 18 and older were smokers in 1998, a rate almost unchanged in the 1990's.
                                                                                    Centers for Disease Control

109. The United States has 47 million adult (24 million men and 23 million women) and six million youth smokers.
                                                    2002 National Conference on Tobacco or Health Abstract
                                                    CESS-238 and USA Weekend, November 3-5, 2000

110. In 1964, the year of the first surgeon general's report about the dangers of smoking, 51.2% of men and 33.7% of women smoked. In 1998, 25.9% of men and 22.1% of women smoked.    San Francisco Chronicle, June 6, 2001

111. One of the national health objectives for 2010 is to reduce the prevalence of cigarette smoking among adults to no more than 12%. In 1998, 24.1% of adults were current smokers, an estimated 47.2 million adults. Rates were highest among persons aged 18-24 years (27.9%) and 25-44 years (27.5%).
                                                                                    JAMA, November 1, 2000, p. 2180

112. Almost 4 million Americans ages 65 and older are current smokers, 10.9% of men and 11.2% of women in this age group.                         2002 National Conference on Tobacco or Health Abstract CESS-5

113. While the overall smoking rate in New York City is 21%, 45% of Asian males and 8% of Asian females in the city are current smokers.            2002 National Conference on Tobacco or Health Abstracts D+D-187-53

114. Toledo Ohio has the highest smoking rate of any metropolitan area in the country, 31% of adults, and Orange County, California, the lowest, just 13%. Kentucky leads the nation with 30.5% adult smoking prevalence, and Utah had the lowest rate, 12.9%.                                    Associated Press, December 14, 2001

115. In 1999, only 13% of Californians were daily smokers; only 7.7% of adolescents and 6.4% of California college graduates smoked.                         Alameda County Tobacco Control Coalition Review, April 2002

116. 20.5% of adults reported that they smoked in 2000, down only slightly from the 1991 median national smoking rate of 21.8%.                                                    2003 AMA Annual Tobacco Report

117. The annual per capita consumption of cigarettes in the United States declined from 2810 in 1980 to 1633 in 1999, a decrease of 42%.                                                    JAMA, August 9, 2000, p. 753

118. 29% of college students smoked in 1999. Most colleges now ban smoking in indoor public areas and classrooms, and many have banned or restricted smoking in dormitories and stadiums.
                                                                                    Associated Press, December 14, 2002

119. In a 1999 survey of US colleges, the prevalence of current (past 30 day) smoking was 28.5%. Among this group, 32% did not smoke every day, 43.6% smoked 1 to 10 cigarettes a day, and only 12.8% smoked one or more packs a day. Current (past 30-day) cigar use was 8.5%, smokeless tobacco, 3.7%, and pipes, 1.2%. Most cigar use was occasional. *JAMA, August 9, 2000, p. 699-705*

120. The world's tobacco companies produce an estimated 5.5 trillion cigarettes each year. That's nearly one thousand cigarettes for every person on the planet, as though every child has received an allotment of fifty packs a year at birth. More than 15 billion cigarettes are sold each day to more than 1.1 billion people puffing away around the world. *Quote from Cigarettes (Parker-Pope), p. 1*

121. Global cigarette consumption in billions: 1880, 10; 1890, 20; 1900, 50; 1910, 50 billion; 1920, 300; 1930, 600; 1940, 1000 (one trillion); 1950, 1686; 1960, 2.15 trillion; 1970, 3.11 trillion; 1980, 4.39 trillion; 1990, 5.42 trillion; 2000, 5.5 trillion cigarettes. *The Tobacco Atlas, pp. 30-31*

122. Projected regional increases and decreases for cigarette consumption in 2008 compared with 1998: Americas, no change; Western Europe, -8.0%; Africa and the Middle East, +16.1%; Eastern Europe and the former Soviet Union, +8.7%; and Asia, Australiasia, and the Far East, +6.5%. Predicted consumption increases by country include Brazil, +40%; Zimbabwe, +56%; and Pakistan, +36%. Countries with predicted decreases include the United States, -13%; the United Kingdom, -21.6%; South Africa, -17%; and New Zealand, -25%. *The Tobacco Atlas, p. 89*

123. There were an estimated 1.2 billion smokers worldwide in 2003; by 2020, this number is expected to increase to almost 1.7 billion. *British Medical Association (www.tobaccofactfile.org)*

124. Only 16.6% of adults in California (19.3% of men and 14% of women) smoked in 2002, down from 17.3% in 2001. Per capita cigarette use is down more than 60% since the state's antismoking campaign began in 1988. RJR and Lorillard are suing the state, alleging that California's antismoking TV ads unfairly "vilify" the tobacco industry. *Associated Press, April 5, 2003*

125. In Kentucky, 30% of adults and 40% of high school students are smokers. The Kentucky state cigarette tax, only 3 cents a pack, has not increased since 1970. *New York Times, March 4, 2003, p. A21*

126. In 2001, the median prevalence of current smoking in the 50 states and DC was 23.4%. Prevalence was highest in Kentucky (30.9%), Oklahoma (28.8%), West Virginia (28.2%), Ohio (27.7%), Indiana (27.5%), Nevada (27.0%), South Carolina (26.2%), and Alaska (26.1%), and lowest in Utah (13.3%), California (17.2%), Massachusetts (19.7%), Idaho (19.7%), Nebraska (20.4%), Oregon (20.5%), Hawaii (20.6%), Connecticut (20.8%), and DC (20.8%). In 2001, the proportion of some day (less than daily) smokers was 24.0%. *Morbidity and Mortality Weekly Report, April 11, 2003, p. 203*

# CHAPTER 3
# MORTALITY AND LONGEVITY DATA

1. If current worldwide smoking patterns persist, about half a billion of the world's population alive today will be eventually killed by tobacco, including one quarter billion still in middle age (35-69) who will each lose about 20 years of life. *Mortality from Smoking*, p. A99

2. About half of regular cigarette smokers will eventually be killed by their habit: about one quarter in old age and one quarter in middle age, with those killed by smoking in middle age losing an average of about 20 to 25 years of life expectancy. *Mortality from Smoking*, p. A1

3. Cigarettes are responsible for 30% of the deaths in middle age in the United States and Great Britain. British Medical Journal, October 8, 1994, p. 937

4. In the previous centuries 70 years used to be regarded as humanity's allotted span of life, and only about one in five survived to such an age. In developed countries the situation is now reversed; in the absence of tobacco, only about one in five will die before age 70. *Mortality from Smoking*, p. A5

5. The average loss of life for those killed by tobacco is about 16 years. Since about half of all regular smokers in developed countries are eventually killed by the habit, teenagers or young adults who became regular cigarette smokers are reducing their life expectancy by the substantial amount of about 8 years. *Mortality from Smoking*, p. A5

6. Among a population of women who smoke regularly, tobacco will be a cause of at least half, and perhaps substantially more than half, of all their deaths in middle age. *Mortality from Smoking*, p. A50

7. One in four deaths in men in developed countries is attributable to smoking. Smoking now causes about a third of all male deaths in middle age, and on average, those killed by tobacco in this age group (35 to 69 years) lose more than 20 years of life expectancy. Smoking is the cause of about half of all male deaths from cancer in middle age, and about a third of cancers and fifth of deaths of those in old age (70 or older). Tobacco Control, Spring 1995, p.102

8. Every cigarette smoked takes 7 minutes off the life of the smoker, about as long as it takes to smoke the cigarette. Each pack of 20 cigarettes takes 140 minutes to smoke, and subtracts 140 minutes from the life of the smoker. 1994 Surgeon General report *Youth and Tobacco*

9. Smokers are three times more likely than nonsmokers to die before the age of 70. 30 out of every 200 nonsmokers will survive until the age of 90, but only three of every 200 people who smoke a pack a day or more will live to age 90. Associated Press, February 1, 1993, and American Medical News, March 8, 1993

10. 60% of smokers survive to age 70 years, compared with 83% of never-smokers. Only 12% of current smokers survive to age 85, compared with 35% of never-smokers. British Medical Journal, October 8, 1994, p.907

11. In a study of 7700 British men, only an estimated 42% of 20 year olds who were lifelong smokers would be expected to live to age 73, compared with 78% of lifelong non-smokers. British Medical Journal, October 12, 1996, p. 907

12. A 50-year-old male smoker has a 31% chance of dying before age 70. A 50 year old nonsmoker has only an 11% chance of not living until age 70. *Deadly Choices*, p. 162

13. A male age 55 to 59 who smokes a pack a day or more has a 46% chance of dying in the next decade and a half. A male lifelong nonsmoker of the same age has only an 18% chance of dying in the next decade and a half. American Cancer Society, Cancer Prevention Study II (1982-1986)

14. 10% of all smokers die before reaching age 55, but only 4% of nonsmokers. By age 65, 28% of smokers are dead, but only 11% of nonsmokers. By age 75, 57% of the smokers are dead, and 30% of the nonsmokers.

    *Smoking Tobacco and Health*, Centers for Disease Control, 1989

15. An adult male nonsmoker has an 89 percent chance of living to age seventy; a smoker reduces his chances of surviving this long to 69 percent, or almost triple the risk of premature death.        *Deadly Choices*, p. 162

16. A male cigarette smoker at age 32 has an 80 percent chance of surviving to age 60, while a nonsmoker has a 93 percent chance.        *Strategies to Control Tobacco Use,* p.23

17. A 40 year prospective study of a male British physicians examined the effects of cigarette smoking on survival to age 70 and to age 85. Never-smokers had an 80% chance of survival to age 70, and a 33% chance of survival to age 85. In smokers of 25 or more cigarettes per day, 50% survived to age 70, and only 8% to age 85.

    *Mortality from Smoking*, p. A16

18. Male heavy smokers in a survey expected a 67% chance that they would live to age 75 or older, while medical studies and actuarial predictions suggest that they have only a 26% chance of living to age 75. (Never-smoker males have a 68% chance of living to age 75.) In women, 83% of never-smokers will live to age 75, compared to only 31% of women who smoke more than 25 cigarettes a day.

    Reuters Health e line, June 13, 1997, and San Francisco Chronicle, June 14, 1997

19. A 35-year-old male never-smoker has an 87% chance of surviving to age 65 (vs. 73% chance for a smoker), a 69% chance of living to age 75 (vs. 47%), and a 34% chance to age to age 85 (vs. 16% for a smoker). For women, the percentages are 90% compared with 83% to age 65, 76% vs. 63% to age 75, and 45% vs. 29% to age 85.        Milbank Quarterly, Vol. 70 No 1, 1992, p. 91

20. At age 70, 78% of male nonsmokers are still alive, as compared to only 57% of smokers; for women, the figures are 86% and 75%. At age 80, the survival for males in 50% and 21% for nonsmokers and smokers, respectively, and among women, 67% and 43%.        NEJM, October 9, 1997, pp. 1053-54

21. A study reported in the May/June 1990 issue of Contingencies found that a 30-year-old smoker could expect to live another 34.8 years, compared with another 52.7 years for a 30-year-old who had never smoked. This was a difference of 17.9 years in life expectancy.

22. A 65-year-old never-smoker can expect a life expectancy of an additional 17 years to age 82. A 65-year-old smoker has a predicted expectancy to age 76, but by stopping at age 65, life expectancy is 80 years, a gain of 4 years.        Clinics in Geriatric Medicine, May 1986, p.338

23. The increase in life expectancy of a man who quits smoking between the ages of 35 and 39 is 5 years; for a woman it is 3 years.        U.S. News and World Report, November 20, 1993, p.11

24. The harmful effects of continuing to smoke are apparent even among women older than age 75. Compared with nonsmokers, women smokers ages 65 to 74 have a more than two-fold increase in mortality; death from smoking-related cancer is increased 8- to 10-fold. Women smokers over age 75 had more than a 5-fold increased risk of dying from a smoking-related cancer.    Archives of Internal Medicine, March 25, 1996, p. 630

25. About one death in four overall in the United States and one death in two designated as "premature," is attributable to smoking. Among people admitted for inpatient treatment of alcoholism, tobacco-related causes of death are significantly more frequent than alcohol-related causes.

    Journal of the American Medical Association 1996; 275:1097

26. "Each year the tobacco companies have to replace two million American smokers. A million and a half kick the habit annually. Another half-million or so are bulldozed into early graves because they couldn't quit."

    New York Times, October 21, 1996, p. A17 (Bob Herbert)

27. Since the poor are more likely to smoke than the rich, their risk of premature death is also greater. In high and middle income countries, men in the lowest socioeconomic groups are up to twice as likely to die in middle age as men in the highest socioeconomic groups, and smoking accounts for at least half of their excess risk.

*Curbing the Epidemic*, executive summary

28. Life expectancy for smokers who quit at age 35 exceeds that of continuing smokers by an average of 8.5 years for men and 7.7 years for women. As support for the adage "it is never too late to quit", even among smokers who quit at age 65, men could expect to gain 2.0 years of life, and women, 3.7 years, relative to those who continued to smoke, and after adjustment for the subsequent quit rate among current smokers at baseline. Estimates from Great Britain show that about 90% of the excess mortality attributable to cigarette smoking can be avoided if persons stop smoking before middle age.

American Journal of Public Health, June 2002, pp. 990-996

29. Half of all chronic smokers are killed by a tobacco-related disease, with half of those deaths occurring between ages 35 and 69, when those killed by tobacco lose an average of 20 to 25 years of life expectancy.

International Agency for Research on Cancer monograph, June 2002

30. 14,000 under-18s take up smoking each day in affluent countries; 68,000 under 18s do so in non-affluent countries.

Time, August 6, 2001, p. 15

31. The average loss of life for all smokers whose deaths are attributable to tobacco is about 16 years.

British Medical Association (www.tobaccofactfile.org)

32. Smoking kills about one in ten adults worldwide; by 2030, the proportion will be one in six.

British Medical Association (www.tobaccofactfile.org)

33. Large decreases in life expectancy are associated with overweight (body mass index 25 to 30) and obesity (body mass index over 30), and if this group of people smokes as well, the life expectancy decrements are compounded. Non-smokers who were overweight but not obese lost an average of three years off their lives, and obese people died even sooner; obese female non smokers lost an average of 7.1 years of life, and obese men lost 5.8 years. (About two thirds of American adults are now overweight or obese.) Obese female smokers lost 7.2 years and obese male smokers lost 6.7 years of life expectancy compared with normal weight nonsmokers. There is a severe double burden of obesity and smoking.

Annals of Internal Medicine, January 7, 2003, pp. 24-32

34. Smoking now causes about 442,400 premature deaths a year in the United States, with health costs and lost productivity adding up to $157 billion a year.        American Medical News, May 20, 2002, p. 25

35. During 1995 to 1999, smoking caused an annual average of 124,800 deaths from lung cancer, 82,000 from ischemic heart disease, and 64,700 deaths from chronic obstructive lung disease in the United States.

JAMA, May 8, 2002, p. 2355

36. At present smoking rates, there will be one billion deaths from smoking in this century.

Dean Edell. M.D., ABC radio, January 17, 2002

37. The percentage of deaths worldwide attributable to tobacco use was 6% in 1990, and is expected to increase to 12.3% of all worldwide deaths in 2020.        American Journal of Public Health, February 2001, p. 191

38. AIDS deaths in the United States dropped from 50,610 in 1995 to 16,273 in 1999. There are 40,000 new cases each year in the U.S. 36 million people in the world are HIV-positive, 26 million of them in sub-Saharan Africa alone.        Time, August 20, 2001, p. 46

39. Every cigarette smoked shortens lifespan by about 11 minutes.

ASH Smoking and Health Review, July-August 2002, p. 6

40. Adult male and female smokers lose an average of 13.2 and 14.5 years of life, respectively, because of their habit.        JAMA, May 8, 2002, p. 2356

# CHAPTER 4
# HISTORY OF TOBACCO
### in chronological order

**Comprehensive (several hundred pages) data on the history of tobacco is found online at www.tobacco.org--click on heading The Tobacco Timeline**

**References in this section (unless otherwise noted) are from the following sources:**
1. *The Story of Tobacco In America*, Joseph C. Robert, University of North Carolina Press, 1949
2. *Sold American*, American Tobacco Company, 1954
3. *Tobacco and Americans*, Robert K. Heimann, McGraw Hill, 1960
4. Gordon Dillow: Thank you for not smoking: the hundred-year war against the cigarette, American Heritage, February-March 1981
5. *They Satisfy: the Cigarette in American Life*, Robert Sobel, Anchor Books, 1978

**Note: there are additional historical sections in the chapters on cancer, smokeless tobacco, pipes and cigars, nicotine, tobacco and the military, and advertising**

# Before 1500

1. About 8000 years ago, the two species of the tobacco plant, Nicotiana rustica and Nicotiana tobacum, were dispersed by Amerindians throughout both North and South America. *Tobacco in History*, p. 3

2. At an 8000 year old Stone Age archeologic site in Nambia, Africa, a sort of stone pipe was found. A previously type of unknown, "indigenous" wild tobacco was discovered in this area in 1965, "nicotiana africana." Reported by Paul Nordgram, National Institute of Public Health, Stockholm, Sweden

3. The tobacco plant (genus Nicotiana) is one of the divisions of the nightshade plant family, which also includes the potato and the pepper. Species of the genus Nicotiana are native to North and South America, Australia and the Pacific, but not to Europe, Asia, or Africa. *Tobacco in History*, p. 3

4. By the 1st century B.C., the Mayans smoked tobacco in religious ceremonies; tobacco use appears in Mayan stone carvings. *Smoke and Mirrors*, p. 29

5. The Aztecs regarded tobacco as holy substance, believing that the body of their chief goddess Cihuacoahuatl was composed of tobacco. Health Education, June 1987, p.6

6. Tobacco gourds and pouches were the insignia of Aztec priesthood, and were described as symbols of divinity. "Tobacco smoking was already well-established among the Aztec upper classes as an after-dinner activity before Europeans first witnessed it." And in the Maya culture, many of the deities in stone monuments, ceramics, and in paintings are depicted as smokers, as are some mythological animals. *Tobacco in History*, p. 31

7. Early information on the smoking of cigars originates from artifacts of the Mayas of the Yucatan region of Mexico. Smoking of tobacco was part of the religious rituals and political gatherings of the natives of the Yucatan peninsula as shown in the artwork on a pottery vessel from the 10th century where a Maya smokes a string-tied cigar. Five hundred years later, in 1492, when Christopher Columbus landed in America, he was presented with dried leaves of tobacco by the House of Arawaks. Columbus and his crew were thus the first Europeans who became acquainted with tobacco smoking. Early in the 16th century, Cortez confirmed that tobacco smoking was practiced by the Aztecs in Mexico. In addition, tobacco was grown in Cuba, Haiti, several of the West Indian Islands, and on the East Coast of North America from Florida to Virginia. Quote from *Cigars*, p. 55

8. Tobacco was used in eastern North America at least 2000 years ago. An Iroquois settlement site more than 500 years old near Toronto yielded over 4000 ceramic and stone smoking pipes and fragments; some pipe bowls still contained nicotine residues *Nicotine and Public Health*, p. 3

9. Plant geneticists have established that tobacco's "centre of origin," ie: the meeting place between a species' genetic origin, and the area in which it was first cultivated, is located in the Peruvian/Ecuadorian Andes. Estimates for its first date of cultivation range from 5000-3000 BC. Tobacco use then spread northwards and by

the time of Christopher Columbus's arrival in 1492 it had reached every corner of the American continent, including offshore islands such as Cuba. Quote from *Tobacco* (Gately), p.3

10. In the pre-Columbian period, tobacco was consumed from Quebec in eastern Canada south to southern Argentina, and on the Pacific coast north to the Aleutian Islands. There were five principal methods of tobacco consumption: smoking, chewing, drinking, snuff and enemas. *Tobacco in History*, pp. 24 and 33

11. At the time that Europeans first arrived in eastern North America, nearly 100% of the aboriginal men were smokers. *Nicotine and Public Health*, p. 5

12. In 1492, Columbus discovered the natives of the West Indies "drinking smoke." Tobacco was unknown in Europe until Columbus brought back samples and plants from the New World. Modern tobaccos are the species nicotiana tabacam, which was not grown north of Mexico until the English colonists introduced it into Virginia. A hardier species, nicotiana rustica, was grown by the tribes of the eastern United States and Canada.

13. A New Yorker cartoon from the 1940s showed Christopher Columbus smoking a peace pipe with the West Indian natives and the comment from one of his men: "Don't worry. If it turns out tobacco is harmful, we can always quit."

14. Christopher Columbus wrote that native Americans carried "a firebrand in the hand, and herbs to drink the smoke thereof, as they are accustomed." Washington Post National Weekly Edition, June 27, 1994, p. 6

15. "The natives wrap the tobacco in a certain leaf, in the manner of a musket formed of paper...and having lighted one end of it, by the other they suck, absorb or receive that smoke inside with their breath." Bartholomio de las Casas, Columbus expedition, 1492

16. The first descriptions of syphilis in Europe appeared at about the time Columbus returned, raising the unproven theory that Columbus introduced syphilis as well as tobacco from the New World.

17. In the era of Columbus, the Carib Indians of the lesser Antilles inhaled or sniffed a fine tobacco powder or smoke through a hollow Y-shaped tube called a taboca or tobago; the name tobacco evolved from this. Health Education, June 1987, p. 6

18. Tobacco use among native tribes was so prevalent that at least 600 words in American aboriginal languages and dialects were used to designate different forms of tobacco. Health Education, June 1987, p. 6

19. Christopher Columbus on his first voyage to the New World brought the tobacco leaf and seeds out of the Caribbean and in 1492 introduced them to Europe. Its use at first in Spain and Portugal was quite limited, however, and seeped deeply of pagan religious mysticism. In fact, tobacco was not received favorably at all by the strongly devout Christian practitioners of the day who did not adapt well to a product that was so new and so strange to them. Indeed, from the beginning the use of tobacco was condemned as wholly evil to any good God-fearing Christian. Rodrigo de Jerez, among the first of Columbus's sailors to inhale tobacco smoke, apparently became dependent on tobacco sometime after his initial encounter of it with the Carib Indians; thereafter he was believed to harbor within him the devil and was imprisoned and condemned during the Inquisition. Quote from *The Tobacco Epidemic*, pp. 15-16 (Gary Huber)

20. Columbus and early European settlers noted that a long, thick bundle of twisted tobacco leaves wrapped in a dried palm or maize leaf was used by Native Americans as a primitive cigar. *Cigars*, p. 1

21. "Among the Hurons of North American, virtually all men, but few if any women, smoked N. rustica leaf, and they did so day in and day out. While women were responsible for growing food crops, men alone had the responsibility for growing tobacco. In one pre-contact Huron village north of present-day Toronto, archaeologists have found 4,000 clay pipes." *The Tobacco Epidemic*, p. 3 (John Slade)

22. Within 150 years of Columbus's finding "strange leaves" in the New World, tobacco was being used in every part of the earth. American Medical News, November 14, 1994, p. 17

23. In 1499, the explorer Amerigo Vespucci reported Indians in Venezuela chewing a "green herb like cattle to such an extent that they scarcely talk." This was probably tobacco mixed with hallucinogenic coca leaves.

*Health Education, June 1987, p. 6*

# 1500

24. "Among other evil practices, the Indians have one that is especially harmful: the inhaling of a certain kind of smoke which they call tobacco, in order to produce a state of stupor. (They) employ a tube shaped like a Y, inserting the forked extremities in their nostrils and the tube filled with the lighted weed; in this way they would inhale the smoke until they became unconscious and lay sprawling on the ground like men in a drunken slumber."

G. Fernandez de Oviedo, 1526 (*Holy Smoke* p. 10)

25. The Jesuit missionary Lalemant in the 16th century said that a Huron's resolution to give up smoking "may pass for one of the most heroic acts of which a Savage is capable, who, it seems, would as soon dispense with eating as with smoking."

*Nicotine and Public Health*, p. 8

26. The Frenchman Lescarbot in the 1500s wrote that the Micmac Indians smoked "almost every hour," and attributed their sexual modesty "partly to their frequent use of tobacco, the smoke of which dulls the senses, and mounting up to the brain hinders the functions of Venus."

*Nicotine and Public Health*, p. 6

27. From September 1535 to May 1536 Cartier visited St. Lawrence Iroquoian communities in the vicinity of modern Quebec City and Montreal. The account of his voyage contains the first description of pipe smoking to appear:
"… they have a plant [i.e. tobacco], of which a large supply is collected in summer for the winter's consumption. They hold it in high esteem, though the men alone make use of it in the following manner. After drying it in the sun, they carry it about their necks in a small skin pouch in lieu of a bag, together with a hollow bit of stone or wood. Then at frequent intervals they crumble this plant into powder, which they place in one of the openings of the hollow instrument, and laying a live coal on top, suck at the other end to such an extent, that they fill their bodies so full of smoke, that it streams out of their mouths and nostrils as from a chimney. They say it keeps them warm and in good health, and never go about without these things. We made a trial of this smoke. When it is in one's mouth, one would think one had taken powdered pepper, it is so hot."

*Nicotine and Public Health*, p. 4

28. "The Indians have a certain herb, of which they lay up a store every summer, having first dried it in the sun. They always carry some of it in a small bag hanging around their necks. They suck themselves so full of smoke that it oozes from their mouths like smoke from the flue of a chimney. They say the habit is most wholesome."

Jacques Cartier on the St. Lawrence River, Quebec, Canada, 1535

29. Cartier noted that tobacco "bit our tongues like pepper." It was not until the 1600's that the strong, native Nicotiana rustica (wild tobacco) was supplanted by mild Nicotiana tabacum (common tobacco) from Central and South America.

30. On Jacques Cartier's second voyage to North America in 1535, he was offered tobacco by the indigenous people he met when he arrived at the island of Montreal. Cartier described this in his diary: "In Hochelaga, at the head of the river in Canada, grows a certain herb which is stocked in large quantities by the natives during the summer season, and on which they set great value. Men alone use it, and after drying it in the sun they carry it around their neck wrapped up in the skin of a small animal, like a sac, with a hollow piece of stone or wood. When the spirit moves them, they pulverize this herb and place it at one end, lighting it with a fire brand, and draw on the other end so long that they fill their bodies with smoke until it comes out of their mouth and nostrils as from a chimney. They claim it keeps them warm and in good health. They never travel without this herb."

*Smoke and Mirrors*, p. 30

31. "A recurrent theory in the history of the use of tobacco is that its use is compulsive and similar to other forms of drug abuse. In the Americas the inability of the Indians to abstain from tobacco raised problems for the Catholic Church. The Indians insisted on smoking even in church, as they had been accustomed to doing in their own places of worship. In 1575 a church council issued an order forbidding the use of tobacco in churches throughout the whole Spanish America. Soon, however, the missionary priests themselves were using tobacco so frequently that it was necessary to make laws to prevent even them from using tobacco during worship."

*Nicotine*, p. 83

32. "… they draw this smoke, and then they speak. The which they do customably one after another in the councils of war… The women use it by no means. If that they take too much of this perfume, it will make them light in the

head, as the smell or taste of strong wine. The Christians that do now inhabit there are become very desirous of this herb and perfume, although that the first use thereof is not without danger, before that one is accustomed thereto, for this smoke causeth sweats and weakness, even to fall into a syncope, the which I have tried myself."

Frere Andre Thevet, *Les Singularites de la France Antarctique, autrement nomme Amerique*, 1557 (trans. Thomas Hacker as *The New Found Worlde*, 1568)

33. A Spanish doctor, Nicolas Monardes, in a 1571 work listed more than twenty ailments, including cancer, that tobacco use could cure. *Faber Book of Smoking*, p. 24

34. "For you see many sailors, all of whom have returned from [the New World] carrying small tubes… [which] they light with fire, and, opening their mouths wide and breathing in, they suck in as much smoke as they can… in this way they say their hunger and thirst are allayed, their strength is restored and their spirits are refreshed; they asseverate that their brains are lulled by a joyous intoxication.

Matthias de l'Obel, botanist, 1570 (*Faber Book of Smoking*, p. 23)

35. Thomas Hariot, a member of the 1585-86 ill-fated Roanoke expedition, was taught to smoke by the North Carolina Algonquians. He later developed cancer of the nose and suffered a "slow, hideous demise."

*Nicotine and Public Health*, p. 8

36. Several 16th century Spanish sources provide possible origins for the word "tobacco." Gonzalo Fernandez de Oviedo, an inspector-general assigned to gold mines in the Antilles, wrote about the "tobago", a Y-shaped tube that was used for tobacco consumption by the Carib Indians of Haiti. A Spanish missionary, Bartolome de las Casas, used the word "tobacco" in 1552 to describe a small cigar-like roll of tobacco leaves that were smoked.

   Sixteenth century Europeans often regarded tobacco as a medicinal plant. Jean Nicot, a French ambassador to Portugal, presented his celebrated gift of N. rustica to the queen mother, Catherine de Medici, around 1560, telling her that this wonderful medicinal herb from the New World was for the royal herb garden. A Spanish physician, Nicolas Monardes, wrote a highly influential treatise on the medicinal uses of tobacco in 1571 that was soon translated into English, Latin, French and Italian. Quote from *The Tobacco Epidemic*, p. 4 (John Slade)

37. From 1500 to 1800, Spain earned more money in the New World from tobacco than it did from gold.

*A Passion for Cigars*, p. 13

38. In about 1550, Jean Nicot, the French ambassador to Portugal, presented his queen, Catherine de Medici, with some powdered tobacco to use in treating her migraine headaches. He popularized the idea that tobacco had curative powers, and distributed seeds in Europe, where tobacco use gained popularity. Nicot's name is the basis for the scientific term for tobacco, nicotiana, and the addictive drug in tobacco, nicotine.

39. By the early and mid-16th century, attempts to grow tobacco throughout Europe had failed, first in Spain and Portugal, and then in Belgium, France, Germany, and eventually, by 1570, in England. Only the strong and harsh varieties, which were not pleasing to the taste and generally were difficult to tolerate upon inhalation, could be grown in these areas, and even then not grown very well or very productively. Therefore, Portugal and Spain, at the early crossroads of the seven seas trade in tobacco, expanded and developed their colonies in the New World, not only in search of gold, but to help supply the growing demand for the New World tobacco leaf, far more highly desired than any variant that would grow in Europe and, ultimately, more economically valuable than gold or silver.

Quote from *The Tobacco Epidemic*, p. 17 (Gary Huber)

40. None of the great explorers of the Orient, including Marco Polo, Vasco da Gama, or any other, described any use of tobacco in the Far East until after it had been introduced there by the trading of these Portuguese and Spanish sailors. Sir John Hawkyns, probably the first English slave trader, brought tobacco from Florida to his own homeland in 1565, as did Sir Francis Drake, returning from Roanoke Island, in Virginia, over a decade later, in 1586. It was Sir Walter Raleigh, however, who won approval from Queen Elizabeth and the English royal court to

smoke tobacco, in the manner modeled after the custom of the American Indian, by burning the dry leaves in a pipe.

Quote from *The Tobacco Epidemic*, p. 16 (Gary Huber)

41. Sir Walter Raleigh perfected a method for curing the tobacco leaf, and helped to popularize smoking among the upper classes in late 16th century England. A servant once mistakenly doused him with water, believing him to be on fire. The Economist, September 15, 1990

42. When Queen Elizabeth in 1584 granted Sir Walter Raleigh a patent entitling him to lands he might discover, he immediately provisioned a small fleet and his mariners soon discovered Virginia, so named upon their return. The following year Raleigh dispatched a second fleet to Virginia, where a colony was established on Roanoke Island. When Sir Francis Drake visited that ill-fated colony in June 1586, Governor Ralph Lane and others returned to England with him, bringing back the tobacco and pipe-smoking practices soon popularized by Sir Walter Raleigh and other members of Queen Elizabeth's court: "So that smoking gained in a little time, a fashionable and polite eclat...and Elizabeth herself was as familiar with a tobacco pipe as with her sceptre." Thus was ushered in "a prosperous time in the history of tobacco; princes, nobles, knights, ladies, the wealthy and fashionable, all numbered themselves among its devotees...and the convenience of a gentleman were considered imperfect without a box of pipes and tobacco." By 1600 tobacco was widely used in all the maritime nations of Europe.

Quote from Population and Development Review, June 1990, p. 214

43. King James and Sir Walter Raleigh, the "father" of tobacco in Great Britain, were sworn enemies, and the king eventually had Raleigh executed. *Faber Book of Smoking*, p. 24

44. "Who has ever found a more sovereign remedy against coughs, rheum in the stomach, head and eyes? ... In few, I think there is nothing that harms a man from his girdle upward, but may be taken away with a moderate use of Tobacco, and in those parts consist the chief reasons of our health, for the stomach and head being clear and void of evil humours, commonly the whole body is the better." Anthony Chute, *Tobacco* 1595

45. In England by 1598, the cost of tobacco was 4 pounds, 10 shillings per pound. "By way of comparison, a mug of ale cost a penny and a young whore with good teeth was less than a shilling a throw." *Tobacco* (Gately), p. 51

46. "[Tobacco] cureth any grief, dolour, imposture, or obstruction proceeding of cold or wind, especially in the head or breast. The fume taken in a pipe is good against rheums, catarrhs, hoarseness, ache in the head, stomach, lungs, breast: also in want of meat, drink, sleep or rest." Henry Buttes, *Dyets Dry Dinner*, 1599

# 1600

47. King James I of England was a prominent early critic of tobacco. He wrote: "A custome loathsome to the Eye, hatefull to the Nose, harmful to the Braine, daungerous to the Lungs, and in the blacke stinking fume thereof, neerest resembling the horrible Stigian smoke of the pit that is bottomelesse." He wrote that tobacco was a "filthie noveltie." *A Counterblaste to Tobacco*, King James I, 1604

48. "What honor or policie can move us to imitate the barbarous and beastly manners of the wilde, godlesse, and slavish Indians, especially in so vile and stinking a custome?..Why do we not as well imitate them in walking naked as they do?" King James I, 1604

49. "For the vanities committed in this filthy custome, is it not both great vanity and uncleanness, that at the table, a place of cleanliness, men should not be ashamed, to sit puffing of the smoke of tobacco, making the filthy smoke and stink thereof, to exhale athwart the dishes, and infect the air, when very often men that abhor it are at their repast?" *A Counterblaste to Tobacco*, King James I, 1604

50. "It makes a kitchen also oftentimes in the inward parts of men, soiling and infecting them with an unctuous and oily kind of Soote, as hath bene found in some great Tobacco takers, that after death were opened." King James I, about 1605 (JAMA, February 26, 1992, p. 1037)

51. "Moreover, which is a great iniquity, and against all humanity, the husband shall not be ashamed to reduce thereby his delicate, wholesome, and clean complexioned wife to that extremity, that either she must also corrupt her sweet breath therewith, or else resolve to live in a perpetual stinking torment." James I, *A Counterblaste to Tobacco*, 1604

52. King James I wrote, "Being taken when they go to bed, it (tobacco) makes one sleep soundly, and yet being taken when a man is sleepy or drowsy, it will, as they say, awake his brain and quicken his understanding." *Nicotine*, p. 41

53. King James raised the tobacco tax from 2 pence to 82 pence per pound, making tobacco more expensive than silver. *Tobacco and Health*, p. 221

54. In the early 17th century, tobacco was so popular in England that it was exchanged for silver ounce for ounce. In 1610, an observer noted: "Many a young nobleman's estate is altogether spent and scattered to nothing in smoke. This befalls in a shameful fashion, in that a man's estate runs out through his nose, and he wastes whole days, even years, in drinking of tobacco." *Licit and Illicit Drugs*, p. 210

55. The English playwright Ben Jonson (1572-1637), called tobacco "the most sovereign and precious weed that ever the earth has tendered to the use of man." Canadian Medical Association Journal, November 1, 1994, p. 1239

56. In Spain in 1614, King Philip III had established Seville as the tobacco center of the world.
The Tobacco Timeline, www.tobacco.org

57. The traditional tobaccos of the New World, those which were spread around the world in the 16th and 17th centuries, are not the predominate tobaccos used in commerce today. Two special varieties of N. tabacum, flue-cured (also called bright or Virginia tobacco) tobacco and Burley tobacco, were developed in the United States in the 19th century. These varieties now dominate the tobacco market. Cigar smoke is harsh compared to cigarette smoke, and this harshness is related to the pH of the smoke. At an alkaline pH, nicotine exists in smoke predominately as the free base and is relatively abundant in the vapor phase of the smoke. Since nicotine is irritating to the mouth and throat, cigar smoke is experienced as harsh and as difficult to inhale. Nicotine is still readily absorbed from cigars, however, because the free base readily traverses the oral mucosa.

In the mid-19th century, a new method for curing tobacco was developed in North Carolina. This new method, flue curing, involved exposing the harvested leaf to high temperatures. The process resulted in a tobacco leaf that burned with an acid pH because of its relatively high sugar content. In an acidic environment, nicotine is predominately in the form of salts and is dissolved in droplets of a smoke aerosol. This results in a milder smoke, one that is easier to inhale. In the lung, nicotine is rapidly absorbed across the vast respiratory epithelium so that a low smoke pH does not limit absorption.

The use of flue-cured tobacco made the inhalation of tobacco smoke easier. Inhalation, in turn, provided a greater boost of nicotine to the brain compared to oral absorption as well as more widespread exposure of the body to the poisons in tobacco smoke. Quote from *The Tobacco Epidemic*, pp. 4-5 (John Slade)

58. "When temperately used, there is not in all the world a medicine comparable to tobacco. All of tobacco is wholesome." William Barclay: *Nepenthes*; or, *The Virtues of Tobacco*, 1614

59. An account regarding Japan in 1616 stated: "It is strange to see how these Japanese men, women, and children, are besotted in drinking that herb; and not ten years since it was in use first." *Faber Book of Smoking*, p. 44

60. There were 7000 tobacco shops in London in 1614. Sir Francis Drake wrote: "The use of tobacco conquers men with a certain secret pleasure, so that those who have once become accustomed thereto can later hardly be restrained therefrom." *Licit and Illicit Drugs*, p. 210

61. "Tobacco, divine, rare, super excellent tobacco, which goes far beyond all panaceas, potable gold, and philosophers' stones, a sovereign remedy to all diseases...But, as it is commonly abused by most men, which take it as tinkers do ale, 'tis a plague, a mischief, a violent purger of goods, lands, health; hellish, devilish and damned tobacco, the ruin and overthrow of body and soul." Richard Burton, English cleric, in *The Anatomy of Melancholy*, 1621

62. Sultan Murad IV considered smokers to be infidels, and decreed the death penalty for smoking tobacco in Constantinople, Turkey in 1633. "Nevertheless, the passion for smoking still persisted...Even the fear of death was of no avail with the passionate devotees of the habit." Ironically, Murad cigarettes were one of the most popular brands of the 1920's. *Licit and Illicit Drugs*, p. 212

63. Turkish smokers under Murad lived under the threat of death by "hanging, beheading, quartering between four strong horses, or being incarcerated in a public cage without food and water until they died."
Journal of the American Dental Association, November 1982, p. 825

64. In Constantinople in 1633 the Sultan Murad IV decreed the death penalty for smoking tobacco. Wherever the Sultan went on his travels or military expeditions, his stopping places were frequently marked by executions of tobacco smokers. Even on the battlefield he was fond of surprising men in the act of smoking: he would punish his own

soldiers by beheading, hanging, quartering, or crushing their hands and feet and leaving them helpless between the lines. In spite of the horrors and insane cruelties inflicted by the Sultan, whose blood lust seemed to increase with age, the passion for smoking persisted in his domain. The first of the Romanov czars, Mihail Feodorovich, also prohibited smoking, under dire penalties, in 1643. "Offenders are usually sentenced to slitting of the nostrils, beatings, or whippings," a visitor to Moscow noted. Quote from *Nicotine*, p. 97

65. In Russia, Czar Michael Romanov (reign 1613-1645) forbade the sale of tobacco and threatened users with dire punishments, including castration and cutting off of noses.
Journal of the American Dental Association, November 1982, p. 825

66. "The Japanese, who had received tobacco courtesy of a shipwreck in 1542, took to the weed with the same unthinking gusto as the English." *Tobacco* (Gately), p. 57

67. By 1603, the use of tobacco was well established in Japan, and an edict prohibiting smoking was pronounced. As no notice was taken of the edict, still severer measures were taken in 1607 and 1609, by which the cultivation of tobacco was made a criminal offense...It was to no avail. The custom spread rapidly in every direction, until many smokers were to be found even in the Mikado's palace. Finally, even the princes who were responsible for the prohibition took to smoking. Tobacco had won again. In 1625 permission was given to cultivate and plant tobacco. By 1639 tobacco had taken its place as an accompaniment to the ceremonial cup of tea offered to a guest.
Quote from *Nicotine*, p. 98

68. The Jamestown settlement established in 1607 had a very difficult first several years. Most of the colony's population starved in the winter of 1610-1611, reducing the population from 500 to only 60. In 1612, John Rolfe experimented with a tobacco seed imported from Trinidad, Nicotiana tobacum, and successfully grew the colony's first crop of tobacco. *Tobacco in History*, p. 134

69. After the establishment in 1607 of the Jamestown colony, John Rolfe was responsible for making tobacco the principal crop and export. The first shipment was in 1613, and amounts increased to 2300 pounds in 1615, 20,000 pounds in 1618, and 40,000 pounds in 1620. Population and Development Review, June 1990, p. 216

70. John Rolfe's Jamestown colony established on the James River in Virginia in 1610 owed its survival and later prosperity to tobacco, its only export to England. Rolfe was the founder of America's oldest industry, and also helped to make peace with the local Indians because of his romance with Pocahontas. In 1619, eager bachelors paid 120 pounds each of tobacco for a shipload of English maidens, "ninety agreeable persons, young and incorrupt." The "golden weed" was worth its weight in wives.
Journal of the American Dental Association, November 1982, p. 826

71. By 1614, Virginia was producing for England 1 lb of tobacco for every 20 lb it obtained from Spain. By 1619, Virginia reached parity with Spain as a supplier of tobacco to England. A year later, in 1620, the amount of Virginia tobacco received in England was twice that received from Spain. In that same year in the more northern settlements of Massachusetts one of the first messages from the newly landed Pilgrims at Plymouth Plantation was, "Send us Virginia." By the 1630s, the Virginia tobacco market was so successful that little else economically mattered. Salaries, including those of the clergy, were paid not in gold or silver, but by poundage of tobacco. So, too, were penalties and fines, such as a levy of 1,000 lb of tobacco for a child born out of wedlock to a white indentured Virginian. A new wife could be obtained from the homeland at much less cost, for about 120 lb of cured leaf. A marriage was paid for with 200 lb of tobacco, a funeral with 400 lb. At one point, tobacco was worth even more, pound for pound, than was silver. Quote from *The Tobacco Epidemic*, p. 18 (Gary Huber)

72. ...the growing of tobacco on tidewater plantations in Virginia and Maryland became the prime source of revenue for the English treasury. The raw tobacco was shipped to England, where it was processed and then sold back to all of the colonies, as well as throughout Great Britain and the British Empire, at substantial profit to the tobacco merchants. Ever-increasing taxes delivered equally ever-increasing revenues to the royal treasury.
The Black slave trade from Africa to America was developed to fulfill the manpower needs that simply could not be met by white indentured servants in the English settlements. In exchange for tobacco, the first ship carrying slaves, delivered by the Dutch, arrived in Virginia in 1626. In a continuing attempt to meet the continuously growing demand, tobacco was over planted, depleting the tidewater basin plantations of their vital soil nutrients. Crop production then began to fall short of promised deliveries and American tobacco planter-farmers fell

progressively further and further into debt to the English tobacco merchants. In attempts to reduce their debts, colonial farmers planted more tobacco seed and went even further into debt to acquire more slaves, sustaining an ever-vicious cycle of economic imbalance. As the American tobacco debts went unpaid, English mercantile houses annexed plantations and seized other colonial assets, fermenting the already percolating strong and growing emotions of dissent.

The taxation burden on American tobacco was economically enormous. Tax revenues from levies on Virginia and Maryland tobacco alone exceeded all other incoming revenues to the royal treasury of any nature from all other British possessions combined. Growing indebtedness and higher taxation led to a progressive loss of autonomy, further eroding individual and economic freedom. The outcome was inevitable. Radical political ideology was fostered and it continually festered. Although certainly not the only issue, tobacco economics, and the closely associated taxations and indebtedness, contributed as much politically and socially as, if not more than, any other factor to the ferment that led ultimately to the American Revolution.

Quote from The Tobacco Epidemic, p. 19 (Gary Huber)

73. John Rolfe, an "ardent smoker", was probably instrumental in importing tobacco seed from Trinidad between 1610 and 1611. He crossed the imported breed with the indigenous tobacco to produce a plant well adapted to the local soil and reportedly of pleasant taste. The English cargo vessel Elizabeth sailed from Jamestown in June 1613, carrying Rolfe's first crop for export.

Jamestown exhibit, National Geographic Society, Washington, D.C., March 1998

74. Tobacco exports from the Chesapeake region to Britain increased from 60,000 pounds in 1620 to 15 million pounds in 1669, 30 million in 1700, and 100 million pounds in 1775 on the eve of the American Revolution.

Tobacco in History, pp. 152 and 205

75. In 1629 at the urging of King James I, Governor Winthrop of Massachusetts banned tobacco sales and public smoking.

Journal of Medical Activism (DOC News and Views), May 1994, p. 6

76. In 1646, the state of Massachusetts made it unlawful to smoke within five miles of any town site.

San Francisco Examiner, September 19, 1999

77. From 1612 to 1803 when cotton became first, tobacco was the American colonies' most valuable export commodity.

78. ". . . in time the American colonies were granted a monopoly on all leaf shipped to England. As the seventeenth century lengthened, every jetty and dockside in the Maryland and Virginia tidewater clattered and rumbled with half-ton hogsheads of the prized leaf being rolled aboard British ships bearing them back to a nation stricken with tobacco mania. Virginia flowered, and tobacco became the mainstay of nearly every phase of the colonists' lives: wages were paid in it, goods bartered for it, wives purchased with it--120 pounds of cured leaf was the going rate for a healthy spouse from the mother country. The only problem was the shortage of hands to tend the demanding crop, and so African slave trade grew under Dutch transport, the dark cargo purchased mostly with the lush harvests of the leaf.

In return for Virginia's privileged status as tobacco supplier to Great Britain, the colonial crop could be shipped nowhere else and only on craft flying the British flag; the growing continental demand for Virginia leaf was gladly satisfied by London merchants who reshipped the leaf at a healthy markup. Still, colonial growers felt sufficiently compensated to expand their tobacco crop at a steady pace--and to the exclusion of any other crop beyond what was needed for subsistence. Thus, their dependency on the exclusively British tobacco market deepened, and with it, their indebtedness to English merchants who supplied them on terms deemed ever harsher by the colonists."

Ashes to Ashes, p. 11

79. French Acadians were "for the most part so bewitched with this drunkenness of tobacco, that they can no more be without it than without meat or drink..." Lescarbot, 1607 (Nicotine and Public Health, p. 9)

80. Paul LeJeune, a Jesuit missionary, in 1634 wrote about tobacco and the Montagnois of Quebec that they "love it to madness." He also noted "Our Savages... made a banquet of smoke...the fondness they have for this herb is beyond all belief. They go to sleep with their reed pipes in their mouths, they sometimes get up in the night to smoke..."

Nicotine and Public Health, p. 2

81. "Tobacco! Divine, rare, super-excellent tobacco! Which goes far beyond all the panaceas, potable gold, and philosopher's stones; a sovereign remedy to all diseases; a virtuous herb, if it be well qualified, opportunely taken,

and medicinally used; but as it is commonly abused by most men, who take it as tinkers do ale, 'tis a plague, a mischief, a violent purge of goods, lands, health, hellish, devilish, and dammed tobacco, the ruin and overthrow of body and soul."  Robert Burton, *The Anatomy of Melancholy*, 1621

82. Roger Williams, who became familiar with the Narragansett [Indians] living in the vicinity of Providence, Rhode Island, from 1636 to 1643, observed that "they generally all take tobacco" and added that those who do not smoke "are rare birds; for generally all the men throughout the country have a tobacco bag with a pipe in it hanging at their back." This corroborates the Cartier account, which suggests that only men smoked.

Quote from *Nicotine and Public Health*, p. 4

83. The Dutch in 1652 bought the peninsula of the Cape of Good Hope in Africa from the natives for "a certain quantity of tobacco and brandy."  *Tobacco* (Gately), p. 89

84. "Whatever Aristotle and all the philosophers may say, there is nothing equal to tobacco. All good fellows like it, and he who lives without tobacco does not deserve to live. It not only exhilarates and clears a man's brains but also teaches virtue, and on learns to become a good fellow through its means. Do you not plainly see that, as soon as we take it, we put on an agreeable manner toward everybody and are delighted to offer it right and left wherever we are?  Moliere, *Don Juan*, 1665

85. "I will summarily rehearse the hurts that tobacco infereth. It drieth the brain, dimmith the sight, vitiate the smell, dulleth and dejecteth both the appetite and the stomach, destroyeth the decoction, disturbeth the humours and the spirits, corrupteth the breath, induceth a trembling of the limbs, exsiccathe the windpipe, lungs, and liver, annoyeth the milt and scorche the heart..."
Dr. Venner of Bathe, 1650 (*Smoking and the Public Interest*, Ruth Brecher, Consumers Union, 1963)

86. In Moliere's *Don Juan* (1665), the character Sganarelle touts tobacco as "the passion of all proper people, and he who lives without tobacco has nothing else to live for. Not only does it refresh and cleanse men's brains, but it guides their souls in the ways of virtue, and by it one learns to be a man of honor."  *Nicotine*, p. 41

87. "Information has lately reach Us from the Dean and Chapter of metropolitan church in Sevilla that in those parts the use of the herb commonly called tobacco has gained so strong a hold on persons of both sexes, yea, even priests and clerics, that – We blush to state – during the actual celebration of Holy Mass, they do not shrink from taking tobacco through the mouth or nostrils, thus soiling the altar linen and infecting the churches with its noxious fumes, sacrilegiously and to the great scandal of the pious… it therefore behooves Us, in order to purge our churches of this shameless abuse, to prohibit and interdict all persons of either sex, clergy or laity, collectively and individually, from using tobacco or snuff in any form whatever in the churches of the said diocese of Sevilla, their vestibules, vestries, or immediate surroundings; and all persons thus offending shall be punished by immediate excommunication, ipso facto, without further ado, in accordance with the terms of the present interdict."
Pope Urban VIII, Papal Bull, 1642

88. Pope Urban VIII issued a formal decree against tobacco in 1642 and Pope Innocent X issued another in 1650, but clergy as well as laymen continued to smoke. "By 1725 even the pope was forced to capitulate. Louis Lewin has written on the subject: 'Benedict XIII, who himself liked to take snuff, annulled all edicts in order to avoid the scandalous spectacle of dignitaries of the Church hastening out in order to take a few clandestine whiffs in some corner away from spying eyes'."  *Nicotine*, pp. 96 and 98

89. "Whatever Aristotle and all the philosophers may say, there is nothing equal to tobacco. All good fellows like it, and he who lives without tobacco does not deserve to live. It not only exhilarates and clears a man's brains but also teaches virtue, and one learns to become a good fellow through its means. Do you not plainly see that, as soon as we take it, we put on an agreeable manner towards everybody and are delighted to offer it right and left wherever we are?"  Moliere, *Don Juan*, 1669

90. Mynheer Van Klaes of 17th century Holland was called the "King of Smokers." When he died at age 81, it was estimated conservatively that his life's consumption of tobacco was four tons, or ten pounds every week of his 60 smoking years.  *Tobacco Advertising*, p. 11

91. It was thought that smoking could help keep the plague in check, "promoting widespread smoking during the Great Plague of 1665. During the plague years, boys at England's Eton College were whipped if they tried to skip their daily smoke."
*Cigarettes*, (Parker-Pope), p.3

92. "I have been told, that in the last great plague at London none that kept tobaconist's shops had the plague. It is certain, that smoking it was looked upon as a most excellent preservative. In so much, that even children were obliged to smoak. And I remember, that I heard formerly Tom Rogers, who was yeoman beadle, say, that when he was that year, when the plague raged, a school-boy at Eton, all the boys of that school were obliged to smoak in the school every morning and that he was never whipped so much in his life as he was one morning for not smoaking."
Thomas Hearne, on compulsory smoking at Eton during the 1721 Plague (*Faber Book of Smoking*, p. 47)

93. In the English-American colonies both visitors and travelers, when commenting on the habits of the colonists, stressed the near-universal use of tobacco. One such traveler reported in 1686 his observations on the backwoods settlement: "Everyone smokes while working and idling. I sometimes went to hear the sermon; their churches are in the woods and when everyone has arrived the minister and all the others smoke before going in. The preaching over, they do the same thing before parting. They have seats for that purpose. It was here I saw that everybody smokes, men, women, girls and boys from the age of seven."
*Tobacco in History*, p. 63

94. A British surgeon on an expedition in Panama in the 1680's wrote an account of an Indian smoke-blowing session: "The End so lighted he puts into his Mouth, and blows the Smoak through the whole length of the Roll into the Face of every one of the Company or the Council, tho' there be 2 or 300 of them. Then they, sitting in their usual posture upon Forms, make, with their Hands held hollow together, a kind of Funnel round their Mouths and Noses. Into this they receive the Smoak as 'tis blown upon them, snuffing it up greedily and strongly as long as ever they are able to hold their Breath, and seeming to bless themselves, as it were, with the Refreshment it gives them."
*Tobacco in History*, p. 34

# 1700

95. The Spanish colonizers of the New World were primarily in South America, where the natives smoked the precursors of cigars, while the British were in North America, where native Americans used pipes. "As a result, for more than 200 years, while the Spanish puffed cigars, smoking in Britain essentially meant pipe smoking.
*Faber Book of Smoking*, p. 18

96. In 1702, a British fleet at Cadiz, Spain, captured thousands of barrels of Spanish snuff. "Back in Britain, the booty was given out to the sailors, who soon spread its fame." By 1720, Johann Cohausen wrote in *Lust of the Longing Nose*:
"The world has taken up a ridiculous fashion – the excessive use of snuff. All nations are snuffing. All classes snuff, from the highest to the lowest. I have sometimes wondered to see how lords and lackeys, High Society and the mob, wood choppers and handymen, broom-squires and beadles, take outwith an air, and dip into them. Both sexes snuff, for the fashion has spread to the women: the ladies began it, and are now imitated by the washerwomen. People snuff so often that their noses are more like a dust-heap than noses…"
*Faber Book of Smoking*, pp. 49-51

97. Tobacco use by the common people in Britain began in 1702 when the British fleet captured from Spain at Cadiz several thousand barrels of choice snuff. This vast quantity was sold at very low prices, and "thus was the general snuff habit born in Britain."
*Licit and Illicit Drugs*, p. 213

98. By the mid-1700's in England, "a gentleman who did not take (nasal) snuff was a contradiction in terms...Ladies snuffed as artistically, vigorously, and conspicuously as men." The first edition of the Encyclopaedia Britannica in 1768 warned that tobacco "dries and damages the brain." Journal of the American Dental Association, November 1982, p. 824, and American Medical News, December 8, 1992

99. "Tobacco profits built England's large merchant marine, afforded the extravagant lifestyles of England's upper class, and financed England's military ventures. Profits from tobacco sales were a major source of funds for the American Revolution." Psychiatric Clinics of North America, March 1993, p. 50

100. "America triumphed over the arrogance of her conquerors by infecting them with her own vices; she hastened on the death of her new masters by giving them venereal disease--and tobacco."
Dr. Fagon, physician to Louis XIV of France (The Practitioner, January 1980, p. 111)

101. As a "revenge of the Indians," the spread of tobacco makes the introduction of syphilis into the new world pale by comparison when the enormous toll in death and disease is considered...Perhaps the most dramatic description of the Indians' revenge was given by "the tobacco fiend" at the court of Lucifer in an 18th century epic:
"Thus do I take in full upon the Spaniards for all their cruelty to the Indians; since by acquainting their conquerors with the use of tobacco I have done them greater injury than even the King of Spain through his agents ever did his victims; for it is both more honorable and more natural to die by a pike thrust or a cannon ball than from the ignoble effects of poisonous tobacco."
Quote from Nicotine, p. 28

102. A physician's description in 1716 of tobacco's effects:
"Tobacco resolves, cleanses, purges, vomits, stupefies the brain, resists poison and is a very great vulnerary. The external application of the leaves (moistened and beat with a little wine) to the head, easeth the megrim, and other pains thereof; to the joints, the pains of gout; to the hips, the sciatica; to the teeth, the toothache; to the skin, it remedies all deformities and beautifies it; to the rib'd heels, it heals them; to the shins, the pains proceeding from the French Disease. Made into an ointment or balsam, it cures all manner of tumors, ulcers, old sores, fistulas, scabs, breakings out, itch, bitings, stingings of venomous beasts, punctures of the nerves and tendons, though made with poisoned weapons, happening in any part of the body from head to foot; it cures scalds, burns, piles, and gouts of all sorts."
Population and Development Review, June 1990, p. 215

103. The Iroquois of New York placed wads of tobacco inside the mouth to ease toothache pain. Other Native Americans made tobacco pastes and poultices to treat burns, sores, colds, dysentery, rheumatism, colic, sciatica, and snake, insect, and mad dog bites.
Health Education, June 1987, p. 6

104. In the American colonies in the 18th century, yearly tobacco consumption averaged between two and five pounds per capita per year.
Reducing Tobacco Use, p. 29

105. In America, almost half of the total export income in 1750 was from tobacco.
Tobacco (Gately), p. 109

106. Tobacco enemas "were used in Europe to loosen the bowels, and to treat cholera until well into the nineteenth century..."
Faber Book of Smoking, p. 17

107. In Boston in 1730, a statue of Pocahontas was reported outside a tobacconist's doorway. After the Civil War, cigar store wooden Indians became common. In the early 1900's, the wooden Indians were no longer fashionable, and most were discarded or burned.
Tobacco Advertising, p. 30

108. Almost life-size, brightly painted wooden cigar store Indians between 1830 and 1890 "were as omnipresent as neon signs are now" before their novelty was over and they were replaced with other kinds of advertising. They stood on the sidewalk in front of tobacco stores, "signaling the wares for sale within," and wore "splendid jewelry, tunic, features, sometimes fringed leggings, the Noble Savage of early-19th-century romantic imagining..."
New York Times, September 7, 1997, p. H93 (Arts and Leisure section)

109. After the American Revolution, the Lorillard brothers Peter and George published the first American advertisements for tobacco. Their American Indian theme developed into the "Red Man" symbol for tobacco, with life-size wooden Indian statues appearing everywhere. The most well known was "Big Chief Me Smoke 'Em."
Health Education, June 1987, p. 7

110. In 1761 a London physician, Dr. John Hill, in his Cautions Against the Immoderate Use of Snuff reported nine cases of cancer of the nostrils and one of cancer of the esophagus among habitual snuff users. This may have been the first report of tobacco as a cause of cancer.
Ashes to Ashes, p. 15, and Smoke and Mirrors, p. 31

111. In 1761, the British physician John Hill described five cases of nasal cancer that he attributed to nasal snuff use. He wrote, "No man should venture upon snuff who is not sure that he is not liable to cancer, and no man can be sure of that."
Pediatrics, December 1985, p. 1009

112. In 1761, the English doctor John Hill related smoking to cancer of the nose. Thirty years later in Germany, Samuel vonSocmmerring noted the same for lip cancer. And in the 1850's, Etienne-Frederick Bousson in France observed that 63 out of 68 patients with mouth cancer were pipe smokers.    *Faber Book of Smoking*, p. 89

113. The first imported cigars from Cuba were brought to Connecticut in 1762 by a British naval officer, Colonel Israel Putnam. "Old Put" later became an American general in the Revolutionary War, and is credited with introducing cigar smoking to the United States.    *A Passion for Cigars*, p. 17 and the Tobacco Timetable, www.tobacco.org

114. In 1775, Percival Pott described an epidemic of scrotal cancer in chimney sweeps in London, an early documentation of the carcinogenicity of chimney smoke.    Population and Development Review, June 1990, p. 218

115. "Sugar, rum and tobacco are commodities which are nowhere necessities of life, which are become objects of almost universal consumption, and which are therefore extremely proper subjects of taxation."
    Adam Smith, *An Inquiry into the Nature* and*Causes of the Wealth of Nations*, 1776 *The Tobacco Atlas*, p. 84

116. In 1769 on his voyage to the Pacific, "Captain James Cook arrives, smoking a pipe. Thought a demon, the natives douse him with water."    The Tobacco Timeline, www.tobacco.org

117. The major export from the American colonies to Great Britain was tobacco; the total was 100 million pounds by 1776. The fact that London merchants unfairly treated tobacco farmers almost as indentured servants was one of the reasons for the American revolution of that year.

118. "I say, if you can't send money, send tobacco."    General George Washington, 1776, appealing to his countrymen during the early stages of the American Revolution

119. "Benjamin Franklin financed the Continental Congresses by swinging a loan from France based on tobacco futures, and the 'royal leaf' virtually paid for the American Revolution."    *A Passion for Cigars*, p. 17

120. Tobacco helped finance the American Revolution, and is mentioned in the Constitution. Its past importance is symbolized by the use of tobacco leaves and flowers as decorations atop columns dating from 1818 in the Old Senate Rotunda of the United States Capitol.  New Jersey Medicine, February 1988, p. 103, and Richard Hurt, M.D.

121. At the end of the Revolutionary War, there were fewer than 800,000 slaves in the United States. By 1860 there were 4 million black slaves, almost all living in southern states as labor for growing tobacco and cotton. "About 400 or more man-hours were required to bring an acre of tobacco from seed to market."
    *The Tobacco Epidemic*, pp. 21-22

122. Benjamin Waterhouse was one of the original professors at Harvard Medical School at its establishment in 1782. (Harvard was the third medical school in the United States, after Penn in 1765 and Columbia's College of Physicians and Surgeons in 1768.) In a lecture for the medical course "Cautions to Young Persons Concerning Health," Waterhouse described the "evil tendency" to use tobacco, especially cigars.
    *Harvard Med*, John Langone, Crown Publishers, 1995, p. 123

123. Until 1800, tobacco enemas were given to surgery patients "to prevent muscular spasms and induce a state of tranquility and a reasonable insensibility to pain."

124. Benjamin Rush, the father of American psychiatry and signer of the Declaration of Independence, condemned tobacco use in his *Essays* written in 1798.    Psychiatric Clinics of North America, March 1993, p. 50

125. In the colonial period until 1800, the pipe was the most popular form of tobacco consumption. Nasal snuff also became very fashionable in the upper classes at this time, while chewing tobacco led all modes of consumption form 1800 to 1900. Cigar smoking had a period of great popularity also in the mid-1800's, where it almost equaled chewing tobacco.    Health Education, June 1987, p. 8

126. "Until the mid to late 19$^{th}$ century, tobacco was consumed almost entirely by pipe smoking and snuff." Snuff was thought to be a "sovereign remedie for the dripping and clogging of ye nose."    *The Tobacco Epidemic*, p. 22

127. English romantic poet Lord Byron (1788-1824) and national poet of Scotland Robert Burns (1759-1796) were tobacco chewers. From "The European Experience with Native American Tobacco," Bill Drake, 1996

# 1800

128. George Washington, Thomas Jefferson, and four of the first five American presidents were tobacco farmers.

129. Tobacco was replaced by cotton as the nation's chief export around 1800. *Tobacco Advertising*, p. 17

130. Lewis and Clark acquired a Mandan Indian ceremonial pipe near present day Bismark, North Dakota on their journey in 1804. "Smoking the pipe was a common goodwill gesture among the tribes Lewis and Clark encountered." *The Saga of Lewis and Clark* Thomas and Jeremy Schmidt, Tehabi Books, 1999, p.77

131. "Among our other difficulties, we now experience the want of tobacco. We use crabtree bark as a substitute." From the diary of Lewis and Clark expedition member Patrick Gass, March 7, 1806, in the winter camp at Ft. Clatsop at the mouth of the Columbia River. Gass died near the age of 99 in 1870, the last surviving member of the expedition. Lewis and Clark, PBS television, 1997

132. "It is a culture of infinite wretchedness. Those employed in it are in a continual state of exertion beyond the power of nature to support. Little food of any kind is raised by them: so men and animals on these farms are ill fed, and the earth is readily impoverished." Thomas Jefferson (1743-1826), *Tobacco in History*, p. 127

133. Dolly Madison passed out samples of snuff to White House guests, and was known to carry a lace handkerchief to wipe telltale tobacco grains from her nose. Health Education, June 1987

134. The first U.S. cigar factory was established in Connecticut in 1810. By 1900, tobacco used in the form of cigars accounted for 2.0 of the 7.5 pounds of tobacco consumed per adult in the U.S., second only to chewing tobacco's 3.5 pounds per adult. *Cigars*, p. 1

135. "Turks are perpetually smoking; Spaniards and Portuguese use tobacco profusely" The Lancet, December 10, 1825, p. 392

136. The English poet Lord Byron (1788-1824) was a strong proponent of smoking. *Tobacco* (Gately), p. 55

137. "Sublime Tobacco! Which from east to west cheers the tar's labour or the Turkman's rest; which on the Moslem's ottoman divides his hours and rivals opium and his brides... yet thy true lovers more admire by far thy naked beauties -- give me a cigar!" Lord Byron, *The Island*, 1823

138. Andrew Jackson (president 1829-1837) installed 20 spittoons in the elegant East Room of the White House. The American President, Public Television series, 2000

139. The German writer Johann Wolfgang von Goethe (1749-1832), the author of *Faust*, was an ardent crusader against smoking. He was among the first to observe and describe the evils of passive smoking. JAMA, November 27, 1996, p. 1630

140. Goethe, the German poet and naturalist who died in 1832, is best known for writing *Dr. Faust*, but among many other interests he was an early tobacco control advocate. He wrote: "Smoking is a wicked impoliteness, an impertinent, antisocial act. Smokers poison the air for miles around and suffocate respectable citizens who don't deign to defend themselves by retaliating in kind. Who could ever enter the room of a smoker without feeling ill?" Tobacco Control, Winter 1995, p. 332

141. Former president John Quincy Adams wrote in 1845 of how he had, as a young man, been addicted to tobacco smoking and chewing before he had successfully stopped. "I have often wished that every individual... afflicted with this artificial passion could force it upon himself to try but for three months the experiment which I made, sure that it would turn every acre of tobacco land into a wheat field, and add five years to the average of human life." *Smoking: The Artificial Passion*, p. xvi

142. In 1843, the French tobacco monopoly began manufacturing tobacco in paper tubes, and named them cigarettes.

143. The Egyptians had begun rolling tobacco in paper in the early 1830's, creating the first cigarettes. Following the Crimean War in 1856, French and British soldiers took these "tobacco cylinders" back to Europe from where they also were sent to the United States. Annals of Allergy, November 1994, p. 381

144. Frederic Chopin's mistress, the Baroness de Dudevant, in 1840 in Paris became the first woman to smoke in public. JAMA, January 23, 1994, p. 629

145. "In France, the cigarette was taken up during the Revolution by the antiroyalist masses as the tobacco product least like snuff, that elaborately boxed and ceremoniously taken powder so beloved by the monarchists. There was nothing fancy about French cigarettes, notorious there as elsewhere for being cheap and made from the leavings of other tobacco products--and further adulterated, it was rumored, by spit, urine, and dung. By the time the government began licensing their manufacture around 1840, cigarettes had been sufficiently improved to have a bourgeois appeal as well. A new, much whiter kind of wrapper, extracted from rice straw, was developed that did not stick to the lips the way earlier cigarette paper had, and a tasteless vegetable paste made the rolling quicker and easier. By mid-century, the prominent tobacco merchant Baron Joseph Huppmann had opened a factory in St. Petersburg and brought the cigarette in quantity to the Russian upper class and intelligentsia, always keen on French style and objects.

"The cigarette was little seen in England until after the Crimean War (1854-56), when its soldiers had been heavily exposed to the short smokes, which seemed ideally suited to wartime use, by their French and Turkish allies and were even proffered them by captured Russian officers. The English veterans of Crimea took their new yen for the cigarette home, where the product had previously been degraded as suitable mainly for the poor and so weak-tasting as to invite the suspicion that those smokers who preferred it were effeminate."
*Ashes to Ashes*, p. 13

146. "This vice brings in one hundred million francs in taxes every year. I will certainly forbid it at once--as soon as you can name a virtue that brings in as much revenue." Napoleon III (1808-1873), *Tobacco in History*, p. 191

147. "British soldiers returning from Wellington's Napoleonic campaigns in the Iberian Peninsula (1808-14) introduced cigarette smoking to England... Likewise, veterans returning from the Crimean War (1853-56) increased cigarette smoking in Britain--a practice soon brought to the United States by returning tourists." Population and Development Review, June 1990, pp. 218-219

148. "Although popular in England, where it had been introduced from Russia after the Crimean War, the cigarette had been slow to take hold in America. Up until the late 1860's it was looked upon as an exotic, imported in very small quantities from Turkey." Less than 2 million cigarettes were made in the United States in 1869, increasing to 238 million by 1879 as use of milder bright tobacco produced a boom. An experienced worker could hand roll 2500 a day. *Tobacco Tycoon*, pp. 47-48

149. Zachary Taylor (president 1849-1850) was a confirmed tobacco chewer, and visitors said that he had perfect spitting aim, never missing the sand-filled box across his office. The American President, PBS television, April 2000

150. Dr. R.T. Trall in 1854 reported that the United States had the highest per capita use of tobacco in the world. *Tobacco Advertising*, p. 16

151. A quotation from the 1854 book *Nature in Disease* by J. Bigelow (reported in Tobacco Control, Winter 1996, p. 279):

"Like all other narcotics its excessive use or abuse must impair the health and engender disease.
Of the different modes of using tobacco, it is probable that smoking is the most injurious, and the most capable of abuse, since in this process the active principles of the tobacco are volatilized with the smoke, and are extensively applied to the lungs as well as the mouth and nose and fauces...Notwithstanding the common use and extensive consumption of tobacco in its various forms, it must unquestionably be ranked among narcotic poisons of the most active class."

152. In the pre-Civil War era, clergymen, educators, and physicians denounced tobacco. They included P.T. Barnum, Hartwell Cocke, the co-founder of the University of Virginia, Reverend Orson Fowler, who attributed insanity, impotence, and cancer of the mouth to the weed ("cast this sensualizing fire from you"), Reverend George Trask of Massachusetts ("tobacco is a poison; it injures health and abridges life"), and Dr. Joel Shew, who listed 87 ailments caused by tobacco, including impotence.                    *Tobacco Advertising*, pp. 14-15

153. Charles Dickens wrote in *American Notes* (1842): "In the hospitals, the students of medicine are requested to eject their tobacco-juice into the boxes provided for that purpose, and not to discolour the stairs." He declared that he could not understand how Americans had won their reputation as riflemen, judging their poor aim when spitting tobacco. Another British writer sardonically commented that the national American symbol should not be the bald eagle, but rather the spittoon.                    Health Education, June 1987, p. 8

154. As Washington may be called the head-quarters of tobacco tinctured saliva, the time is come when I must confess, without any disguise, that the prevalence of those two odious practices of chewing and expectorating began about this time to be anything but agreeable, and soon became most offensive and sickening. In all the public places of America, this filthy custom is recognized. In the courts of law, the judge has his spittoon, the crier his, the witness his, and the prisoner his; while the jurymen and the spectators are provided for, as so many men who in the course of nature must desire to spit incessantly. In the hospitals, the students of medicine are requested by notices upon the wall, to eject their tobacco juice into the boxes provided for that purpose, and not to discolour the stairs. In public buildings, visitors are implored, through the same agency, to squirt the essence of their quids, or 'plugs', as I have heard them called by gentlemen learned in this kind of sweetmeat, into the national spittoons and not about the bases of the marble columns.

Quote from *American Notes*, Charles Dickens, 1842

155. On an American visit, Charles Dickens called Washington, D.C. the "headquarters for tobacco-tinctured saliva," and another British author remarked that the national emblem of the United States should be the spittoon rather than the bald eagle because of the widespread use of chewing tobacco.

*Drugs and Behavior*, W.A. McKim, Prentice Hall, 1986

156. Charles Dickens wrote while on a boat trip in the United States: "You never can conceive what the hacking and spitting is. I was obliged to wipe the half dried flakes of spittle from my coat." The boat passengers had "yellow streams from half-chewed tobacco tricking down their chins."                    *American Notes*, 1842

157. "A veritable stream of tobacco juice filled the American air throughout much of the nineteenth century, targeted at the ubiquitous cuspidor but at least as frequently darkening carpets, walls, draperies, and trousers, demonstrating to foreign visitors that they were among a slovenly people...The cigar did not seriously awaken American smoking tastes until after the war against Mexico (1846-48), with its exposure to that strong form of tobacco preferred by Latin cultures."                    *Ashes to Ashes*, p. 14

158. "By the midpoint of the nineteenth century, cigars were a goodly manufacturing business in New York and Philadelphia, another 100 million of them a year were being imported from Cuba, and among those sturdy pioneers trailblazing westward, foot-long cigars called 'stogies' after the Conestoga wagons in which they rode were a prized time killer. As for the cigarette, it was scarcely more than an American curio at mid-century, and while it began to show up occasionally on the streets of New York in the ensuing decade as travelers abroad brought the custom home with them, the little smokes did not begin to exert any real appeal until the Civil War."                    *Ashes to Ashes*, p. 14

159. In the mid-1800's, Pennsylvania became well known for a type of cigar named the "stogie" because the makers used the famous Conestoga wagon manufactured in the same region, as an advertising tie-in.
                    *A Passion for Cigars*, p. 18

160. Two prominent chewing tobacco manufacturers in the 1850's were Pierre Lorillard in New York and Joseph Liggett in St. Louis.

161. A physician in 1850 described an "intemperate South American who placed snuff up his nostrils, then stuffed shag tobacco after it, put a coil of pigtail tobacco in each cheek, and lit a Havana cigar. The gentleman was frightfully nervous."

162. In the 1800's an American national characteristic was a distended cheek, the identifying mark of the tobacco chewer. In a Lorillard ad, a happy farmer with a swollen jaw exclaims, "It ain't toothache – it's Climax."

Health Education, June 1987, p. 8

163. "The constitutional effects of Tobacco...are numerous and varied, consisting of giddiness, sickness, vomiting, dyspepsia, vitiated taste of the mouth, loose bowels, diseased liver, congestion of the brain, apoplexy, mania, loss of memory, amaurosis [blindness], deafness, nervousness, palsy, emasculation and cowardice."

John Lizars, senior operating surgeon to the Royal Infirmary of Edinburgh,
*Practical Observations on the Use and Abuse of Tobacco*, 1853

164. In 1856 and 1857, The Lancet published "an avalanche of correspondence from doctors all over the world, in what was initially called 'The Tobacco Controversy: Is Smoking Injurious?' and soon became 'The Great Tobacco Question'." *Faber Book of Smoking*, p. 67

165. "This tobacco controversy may – I sincerely trust it will – lead to directors of Insurance companies taking the precaution of inquiring from the party proposing an insurance, or through his agents and medical referees,--if he is an habitual and inveterate smoker?" J.B. Neil, *The Lancet*, 10 January 1857

166. Sir,--Having had much experience of the baneful effects of smoking in my own country, Germany, which is affected by her reeking atmosphere in many ways, I trust that my opinion may have some weight with your readers.

The tendency of Germans to disease of the lungs may be traced to their incredible passion for smoking; and our principal medical men and physiologists compute that, out of twenty deaths of men between eighteen and twenty-five, ten originate in the waste of the constitution by smoking. So frequently is vision impaired by the constant use of tobacco, that spectacles may be said to be as much a part of parcel of a German as a hat is of an Englishman. J.G. Schneider, Letter to *The Lancet*, 31 January 1857

167. In 1851, Sir James Paget saw a patient with leukoplakia of the tongue from pipe smoking, and "told him he certainly would have cancer of the tongue if he went on smoking." In 1859, Bouisson reported that of 68 cases of patients with mouth cancer at a French hospital, 66 smoked tobacco and one chewed tobacco. He also noted that cancer of the lip usually occurred at the spot where the pipe or cigar was held.

Population and Development Review, June 1990, pp. 219-220

168. Before colonization of the area by white settlers, the Kootenai Indians in northwest Montana grew tobacco in what it now called the Tobacco Valley. *Montana Handbook*, W.C. McRae, Moon Publications, 1996, p. 401

169. Tobacco is a very labor-intensive crop requiring 250 man-hours per acre to harvest, in contrast to 5 hours for wheat. Many of the four million slaves in the South in 1860 were utilized in the tobacco harvest.

170. The first federal excise tax on tobacco was imposed in 1862 to help finance the Civil War (it yielded $3 million that year), and tobacco taxes were the chief source of government revenue until the imposition of the income tax in 1913. American Medical News, November 14, 1994, p. 16 and *The Tobacco Timeline*, www.tobacco.org

171. "Cigars helped the Union win the bloody battle of Antietam. A Rebel officer used a piece of paper containing General Robert E. Lee's orders to bundle his cigars, and when the cigars fell into the hands of Union soldiers, so did the Confederate battle plans." *A Passion for Cigars*, p. 21

172. During the Civil War, the Confederacy issued tobacco rations to its soldiers, the first time a government had ever done so. *Cigarettes* (Parker-Pope), p. 9

173. Tobacco was given with rations to Union and Confederate soldiers in the Civil War, and many Northerners were introduced to tobacco this way. www.uchsc.edu

174. During lulls in fighting in the Civil War, the soldiers of the opposing armies would mingle and trade goods. The Confederates usually wanted food and coffee, and the Union troops were most interested in tobacco.

*They Satisfy*, Robert Sobel, Anchor Books, 1978, p. 14

175. Abraham Lincoln had several spittoons placed in the White House for the use of his friends and visitors.

176. Richmond Virginia in 1860 had more than 50 tobacco factories. During the Civil War, tobacco was often included in the regular food rations of Confederate soldiers. *Ashes to Ashes*, p. 17

177. "Ulysses S. Grant smoked and chewed cigars incessantly. Following victory at Vicksburg in 1963, a grateful Union sent Grant 11,000 cigars, increasing his consumption to 25 daily. In 1884, when he felt a painful lump in the roof of his mouth that became more troublesome day by day, his physicians advised limiting his indulgence to three cigars daily; but Grant died the following year, a few days after completing his autobiography. His son, General F.D. Grant, also an inveterate cigar smoker, died similarly of cancer of the mouth in 1916. Likewise, Prussia lost a famed military leader and sovereign to tobaccosis when, in 1888 at age 56 and after just 99 days of rule, Kaiser Frederick III, anglophile husband of Queen Victoria's eldest daughter, died of cancer of the larynx. Had he instead lived to age 91 as did his father, European and world history might have been greatly different." Population and Development Review, June 1990, p. 220 (R.T. Ravenholt)

178. Provisions were scarce during the winter of 1864-65 at a new gold mining site at "Yellowstone City" near present day Gardiner, Montana, and "tobacco was literally worth its weight in gold."
Montana historical highway marker

179. Tobacco chewing was common among certain American Indian groups. After 1815 it became almost a distinctive mode of tobacco usage in the United States, replacing pipe smoking. Partly the switch was a chauvinistic reaction against European snuff-taking and pipe-smoking; partly it was a matter of convenience for pioneering Americans on the move, since chewing was easier than lighting up a cumbersome pipe. The symbol of the change was the spittoon or cuspidor, which became a necessity of 19th-century America. Manufacturing statistics are revealing: of 348 tobacco factories listed by the 1860 census for Virginia and North Carolina, 335 concentrated wholly on chewing tobacco, and only 6 others even bothered with smoking tobacco as a sideline, using scraps from plug production. The rising popularity of manufactured cigarettes by the beginning of the 20th century spelled the decline of chewing tobacco. After World War I, plug-taking fell off abruptly.
Quote from Encyclopedia Britannica, 1985 Edition, Volume 3, p. 185

180. Three Questions:
(1) "As the discovery of this country," says an English statesman, "cursed Europe with Tobacco, who can tell whether the discovery has been more of a blessing or a curse?"
(2) "As the white man gave the red man rum, and the red man give the white man tobacco, which got the best end of the bargain?"
(3) "Which is toughest, for an old'un to take his last quid, or for a young'un to take his first quid?"
From the Anti-Tobacco Journal, July 1860 (reported by John Slade, Tobacco Control, Summer 1994, p. 144)

181. Between 1857 and 1872, George Trask published the *Anti-Tobacco Journal* in Fitchburg, Massachusetts, attacking the filth (especially of chewing tobacco), the dangers to health, and the costliness of tobacco.
Quote from *Reducing Tobacco Use*, 2000 Surgeon General report, p. 31

182. The first U.S. marketed cigarettes were by F.S. Kinney and Company in 1869, employing a mostly female force of hand-rollers. In the following decade, Allen and Ginter, W.S. Kimball and Co., and Goodwin and Co. also entered the market. *Tobacco in History*, p. 229

183. "Nicotine had been identified and accepted as the cause of tobacco's toxic properties as early as the 1860s. Laboratory experiments had graphically proven its poisonous qualities: A few drops of pure nicotine injected into a small animal was enough to kill it, and as an insecticide, nicotine had few equals."
*Tobacco Advertising*, p. 238

184. "The habit once established gives rise to more or less craving for this form of indulgence."
Ralph Waldo Emerson, about 1870 (*Ashes to Ashes*, p. 38)

185. Until the late 1860's, cigarettes were looked on as an "exotic", but then a rapid increase in manufacture and consumption began: 1869, 2 million; 1879, 238 million; 1885, one billion; and 1889, 2.1 billion.

186. In 1870 in the U.S. there were 1.2 billion cigars manufactured, compared to only 16 million cigarettes.
*Tobacco in History*, p. 236

187. In 1871, R.A. Patterson founded the "Lucky Strike" company, named for the 1849 California gold rush.
The Tobacco Timeline, www.tobacco.org

188. In 1875, Allen and Ginter cigarettes began using picture cards to stiffen the pack and protect cigarettes. The cards had pictures of actresses, Indian chiefs and baseball players and were extremely successful, representing the first modern promotion scheme for a manufactured product.
www.uchsc.edu

189. The Palace Hotel in San Francisco, the grandest in the city, opened in 1875 and had 800 rooms and 9,000 cuspidors. It burned in the 1906 earthquake.
*The Pacific States: Smithsonian Guides to Historic America*, William Logan, Stewart, Tabori and Chang, 1998, p. 217

190. The superintendent of the Naval Academy at Annapolis, Commodore Parker, in 1879 lifted a regulation that had barred the use of tobacco by midshipmen.
*Tobacco Advertising*, p. 16

191. In 1880, cigarettes constituted only 3% of the tobacco consumed in the United States, most of the consumption being chewing tobacco. In this year, tobacco taxes accounted for 31% of all federal tax revenues.

192. Prior to 1880, cigarettes were made by "hand rollers." A fast worker could hand roll four cigarettes a minute, or 2000 in a day. In 1881, Virginian James Bonsack invented a machine that could mass-produce cigarettes at the rate of 120,000 per day, and the "cigarette age" had begun.
New York Times, August 28, 1994

193. But in North Carolina the flue-cured Bright tobacco that made possible the triumph of cigarettes was already gaining popularity. This tobacco led to a much gentler smoke, as the Northerners passing through during the Civil War soon recognized. Next, from a small farmstead in the same state came James Buchanan Duke. Realizing that the neighbouring Bull Durham brand had cornered the pipe-tobacco market, in the early 1880s Duke took the apparently foolhardy step of putting all his energy into cigarettes. Within 20 years, his annual sales were around $125m a year, his workforce numbered 100,000 and he was controlling almost the whole of the American tobacco industry.

Duke's first breakthrough was to spot the potential of the new Bonsack automatic rolling machine. While others were still arguing that hand-rolling was the essence of the cigarette's appeal, he bought up all the Bonsacks available, also securing a deal whereby he received 25 percent royalties on every machine bought by anybody else. Now he just needed to create a market for all the cigarettes he could produce so cheaply. He began with aggressive selling – including the introduction of cigarette cards, 'sweeteners' paid to tobacconists and giving out Duke cigarettes to immigrants as they landed. Once this was successful, he moved on to aggressive buying – of nearly all of his competitors.

The result was the American Tobacco Company which made 90 percent of the country's cigarettes and soon set about undermining those who made the rest. The company was broken up in 1911 by the same kind of government trustbusting that also did in Rockefeller's Standard Oil.
*The Faber Book of Smoking*, p. 76

194. "One of Bonsack's early machines could produce 70,000 cigarettes per shift, equivalent to what 40-50 workers could generate during the same time."
*The Tobacco Epidemic*, p. 23

195. After James Bonsack patented his cigarette-making machine that manufactured up to forty times what the best skilled workers could produce by hand, the cost of producing a cigarette was reduced dramatically. When James Buchanan Duke turned exclusively to machine production in 1885, he quickly saturated the American market. A single Bonsack machine working for 55 hours a week could turn out as many cigarettes as all the hand rollers in America combined.
*Advertising*, p. 185, and *They Satisfy*, p. 34

196. The maximum output for a Bonsack machine was 212 cigarettes per minute, or more than 12,000 per hour.
*Tobacco* (Gately), p. 207

197. "Buck" Duke spent 20 percent of his cigarette sale profits on advertising. In 1889, this amounted to "an unheard of $800,000 in billboard and newspaper advertising."
*Tobacco* (Gately), p. 208 and The Tobacco Timeline, www.tobaco.org

198. The first mass marketed and nationally advertised cigarette brand was James B. Duke's Duke of Durham in 1881. *Tobacco in History*, pp. 101-102

199. With the introduction of the Bonsack machine, U.S. cigarette production reached 1 billion in 1885, 2.1 billion in 1889, and 8.6 billion in 1910. Buck Duck's leading competitor, Allen and Ginter, first adopted the Bonsack machine in 1887. *Tobacco Tycoon*, pp. 62 and 258

200. Before mass production, cigarettes sold for 20 for 10 cents as a luxury item. The Bonsack machine reduced the unit cost by 90%, and Duke soon cornered the market. He was able to cut the price in half to a nickel for a pack of ten and still make nearly a 100 percent profit. *Ashes to Ashes*, p. 23

201. By 1884, each Bonsack machine operating at full capacity produced the output of 48 hand rollers, and Duke's manufacturing costs dropped immediately from eighty to thirty cents per thousand cigarettes.
*Cigarette Confidential*, p. 101

202. "Buck" Duke controlled more than 50% of the cigarette market by 1889, marketing brands called Duke of Durham, Cameo, Cross Cut, and Pin Head. He never used his product himself.

203. "...the decadence of Spain began when the Spaniards adopted cigarettes. If this pernicious practice continues among Americans, the ruin of the republic is close at hand." New York Times editorial, 1883

204. Victorian England presumed smoking to be impolite when practiced in public. In Great Britain municipal ordinances prohibited smoking on city streets, generally limiting the practice to smoking rooms and to men-only gatherings. In the 1840s British men's clubs became the principal havens of cigar smokers; in 1868 Britain enacted a law that trains would include smoking cars. Smoking in the Victorian era could be generalized by the statement "Men did it, women objected." Queen Victoria's son Edward, Prince of Wales, was a passionate cigar aficionado. When, upon his accession to the throne in 1901, he spoke the memorable line "Gentlemen, you may smoke," cigars finally gained their rightful place in social settings. Quote from *The Cigar Connoisseur*, p. 11

205. In 1884, the superintendent of the Department for Overthrow of Tobacco Habit acknowledged the difficulty of the task before her: "With a spittoon in the pulpit and the visible trail of the vice in countless churches, with its entrenchments bearing the seal of respectability, its fortifications so long impregnable will yield slowly and unwillingly to the mightiest opposing forces."
Quote from *Reducing Tobacco Use*, 2000 Surgeon General report, p. 31

206. "Cases are given in medical works in which excessive smoking has caused death; in other cases, it has caused paralysis, and, in general, the use of tobacco tends to bring about dyspepsia, palpitation of the heart, and various diseases of the nerves." *Primer of Physiology and Hygiene*, William Thayer Smith, 1885

207. In 1886, Vincent Van Gogh painted "A Skull with Cigarette", probably intended as a covert self-portrait. This painting has been on the cover of the JAMA four times. JAMA, February 28, 1986, p. 1054

208. Dr. John Harvey Kellogg in the 1870s and 1880s argued that tobacco was a principal cause of heart disease and other illnesses and that it adversely affected both judgment and morals.
*Reducing Tobacco Use*, 2000 Surgeon General report, p. 31

209. "Many a young man finds himself as old at twenty or twenty-five years of age as he ought to be at sixty or seventy. His constitution has been dissipated in smoke at the end of a cigarette."
John H. Kellogg, M.D. (1852-1943), inventor of cornflakes who believed that cigarettes were "the most common cause of premature decrepitude in America" *Tobacco* (Gately), p. 216

210. "A million surplus Maggies are willing to bear the yolk; and a woman is only a woman, but a good Cigar is a Smoke." Rudyard Kipling, 1888

211. President Grover Cleveland, a heavy smoker, was diagnosed with a malignant tumor of the mouth during his second term (1893-1897). He was operated on by five surgeons and a dentist with ether and nitrous oxide

anesthesia, and a large sarcoma was successfully removed, along with his entire left upper jaw, which was replaced with a rubber prosthetic jaw. He died in 1908 at age 71.

*The American President, PBS television, April 2000*

212. "I smoke in moderation – only one cigar at a time."                    Statement attributed to Mark Twain

213. "As an example to others, and not that I care for moderation myself, it has always been my rule never to smoke while asleep, and never to refrain when awake. And I have made it a rule never to smoke more than one cigar at a time."                                           Mark Twain, Ken Burns, PBS television, 2002

214. "To cease smoking is the easiest thing I ever did; I ought to know, because I've done it a thousand times."
Attributed to Mark Twain

215. "I had not smoked for three full months, and no words can adequately describe the smoke appetite that was consuming me."                                                              Mark Twain, *Autobiography*, 1906

216. "It has been my rule never to smoke when asleep and never to refrain when awake. It is a good rule."
Mark Twain (*Tobacco Advertising*, p. 201)

217. "If I cannot smoke in heaven, then I shall not go."
Mark Twain (Los Angeles Times Magazine, August 10, 1997, p. 9)

218. Mark Twain in 1900 turned down several lucrative offers for tobacco endorsements. In 1909 at age 73, he began to suffer from chest pain. He called it his "tobacco chest," and cut back from 40 cigars a day to four.
Mark Twain, Ken Burns, PBS television, 2002

219. "A cigarette is the perfect type of a perfect pleasure. It is exquisite, and it leaves one unsatisfied. What more can one want?"                                          Oscar Wilde, in *The Picture of Dorian Gray*, 1891

220. "A passing but dangerous smoking fad of the 1880s was Cocarettes, a product of the Cocabacco Tobacco Company of St. Louis. These lethal smokes contained shredded leaves of the Bolivian coca plant, the source of cocaine. Preposterous and inaccurate statements filled the wordy advertising pamphlet extolling the safety and virtues of this new and exciting smoking adventure. The same company also marketed a companion product, Coca Plug, for those who preferred to get their kicks from chewing, not smoking. Products like these lent credence to tobacco opponents who claimed that American-made cigarettes contained opium and were addicting."                                                                    *Tobacco Advertising*, p. 245

221. Under "Reasons Why Cigarettes Should Be Used By All Smokers," the Cocarette company ad included:
They are not injurious.
The Coca neutralizes the depressing effects of the Nicotine in the tobacco.
Coca stimulates the brain to great activity and gives tone and vigor to the entire system.
Cocarettes can be freely used by persons in delicate health without injury, and with positively beneficial results.
Coca and Tobacco combined is the greatest boon ever offered to smokers.
Quote from *Tobacco Advertising*, p. 245

222. In the late 1880's, some names for cigarettes and tobacco products were the following: Pin Head, Country Doctor, Old Rip, Catarrh, Hunkidori, Cyclone, Piper Heidsieck, Ole Varginy, Battle Ax, Nosegay, Jolly Tar, Sailor Jack, Motor, Fatima, Mecca, Coal Smoke, Befoe deWar, Pigs Foot, Gloomy Gus, Catch Me Willie, Wah Hoo, Total Eclipse, Jack the Giant Killer, Bogaboo, Peoria Sweepers, Mayer Rat Tail, Ham Bone Granulated, Little Red Riding Hood, and Huchy Kuchy.

223. Connorton's Tobacco Brand Directory listed 108 cigarette brands in its 1885 edition. By 1903, the directory listed 2124 cigarettes, 7046 smoking tobaccos, 3616 different kinds of snuff, 3625 fine cut chewing tobaccos, and 9005 brands of plug and twist.                                                      *Sold American*, 1954

224. In 1889 the *New York Times* carried the following observation about tobacco:
"Whatever be its merits or demerits, one thing is certain--namely, that there is an ever-increasing subjection to the influence of this narcotic, whose soothing powers are requisitioned to counteract the evil effects of the worry, overpressure and exhaustion which characterize the age in which we live." *Tobacco in History*, p. 121

225. During the period from 1880 to 1896, tobacco consumption in the United States increased six-fold, mostly attributable to the increased popularity of cigarettes. Health Psychology 14:504, 1995

226. Cigarette production in the United States increased from 20 million in 1869 to 250 million in 1879, a billion in 1885, and two billion in 1889. *Cigarette Confidential*, pp. 99 and 104

227. Between 1865 and 1915, American cigarette production increased one thousand fold as the Bonsack machine made mass production possible, and cigarettes became more fashionable than chewing tobacco. By 1921, cigarettes had surpassed all other forms of tobacco usage. *Sold American*, p. 93

228. In 1888, Americans consumed 3.6 billion cigars. *They Satisfy*, p. 42

229. Robert Louis Stevenson died in Samoa in 1888 at the age of 44 of a sudden "apoplectic fit," or stroke. He had been a lifelong smoker. JAMA, April 26, 1996, p. 1226

230. In 1890, Key West was the largest city in Florida, with a population of 18,786. Its largest industry, employing 2000 workers, was the manufacture of cigars. The Tobacco Timeline, www.tobacco.org

231. In the late 1800's, and early 1900's, H.J. Heinz allowed no smoking in his food processing factories. Biography, A & E television, 1999

232. Queen Victoria disapproved of tobacco, and banned smoking in the royal residences. The youthful Prince of Wales (later Edward VII), who smoked, learned that his mother planned to inspect every room in Windsor castle. He escaped by putting "WC" on his smoking room.

233. The development of book safety matches in 1892 helped to popularize cigarette smoking. The phosphorus fumes from matches prior to this had been so dangerous that no one routinely carried matches. Instead, smokers lit up from a fireplace or an oil or gas lamp. This cut down on the number of cigarettes smoked. Soon after the new matchbooks were distributed free with cigarette purchases, the consumption of cigarettes doubled. *Tobacco Biology and Politics*, Stanton Glantz, p. 6

234. In 1893, a smoking tobacco called Dental was advertised to cure "Asthma, Neuralgia, Bad Colds, Toothache, Headache, and Catarrh. It deodorizes the Breath and preserves the teeth." Its trademark was a large denture.

235. "Nicotine is a virulent poison and the chief ingredient of tobacco. It is the cause of all the nervous troubles and general debility of smokers." Ad for an unnamed product in the Sears Roebuck catalogue labeled as "Sure Cure for the Tobacco Habit" (Reported in JAMA, February 26, 1992, p. 1037)

236. "If you will study the history of almost any criminal you will find that he is an inveterate smoker." Thomas Edison

237. Chewing tobacco brand names from the late 1800's included Big Gun, Big Lump, Climax, Green Turtle, Red Meat, Early Bird, Brown's Mule, Good Luck, Honey Dip, No Tax, and Happy Thought.

238. Sir William Osler of Johns Hopkins devoted only three sentences in 1000 pages to the effects of tobacco in his classic 1892 textbook, *The Principles and Practice of Medicine*. Osler himself was a smoker, and died from "chronic bronchitis" in 1919; he also suffered from what he termed "tobacco angina." Population and Development Review, June 1990, pp. 219-220

239. In April 1896, Sir William Osler described chest pain related to tobacco consumption as "tobacco angina." Osler himself had been a smoker for 24 years at the time, and write that "in moderation it soothes physical irritability and corrects mental and moral strabismus." Canadian Medical Association Journal, November 1, 1994, p. 1238

240. "A woman is a woman, but a good cigar is a smoke."                    Rudyard Kipling, about 1895

241. In 1898, Surgeon General Rixey of the U.S. Navy expressed alarm at the increased cigarette smoking by sailors during the Spanish-American War. He threatened to ban cigarettes aboard ships, but backed down in the face of a possible mutiny.                    *Tobacco Advertising*, p. 115

242. Chewing tobacco comprised 44% of the American market in 1900, and spittoons were not removed from federal buildings until 1945.                    *The Faber Book of Smoking*, p. 59

243. At the beginning of the 20th century, more tobacco was consumed in the form of chewing tobacco than nearly all other forms of tobacco combined. Of the 7.43 pounds of tobacco consumed per adult in 1900 (ages 14 years and older), 3.5 pounds were consumed as chewing tobacco, 2.0 pounds as cigars, 1.4 pounds as smoking tobacco (for pipes and roll-your-own cigarettes), and 0.30 pounds as snuff. Less than 0.20 pounds of tobacco was consumed per adult in the form of machine-made, mass produced cigarettes.
                    Quote from *Nicotine and Public Health*, p. 179

244. In the United States in 1901, 3.5 billion cigarettes and 6 billion cigars were sold; four out of five American men smoked at least one cigar each day.                    The Tobacco Timeline, www.tobacco.org

245. In 1900, cigarettes were banned in the U.S. Navy at the same time that the cigar was widely accepted. The cigarette was regarded as "a debasement of manhood."                    *Advertising, the Uneasy Persuasion*, p. 184

246. "At the turn of the century, it was discovered that tuberculosis was transmitted through expectoration, and the practice of chewing and spitting quickly became socially unacceptable and illegal in many public places. With the invention of the cigarette-rolling machine, it was possible to produce a cheap new tobacco product. By the early 1920's, cigarettes had replaced smokeless tobacco. Per capita consumption of cigarettes in the United States rose dramatically, from 50 cigarettes per year in 1900 to 4200 by 1965."    NEJM, May 12, 1988, p. 1281

247. At the end of the nineteenth century, nicotine was isolated and its toxicity confirmed; it was in general use as an insecticide until the production of DDT until the early 1940's.                    *Tobacco in History*, pp. 121-122

248. "The cigarette in modern life is as ubiquitous as the bacillus, and...it is as mischievous as the most truculent of those invisible enemies."                    British Medical Journal, February 15, 1896, p. 424

249. "In the late 19th century, chewing tobacco and pipes were considered safe and traditional, while the newly popular cigarettes were viewed as dangerous and disreputable... At the same time, narcotics such as opium, morphine and heroin were sold over the counter and from mail order catalogues... In 1899, the Bayer Co. of Germany developed two pain medications that proved instantly popular. One was sodium acetylsalicylic acid and was named Aspirin. The other, diacetylmorphine, was added to cough syrups. It was named Heroin. Cocaine was commonly found in tonics and was the recommended treatment for those with hay fever and sinus trouble. Until 1903, it was added to the newly popular soda know as Coca-Cola. By the 1920's, however, the tides had reversed," and the sale of narcotics was banned under federal law.
                    Los Angeles Times, December 26, 1999 (David Savage)

250. By 1900, an estimated four out of five men smoked cigars, and cigars accounted for nearly 60% of all tobacco sales. In 1903 in the US, there were twice as many cigars smoked as cigarettes, a total of 6.7 billion.
                    *Tobacco Advertising*, p. 81

251. In 1900 cigarette sales were illegal in 14 states. In upholding a prohibition on sales in Tennessee, the Supreme Court commented in a 6-3 decision that cigarettes are a "noxious" product, and "a belief in their deleterious effects, particularly among young people, has become very general." Earlier the Tennessee Supreme Court said that cigarettes "possess no virtue but are inherently bad and bad only."
                    Los Angeles Times, December 26, 1999

252. 14 states in 1900 prohibited the sale of tobacco to anyone of any age. San Francisco Examiner, August 22, 1999

253. In 1901, it was illegal in twelve states to sell or use cigarettes. By 1927, all these laws had been repealed. At the same time, all states except Texas banned cigarette sales to minors.
American Medical News, November 14, 1994, p. 17, and Health Education, May 1984, p. 3

254. In 1898, the Tennessee Supreme court upheld a total ban on cigarette sales, ruling cigarettes "not legitimate articles of commerce, because wholly noxious and deleterious to health. Their use is always harmful."
American Medical News, November 14, 1994, p. 16

255. In 1900 the Supreme Court, which in 2000 ruled that the FDA did not have the power to regulate tobacco, upheld a Tennessee law forbidding the sale of cigarettes. A state court had concluded: "They possess no virtue but are inherently bad and bad only." At the turn of the century, cough syrups contained heroin, and Coca-Cola had cocaine.
Newsweek, July 31, 2000 p. 68 (Anna Quindlen)

256. More than 100 years ago, the Tennessee Supreme Court upheld the conviction of a person for selling cigarettes, saying that cigarettes were "wholly noxious and deleterious to health. Their use is always harmful, never beneficial. They possess no virtue, but are inherently bad, and bad only. They find no true commendation for merit or usefulness in any sphere." At the turn of the 20th century, 14 states outlawed the sale, the manufacture, or the possession of cigarettes; 21 other states had considered such a ban; and 2 states had passed laws that declared cigarettes to be narcotics.

Henry Ford and Thomas Edison condemned cigarettes and their users in a book entitled *The Case against the Little White Slaver*. In the book, Edison wrote that cigarettes produce "degeneration of the cells of the brain, which is quite rapid among boys. Unlike most narcotics this degeneration is permanent and uncontrollable. I employ no person who smokes cigarettes."    Quote from NEJM, December 14, 2000, p. 1802

257. In 1899, Norway adopted a law prohibiting tobacco sales to children.
*Smoking: Third World Alert*, Uma Nath, 1986

258. At the end of the nineteenth century, brand names for smoking and chewing tobacco proliferated. The included Mail Pouch, Open Book, Day and Night, Bagpipe, Sure Shot, Silver Cup, Pick, Polar, Green Goose, Dark Horse, Dixie Queen, Pony Boy, Ace High, Gold Crumbs, Hilly Billy, Greenback, Recruit, Commander, Red Indian, Nic Nac, Cut and Slash, Yale, Royal Bengal, Ty Cobb, Cy Young, Home Run, Shogun, Yacht Club, Honey Moon, Whip, Stetson, Picayune, Bagdad, Hindoo, Mastiff, Orphan Boy, Big Ben, Stud, Stag, Navy Blue, G I Joe, Cowboy, Poker, Snowball, Boomerang and Daily Double.    *Tobacco Advertising*, pp. 124-125

259. Lucy Page Gaston in 1899 founded the Anti-Cigarette League with the goal of "Abolition of the Cigarette in America." She campaigned tirelessly until her death in 1924. Cigarette consumption in the United States had increased fifty-fold between 1899 and 1924.
*Tobacco Advertising*, p. 205.

260. There were a few forces developing against the rising popularity of cigarettes that only transiently tempered their expanding economic impact. In 1898, in part in the face of a growing national mood against what more and more was called the "dirty weed" and "sinful tobacco", Congress increased taxes on cigarettes by 200%, primarily (once again as a consequence of military conflict) to meet the need for revenues generated by the cost of the Spanish-American War. The price of a package of 10 cigarettes was raised from USD 0.05 to 0.20. Also during this period, an abolitionist and temperance crusader, a spinster school teacher named Lucy Page Gaston from Illinois, mounted a strong and evangelistic national crusade against the ills of tobacco. This "Gastonite movement" led to the banning, at least temporarily, of all cigarette sales in the states of North Dakota, Iowa, and, almost unbelievably for a "tobacco state", in Tennessee and in 12 other states.

The United States Senate Finance Committee, whose chairman, Nelson Aldrich of Rhode Island, owned over a million dollars in tobacco stock, instituted two measures that greatly countered the growing national sentiments against cigarettes. First, the Federal excise tax on cigarettes was reduced again, opening the way for greater profits in what had become a dwindling profitable margin for cigarettes sales. Second, and for what was to prove far more important to the century of growing cigarette consumption that was ahead, tobacco itself and cigarette additives were excluded from the Pure Food and Drug Act of 1906. Tobacco and nicotine were also removed from the US Pharmacopeia, excluding them as part of the pharmacological compendium. They were to remain outside of this legislation, and also thus outside the regulatory control of the FDA, until 1997, when a

Federal court in North Carolina ruled that nicotine-containing tobacco could, in fact, for the first time be regulated; not surprisingly, that ruling currently remains as yet not enforced and on litigated appeal.

Quote from The Tobacco Epidemic, pp. 26-27 (Gary Huber)

261. A turn of the century poem by James Harvey satirized the cigarette (from *Nicotine*, p. 56):

> Sing the song of the cigarette
> The nineteenth century dudelet's pet.
> With its dainty white overcoat,
> Prithee, now, make a note,
> How your affections entangled get
> The Machiavelian power I sing,
> Of the stealthy, insidious, treacherous thing.
>
> What odors unpleasant our nostrils fret!
> That subtle aroma we ne'er forget.
> But wherefore complain of it
> Spite of the pain of it,
> We too, indulge in our cigarette.
> The skeletonizing power I sing,
> Of the mind-paralyzing, perfidious thing.
>
> Shades of the past, that linger yet!
> Is there no land where laws beset
> Those who lay sense aside,
> Puffing slow suicide,
> Into themselves from a cigarette?
> Thither I'd fly and forever sing
> The praise of the land that is free from the thing.
>
> What sinner without and beyond the pale
> Of civilization, began to inhale,
> Sealing his own sad fate,
> Telling us, oh! too late!
> Gibbering lunacy ends the tale,
> Husky my voice, I must cease to sing,
> I'm puffing, myself, at the poisonous thing.

# 1900

262. In 1900, the average life expectancy in the United States was 47 years (49 for women, 45 for men), and only 3% of the population of 78 million was over age 65 (compared to 13% over age 65 in 1996). Mortality from tobacco was very small, although there are no good estimates; the average adult yearly per capita cigarette consumption was only 50, but it was about to increase rapidly, peaking at 4340 in 1963 and declining to 2500 by 1994.

263. In 1900, only one American in ten lived to age 65. Two thirds were dead by age 50, and half before age forty. A third of babies born died before age five, including 20% before their first birthday.

Dean Edell, M.D., KGO TV news, San Francisco, March 7, 1997

264. In 1900, less than 1% of the world's population was older than age 65; this had increased to 6% by 1996.

265. At the turn of the century, cigarette smoking by women was seen as the symbol of the prostitute, and men's use was viewed as effeminate.

Cigarettes, p. 35

266. In 1900, cigarettes accounted for only 3% of all U.S. tobacco consumed; this increased to 50% in 1937, 77% in 1967, and close to 90% at present. (The 1980 global figure was 70%).

Tobacco in History, p. 235

267. "Coffin nails" and "Little White Slavers" were commonly used names for cigarettes at the turn of the century.

268. "One of the first acts of Britain's new king, Edward VII, who appeared in front of a gathering of friends in a drawing room in Buckingham Palace after the death of his tobagophobe mother Queen Victoria in 1901, carrying a cigar, and announced 'Gentlemen, you may smoke.'" *Tobacco* (Gately), p. 219

269. "The etiquette in this, as in many other matters, has quite altered during the last few years. At one time it was considered a sign of infamously bad taste to smoke in the presence of women in any circumstances. But it is now no longer so. So many women smoke themselves, that in some houses even the drawing room is thrown open to Princess Nicotine. The example of the Prince of Wales has been largely instrumental in sweeping away the old restrictions. He smokes almost incessantly. On one occasion, I noticed that he consumed four cigars in rapid succession, almost without five minutes' interval between them…"*Manners for Men*, C.E. Humphrey, 1898

270. At the turn of the century, Red Cross cigarettes, featuring a red cross on a white background, were one of the most heavily advertised brands in Canada. *Smoke and Mirrors*, p. 39

271. In 1900, tobacco sales consisted of 60% cigars, 23% chewing tobacco, 10% pipes, 5% cigarettes, and 2% snuff.

272. "The cigarette is a most insidious and potent enemy of health and morality among young men and boys. It undermines both the health and morals in a most certain and effective way. Many a young man finds himself as old at twenty or twenty-five years of age as he ought to be at sixty or seventy. His constitution has been dissipated in smoke at the end of a cigarette or cigar. His lungs, liver, kidneys, and other internal organs are almost as densely saturated with smoke as a ham from a smoke house. The 'bouquet' of such a man has a whiff of perdition in it…
    "It is clearly the duty of all intelligent men and women to take a strong stand against this evil, and to make earnest efforts to secure such legislation as will prohibit the manufacture, sale, and public use of this most pernicious drug." J.H. Kellog, *The Living Temple*, 1903

273. The 1901-3 British Discovery expedition to Antarctica carried 1800 pounds of tobacco for its 47 men.
*A First Rate Tragedy*, Diana Preston, Houghton Mifflin, 1998, p. 39

274. In 1905, Ernest Shackleton between his Antarctic voyages started a cigarette company.
Biography, A & E television, 2002

275. The dominating force in cigarette promotion up until the age of radio advertising had been the premiums. A 1901-catalog of premium merchandise redeemable from a Richmond Virginia tobacco distributor contains a wide variety of items; including handguns. For one thousand coupons, you could get an "Iver Johnson .32 Special Safety Hammer Automatic Revolver." Quote from *Cigarette Confidential*, p. 128

276. In 1904, cigar sales peaked at 7 billion in the U.S., and represented 60 percent of the total value of all tobacco products that year. *Ashes to Ashes*, p. 37

277. In 1905, the cheapest American cigarettes, Home Run, King Bee, and Coupon, sold at twenty for a nickel. The best Turkish blends were as much as a quarter for ten.

278. One 1905 cigar brand name was Rotten, with the logo in ads, "Rotten, But What's in a Name?"
Cigar Aficionado, October 1997, p. 142

279. Finnish composer and dedicated cigar smoker Jean Sibelius developed a malignant throat tumor at age 42. After two operations, he was given a gloomy prognosis, but went on (despite continuing the habit) to live another 49 years, dying in 1957 at age 91. San Francisco symphony program notes (Michael Steinberg), April 14, 2000

280. In the early 1900's, pioneer botanist Luther Burbank remarked that smoking is "nothing more or less than a slow, but sure, form of lingering suicide." Mother Jones, May-June 1996, p. 40

281. A tuberculosis epidemic in 1905 indirectly contributed to a decline in chewing tobacco use and an increase in cigarette sales. It was realized that disease could be spread through contaminated dust aerosols (Robert Koch

had discovered the tuberculosis bacillus in 1882), and public outcry against unsanitary American spitting practices caused the habit to become socially unacceptable. *Health Education, June 1987, p. 10*

282. Tobacco magnate James Buchanan Duke from the turn of the century until 1905 posted company agents at Ellis Island in New York harbor, the first stop for millions of immigrants to the United States. Every man who entered was given a bag of free cigarettes. *World Watch, July-August 1997, p. 21*

283. In 1905, tobacco state congressmen and tobacco magnate "Buck" Duke successfully lobbied to have the word tobacco removed from the 1905 edition of the US Pharmacopoeia. This was significant because the FDA, which was created by the Food and Drug Act of 1906, could only regulate drugs that appeared in the US Pharmacopoeia. Tobacco had been in the 1890 edition. *Joel Dunnington, MD*

284. By 1906, the American Tobacco Company controlled 80% of the entire domestic tobacco industry except for cigars. It had 82% of the cigarette and chewing tobacco business, 96% of the snuff consumed, but only 15% of the cigars produced. *Tobacco Tycoon, p. 180*

285. In 1910, James B. Duke controlled 86% of the U.S. cigar market, 85% of the plug tobacco market, and 76% of the cigarette market. *Psychiatric Clinics of North America, March 1993, p. 50*

286. In 1907, the American Tobacco Company signed a contract with the operator of a horse-drawn stage line in New York to lease advertising space. One very controversial ad appeared for "Bull" Durham, the nation's leading tobacco brand. "Onlookers were shocked at the sight of the bull's well-endowed maleness so graphically rendered, and had the driver of the first stage that appeared on the street arrested." The City of New York sued the coach company and its client, the American Tobacco Company, to ban the ads. The case went all the way to the Supreme Court in 1911, which upheld New York's ban. Ironically, this case ruling took place the day after the same court handed down a historic verdict ordering the dissolution of Buck Duke's $240 million-a-year American Tobacco Company monopoly, which the court deemed in violation of the Sherman Antitrust Act. *Tobacco Advertising, pp. 110 and 140*

287. Buck Duke's American Tobacco aggressively looked for export markets, and in 1898 exported 1.2 billion cigarettes, a third of its total production. *Tobacco Tycoon, p. 129*

288. Duke pursued the same strategies overseas as today's cigarette industry: expand foreign trade, and recruit new smokers. By the end of his life, he had 25,000 cigarette salesmen in the Far East alone. *Cigarette Confidential, p. 102*

289. The efforts of American cigarette manufacturers to hook the Chinese on their products are nothing new. Until the tobacco magnate, James B. Duke, led his American Tobacco company into China a century ago, only a few Chinese, mostly older men, smoked a bitter native tobacco, usually in pipes.

Duke sent experts to Shantung Province with bright leaf from North Carolina to cultivate a milder tobacco. His minions hired "teachers" to walk the streets of villages showing curious Chinese how to light and hold cigarettes. Not only did Duke install the first mechanical cigarette-rolling machines in China, but he also unleashed a panoply of promotional devices.

One involved adorning cigarette packs with pictures of nude American actresses, which proved to be a big hit with Chinese men. Later, Duke successfully persuaded President Theodore Roosevelt to get the Chinese government to drop its ban on imported cigarettes. *Quote from letter to the editor by Richard Grayson, New York Times, September 14, 1997, p. 14*

290. Buck Duke's cigarette monopoly, the American Tobacco Company, produced 10 billion cigarettes in 1911 (up from a billion in 1889). In 1911, it was broken up when the Supreme Court found it to be in violation of the Sherman Antitrust Act. Until 1911, American Tobacco was the third largest company in the United States, behind only U.S. Steel and Standard Oil. *Science 80, September 1980, p. 43, and Nicotine Addiction, p. 7*

291. "500,000 youths today are habitual cigarette smokers. Few can be educated beyond the eighth grade, and most are destined to become mental and physical dwarfs." *Education magazine, 1907*

292. By 1909, 17 states had adopted prohibitions on the sale of tobacco. However, these were overturned during World War I with the tremendous popularity of tobacco with the United States military forces.

*Cancer Wars*, p. 295

293. "The right of each person to breathe fresh and pure air – air uncontaminated by unhealthful or disagreeable odors and fumes is a constitutional right, and cannot be taken away."    New York Times, November 10, 1911

294. Turkish cigarettes, also called Egyptian cigarettes, were a popular fad between 1890 and 1920. "Creative minds conjured up a long list of intriguing brand names, putting a final touch to the suggestive imagery." Murad, Fatina, and Mecca were the most popular; other brands were Egyptian Deities, Egyptian Mysteries, Turkish Trophies, Turkey Red, Red Kamel, Rameses, Helmar, Tasha, Arabs, Fez, Minaret, Sultan, Delhi, Durbar, Soudan, Otez, Omar, Reyno, Mogul, Hassan, and Zubelda..

*Tobacco Advertising*, pp. 179-180, and *They Satisfy*, p. 81

295. Elinor Glyn was an ally of Lucy Gaston of the National Anti-Cigarette League about 1910 and an exponent of sexual freedom. She thought that smoking robbed men of their virility. "Every smoke is a tiny drop of old age, so small that for a long time it is unnoticed."

*They Satisfy*, p. 61

296. English women of high social class began to smoke cigarettes in public in the 1880's, and in 1906, English railroad officials adopted special smoking cars for women. At about this time, the "new spirit of liberation" spread to upper class women in the United States. In 1910, Alice Roosevelt Longworth, President Roosevelt's daughter, was scolded for smoking in the White House and retorted she would smoke on the roof. She would later appear in an advertisement for Lucky Strikes.    NY State Journal of Medicine, July 1985, p. 335

and *Tobacco Advertising*, p. 212

297. In 1910 a picture of Alice Roosevelt Longworth appeared on the front page of the Woman's Daily, as she was accused of the dastardly act of smoking in public. In 1927, society had changed, and she posed for an ad for Luckies.    *Tobacco Advertising*, p. 218

298. A rapid rise in per capita cigarette consumption that began around 1910 provided one of the first demonstrations that advertising and mass marketing could create demand for a product where no previous demand existed.

"Shortly after the court-ordered break-up of the tobacco industry monopoly in 1911, the R.J. Reynolds Tobacco Company introduced the Camel brand of cigarettes, which contained a sweeter blend of tobaccos than other brands of the time. The marketing campaign that launched this brand was undertaken with an expensive town-by-town promotional approach. The teaser ('Camels are Coming!') was followed by unprecedented advertising of the brand in print and billboard media. In 1913, the R.J. Reynolds Tobacco Company spent nearly $800,000 on advertising and promotion; this amount increased to $2.2 million by 1916 and to $8.7 million by 1921. The money spent on marketing leveled off at about 60% of total profits. From 1913 to 1921, the R.J. Reynolds Tobacco Company's market share rose from 0.2%, representing the sale of 1.5 million Camel cigarettes, to 50% of all cigarette sales, or 18.3 billion Camel cigarettes.

"In 1915, Reynolds was interviewed on how he came by his strong beliefs in advertising. He responded that he started with a small advertising budget for plug tobacco in 1894 and observed that his sales rose considerably. A fourfold increase in his advertising budget in the following year was associated with a doubling of his sales. According to the Winston-Salem Journal in 1915, he said that, after that, he did not need any more proof of the power of advertising."    Health Psychology 1995;14:505 (John Pierce)

299. R.J. Reynolds introduced Camel in 1913 as the first national brand, and sold it for 10 cents a pack, two thirds of the price of competing brands, which were primarily Chesterfield and Lucky Strike. By 1927, more than half the tobacco consumed in the United States was in the form of cigarettes.    *The Tobacco Epidemic*, p. 7

300. "The time will come when cigarette smoking will be condemned by public sentiment and prohibited by law just as the use of opium is today."    Lucy Page Gaston, Founder, Anti-Cigarette League of America, 1911

301. Early objections to smoking did not distinguish between moral and health hazards. "The dirty habit, like alcohol, was associated with idleness, immorality, and sin. Women's groups encouraged young women to pledge abstinence from tobacco, as well as from jazz dancing and petting."

*Harvard magazine*, July-August 1996, p. 19

302. In her book *The Coldest March* (Yale, 2001), author Susan Soloman (p. 217) describes the ill-fated Scott party at the South Pole (elevation 9200 feet) in 1912, where they arrived a month after Roald Amundsen. "Where Amundsen had celebrated his triumph with a cigar, Scott, Oates, and Seaman Evans enjoyed cigarettes that Wilson had bought. The three smokers probably had increased difficulty breathing the thin air, but like today's visitors to the Pole, they nevertheless enjoyed the tobacco."

303. "The cigarette, however, did not rise unopposed. Although the anti-tobacco movements were much smaller than they had been, on both sides of the Atlantic, the cigarette was greeted with the most hysterical attacks yet. And victories were won. In Britain – where, as you might imagine, the tobacco companies had soon followed Duke's lead – the 1908 Children's Act made it illegal to sell tobacco to anybody under 16. (The relative cheapness of cigarettes and their ease of use had made the new craze highly attractive to children.) More dramatically, between 1895 and 1909, 12 American States banned cigarettes entirely – Compton Mackenzie could remember being on a train where the passengers were told to stub out all cigarettes as it crossed into Indiana. (Kansas was the last to repeal such legislation, in 1927). Most dramatically of all, Lucy Page Gaston, the editor of Coffin Nails, stood for the American presidency in 1920 on an anti-smoking ticket, denouncing the eventual winner, Warren Harding, as 'a cigarette-face.' (As pro-smoking writers invariably point out with some glee, Gaston died four years later of throat cancer.)"     *The Faber Book of Smoking*, p. 77

304. The first baseball cards promoted cigarettes, and a 1909 card of Honus "the Flying Dutchman" Wagner sold for $450,000 in 1991. Wagner, a nonsmoker, had ordered all the cards destroyed because of his disapproval of tobacco, but a few survived.

305. "...in 1909, the baseball star Honus Wagner had ordered the American Tobacco Company to take his picture off their 'Sweet Caporal' cigarette cards, fearing they would lead children to start smoking. The shortage made the Honus Wagner cigarette card the most valuable of all time, and children hoarded their pocket money or pestered their fathers to buy Sweet Caporals in the hope of obtaining one. The card is now worth nearly $500,000."     *Tobacco* (Gately), p. 223

306. In 1909, baseball great Honus Wagner ordered American Tobacco Company to take his picture off their Sweet Caporal cigarette packs, fearing that it might cause children to smoke. The resulting scarcity made the Homus Wagner baseball card the most famous and rarest of all time.     www.uchsc.edu

307. In 1999 American Tobacco Company baseball card Hall of Fame Pittsburg Pirate shortstop Homus Wagner was sold on eBay online auction house for $1.1 million to an anonymous bidder. It is the first known specimen of 50 Wagner cards known to exist from the 1909 set. The card was sold by a Chicago collector, who had paid $640,500 for it in 1996, at the time the record for a sports card. Hockey star Wayne Gretzky previously bought it for $461,000 in 1991.     Associated Press, July 16, 2000

308. In 1910 the most popular cigarette brands were Pall Mall, Sweet Caporal, Piedmont, Helmar and Fatima.

www.uchsc.edu

309. In 1912, Dr. Isaac Adler in a monograph was the first to strongly suggest that lung cancer is related to smoking.

The Tobacco Timeline, www.tobacco.org

310. Janet Stancomb-Wills, daughter of a tobacco tycoon, was a major benefactor of the 1914 Shackleton Endurance expedition to Antarctica.     *The Endurance*, Caroline Alexander, Knopf, 1999, p. 10

311. In 1914, Henry Ford published and distributed a book entitled *The Case Against the Little White Slaver*.

*Cigarettes*, p. 37

312. "If you will study the history of almost any criminal you will find that he is an inveterate cigarette smoker."

Henry Ford in *The Case Against the Little White Slaver*, 1914

313. "With every breath of cigarette smoke, they inhale imbecility and exhale manhood."

Henry Ford (Harvard magazine, July-August 1996, p. 19)

314. "The cigarette has a violent action in the nerve centers, producing degeneration of the brain, which is quite rapid among boys. Unlike most narcotics, this degeneration is permanent and uncontrollable. I employ no person who smokes cigarettes." Thomas A. Edison to Henry Ford, 1914 (JAMA, June 25, 1997, p. 1920)

315. Edison was himself addicted to cigars, but alleged that cigar smoke was not as harmful as was inhaled cigarette smoke. *Licit and Illicit Drugs*, p. 230

316. Yearly US per capita cigarette consumption was only 0.36 in 1870, increasing to 8 in 1880, 35 in 1890, 53 in 1900, 85 per capita in 1910, and then a rapid rise to 471 in 1920, 977 in 1930, 1550 in 1940, and 2027 in 1945.

317. In 1909, the legislatures of 15 states had banned the sale of cigarettes. During World War I, however, General cabled Washington to say that "tobacco is as indispensable as the daily ration" for his troops. Those speaking out against tobacco during the war were threatened with prosecution under the Espionage Act of 1917, so unpatriotic was their stand seen to be. By 1927, all state statutes prohibiting cigarette sales had been repealed. *No Smoking*, RE Goodin, University of Chicago Press, 1989, p. 125

318. One cigarette brand launched in 1914 in Norway and still sold is "Teddy" cigarettes, featuring a picture of Theodore Roosevelt. Tobacco Control, Fall 1993, p.194

319. "Smoking is perfectly innocuous. It is on a par with tea drinking." Encyclopedia Sinica, 1917, 9th World Conference on Tobacco or Health, Paris, 1994 (F.Lam)

320. In 1913 a chewing tobacco firm called RJ Reynolds, which had not previously manufactured cigarettes, introduced a new brand called Camel, along with an advertising and promotional campaign rising from $800,000 in 1913 to $8 million in 1924. The famous slogan "I'd walk a mile for a Camel" was first used on billboards in 1921. Camel sales increased from a million cigarettes in the 1913 inaugural year to 400 million in 1914 and 20 billion in 1919, in the latter year accounting for almost 40% of the cigarettes sold in the United States. Camel's market share as the most popular brand in America fluctuated from 23% to 42% until its decline in the 1950's. The other major brands of the 1920 to 1950 era were Lucky Strike and Chesterfield; together with Camel, they accounted for about 65% of the market. *Tobacco in History*, pp. 104-105

321. In 1913, R.J. Reynolds first marketed Camel, the first nonregional cigarette, accompanied by a then massive $1.5 million national advertising campaign. Consumption of Camel cigarettes immediately increased, providing one of the first documented cases demonstrating that advertising could create demand for a product where no previous demand existed. Other manufacturers followed by introducing such brands as Lucky Strike and Chesterfield; for decades these brands dominated the domestic U.S. market.

*Smokeless Tobacco or Health*, p. xxxix

322. R.J. Reynolds introduced Camel in 1913 with immediate success. To meet the challenge, American Tobacco in 1916 brought out Lucky Strike, while Liggett and Myers entered the advertising race by pushing its Chesterfield brand. *Tobacco Tycoon*, p. 260

323. Camel cigarettes were introduced by R. J. Reynolds in 1913, when 1.1 million were manufactured, and was the first nationally advertised brand. Sales increased to 2.3 billion in 1915 and 20.8 billion in 1919, accounting for 40% of the US market share that year.

*They Satisfy*, p. 78, and Joe DiFranza, June 22, 1995, STAT conference, San Jose

324. In 1915, a Dr. Abbe described a series of oral cancer patients who were tobacco chewers, and postulated tobacco use as a risk factor.

*The Health Consequences of Using Smokeless Tobacco*, 1986 Surgeon General report, p. xix

325. Sir Ernest Shackleton in his book *South* (p. 221) describes the rescue of his comrades from the Endurance Antarctic expedition on Elephant Island in 1916. "As I drew close to the rock I flung packets of cigarettes

ashore: they fell on them like hungry tigers, for well I know that for months tobacco was dreamed of and talked of."

Frank Wild, the leader of the shore party, gave this account (p. 242): "Before he could land, he threw ashore handfuls of cigarettes… and these the smokers, who for two months had been trying to find solace in such substitutes as seaweed… and sennegras, grasped greedily."

326. In 1917, First Lady Edith Wilson helped to pass out free cigarettes to thousands of soldiers departing for Europe at Washington's Union Station.          Woodrow Wilson, American Experience, PBS television, 2002

327. During World War I, the three dominant cigarette brands became Camel (R.J. Reynolds), Lucky Strike (American Tobacco Co.), and Chesterfield (Liggett and Myers). During the first and second World Wars, tobacco companies gave away millions of free cigarettes to the troops. This practice coincided with the most rapid increases in overall smoking prevalence and in cigarette sales at any time in the United States.

328. "You ask me what we need to win this war, I answer tobacco, as much as bullets. Tobacco is as indispensable as the daily ration. We must have thousands of tons of it without delay."
General John J. Pershing, Commander of U.S. troops in Europe, 1918

329. American soldiers first received tobacco rations (0.4 ounces with 10 cigarette papers) in World War I. When the War Department approved the rations, "a wave of joy swept through the American Army." Until 1975, cigarettes were included in all k-rations and c-rations provided to soldiers and sailors.
*Advertising, the Uneasy Persuasion*, p. 186 and *Reducing the Health Consequences of Smoking*, p. 278

330. In World War I, wounded soldiers were allowed to smoke while being operated on. An army surgeon described the calming effect of cigarettes. "Wonderful. As soon as the lads take their first wiff, they seem eased and relieved of their agony."          *Tobacco Advertising*, p. 184

331. "...cigarette consumption doubling during World War I when cigarettes were included in soldier's rations sent to France; a further doubling of cigarette consumption during the 1920s, propelled by innovative advertising campaigns, augmented by radio and cinema; decreased cigarette consumption during the early years of the economic depression of the 1930s; and increasing consumption during the late 1930s, in response to intensified advertising in magazines, on billboards, and on radio ('Lucky Strike Hit Parade') and to the incessant smoking of enormously popular film stars.

"Again during World War II, when cigarettes were made freely available to many military and some civilian groups (including women), consumption almost doubled--from 1,976 cigarettes per adult in 1940 to 3,449 in 1945."          Population and Development Review, June 1990, p. 221 (R.T. Ravenholt)

332. In 1917, there were an estimated 580,000 cigar and tobacco shops operating in the United States.
*Tobacco Advertising*, p. 71

333. In 1918, the US military contracted for the entire Bull Durham smoking tobacco output to be shipped to the doughboys in Europe.

334. 100 boxcars with 36 million sacks of "Bull" Durham were shipped to Europe each month, but the government wanted more. In April 1918, federal authorities commandeered all factory stores of "Bull" Durham and requisitioned all future production. "Considerable promotional hay was made during the seven-month period that production of 'Bull' Durham was taken over. The American Tobacco Company played up the mistaken notion that they had made the sacrifice willingly and with patriotic intent."          *Tobacco Advertising*, p. 188

335. During World War One, an advertising campaign featured an American soldier in France leaning wearily against the side of trench as he smoked a cigarette. The message beneath the picture read, "After the Battle, the Most Refreshing Smoke is Murad. 20 cents for 20."          *They Satisfy*, p. 83

336. In May 1918, it was announced that daily tobacco rations would be issued to every soldier, sailor, and marine. In November 1918, the War Department placed orders for three billion cigarettes to meet military demands for the following two months.          *Tobacco Advertising*, p. 187

337. A 1921 article indicated that of 160 persons with cancer of the tongue, all but two were tobacco users.

JAMA, February 28, 1986, p. 1041

338. The first cigarettes marketed specifically to women appeared between 1910 and the early 1920's. They included Milo Violets, Blue Peter, Ulissa, Gold Tip and Marlboro. *Tobacco Advertising*, p. 221-223

339. The first ad showing women smoking was in 1919 for Helmar's cigarettes. *Tobacco in History*, p. 107

340. In 1924 women accounted for only 5% of national cigarette consumption. This rose to 12% by 1929.

*Tobacco in History*, p. 106

341. "Women--when they smoke at all--quickly develop discriminating taste…That is why Marlboros now ride in so many limousines, attend so many bridge parties, repose in so many hand bags."

1927 ad for Marlboro, a new women's cigarette

342. From 1910 to 1919, cigarette production increased more than six-fold, from 11 billion to 70 billion per year.

343. Reynolds Aluminum started out in 1919 as the U.S. Foil Co. to produce tin foil to wrap cigarette packs.

San Francisco Chronicle, April 5, 1998, p. 8

344. Cigarette tobacco outsold pipe tobacco for the first time in 1919; it passed cigars in 1921 and outsold chewing tobacco in 1922. *Advertising, the Uneasy Persuasion*, p. 184

345. Between 1918 and 1940, American consumption of cigarette tobacco grew from 1.70 to 5.16 pounds per adult each year. *Advertising, the Uneasy Persuasion*, p. 183

346. Yearly U.S. adult per capita cigarette consumption more than doubled from 610 in 1920 to 1370 in 1930. It increased again to 1976 in 1940 and 3552 in 1950. *Tobacco in History*, pp. 105 and 125

347. The chairman of the department of medicine at Barnes Hospital, St. Louis, in 1919 asked all third- and fourth-year medical students to observe an autopsy of a man who died of lung cancer. The disease was so rare, he said, that most of them would never see it again.

348. One of the 1919 students, Dr. Alton Ochsner, wrote years later: "I did not see another case until 1936, when in 6 months, I saw nine patients with cancer of the lung. This represented an epidemic for which there had to be a cause. All the afflicted patients were men who had smoked heavily since World War I. …I had the temerity, at that time, to postulate that the probable cause of this new epidemic was cigarette use."

Medical Journal of Australia, March 5, 1983, p. 230

349. In 1928, an article in the Lancet from English medical experts assured smokers that cigarette smoking did not cause lung cancer. A New York Times headline read "Clears Cigarettes as Cancer Source."

*Tobacco Advertising*, p. 262

350. In 1921, RJR inaugurated the famous "I'd walk a Mile for a Camel" slogan, and spent $8 million on advertising, mostly for its Camel brand. The Tobacco Timeline, www.tobacco.org

351. In the 1920's, Tuxedo smoking tobacco was flavored with chocolate.

352. In the post World War I era, a cigarette brand called Coffee-Tone attempted to combine coffee and tobacco by marrying "the flavor and aroma of selected coffees with the finest domestic and imported tobaccos."

Smithsonian, October 2002, p. 29

353. In 1921, total consumption of tobacco products by British men was 67,000 tons, compared to a total of only 300 tons for British women. *Tobacco* (Gately), p. 238

354. The original Marlboros introduced in 1924 as a woman's cigarette were called Marlboro Beauty Tips and had their end colored red "to conceal those tell-tale lipstick traces." It was advertised with the slogan "Mild as May."

*Holy Smoke*, p. 101

355. In 1924 the United States was the world's leading tobacco producer, with 450,000 farms growing the crop on two million acres.

*Tobacco Advertising*, p. 254

356. Of males born in the United States between 1910 and 1930, almost 80% were smokers at some point in their lives.

David Burns, M.D.

357. In the 1920's, "when a teenager took to cigarettes, he might be a customer of the same brand for a half century. Figured at a pack per day, that came to 17,800 packs in a lifetime, and at fifteen cents each, $2670, or close to three years' salary for the average worker of that decade. It was a pleasing prospect." *They Satisfy*, p. 105

358. "What this country really needs is a good five cent cigar."

Thomas Riley Marshall, Woodrow Wilson's former vice president, 1925

359. Trinity College in Durham, North Carolina changed its name to Duke in 1924 after tobacco king James Buchanan Duke gave the school forty million dollars.

*America's South*, p. 114

360. "Gentlemen, the motto of Trinity College should be changed from 'Eruditio et Religio' to 'Eruditio et Cherooto et Cigaretto.'"   Cyrus B. Watson, remarking on the school that would later change its name to Duke University

*Cigarette Confidential*, p. 89

361. "Short, snappy, easily attempted, easily completed or just as easily discarded before completion – the cigarette is the symbol of the machine age."

New York Times, 1925 (*The Tobacco Atlas*, p. 30)

362. In 1926, Liggett and Myers ran a Chesterfield ad showing a man and a woman seated in a romantic setting by a riverbank at dusk. The man is lighting up and the woman looks at him with admiration mixed with wistful envy. "Blow some my way," she coaxes as the gender taboo begins to be broken.   *They Satisfy*, p. 99

363. In the late 1920's, a series of celebrated Metropolitan Opera Singers gave testimonials for Lucky Strike cigarettes, with slogans like "Cigarettes are kind to your throat", and "I protect my precious voice with Lucky Strikes."

*Taken at the Flood*, p. 168

364. The Lucky Strike "Reach for a Lucky instead of a Sweet" campaign resulted in a rise in sales from 13.7 billion cigarettes in 1925, when it was the third ranked brand, to over 40 billion in 1930, when it became the top-ranked brand.

New York Times, January 1, 1996, p. 21 (Bob Herbert column).

365. In 1928, the advertising expert Albert Lasker developed the slogan "Reach for a Lucky instead of a Sweet." He began the association of cigarettes with the attribute of slimness with the principal selling idea of smoking as an aid to dieting and weight control.

*Preventing Tobacco Use Among Young People*, 1994 Surgeon General report, p. 165

366. "In the 1920s, the cigarette industry was dominated by three brands (Camel, Chesterfield, and Lucky Strikes) that appeared indistinguishable from each other on blindfolded consumer testing. Furthermore, the industry maintained a price equivalence between these brands, focusing competition only in their marketing strategies. In the first 40 years of the cigarette industry, cigarette smoking had been characterized as a habit to be pursued only by men. In 1919, the Lorillard Company produced a cigarette ad aimed specifically at women, but public outcry led to its prompt withdrawal. Apparently the public was not yet ready to accept the idea of women smoking.

"This situation had changed by the mid-1920s when Chesterfield cigarettes produced an acceptable and effective marketing campaign aimed at women with the 'Blow Some My Way' message in 1926. The conduct of this campaign was associated with a 40% increase in sales over the 2-year period. However, the major success story was the marketing campaign for Lucky Strike cigarettes developed by Albert Lasker for the American Tobacco Company. Lasker's selection as campaign director was based on his track record of successful promotion to women. This 'Reach for a Lucky Instead of a Sweet' campaign focused very pointedly on women's fear of gaining weight and was associated with a rapid rise in sales, taking the brand from sales of 13.7 billion cigarettes in 1925 (third-ranked brand) to over 40 billion and market leadership by 1930."

Health Psychology 1995; 14:505 (John Pierce)

367. Camel, Chesterfield and Lucky Strike between them accounted for 82% of all cigarette sales in 1925. By 1930, Luckies with their "Reach for a Lucky instead of a Sweet" slogan became the market leader. 20,679 physicians endorsed Luckies as a healthy brand after the opinions of doctors across America were solicited; five free cartons were offered for everyone who answered the question correctly. *Tobacco* (Gately), pp. 244-245

368. In the 1920's, American Tobacco Company's Lucky Strike was changed from a chewing tobacco to a cigarette. In these days, it was comparatively rare for women to smoke, and almost unknown for them to smoke in public. The advertising genius Albert Lasker recognized that cigarettes served as an appetite suppressant, and Lucky Strike sales (mostly to women) increased 312% in a year and six-fold in three years after his popularization of the slogan "Reach for a Lucky instead of a sweet", one of the most successful slogans in advertising history.

*Taken at the Flood*, p. 169

369. In the United States, Lucky Strike's well-known campaign that began in 1928 encouraged women to "Reach for a Lucky instead of a sweet," deliberately zeroing in on weight concerns. Candy manufacturers protested, so the slogan was changed to "When tempted Reach for a Lucky instead," but the message was still the same. One ad, featuring the shadow of a woman with a double chin, contained the following text:
   Avoid that future shadow by refraining from overindulgence, if you would maintain the modern figure of fashion. We do not represent that smoking Lucky Strike cigarettes will bring modern figures or cause the reduction of flesh. We do declare that when tempted to do yourself too well, if you will 'Reach for a Lucky' instead, you will avoid overindulgence in things that cause excess weight and, by avoiding overindulgence, maintain a modern, graceful form. Quote from *Smoke and Mirrors*, p. 176

370. "Reach for a Lucky--instead of a sweet."
"Pretty curves win! When tempted to over-indulge, reach for a Lucky instead." 1928 ads for Lucky Strike

371. Lucky Strike sales tripled within a year of the start of the campaign, and by 1930, Luckies passed Camels as the market leader. *Tobacco Advertising*, p. 260

372. "20,679 physicians have confirmed the fact that Lucky Strike is less irritating to the throat than other cigarettes." 1929 ad

373. In 1928, Babe Ruth was paid by Lorillard for declaring that it was possible to recognize Old Gold cigarettes while smoking blindfolded. *Tobacco Advertising*, p. 254

374. Babe Ruth proclaimed in ads in the 1930's that Old Gold cigarettes had "Not a cough in a carload."
Journal of the American Medical Women's Association, January 1996, p. 67

375. Federal tobacco taxes totaled $387 million in 1927. *Tobacco Advertising*, p. 254

376. From 1925 to 1930, American cigarette production and sales increased by 50 percent, from 82 to 124 billion cigarettes. *They Satisfy*, p.103

377. Reed Smoot, the Republican senator from Utah, was a leading anti-smoking activist in the 1920s. In 1921, he introduced a bill prohibiting smoking in all buildings belonging to the executive branch of the government. It did not pass. Neither did his proposal in 1929 to place tobacco under the supervision of the Pure Food and Drug Act, and to make all tobacco advertising subject to the same regulations as patent medicines.

*Tobacco Advertising*, p. 209

378. "Not since the days when public opinion rose up in its might and smote the dangerous drug traffic has the country witnessed such an orgy of buncombe, quackery, and downright falsehood and fraud as now marks the current campaign promoted by certain cigarette manufacturers to create a vast woman and child market for the use of their product." Address to the Senate on June 10, 1929 by Senator Reed Smoot

379. The president of the American Tobacco Company, George Washington Hill, paid himself $826,000 in 1932, the worst year of the depression. In the same year, the average annual wage of a full-time worker in the tobacco industry was $614.                                                                                    *Taken at the Flood*, p. 166

380. The first mentholated cigarette, Spud, was introduced in 1927 and, because of the local anesthetic quality of menthol, promoted as an ideal cigarette for the smoker who had a sore throat. Kool, long the most popular menthol brand, was introduced in 1932.                                                    *Nicotine Addiction*, p. 8

381. "Spuds do for hot weather smoking what a refreshing shower does for a July afternoon."
Ad in Time for Spuds, an early menthol cigarette, July 9, 1934, p. 29

382. In 1933, B&W brought out a mentholated brand to compete with Spud, marketed by its Louisville neighbor, Axton-Fisher. Menthol, a chemical compound extracted from the peppermint plant and classified by medical science as a mild local anesthetic sometimes used in veterinary medicine, served to mask the harsher taste of nicotine and other elements in cigarette smoke by, in effect, numbing the throat to the irritating effects without diluting them. The menthol additive gave Spud's taste a kind of cooling, faintly medicinal quality that some buyers believed made smoking a less unhealthy habit. Brown & Williamson's new menthol entry, at fifteen cents, was a nickel cheaper than Spud and had a much more suitable name--Kool. Its ads featured a playful penguin and copy that narrowly skirted the sort of blatant malarkey peddled by the big brands. "GIVE YOUR THROAT A KOOL VACATION!" a typical ad was headlined, and its text followed up: "Like a week by the sea, this mild menthol smoke is a tonic to hot, tired throats. The tiny bit of menthol cools and refreshes, yet never interferes with the full-bodied flavor..."                                      Quote from *Ashes to Ashes*, p. 93

383. Popular cigarette brands from the 1920's included Ramrod, Zipper, Cookie Jar, Salome, Turkey Red, El Ahram, Yankee Girl, Sunshine, Sweet Caps, King Bee, Dog's Head, Egyptian Oasis, Clown, Go, Home Run, Cake Box, Old Mill, Jeep, Ski, and Hed Kleer.

384. The first filter cigarette was DuMaurier, marketed in Great Britain in 1930.         *Nicotine Addiction*, p. 11

385. In the 1930s, low nicotine cigarettes such as O-Nic-O and Sano were introduced, but they proved unprofitable and were discontinued from production.                                                       *Tobacco Advertising*, p. 247

386. During the Great Depression, American families spent on average almost 7% of their income on tobacco products.                                                                                              *The Tobacco Epidemic*, p. 29

387. In 1934, the most popular cigarette brands (Lucky Strike, Chesterfield, Old Gold and Camel) were advertised for 25 cents for two packs, or a carton of ten for $1.20                      The Tobacco Timeline, www.tobacco.org

388. In 1935, tobacco caused about 5000 deaths per year in the United States.

389. Sigmund Freud (1856-1939), the founder of psychoanalysis, was an early prototype of tobacco addiction as he struggled for over 45 years to stop smoking. In his last 16 years of life, he endured 33 operations for cancer of the jaw and mouth, which finally killed him in 1939.                                          *Licit and Illicit Drugs*, p. 215

390. In 1933, Dr. Evarts Graham of Barnes Hospital, St. Louis, performed the world's first successful surgical removal of an entire lung for cancer. His patient lived until 1962. Dr. Graham was the co-author of a landmark 1950 study linking smoking to lung cancer, and he himself stopped smoking that year, but it was too late. He died of small-cell lung carcinoma in 1957.

391. In 1934, Eleanor Roosevelt smoked a cigar in public, the first First Lady to do so.         *Tobacco* (Gately), p. 252

392. The Journal of the American Medical Association (JAMA) published cigarette ads from 1933 to 1953.
www.uchsc.edu

393. Beginning in 1936, Camels were advertised in ads that featured health claims such as aiding digestion and relieving fatigue. One assertion was "More doctors smoke Camels than any other cigarette." Since Camels were

the most popular brand, this claim could have been made for any occupational group.

Reader's Digest, April 1992

394. "For a good sense of deep-down contentment – just give me Camels. After a good man-sized meal, that little phrase 'Camels set you right' covers the way I feel. Camels set me right whether I'm eating, working – or just enjoying life. All the years I've been playing, I've been careful about my physical condition. Smoke? I smoke and enjoy it. My cigarette is a Camel." Baseball legend Lou Gehrig, the Saturday Evening Post, April 24, 1937

395. In 1924, *Reader's Digest* published an article entitled "Does Tobacco Injure the Human Body?" The author, Irving Fisher, concluded, "from every indication, it behooves the man who wishes to remain fit to omit tobacco from his daily schedule." In 1938, *Science* published the results of a study by Johns Hopkins University biostatistician Raymond Pearl. After looking at the longevity of 6813 men, Pearl concluded that 45% of smokers lived until age 60, compared with 65% of nonsmokers, and that a reduction in longevity was found at every age until age 60. Quote from *Smoke and Mirrors*, p. 42

396. In 1938, Raymond Pearl, a biology professor at Johns Hopkins University, reported that in a sample of 6800 people, 66% of the nonsmokers lived beyond age 60, while only 46% of the heavy smokers did. This report in the journal Science was the first published connection of smoking to reduced life span.

Reader's Digest, April 1992

397. In 1938, Raymond Pearl published one of the first studies that indicated smoking to be "statistically associated with an impairment of life duration." *Reducing Tobacco Use*, p. 38

398. In the 1930's and 1940's, Nazi scientists amassed important evidence linking smoking to cancer, and the first laws against smoking in some public places and by pregnant women were enacted in Germany at this time. The head of the project committed suicide at the end of the war, and the research was not rediscovered until 1995.

*Cancer Wars*, PBS television, 1998

399. "The marketing concept of redeemable cigarette premium coupons reached an all-time low when, in 1936, a German cigarette manufacturer, Cigaretten Bildendienst, used this coupon-redemption scheme to promote the early propaganda of Adolph Hitler. The way it worked was smokers collected coupons from packages of cigarettes to exchange for a coffee-table book on Hitler… The photo book was an important part of the Nazi war machine, intended to show Hitler in a sympathetic light at a crucial time for him politically. The fact that it was sponsored by a cigarette company is ironic because of the Fuhrer's fevered loathing of smokers and anything to do with cigarettes." *Cigarette Confidential*, p. 128

400. Adolf Hitler was a fanatical opponent of tobacco; and signs declaring Deut Sche Weiber Rauchen Nicht (German women do not smoke) were posted throughout the Third Reich during World War II.

Time, April 18, 1994, p. 60

401. The German "government commenced a war against smoking, attacking the habit with propaganda and taxes. It began with a poster campaign, which featured a smoker's head being crushed under a jackbooted heel. Hitler supported his pet crusade with rhetoric: Tobacco was the 'wrath of the Red Man against the White Man for having been given hard liquor'. Hitler was particularly opposed to cigarettes appearing between the lips of the fairer sex…

Germany's cigarette manufacturers decided the best form of resistance to the onslaught was collaboration and donated large sums to the Nazi party. Some made pathetic attempts at appeasement, including the market leader, Cigaretten Bildendienst, which offered coupons with its cigarettes that could be exchanged for a coffee-table book on Hitler.

Hitler's scientists, meanwhile, had come up with some disturbing theories about smoking. In 1939, Franz H. Müller was the first to use case-control epidemiological methods to document a relationship between smoking and lung cancer. Müller concluded that the 'extraordinary rise in tobacco use' was 'the single most important cause of the rising incidence of lung cancer'." *Tobacco* (Gately), pp. 254-255

402. Hitler characterized tobacco as "the wrath of the Red Man against the White Man, vengeance for having been given hard liquor." (*The Nazi War on Cancer*, Robert Proctor, 1999)… "the fact remains that the man who brought more misery to the world than any other human being hated smoking, as in medieval days the Devil

was said to hate holy water." (*Sublime Tobacco*, Compton Mackenzie, 1957.) There were bans on smoking in buses and trains in Germany, as well as on SS and police officers smoking in public when in uniform.

*Faber Book of Smoking*, p. 89

403. "The cigarette was well on the way to its status as the twentieth century's most successful consumer product. The rations for soldiers in the First World War had introduced a new generation to its delights, as well as removing any doubts about its unmanliness. And in the Second World War the British government spent more on tobacco for the troops than on tanks, ships or planes. By 1945, around 80 percent of British men smoked, with women catching up fast." *Faber Book of Smoking*, p. 77

404. A World War II Pall Mall cigarette ad: "...in cigarettes, as in armored scout cars, it is modern design that makes the big difference." *Tobacco* (Gately), p. 264

405. When Montgomery told Churchill, "I do not drink. I do not smoke. I sleep a great deal. That is why I am 100 percent fit," Churchill responded, "I drink a great deal. I sleep little, and I smoke cigar after cigar. That is why I am 200 percent fit." *Tobacco* (Gately), p. 257

406. In fact, hardly a photograph of Churchill exists without his trademark cigar, documenting his very real passion for smoking. After a German blitz damaged the Dunhill store, Churchill anxiously waited to learn whether his cigars had escaped harm, especially his favorite Havana Double Coronas. At another time, Field Marshal Montgomery was claiming to be in 100 percent good shape because he did not smoke or drink and got plenty of rest. Churchill shot back, "I drink a great deal, I sleep little, and I smoke cigar after cigar. That is why I am in 200 percent form." Quote from *The Cigar Connoisseur*, p. 113

407. In 1940, Old Golds continued to boast "not a cough in a carload", and Kools claimed to protect against the common cold. Reader's Digest, April 1992

408. By 1940, yearly adult cigarette consumption was 2558 per capita, nearly twice the 1930 level.

*Ashes to Ashes*, p. 110

409. In 1940, top cigarette brands and their market share were Camel, 24%, Lucky Strike, 23%, Chesterfield, 18%, Raleigh, 5%, Old Gold, 3%, and Pall Mall, 2%. *Ashes to Ashes*, p. 105

410. In 1941, retired world heavyweight boxing champion Gene Tunney, then head of the US Navy's physical fitness program, wrote an article in *Reader's Digest* entitled "Nicotine Knockout, or the Slow Count." Tunney strongly criticized smoking, writing that "I can bluntly say that few things could be worse for physical fitness than promoting the cigarette habit." Tunney described tobacco advertising as a "national menace," recalling that when he was a boxer, he declined an offer of US $15,000 to endorse a brand of cigarettes.

Quote from *Smoke and Mirrors*, p. 43

411. "In the United States, President Roosevelt declared tobacco an essential wartime material and granted military exemptions to those who grew it." *Tobacco* (Gately), p. 257

412. President Roosevelt in a 1941 executive order listed tobacco as an essential crop, and local draft boards were directed to give tobacco farmers draft deferments to ensure continued output. Reader's Digest, April 1992

413. Franklin D. Roosevelt as a college student wrote an editorial in the Harvard Crimson in 1903 about the problem of smoking at football games, requesting a separate section for women "without fear of being asphyxiated" and for others who objected to smoking. FDR smoked Camels, and after he was president was offered a large amount of money to act as spokesman for Camels. "Roosevelt responded by letter...that stated he had smoked the company's cigarettes since the age of 13 and had been coughing ever since. The company subsequently withdrew its offer." Tobacco Control, Winter 1996, p. 313

414. Joe DiMaggio was a heavy smoker during his record 56-game hitting streak in 1941.

*Baseball*, Ken Burns, PBS film, 1995

415. In 1942, Lucky Strike eliminated the gold panels on the pack and the solid green used on Lucky labels. The gold ink base was copper powder, and copper was way up on the critical metals list. Soon afterward, chromium used in the green ink also began to run low. They promoted their loss as a contribution to the war effort, claiming that their sacrifice had released enough copper to build many light tanks. New ads had a pack next to a tank and read: "Lucky Strike Green has gone to war! So here's the smart new uniform for fine tobacco."

*Nicotine*, p. 62

416. Winston Churchill claimed to have smoked a quarter of a million cigars in his 91 years. "During the Nazi blitz of London in 1941, one of the Luftwaffe's raids destroyed the Dunhill tobacco shop on Drake Street, in which was stored a portion of the prime minister's treasured cache of Havanas... the store manager made a careful survey of the damage and rushed to the phone to report 'your cigars are safe, Sir.'"  *A Passion for Cigars*, p. 24

417. After a German bombing raid destroyed Winston Churchill's favorite tobacconist shop during the London Blitz of 1941, an aide telephoned the prime minister at 2 a.m. to tell him, "Your cigars are safe, sir."

*The Cigar*, Barnaby Conrad, Chronicle Books, 1996

418. World War II Supreme Allied Commander Dwight D. Eisenhower puffed Camels at the rate of four packs a day. The corncob pipe was the trademark of General Douglas MacArthur.

U.S. News and World Report, March 16, 1998, p. 60

419. "During World War II close observation noted another farce--that of sending cigarettes to our armed forces both in training and actual combat. Good strategy would have been to have done the reverse; namely ship all the cigarettes to our enemies, who would have been slowed up by their toxic effects, and thereby the war's duration may have been shortened. Had such an event occurred, who knows how many lives would have been spared."

*Stop Smoking Before It Stops You*, Emil Alban, Christopher Publishing, 1949, p. 23

420. When the supply of cigarettes is limited, cigarette smokers behave much like heroin addicts. During extreme deprivation in Germany after World War II, "the majority of the habitual smokers preferred to do without food even under extreme conditions of nutrition rather than forego tobacco. Thus, when food rations in prisoner-of-war camps were down to 900-1000 calories, smokers were still willing to barter their food rations for cigarettes."  *Licit and Illicit Drugs*, p. 226

421. A British former World War II prisoner of war wrote: "The one thing that men were unable to give up was cigarette smoking. There was a very active market in bartering the handful of rice we received daily for the two cigarettes we were given. I have actually seen men die of starvation because they had sold their food for cigarettes."  *Smoking: the Artificial Passion*, David Krogh, W.H. Freeman, 1991

422. A series of ads for Philip Morris cigarettes in the New England Journal of Medicine in 1944 stated: "Doctor, have you ever suffered from throat irritation due to smoking?" and "Clinical test showed that when smokers changed to Philip Morris cigarettes every case of irritation of the nose and throat due to smoking cleared completely or definitely improved."

423. In the first 45 minutes of the movie Casablanca, Humphrey Bogart smoked ten cigarettes.

Modern Maturity, June 1994, p. 58

424. Humphrey Bogart and Lauren Bacall between them smoked a total of 21 cigarettes "on camera" in the 1944 movie "To Have and Have Not." Bogie died of esophageal cancer at age 57.

425. After World War II, American cigarettes were accepted as currency "from Paris to Peking."

New York Times, August 28, 1994

426. As part of the Marshall Plan for the reconstruction of Europe, the US government sent a gift of 210 million cigarettes to Germany.  *Tobacco* (Gately), p. 267

427. In 1949, 81% of British men and 39% of women were smokers.  *Tobacco* (Gately), p. 268

428. Cuspidors and spittoons were eliminated from federal buildings in 1945.

429. In 1945, Drs. Ernest Wynder and Evarts Graham of Washington University Medical School found that of 605 men with bronchogenic cancer of the lung, almost all were smokers for more than twenty years. Graham stopped smoking in 1952, but died of lung cancer in 1957.                    *They Satisfy*, p. 164

430. "I have never smoked in my life, and look forward to a time when the world will look back in amazement and disgust to a practice so unnatural and offensive."
                    George Bernard Shaw, the New York Herald Tribune, April 14, 1946

431. A Camel man in Times Square, New York City, blew giant smoke rings (steam actually) one every four seconds from 1941 until 1966 when it was torn down.                    Smithsonian, February 1998, p. 41

432. "I've smoked Camels for 8 years. They have the mildness that counts with me."
                    Joe DiMaggio, advertising Camels in the late 1940's (*Cigars*, p. 15)

433. Henry Fonda appeared in a 1940's ad for Camels where the claim was made of "not one single case of throat irritation from smoking Camels."                    Information courtesy of Dean Ornish, M.D.

434. The number of smokers doubled in Germany between 1940 and 1950, and almost doubled in the United States in this time period.                    *Cancer Wars*, PBS television, 1998

435. In the late 1940's, Ronald Reagan, a non-smoker, served as a spokesman for Chesterfield cigarettes.

436. "My cigarette is the mild cigarette… that's why Chesterfield is my favorite."
                    Ronald Reagan appearing in a Chesterfield ad in 1948

437. In 1947, one of the year's biggest hit songs was "Smoke! Smoke! Smoke!" by Tex Williams. One of the lines went "I've smoked all my life, and I ain't dead yet."                    Reader's Digest, April 1992

438. As late as 1948, the Journal of the American Medical Association reported that smoking reduced stress and that it did not cause health problems.                    *Nicotine*, Judy Monroe, Enslow Publishers, 1995, p. 12

439. In the 1940's, the J.H. Guild Company in Rupert, Vermont marketed "Dr. Guild's Green Mountain Asthmatic Cigarettes to Relieve Attacks and Paroxysms of Asthma" (from the cigarette pack label). The ingredients were listed as stramonium, belladonna, and potassium nitrate.
                    From the American Academy of Allergy, Asthma, and Immunology
                    exhibit "Treasures from the Archives," San Diego, March 2000

440. In 1949, Camel advertised a group of "noted throat specialists" who had found "not one case of throat irritation due to smoking Camels!" This ad ran in many issues of the JAMA until late 1953, when the journal stopped accepting tobacco advertisements.

441. In 1950, Camels were the most popular cigarette with a 27 percent market share, leading Luckies with 23 percent. The market share for Marlboro was less than one half of one percent.   *Tobacco and the Clinician*, p. iii

442. C.H. Long was "just another cowboy" in the Texas panhandle until a picture of him smoking a cigarette appeared on the cover of Life magazine on August 22, 1949. "Advertising mogul Leo Burnett saw the picture and was inspired to create a mythic hero who could be used to sell cigarettes: the Marlboro Man. Advertising changed a cowboy into the cowboy, a noble archetype into a sales pitch."
                    Life magazine 60th Anniversary issue, October 1996, p. 132

443. In the early 1950's Marlboro was a brand aimed at women, much like Virginia Slims today. Marlboro sales were one quarter of one percent of the American market, and Philip Morris was last among US cigarette makers. In 1954, the brand's packaging and image were redesigned to appeal to men. They cowboy was introduced in newspaper ads, and the slogan was "Delivers the goods on flavor." The next year, the campaign featured a Marlboro man with tattoos and the slogan: "Filter, flavor, flip-top box – you get a lot to like." Sales

jumped to 5 billion, a 3241 percent increase over 1954. By 1957, sales had increased to 20 billion for that year, which meant that Marlboro sold three times as many cigarettes every day as it did in the entire year of 1954.

New York Times, August 27, 1995, p. F11

444. In the early 1950's, celebrities advertising Chesterfield cigarettes in the Journal of the American Medical Association included Bing Crosby, Gregory Peck, Kirk Douglas, Ben Hogan, Gene Tierney and Barbara Stanwyck.

445. The TV series "I Love Lucy" was introduced in the fall of 1951, and was the top rated show in four of its first six seasons. It was sponsored by Philip Morris, and the "animated titles that opened the show each week featured stick figures of Lucy and Desi climbing a giant pack of Philip Morris cigarettes."

The Tobacco Timeline, www.tobacco.org

446. In 1951, Herbert Brean published the book *How to Stop Smoking* which sold 750,000 copies. His major argument was that smoking wastes time, and that a pack and a half a day (30 cigarettes) smoker "blows away" a week every year by smoking.                                                Modern Maturity, June 1994, p. 78

447. "Just what the doctor ordered."                                                Slogan for L&M Filters, 1954

448. Marlboro, formerly a woman's cigarette, was relaunched in 1954 with a new red and white pack with cowboys among its mix of macho images. By 1963, the "Marlboro Man" was exclusively a cowboy, and the slogan, "Come to Marlboro Country" was created. Marlboro sales began growing by 10% per year.

Wall Street Journal, October 18, 1995, p. A8 and The Tobacco Timeline, www.tobacco.org

449. In 1954, Marlboro's market share of the U.S. market was one quarter of 1%.

450. In the 1950's Arthur Godfrey would sign off at the end of his Chesterfield-sponsored variety show by saying "This is Arthur Buy-em-by-the-carton Godfrey!" The message was dropped in 1959 when he was diagnosed with lung cancer.

451. In the 1950's when John Cameron Swayze anchored "The Camel News Caravan," RJ Reynolds required him to have a burning cigarette visible whenever he was on camera.

452. In the 1950's, filters were advertised with unsubstantiated promises of health protection. In addition, the tobacco industry in full page nationwide newspaper ads professed to have "an interest in people's health as a basic responsibility, paramount to every other consideration in our business."                *Nicotine Addiction*, p.12

453. In the 1950's, Philip Morris proclaimed "The cigarette that takes the fear out of smoking."

*Smoke and Mirrors*, p. 46

454. The tobacco industry published in January 1954 "A Frank Statement to Cigarette Smokers." Just before publication, the sentence, "We will never produce and market a product shown to be the cause of any serious human ailment," was deleted.                                                JAMA, October 7, 1998, p. 1173

455. In 1952, Lorillard introduced Kent cigarettes with the "Micronite" asbestos filter. "Kent and only Kent has the Micronite filter. Made of a pure, dust-free, completely harmless material that is not only effective but so safe that it actually is used to help filter the air in operating rooms of leading hospitals." (Life Magazine). The filter offered "the greatest health protection in cigarette history." The filter was discontinued in 1956.

The Tobacco Timeline, www.tobacco.org

456. A 1954 Life magazine ad for the Kent Micronite filter (made with crocidolite asbestos fibers) stated that the filter is "made of a pure, dust-free, completely harmless material that is...so safe that it actually is used to help filter the air in operating rooms of leading hospitals."                Tobacco Control, Spring 1994, p. 64

457. The 1956 campaign for Kent cigarettes containing the asbestos Micronite filter implied that the filter solved the health problems of cigarettes and that it was endorsed by the AMA.        Tobacco Control, Summer 1994, p. 136

458. Kent cigarettes promised, "the greatest health protection ever developed" by virtue of its new crocidolite asbestos filter. A lawsuit by a former Kent smoker who developed mesothelioma, an asbestos-related lung cancer, was dismissed in 1992 because he could not prove that he smoked Kents in the 1950's.

*Journal of Psychoactive Drugs*, July 1989, p. 281

459. A jury ordered Lorillard, maker of Kent cigarettes, to pay former smoker Charles Conner $2.2 million after he discovered that he had mesothelioma, a cancer linked to asbestos. Kent cigarettes were manufactured with asbestos-containing micronite filters from 1952 to 1956. Connor was a Kent smoker in the 1950's before quitting in 1962. Kent ads at the time said that it was "the one cigarette that can show you proof of greater health protection."

Associated Press, April 20, 1999

460. Lyndon Johnson was a heavy smoker until he suffered a serious heart attack while serving as a Senate majority leader. He died suddenly of another heart attack at age 64 at his Texas ranch in 1973.

*Ashes to Ashes*, p. 265 and google.com

461. In 1959, Surgeon General Leroy Burney wrote in the Journal of the American Medical Association that "the weight of evidence at present implicates smoking as the principal etiological factor" in the increased incidence of lung cancer. To Burney's surprise, two weeks later the A.M.A. published an editorial which insisted that there were not yet enough facts to "warrant the assumption of an all-or-none authoritative position" on causation.

Mother Jones, May-June 1996, p. 45

462. By 1960, the distribution of free cigarettes at medical and public health meetings had stopped.

The Tobacco Timeline, www.tobacco.org

463. When Time magazine featured RJR chairman Bowman Gray on its April 21, 1960 cover, he was quoted as saying about tobacco and cancer: "I just don't believe it. People are hearing the same old story, and the record is getting scratched." Bowman Gray later had a medical school named after him.     *Ashes to Ashes*, p. 212

464. In the 1960's, popular television shows such as the "Ben Casey, M.D." and "Dr. Kildare" medical dramas were brought into millions of homes each week via cigarette sponsorship, and health protection was a commonly implied theme.

*Tobacco and the Clinician*, p. vi

465. In 1961, President John F. Kennedy ordered Pierre Salinger to purchase 1200 of Cuba's finest Petit Upmann cigars just before ordering a trade embargo on all imports from Castro's Cuba.

San Francisco Chronicle, January 25, 1993, p. B3

466. In 1961, "Dr. Kildare" played by Richard Chamberlain offered cigarettes to one of his troubled patients, and "on the show, cigarettes convey the pervasive assumption that all good doctors smoke...Whenever Dr. Kildare is faced with a grim alternative, he pulls out a cigarette." In the 1950's, Lucille Ball's character on "I Love Lucy" smoked right through her television pregnancy.     New York Times, August 24, 1997, Section 2, p. 31

467. "It is even more surprising, today, looking at early television, to see the title character of 'Dr. Kildare' offering a light to one of his troubled patients. In the very first scene of the premiere show, in 1961, Dr. Kildare, played handsomely by Richard Chamerlain, bounds up the hospital stairs and puts quarters in a cigarette machine in the lobby. On the show, cigarettes are practically his signature and convey the pervasive assumption that all good doctors smoke. Offering a light or a cigarette, in the hospital, is a sign of sympathetic attention, a gesture of conviviality and sociality that made Dr. Kildare's hospital, before HMO's, a close-knit community."

Richard Klein, "After the Preaching, the Lure of Taboo," New York Times, August 24, 1997

468. In 1964, the American Medical Association accepted a $10 million grant from the tobacco industry for a five-year study of smoking.

*Ashes to Ashes*, p. 286

469. Dr. Luther Terry smoked in the car as he reviewed his notes on the way to the press conference to announce the results of the first Surgeon General's Report on smoking in 1964. In the question period, a reporter asked: "Dr. Terry, do you smoke?"

He replied:     "No sir, I do not."

"Dr. Terry, have you ever smoked?"

"Yes, I used to."

"Dr. Terry, when did you quit?"

"About ten minutes ago."

The Surgeon General never smoked again.

from A Science Odyssey with Charles Osgood,
PBS television, January 11, 1998

470. For decades the AMA (American Medical Association) was a loyal ally of the tobacco industry. When the Surgeon General's report condemning smoking was published in 1964, the AMA refused to endorse it, saying instead that "more research" was needed. An AMA research program on tobacco received $18 million from the tobacco companies over the next nine years, during which the association kept silent about the dangers of smoking.

The Nation, January 1, 1996, p. 16

471. In the 1960's and 1970's, Lorillard tried unsuccessfully to find a counterpart to Marlboro, a full-flavored smoke with a western motif. It marketed Maverick, Redford, Luke, and Zach, all of which failed. *They Satisfy*, p. 227

472. Kent Cigarettes sponsored the famous Ed Sullivan Show in 1965 marking the American television debut of the Beatles.

1994 Surgeon General report, p. 169

473. Market share for filter cigarettes increased from less than 1% in 1950 to 19% in 1955, 51% in 1960, 80% in 1970, 92% in 1980, and 95% in 1990. Low tar and nicotine brands increased from 2% in 1965 to 45% in 1980, 56% in 1989, and 69% in 1992. The latter products were offered as an alternative between smoking conventional brands on one hand and quitting altogether on the other hand. *Nicotine Addiction*, p. 12

474. In 1966, Congress voted to send a gift of 600 million cigarettes to flood disaster victims in India.

The Tobacco Timeline, www.tobacco.org

475. The Cigarette Labeling and Advertising Act of 1965 was an important victory for the tobacco industry. In return for the weak warning label "cigarettes may be hazardous to your health," federal preemption of state and local regulation on advertising went into effect. This meant that no state or local government could pass a more restrictive advertising ban than the federal government; the ban continues in effect more than 30 years later.

Joel Dunnington, MD

476. The banning of cigarette ads on TV in 1970 was at the request of and with the support of the tobacco industry, and was followed by a rise in cigarette sales. The industry had just seen the most dramatic drop in smoking ever due to the anti-smoking public service announcements required by the Fairness Doctrine of 1967. The rise in sales came immediately following the removal of anti-smoking public service announcements from television, strong evidence that counter advertising is effective in altering behavior.

477. In 1969, America's two most popular medical shows, Ben Casey and Dr. Kildare, were both sponsored by tobacco companies. *Smoking and the Public Interest*, Ruth Brecher, Consumers Union, 1963, p. 163

478. In 1970, the top five US cigarette brands and sales in billions were Winston (82 billion), Pall Mall (58 billion), Marlboro (51 billion), Salem (44 billion) and Kool (40 billion). The Tobacco Timeline, www.Tobacco.org

479. In 1970, American cigar consumption peaked at about 9 billion per year.

The Tobacco Timeline, www.tobacco.org

480. "12 Dogs Develop Lung Cancer in Group of 86 Taught to Smoke" February 6, 1970, front page headline in the New York Times

481. A researcher named Dr. Auerbach did tracheotomies on 86 beagles in order to pump cigarette smoke into their lungs. The Tobacco Timeline, www.tobacco.org

482. Phillip Morris CEO Joseph Cullman in an appearance on "Face the Nation" in 1971 when asked about "invasive lung tumors" in smoking beagles said that this was not the same thing as cancer. When he was asked to comment about a study that found smoking mothers gave birth to smaller babies, he said, "Some women would prefer having smaller babies." *Ashes to Ashes*, p. 358

483. In 1972, 65% of men and 42% of women in Great Britain were smokers.     *Faber Book of Smoking*, p. 103

484. Partly at the urging of the tobacco companies, President Nixon in 1973 at the beginning of his second term did not reappoint his anti-tobacco Surgeon General Jesse Steinfeld. The post of Surgeon General went unfilled for four years.     *Ashes to Ashes*, p. 367

485. Arnold Palmer quit smoking in 1975, as did Jack Nicklaus in 1982.

486. In 1978, Secretary of Health, Education, and Welfare Joseph Califano labeled cigarettes "Public Health Enemy No. 1" and said that their users were committing "slow-motion suicide."     *Ashes to Ashes*, p. 436

487. Two years earlier, Jimmy Carter had appointed a Philip Morris board member as the head of the President's Council on Physical Fitness and Sports.     *Dying for a Smoke*, Pyramid Video, 1993

488. In 1990, the top five U.S. cigarette brands and sales in billions were Marlboro (134 billion), Winston (46 billion), Salem (32 billion), and Newport (24 billion).     The Tobacco Timeline, www.tobacco.org

489. Total per capita consumption of tobacco (in pounds of tobacco) peaked in the early 1950's at just under 13 pounds per adult. Of that amount, cigarettes accounted for nearly 10.5 pounds and cigars 1.26 pounds. In 1997, each adult in the United States consumed, on average, approximately 4.55 pounds of tobacco, 4.0 pounds as cigarettes, 0.31 pounds as snuff, 0.28 pounds as large cigars and cigarillos, and .32 pounds as chewing tobacco.     Quote from *Nicotine and Public Health*, p. 180

# CHAPTER 5
## ENVIRONMENTAL TOBACCO SMOKE (ETS)

## General

1.  "For the vanities committed in this filthy custome, is it not both great vanity and uncleanness, that at the table, a place of cleanliness, men should not be ashamed, to sit puffing of the smoke of tobacco, making the filthy smoke and stink thereof, to exhale athwart the dishes, and infect the air, when very often men that abhor it are at their repast?"
    *A Counterblaste to Tobacco*, King James I, 1604

2.  A detailed reference on passive smoking is *Health Effects of Exposure to Environmental Tobacco Smoke,* Amy Dunn and Lauren Zeise, editors, California Environmental Protection Agency, Office of Environmental Health Hazard Assessment, 1997. The executive summary for this may be found in Tobacco Control, Winter 1997, pp. 346-353.

3.  A study by the California Office of Environmental Health Hazard Assessment and the Air Resources Board estimated death and disease among nonsmokers exposed to secondhand smoke. Up to 188,000 cases of ear infections, 36,000 cases of bronchitis or pneumonia, and 3100 cases of asthma each year among California children were attributed to the effects of secondhand smoke, as were an estimated 4700 to 7900 deaths in California, including 136 infants.
    Associated Press, October 24, 1997

4.  A California Environmental Protection Agency report estimates that secondhand smoke causes between 35,000 and 62,000 deaths nationwide each year from heart attack and stroke, and between 4,200 and 7,440 such deaths in California alone. In comparison, environmental tobacco smoke is responsible for lung cancer that kills 3,000 Americans each year, 360 of them Californians. The study also blames secondhand smoking for up to 3,000 new childhood asthma cases in California each year and for as many as 188,000 doctor visits for middle-ear infections.
    Associated Press, March 3, 1997

5.  Passive smoking in the US causes 53,000 deaths per year: 37,000 from heart disease, 4000 from lung cancer, and 12,000 from other cancers.
    Circulation, January 1991, p. 1

6.  Passive smoking, or second-hand smoke, kills about the same number of Americans each year as died in the Vietnam War. One American dies from second-hand smoke for every eight who die from active smoking.
    Circulation, January 1991, p. 1

7.  Environmental tobacco smoke (ETS) is a cause of illness and death in nonsmokers. The data that establish this are more extensive and more compelling than the data that are the scientific basis for stringent environmental controls on other pollutants such as asbestos, benzene, radon, and formaldehyde.
    Adolescent Medicine, June 1993, p. 308

8.  "Environmental tobacco smoke (ETS) consists of the sidestream smoke emitted from smoldering tobacco between puffs and mainstream smoke exhaled by the smoker. The major portion of ETS, 80-90%, is derived from sidestream smoke."
    *The Tobacco Epidemic*, p. 108

9.  Two thirds of the total smoke in each cigarette ends up in the environment. This "sidestream" smoke has higher concentrations of poisons and carcinogens than the "mainstream" smoke that the smoker inhales, and 2.5 times higher levels of carbon monoxide.
    American Journal of Public Health, February 1989, p. 209

10. Another estimate is that 55% of cigarette smoke is not inhaled and ends up in the air directly, and another 20% is exhaled by the smoker, making 75% total sidestream smoke. Smoking is the major cause for indoor air pollution, and overwhelms any other source.
    Audio Digest Internal Medicine, November 3, 1993 (Neal Benowitz)

11. Sidestream smoke accounts for 85% of the total smoke in a cigarette. It burns at lower temperatures than mainstream smoke, so is "dirtier" and more carcinogenic with increased tar, benzopyrene, benzene, ammonia, nitrosamines, hydrazine, and cadmium than mainstream smoke.

    Seminars in Respiratory Medicine, January 1990, p.87 and Consumer Reports, January 1995, p. 31

12. Sidestream smoke has higher concentrations of many toxic chemicals than does mainstream smoke, because it is not filtered and because cigarettes burn at a lower temperature when they are smoldering, leading to a less complete and dirtier combustion. *The Cigarette Papers*, p. 392

13. Many toxic gases are more concentrated in sidestream than in mainstream smoke, and nearly 85% of the smoke in a room results from sidestream smoke.

    UICC Tobacco Control Fact Sheet 7, International Union Against Cancer, 1996

14. Sidestream smoke contains twice the tar and nicotine compared to the mainstream smoke inhaled by the smoker, and five times more carbon monoxide.

    *250 Reasons to Quit Smoking*, Molli Nagel, Vision Books, 1994, items 221 and 222

15. "The ETS exposures in workplaces that allow smoking is comparable with, and often greater than, the ETS exposures in smokers' homes as well as the personal exposures of nonsmokers married to smokers, who have been shown to be at an increased risk for lung cancer and heart disease compared with nonsmokers married to nonsmokers...

    "Were 'cigarette equivalents' calculated on the basis of carcinogens in ETS, rather than nicotine, the cigarette equivalents would be much higher. This seeming anomaly results from the differences between mainstream and sidestream smoke...

    "For example, although twice as much nicotine is emitted in sidestream as mainstream smoke, the ratio for benzene is approximately 10 to one; sidestream smoke is even more enriched in many other carcinogens: e.g., more than 30 times as much 4-aminobiphenyl and 100 times as much N-nitrosodimethylamine is emitted in sidestream as in mainstream smoke. Thus, the complex chemistry of tobacco smoke leads to different numbers of 'cigarette equivalents' depending on which compound is examined." JAMA, September 27, 1995, p. 960

16. A father's smoking contributes the equivalent of 30 cigarettes per year in passive smoking to a child's lungs, and a mother's smoking contributes 50 cigarettes per year. A child would then inhale, as if he or she smoked "actively," about 80 cigarettes a year. American Journal of Diseases of Children, November 1985, p. 1101

17. Another study estimated that a child both of whose parents smoke, is the equivalent of the child actively smoking between 60 and 150 cigarettes per year. The Lancet, June 6, 1987, p. 1325

18. If a nonsmoker works next to smoking coworkers for eight hours, it has the same effect as smoking three cigarettes." Tobacco IQ," American Cancer Society, September 1991

19. In the United States, an average worker in an average office where smoking is permitted will inhale nicotine, tar, carbon monoxide, and other carcinogens at levels equivalent to the active smoking of two to three cigarettes per day. Chest, July 1991, p. 39

20. Jacob Sullum, the former managing editor of Reason magazine, wrote an article widely reprinted in tobacco industry ads where he criticized the EPA report on secondhand smoke. But the Reason Foundation received $10,000 from Philip Morris, and Sullum himself was paid $5000 from RJ Reynolds for another article he wrote about secondhand smoke. Sullum later admitted that the "vast majority" of epidemiologists would find the methods the EPA used "perfectly legitimate." ASH Review, November 1994, p. 3

21. Referring to the EPA report, a column by Richard Daynard in the New York Times, stated, "This basically marks the end of any debate about whether ETS causes serious, fatal diseases among nonsmokers."

    New York Times, January 8, 1993, p. A16

22. Passive smoking has been identified as a Group A carcinogen by the Environmental Protection Agency. This category includes only the most potent cancer-causing agents such as benzene, asbestos, arsenic, and vinyl

chloride. *Respiratory Health Effects of Passive Smoking*, Environmental Protection Agency report, January 1993

23. The particulate matter from a single cigarette smoked in a large room would violate the federal standard in the Clean Air Act for outdoor air.
Stanton Glantz, Ph.D., University of California, San Francisco lecture, February 24, 1994

24. Ventilation systems in buildings are designed to recirculate air, not to filter it. For this reason, they are often responsible for bringing polluted air from smoking areas into designated "smoke-free" areas.

25. Nonsmoking workers and their employers incur significant financial losses because of missed work secondary to illness resulting from exposure to second-hand tobacco smoke. Workers exposed to passive smoke experience greater carbon monoxide levels, greater eye irritation, more cough, more phlegm production, and more chest colds than workers not exposed to passive smoke.
Chest, July 1991, p. 39

26. A study made measurements of two markers of environmental tobacco smoke, respirable suspended particles and nicotine, in the smoking and nonsmoking sections of seven restaurants. The concentration of respirable suspended particles and nicotine were 40% and 65% lower, respectively, in the no-smoking than in the smoking sections, indicating incomplete protection against smoke exposure.
American Journal of Public Health, September 1993, p. 1339

27. "To have a nonsmoking section in a restaurant... is like having a non-chlorinated space in a chlorinated pool. The cigarette smoke knows no boundaries."
Mark Pertschuk, Americans for Nonsmokers' Rights

28. The United States Occupational Health and Safety Administration, which regulates workplace and worker safety, regards a mortality risk on the job of greater than one per thousand as "very hazardous." This assessment is shared by the EPA (Environmental Protection Agency) and FDA (Food and Drug Administration). A study by the Direction de la Sante Publique de la Monteregie in Quebec reported on the health risks for nonsmoking restaurant workers exposed to environmental tobacco smoke in the workplace. The conclusion was that this smoke exposure creates a lifetime risk of 1% of dying from lung cancer for the average worker, and a 10% risk of dying from heart disease, over and above the likelihood of dying from these diseases for the general population.

29. Restaurant workers are exposed to three to five times more ETS than other workers, and consequently have about four times the expected lung cancer mortality and 2.5 times the expected heart disease mortality.
*Tobacco Use: An American Crisis*, p. 49

30. 400 billion cigarettes, 4 billion cigars, and 11 billion pipefuls of tobacco adding up to 467,000 tons of tobacco are burned indoors each year in the US.
Advocacy Institute, May 4, 1992, and Indoor Air Facts, US EPA, 1989

31. Because tobacco smoke is exempt from regulation under the Toxic Substances Control Act of 1976, the Environmental Protection Agency (EPA) is prohibited from doing anything to control exposures to it.
Journal of the National Cancer Institute, April 1, 1992, p. 481

32. In a 7 to 2 Supreme Court decision, William McKinney, a nonsmoker serving a life sentence for murder in Nevada, won the right not to be subjected to a 4 pack a day cellmate's secondhand smoke, and was granted his own cell. The dissenting justices were Clarence Thomas and Antonin Scalia.
New York Times, June 20, 1993

33. "This moment of silence is brought to you by the California Department of Health Services in memory of the 14 Californians who died today because they were forced to breathe someone else's tobacco smoke."
California television message about passive smoking, 1993

34. A study from the Centers for Disease Control found that 100% of 800 people tested, ages 4 to 91 and most of them nonsmokers, had measurable serum levels of cotinine, a byproduct or metabolite of nicotine.
Morbidity and Mortality Weekly Report, January 29, 1993, p. 37

35. 60,000 current and former flight at[...]it against a number of tobacco
companies because of illnesses cau[...]n flights before the 1989
smoking ban. Exposure was equival[...]r flight.
November 6, 1994, p. A11, and
[...]mber 3, 1993 (Neal Benowitz)

36. During the era before the airline smoki[...]ht attendant, whether she
wanted to or not, smoked two to three c[...]
[...]uis Times, July 1996, p. 15)

37. Passive smoking is responsible for 22,000[...]0 from lung cancer and
20,000 from cardiovascular disease. About[...]xposed to environmental
tobacco smoke, and inhale the equivalent o[...].
[...]al, January 3, 1998, p. 9

38. In Australia, a patient with asthma won a $85[...]f passive smoke
exposure at work, which worsened her conditi[...]
[...]une 6, 1992, p. 138B

39. In a study on upper respiratory sensitivity to sid[...]subjects underwent
controlled 15 minute challenges with clean air fo[...]cco smoke (45 ppm carbon
monoxide). Nasal airway resistance increased mo[...]8% of subjects, and 75% of them had a more
than 10% drop in maximum inspiratory flow meas[...]ements and/or a more than 50% increase in nasal airway
resistance. Today in Medicine Respiratory Disease, April 1990, p. 138B

40. Each year in Australia, passive smoke exposure leads to more than 5400 extra hospital admissions and costs the
country about $21 million. The excess morbidity includes 51,000 episodes of asthma (about 9% of all cases) in
children under age 15, and about 2000 hospital admissions for babies under age 18 months because of chest
illness. Medical Journal of Australia, March 4, 1996, p. 260

41. In a study from China, nonsmoking adults exposed to passive smoke had a significant decrement in lung function
tests (average 102-ml reduction in FEV1 and 151-ml reduction in forced vital capacity) compared to nonsmoking
adults without exposure to environmental tobacco smoke at home or at work.
American Journal of Respiratory and Critical Care Medicine, January 1995, p. 41

42. Passive smoking is reported by 53.5% of adult nonsmokers in China.
Abstract S 15/1, 10th World Conference on Tobacco or Health, Beijing, 1997

43. Among bartenders in California, pulmonary function improved and respiratory symptoms declined rapidly after a
smoking ban in bars and taverns. JAMA, August 18, 1999, p. 629

44. Levels of toxic chemicals produced in nonsmokers' blood by second hand smoke exposure have fallen more than
75% on average compared to 10 years ago (CDC data). Time, January 21, 2002, p. 123

45. In England, King James I published an anti-tobacco tract in 1604 that, among other things, offered an early
critique of second hand smoke: the royal author expressed his concerns that a husband who smoked might
"reduce thereby his delicate, wholesome, and cleane complexioned wife to that extremitie, that either shee must
also corrupt her sweete breath therewith, or else resolve to live in a perpetuall stinking torment."
Quote from *Reducing Tobacco Use*, 2000 Surgeon General report, p. 29

46. Speaking of ETS inside homes with smokers, Stanford researcher Wayne Ott says: "The concentration of
particulate pollution [fine particles emitted by burning objects that go deep into the lungs where they're trapped]
is incredibly higher than what we would expect to find outside on the very worst day in the most polluted U.S.
city." U.S. News and World Report, December 2, 2002, p. 15

47.  In 1928, an editorial in the American Journal of Public Health complained that cigarette smoke at medical meetings was so thick that it was difficult to see the lantern slides.

American Journal of Public Health, Vol. 18, 1928, pp. 1285-1286

# ETS and Children

1.  More than 752,000 children in the United States are at risk for environmental tobacco smoke exposure in licensed day care centers. In the early 1990's, Alaska, Arkansas, and Minnesota were the only states that required completely smoke-free day care centers. 19% of the centers allowed smoking indoors.

Pediatrics, February 1993, p. 460

2.  Over 50% of pregnant women in China are exposed to environmental tobacco smoke, usually from their husbands. Nonsmoking women in households with ETS delivered babies that averaged 30 grams (one ounce) less in birth weight compared to babies from households with no ETS exposure.

American Journal of Public Health, February 1993, p. 207

3.  A study from Norway concluded that pregnant nonsmokers exposed to ETS in the home increased the risk for low birth weight (small-for-gestational-age) babies.    American Journal of Public Health, January 1998, pp. 120-124

4.  Children with high exposure to tobacco smoke had a 38% higher rate of middle ear infection, 9 more days of infection and more prolonged ear infections, than those with no smoke exposure. Exposure to second hand smoke was responsible for 18% of the children's annual sick days.    Journal of Respiratory Disease, August 1994, p. 719

5.  In children, 8% of cases of otitis media with effusion may be attributable to exposure to tobacco smoke in the home.

Pediatrics, August 1992, p. 228

6.  Having a mother who smokes triples the risk for recurrent otitis media (ear infection) in babies in the first year of life.

Pediatrics, May 1995, p. 670

7.  Children under age three who breathe ETS at home are twice as likely to get persistent middle ear infections as children who are not exposed.

Time, February 23, 1998, p. 24

8.  In a study from Calgary, Alberta, environmental tobacco smoke was an important risk factor for middle ear disease in preschool age. Children who lived with two smokers had an 85% higher risk of ear infections compared to children from smoke-free homes.    Archives of Pediatric and Adolescent Medicine 1998; 152:127

9.  Children undergoing myringotomy surgery for serous otitis media, or glue ear, were about 50% more likely to live in a household where someone smoked, than were control subjects.

International Journal of Pediatric Otorhinolaryngology 1985; 9:121

10.  Exposure to tobacco smoke increases the risk of chronic infections and fluid in the middle ear. ETS-exposed children also undergo more tonsillectomies and adenoidectomies. ETS-exposed children who develop pneumonia have a 20-40% increased risk that hospitalization will be needed for treatment.    *Cigarettes*, p. 72

11.  The Royal College of Physicians estimates that each year in Britain, 17,000 children under age 5 were admitted to the hospital because of illness caused by exposure to parents' smoke.    Thorax 1994; 49:733

12.  Children exposed to household smoke have four times the risk of being hospitalized for a bacterial or viral infection than babies and children from smoke-free households.

American Journal of Public Health, February 1989, p. 209

13.  In children ages 3 to 5 years, passive smoke exposure increases the risk of serious infectious illnesses requiring hospitalization almost four-fold.    American Journal of Epidemiology 1991; 133:154

14.  Smoking in the presence of infants and children has been termed the most prevalent yet least reported form of child abuse.    New York State Journal of Medicine, December 1983, p. 1255

15. Mothers who smoke can pass on the chemicals in tobacco smoke to their babies through breast milk. A study from Massachusetts General Hospital also found that babies may get more exposure to tobacco toxins through breast milk than by breathing secondhand smoke.

Reuters, June 10, 1998 from American Journal of Public Health

16. Children from families where one or both parents smoke are twice as likely to be in poor or only fair health as children who live in smoke-free households.                    US News and World Report, June 24, 1991 p.22

17. In patients with cystic fibrosis and heavy exposure to passive smoke at home, pulmonary function tests were significantly poorer, and there was a fivefold increase in the number of pulmonary-related hospitalizations.

NEJM, September 20, 1990, p. 782

18. More than a quarter of the nation's children are exposed to cigarette smoke, rising to 43% of children in families below the poverty level. Another estimate is that two-thirds of children from families below the poverty level have household smokers, compared with one-third of children with family incomes over $40,000.

Tobacco Free Youth Reporter, Spring 1993, and Los Angeles Times, June 30, 1991

19. In the early 1990's, 45% of children younger than age 6 in the United States, a total of 10 million, lived in households with one or more smokers.

Tobacco Control, Winter 1993, p. 514 and 1994 Cancer Facts and Figures (ACS)

20. 63 million nonsmoking adults and 9 to 12 million children younger than age 5 years in the United States have exposure to secondhand or sidestream smoke, which contains 2.5 times more nicotine, carbon monoxide, and benzopyrene that mainstream smoke.                       Journal of Respiratory Disease, August 1994, p. 716

21. In a study of 7680 children ages 2 months through 5 years of age, 38% were presently exposed to ETS in the home, and 23.8% were exposed by maternal smoking during pregnancy. The increased risk in children 2 months to 2 years old in homes with ETS for three or more episodes of wheezing was 2.7-fold, and for a diagnosis of asthma in children 2 months to 5 years old was 2.1 times the risk compared to homes without ETS. Overall, in the babies and younger children, 40% to 60% of the cases of asthma and three or more episodes of wheezing were attributable to ETS exposure, and for diagnosed asthma, there were an estimated 133,800 to 161,600 excess cases from ETS.                                                                Pediatrics, February 1998, p. 302

22. In a study of 4000 children ages 5 to 7 in England and Wales, 53% were exposed to cigarette smoke as determined by salivary cotinine levels.               British Medical Journal, February 4, 1994, p. 384

23. A 1998 study found that 47% of children in Canada were exposed to ETS in the home.

Tobacco Control, Spring 1998, p. 1

24. Of the estimated 54.1 million US children under age 15, 21.1 million (39%) are exposed to environmental tobacco smoke in the home. In children in households with less than $20,000 income, ETS exposure was reported in 51%. ETS exposure was associated with 24% more hospitalization days and 43% more lost school days.

9th World Conference on Tobacco or Health, Paris, 1994 (D. Mannino)

25. In a study from Shanghai, low birth weight babies living in households where there was a heavy smoker (a pack a day or more) had 4.48-fold increased risk for requiring hospitalization for a respiratory illness.

American Review of Respiratory and Critical Care Medicine, January 1994, p. 54

26. Children with exposure to environmental tobacco smoke have elevated levels of carcinogenic polyaromatic hydrocarbons, as well as of cotinine, a metabolite of nicotine. Exposure to environmental tobacco smoke for nonsmokers is estimated to be roughly one percent of the amount from direct exposure from active smoking.

New York Times, September 21, 1994, p. A16

27. After the first month of life, infants of parents who smoke have higher mortality rates through the first year of life, mostly because of an increased risk for sudden infant death syndrome and respiratory conditions such as bronchiolitis.                                                                       Pediatrics, November 1994, p. 750

28. In children, there is a highly significant association between the incidence of snoring and exposure to passive smoking in the household.                                                  British Medical Journal, December 16, 1989, p. 1491

29. In a study from France, 42% of children with one smoking parent and 51% of children with two smoking parents had had a tonsillectomy or adenoidectomy (or both), compared with 28% of the children of nonsmokers.
                                                                       Journal of Epidemiology and Community Health 1978; 32:97

30. States now consider parental smoking as a factor in deciding child custody cases, especially if the child has asthma.                                                                                               ASH Review, May-June 1996

31. Infants whose mothers smoke cigarettes have a hospital admission rate for bronchitis and pneumonia that is 28% higher than that for infants of nonsmoking mothers.                                Journal of Respiratory Disease 1993; 14:950

32. In a study from Greece, children exposed to ETS had a 3.5-fold increased risk of increased "respiratory morbidity" (three or more episodes of upper or lower respiratory infection in the preceding year) compared to children not exposed to ETS.                                                            The Lancet, July 29, 1995, p. 280

33. "Forty percent of American children are exposed to household tobacco smoke. The levels of household smoke to which 20 million children are constantly exposed throughout childhood are high enough to produce both measurable levels of blood cotinine and serious health damage. That 75% of all teenagers who smoke have parents who smoke continues to be the most consistent and most ignored factor in youth smoking. Though youths and adults (each for their own reasons) would deny parental influence, evidence is compelling that teenage smoking is largely the active continuation of a childhood of passive smoking."       JAMA, June 24, 1992, p. 3282

34. Passive smoke exposure is responsible for 19% of all expenditures for treatment of childhood respiratory disorders, or $661 million each year.                                                Dean Edell, MD, ABC radio, March 18, 1997

35. Each year among American children, tobacco is associated with an estimated 284 to 360 deaths from lower respiratory tract illnesses and fires initiated by smoking materials, more than 300 fire-related injuries, 5200 to 6500 tympanostomies, 1.3 million visits for coughs, and in children younger than 5 years of age, 260,000 to 436,000 episodes of bronchitis and 115,000 to 190,000 episodes of pneumonia. Out of 17 million ear infections children get each year, between 354,000 and 2.2 million are linked to second-hand smoke. Parental smoking doubles the chances that children will need their tonsils or adenoids removed, and at least 16% of these procedures, from 14,000 to 21,000 each year, are attributable to parental smoking. Finally, childhood asthma is caused by household smoking in 8% to 13% of all cases in children under 15, or 307,000 to 522,000 cases per year. Household smoking increases the overall prevalence of asthma by about 12%, and 529,000 office visits for asthma each year in children are attributable to household smoking. The authors of the meta-analysis believe that the true risk is probably closer to the worst-case than the best-case estimates above.  Pediatrics, April 1996, p. 560

36. American children ages 1 to 10 exposed to ETS in the home had 10% more respiratory illnesses than children not exposed, an additional 1.7 million cases annually. Children who were exposed to ETS had, on average, 1.87 more days per year of restricted activity, 1.06 more days of the confinement (20% more than children not exposed), and 1.45 more days of school absence (a 35% increase) than children who were not exposed.
                                                                                       Tobacco Control, Spring 1996, pp. 13-18

37. In West Virginia, where 26% of children live below the poverty level, a study showed that 69% of children of lower socioeconomic status had exposure to tobacco smoke at home, compared with 38% of children of higher socioeconomic status.                                         Journal of Allergy and Clinical Immunology, January 1996, p. 377

38. In a study of 16,800 people, 87.9% of the non-tobacco users had detectable levels of serum cotinine, indicative of exposure to environmental tobacco smoke. Of all US children ages 2 months to 11 years, 43% lived in a home with at least one smoker, and 37% of adult non-tobacco users lived in a home with at least one smoker, or

reported environmental tobacco smoke exposure at work. And overall, 91.7% of the US population age 4 years and older have detectable levels of cotinine, presumably from active smoking or exposure to ETS.

JAMA, April 24, 1996, p. 1233

39. 15 million American children, or one in five nationwide, were exposed to secondhand smoke in the household in 1996. About 41% of adult smokers live with children, and in most of the homes, smoking was permitted, the Centers for Disease Control and Prevention said. Associated Press, November 6, 1997

40. In a study from Australia of very low birth weight children, those who had been exposed to tobacco smoke since birth had worsened respiratory function (reduced airflow and air trapping) than non-exposed peers when tested at 11 years of age. Medical Journal of Australia, March 4, 1995, p. 260

41. Maternal smoking is associated with a permanent 7 to 11 percent reduction in their children's lung capacity as measured by FEV1 (forced expiratory volume in one second). Among school age children, the decrement in pulmonary function associated with maternal smoking appears to be related both to exposure during pregnancy, and an additional deficit related to continued exposure after birth.

American Journal of Respiratory and Critical Care Medicine,
June 1994, p. 1424 and Pediatric Pulmonology 1992; 12:37

42. Lung function in newborn infants measured by respiratory inductance plethysmography showed a significant decrement in babies whose mothers smoked ten or more cigarettes a day. This study from Perth, Australia demonstrated that smoke exposure in utero (before birth) reduces respiratory function and lung development, independent of direct harm from passive smoke after birth. The Lancet, October 19, 1996, p. 1060

43. Passive smoking exposes children to lead, a component of tobacco smoke, and children of heavier smokers have higher lead levels than children of lighter smokers. *Cigarettes*, p. 74

44. Children exposed to ETS after birth have a 5.3 times increased risk of Crohn's disease, an inflammatory bowel condition leading to pain, diarrhea, and bleeding. ETS exposure also doubles the risk in children for ulcerative colitis, another chronic large intestinal condition. *Cigarettes*, pp.74-75

45. The annual direct medical expenditure for childhood respiratory illness attributable to maternal smoking in children under the age of six totaled $661 million in 1987. This represented 19% of all expenditures for childhood respiratory conditions. Maternal smoking was associated with increased health care expenditures averaging (in 1995 dollars) $120 per year for children age 5 and under and $175 per year for children age 2 years and under.

American Journal of Public Health, February 1997, p. 205

46. In a survey from Hebei, China, the passive smoke exposure rate was 58% for a group of 1469 pregnant women. Abstract PO 231, 10th World Conference on Tobacco or Health, Beijing, 1997

47. In China, at least 65%, or 10,400,000 pregnant women, as well as 16 million babies born each year, are heavily exposed daily to passive smoke in the household.

Abstract PO 140, 10th World Conference on Tobacco or Health, Beijing, 1997

48. Passive smoking is a risk factor for airway complications in children having a general anesthetic. In a study of 499 children from Columbia-Presbyterian hospital in New York, airway complications occurred in 42% with urinary cotinine values greater than 40 ng/ml, compared to only 24% of children with levels less than 10 ng/ml.

Anesthesiology 1998; 88:1144-53

49. Children exposed to secondhand smoke who undergo surgery and general anesthesia experience serious perioperative complications compared to children from smoke-free households. Children who reside with smokers have a 10-fold greater risk of laryngospasm during anesthesia, and are three times more likely to require unexpected hospital or intensive care unit admission after surgery. Pediatrics, October 1997, p. 731

50. A study from the July 1997 issue of *Archives of Pediatrics and Adolescent Medicine* estimates that parents who smoke contribute to the deaths of at least 6200 children in the United States each year. The deaths include 2800

from low birth weight from mothers who smoke during pregnancy, 2000 from sudden infant death syndrome caused by secondhand smoke, 1100 from respiratory infection (bronchiolitis, respiratory syncytial virus), 250 from burns, and 14 from asthma. In addition, 5.4 million children each year have ailments such as asthma and ear infections caused by smoke exposure, costing $4.6 billion to treat. Associated Press, July 15, 1997

51. Children less than 18 years old whose mothers smoke have a 3.8 times greater risk for developing bacterial meningitis. 37% of all cases of meningococcal disease in this age group have maternal smoking as a risk factor.
Pediatric Infectious Disease 1997; 16:979

52. Children exposed to tobacco smoke in the home miss 33% more school days and have 10% more colds and acute respiratory infections than children not exposed. Nationwide in the United States, 31% of children are exposed to cigarette smoke daily in the home. There are wide regional, income and educational differences. 48% of children in homes of low income and education levels were exposed, compared to 25% in higher income and education homes. Regionally, almost 40% of parents in the Midwest exposed their children to passive smoke, compared to 24% of California parents.
Tobacco Control, Spring 1996, pp. 13-18

53. In a study from Canada, in infants of mothers who smoked, urinary cotinine levels of breast fed babies were 5 times higher than those of smoking mothers who were not breastfed. Breast milk cotinine levels were high, and breast milk was the major contributor to the infant's urinary cotinine level.
Archives of Pediatric and Adolescent Medicine, July 1999, pp. 689-691

54. "Smoke a pack a day at home...your kid inhales 50 packs a year."
California Department of Health Services television message, 1999

55. The child of a parent who smokes doubles the risk for having a serious respiratory infection that requires hospitalization, an association especially pronounced before the age of two.
Pediatric Pulmonology, January 1999, p. 11

56. Exposure to ETS increases the risk of respiratory illness in children by about 20%, and the risk of middle ear disease by about 60%.
Thorax 1999; 54: 357-366

57. A pregnant woman who smokes a pack a day triples the risk that her child will develop an ear infection serious enough to require surgical drainage.
Time, August 16, 1999, p. 73 (from Pediatrics)

58. "Each year, more than 17,000 children aged under five are admitted to UK hospitals because of exposure to other people's cigarette smoke."
British Medical Association (www.tobaccofactfile.org)

59. About 42% of children in the UK are exposed to secondhand smoke in the home.
British Medical Association (www.tobaccofactfile.org)

60. In a study from Rochester, New York, ETS exposure was associated with an increased risk of dental caries (cavities) in children.
JAMA, March 12, 2003, p. 1258

61. 35% of American children, or about 21 million, are exposed to ETS in the home.
Archives of Pediatric and Adolescent Medicine 2002; 156:1094-1100

62. A study from Tasmania, Australia, concluded that tobacco smoke exposure greatly increases the risk for babies in the first 12 months of life needing hospitalization for a respiratory tract infection such as bronchitis and pneumonia. "Relative to the infants of mothers who smoked postpartum, but never in the same room with their infants, risk of hospitalization was 56% higher if the mother smoked in the same room with the infant, 73% higher if the mother smoked when holding the infant, and 95% higher if the mother smoked while feeding the infant." For mothers who smoked, "good smoking hygiene," not smoking in the same room with the baby, eliminated more than 70% of the excess risk of hospitalization with respiratory infection associated with maternal postnatal smoking. Overall in the study, the infants of mothers who smoked at the end of the first postnatal month had a 50% higher risk of hospitalization with respiratory infection than did the infants of nonsmokers.
American Journal of Public Health, March 2003, pp. 482-487

63. Almost 40% of U.S. children younger than age 5 live with a smoker, and a recent study from Canada found that 47% of children there are exposed to passive smoke in the home. ETS exposure among children results in direct medical expenditures in the U.S. of $4.6 billion each year.                    Pediatrics, July 2001, p. 18

64. More than 6000 deaths among children each year are linked to parental smoking, most from low birth weights caused by smoking during pregnancy.
                    Robert Wood Johnson Foundation Report on Substance Abuse, March 2001

65. An EPA report showed that the number of U.S. children who live in a home with a smoker declined from 29% to 19% between 1994 and 1999.                    Reuters, February 25, 2003

66. A Cleveland judge has ordered an estranged couple not to smoke around their daughter, a healthy 8-year-old. This is the first known example of a court independently raising the issue of secondhand smoke.
                    Associated Press, September 14, 2002

67. In an unusual potential danger of ETS for children, children exposed to ETS had significantly lower levels of serum ascorbic acid (Vitamin C) compared to children without exposure to ETS in the home.
                    Pediatrics 2001; 107:540-542

68. In a study from Indiana, "an estimate of the expenses associated with "death and illness reveals that secondhand smoke may cost people… $70 per year." More than half of this per capita cost was from expenses from illness in children exposed to ETS.                    Reuters Health, November 14, 2002

69. 700 million children worldwide are exposed to passive smoking in the home.      *The Tobacco Atlas*, p. 90

70. Among inner-city families, ETS exposure is especially problematic. One study that assessed ETS exposure among urban low-income children seen in a pediatric resident practice reported that 75% of the children studied lived in a home with a smoker. Another study of inner-city children in Baltimore, Maryland, reported that 80% of the children in this study had cotinine values of 30 ng/mg or greater, a level commonly associated with household ETS. Up to one third of low-income children who do not live with a smoker spend time in a place with smokers.
                    Quote from Journal of Allergy and Clinical Immunology, July 2002, p. 147

71. 40% of children worldwide are exposed to passive smoking at home.      *The Tobacco Atlas*, p. 28

72. More than 20 million children in the United States are now exposed to ETS in the home.
                    Archives of Pediatrics and Adolescent Medicine, November 2002, pp. 1094-1100

73. Up to 40% of children in the United States live in homes where at least one adult smokes.
                    Allergy Report (American Academy of Allergy), December 2001

74. In the United States, 43% of children ages 2 to 11 years are exposed to ETS.      Pediatrics, April 2001, p. 794

75. 35% to 45% of American children grow up in homes where they are exposed to ETS; in a 2002 study from Colorado, 38% of children had smokers in the household.      Journal of Pediatrics, July 2002, pp. 109-115

# ETS – Political Issues and the EPA Report

1. "At Philip Morris, we believe that secondhand smoke has not been proven to cause disease in nonsmokers."
                    Full-page ad in New York Times, October 27, 1994

2. A 1996 Philip Morris campaign in Europe "promoted the seeming innocuity of second-hand tobacco smoke. For example, the ad tried to show that the risk of lung cancer from ambient tobacco smoke is lower than the risk of cardiovascular disease from eating one cookie a day…The ads provided references to many scientific publications, including the Journal of the National Cancer Institute, in an attempt to confuse the public." A Paris civil court later

banned the advertisements.    Journal of the National Cancer Institute, February 5, 1997, p. 260 (G. Gomez Crespo)

3. In an advertising campaign, Philip Morris said that milk drinkers can run as much of a risk of getting lung cancer as people exposed to second-hand smoke.                                        Associated Press, June 15, 1996

4. "The tobacco companies are treating tobacco smoke pollution as a public relations problem, instead of a public health problem."                Journal of the National Cancer Institute, January 17, 1990, p. 89 (John Slade)

5. "What the smoker does to himself may be his business, but what the smoker does to the nonsmoker is quite a different matter. This we see as the most dangerous development to the viability of the tobacco industry that has yet occurred."                                                                    1978 Roper Poll for the Tobacco Institute

6. "It would take 800 continuous hours of exposure to environmental tobacco smoke for a nonsmoker to breathe enough smoke to equal one cigarette."
                                Tobacco Institute spokesman Tom Lauria (San Francisco Chronicle, March 24, 1994, p. A9)

7. The 1993 EPA report *Respiratory Health Effects of Passive Smoking* concludes that passive smoking causes 150,000 to 300,000 cases per year of lower respiratory infections in babies under age 18 months resulting in 7500 to 15,000 hospital admissions. As well, passive smoking causes a worsening of asthma in 400,000 to one million children, plus 8000 to 26,000 new cases of asthma each year in the United States.

8. The Environmental Protection Agency (EPA) report on passive smoking labeled ETS a Group A (proven human) carcinogen causing approximately 3000 lung cancer deaths in nonsmokers, compared with only 10 to 30 deaths per year from asbestos, benzene, and other Group A carcinogens.

9. The 1993 EPA report declaring environmental tobacco smoke a Group A carcinogen makes businesses potentially liable for smoking-related diseases among nonsmoking workers.        San Francisco Chronicle, July 12, 1993

10. The EPA report is the "torpedo below the waterline that may sink the tobacco industry in the US, since it will lead to a smoke-free workplace."            Lonnie Bristow, MD, President-elect, American Medical Association
                                                                                                        (JAMA, October 27, 1993, p. 1982)

11. The tobacco industry claims that publication bias against negative studies invalidates the risk assessment of environmental tobacco smoke (ETS) conducted by the US Environmental Protection Agency and other reviews of the health effects of ETS. A formal review of 397 articles concluded that there is no publication bias against statistically nonsignificant results on ETS in peer-reviewed medical literature, contrary to the claims of the tobacco industry.                                                                                        JAMA, July 13, 1994, p.133

12. The tobacco industry has attempted to discredit the EPA report on passive smoking released in 1993, and has sued the EPA to have the findings "overturned." However, 24 of the 30 studies in the report did show increased risk; the possibility of that happening by chance is less than 1 in 10 million. The New York Times commented (January 10, 1993, p. A22): "The EPA marshals an enormous array of evidence to build an overwhelming case that tobacco smoke is hazardous to innocent bystanders...The Tobacco Institute...counters with sophistry."
                                                                                                        Advocacy Institute, March 31, 1993

13. The Environmental Protection Agency in their 1993 report on environmental tobacco smoke "calculated extremely low probabilities that the epidemiological findings had occurred by chance: a one in 10,000 probability that 24 of 30 studies would show a positive association between passive smoking and lung cancer; a one in 10 million probability that 17 out of 17 studies characterized by exposure level would show an increased risk at the highest exposure level; and a one in a billion probability that 14 out of 14 studies would show positive dose-response trends."                                            British Medical Journal, October 18, 1997, p. 961 (Ronald Davis)

14. Referring to the tobacco industry suing the EPA over their findings on health hazards of passive smoking, Cliff Douglas of the Advocacy Institute commented: "It's like the Flat Earth Society suing NASA for publishing photographs showing that the earth is round."                                    Wall Street Journal, June 23, 1993, p. B1

15. While Big Tobacco likes to shed crocodile tears in public over America's youth, an industry executive's off the cuff remark on secondhand smoke at a 1996 shareholder meeting is revealing:
"If children don't like to be in a smoky room, they'll leave." When asked about infants, who can't walk out of a smoky room, Harper stated, "At some point, they begin to crawl."
Charles Harper, Chairman, R.J. Reynolds, USA Today, April 18, 1996(quote from ANR Update, Summer 1998)

16. 106 review articles on the health effects of passive smoking were identified. Of these, 94% of those written by tobacco industry-affiliated authors concluded that passive smoking is not harmful, compared to only 13% of the 75 reviews by authors without any tobacco industry affiliation. "These findings suggest that the tobacco industry may be attempting to influence scientific opinion by flooding the scientific literature with large numbers of review articles supporting its position that passive smoking is not harmful to health."
JAMA, May 20, 1998, pp. 1566-1570

17. The tobacco industry has prepared a report "Environmental Tobacco Smoke: A Review of the Literature"... that has been shown to be severely flawed. Many of the industry references (75 out of 331) could not be found in a literature search. Un-refereed research citations were heavily used in the report, including industry-sponsored symposia, letters to the editor, and unpublished conference reports. Evidence about the health effects of environmental tobacco smoke was taken out of context, not cited, or even deliberately misinterpreted.
JAMA, November 20, 1991, p. 2702 (Tom Houston)

18. In terms of secondhand smoke, the tobacco industry is doing exactly what they did with "firsthand" smoke: they are using a bit of scientific uncertainty and a lot of public relations to suggest that there is still a serious debate about the health hazards of breathing ETS. The industry has attempted to recast the issue of ETS as one of individual rights versus an overzealous government agency, the EPA.      Consumer Reports, January 1995, p. 27

19. Consumer Reports magazine in January 1995 commented on the tobacco industry's criticisms of the EPA report on environmental tobacco smoke: "To read this material is to enter into a house of mirrors that endlessly reflects the same set of opinions, voiced by the same few people, again and again."

20. "Exposure to environmental tobacco smoke has not been shown to cause lung cancer in nonsmokers. Such exposure has not been shown to impair the respiratory or cardiovascular health of nonsmoking adults or children or to exacerbate preexisting disease in these groups, or to cause 'allergic' symptoms on a physiological basis."
Tobacco industry statement (JAMA, July 19, 1995, p. 222)

21. The EPA concluded in 1993 that second hand smoke is carcinogenic. "...The EPA findings would provide a brand new weapon to drub your local smoker with. All of this would, possibly, lead to even more quitting."
"So at least two tobacco companies rolled out the guns, including the usual expensive, full-page pleadings. One of the ads which appeared to parody earlier deceits was one from Philip Morris, in July of 1994: 'A large U.S. study published in the American Journal of Public Health, found no overall statistically significant link between second-hand smoke and lung cancer. Why did the EPA not include this study?
"The study, in fact, supported the EPA conclusion. The paper concluded that 'In summary, our study and others conducted during the past decade, suggest a small but consistent elevation in the risk of lung cancer in nonsmokers due to passive smoking. The proliferation of federal, state and local regulations that restrict smoking in public places and work sites is well founded.'
"It would be difficult to imagine advertising that is more deceitful."      *Smokescreen*, p. 106

22. "... the tobacco industry is not committed to learning and disseminating the truth about the health effects of its products. Rather, it has consistently attempted to discredit research even when its own scientists have admitted that the research results are valid. Just as the industry has continued to deny that active smoking has been proven dangerous to health, it continues to deny that the case is proven against passive smoking."
*The Cigarette Papers*, pp. 413-416

23. The following are passages from an article "Passive Smoking and Health: should we believe Philip Morris' experts?" which appeared in the British Medical Journal on October 12, 1996 (pp. 929-933). It dealt with a series of Philip Morris advertisements (or "adverts") in newspapers across Europe which minimized the risk of lung cancer from passive smoking: The central message of the advert is that passive smoking is not "really a

meaningful health risk to people who have chosen not to smoke." Readers were asked to write for a copy of a report "Environmental Tobacco Smoke and Lung Cancer: an Evaluation of the Risk," from a team of authors referred to as "The European Working Group on Environmental Tobacco Smoke and Lung Cancer." The report focused only on the risk of lung cancer, while the adverts referred to an absence of risks of health problems in general with passive smoking. The title of the working group has the ring of authority to it, although unsurprisingly it turns out to be an industry funded enterpris.

Having found a significantly increased risk in its meta-analysis of spousal studies, the working group goes on to attempt to discredit this finding. The working group makes much of the possible confounding of the passive smoking-lung cancer association by dietary factors...

(Peter) Lee is the main authority referred to by the working group, which accepts all his propositions and applies his misclassification model to their data. Nowhere do they point out that Lee is an enthusiastic recipient of tobacco industry financial support.

24. In 1991, a Philip Morris spokesman appearing on PBS TV's Frontline program argued that bird keeping was six times more likely to cause cancer than sidestream smoke. (Birds have mites on their feathers, which may cause cancer.)                                                                                     *Cancer Wars*, p. 108

25. A proposed bill by Rep. Henry Waxman would have banned smoking in all public buildings. It was endorsed by the Clinton Administration, six former Surgeons General, and the National Council of Chain Restaurants. Carol Browner of the Environmental Protection Agency estimated that if the bill became law, the lives of 5000 to 9000 nonsmokers would be spared each year, along with the lives of 33,000 to 99,000 smokers who would quit or cut back on cigarette smoking. The savings in medical costs and lost wages would be $6.5 to $19 billion a year.

New York Times, February 24, 1994, p. A13

26. "Government agencies... are trying to pass laws that outlaw all smoking at all times in all public buildings... Their efforts have one goal in mind: an outright ban... These attacks are another case of excessive government intrusion into the private lives of Americans... They are the 'New Puritans'... There is simply no reason to stand for this new prohibition and the no-smoking statutes sweeping America... We are sick and tired of public officials imposing their value systems upon us."                                                        Editorial, Cigar Aficionado, Winter 1994

27. The tobacco industry paid 13 scientists more that $156,000 to write letters to newspapers and medical journals to criticize a major 1993 government report that said that second hand smoke caused lung cancer. In many instances, tobacco industry lawyers edited the letters before they were published. The fact that the scientists were being paid to write the letters was not revealed until 1998.Journal of the National Cancer Institute, September 2, 1998, p. 1259

28. Philip Morris in 1993 filed a lawsuit against the Environment Protection Agency after the EPA published a report which classified ETS as a known human carcinogen. A decade later, after a federal appeals court let the EPA report stand, Philip Morris dropped out of the case. Philip Morris and other tobacco company plaintiffs had argued that the EPA exceeded its authority and used flawed methods to reach its conclusions. Edward Sweda, Senior Attorney for the Tobacco Products Liability Project at Northeastern University, commented, "They filed this lawsuit not to get compensation for a real grievance... but to use smoke and mirrors to confuse the public about how dangerous secondhand smoke is, and to delay additional regulation."

Richmond Times-Dispatch, January 15, 2003

29. "In Latin America, Philip Morris International and British American Tobacco, working through the law firm Covington and Burling, developed a network of well placed physicians and scientists through their 'Latin Project' to generate scientific arguments minimizing secondhand smoke as a health hazard, produce low estimates of exposure, and to lobby against smoke-free workplaces and public places. The tobacco industry's role was not disclosed... The strategies used by the industry have been successful in hindering development of public health programs on secondhand smoke."                                                        Tobacco Control, December 2002, p. 305

30. The Wall Street Journal has openly questioned antismoking science and government reports. In a 1994 editorial, the paper claimed that "... the anti-smoking brigade relies on proving that secondhand smoke is a dangerous threat to the health of others. 'Science' is invoked in ways likely to give science a bad name... the health effects of secondhand smoke are a stretch."                                   Reported in American Journal of Public Health, June 2002, p. 952

31. The *Journal of Epidemiology and Community Health* (August 2001, p. 588) reported on tobacco industry efforts to discredit research on passive smoking. Searches of tobacco industry documents in both the Minnesota and Guilford (England) depositories found that the industry built up networks of scientists sympathetic to its position that ETS is an insignificant health risk. Industry lawyers had a large role in determining what science would be pursued. The industry funded independent organizations to produce research that appeared separate from the industry and would boost its credibility. Industry-sponsored symposia were used to publish non-peer reviewed research. Unfavorable research conducted or proposed by industry scientists were prevented from becoming public. The conclusion was that tobacco industry documents illustrate a deliberate strategy to use scientific consultants to discredit the science on ETS.                    2002 AMA Annual Tobacco Report

32. An article in the American Journal of Public Health (September 2001, pp. 1419-1423) reviews the tobacco industry's campaign aimed at policies addressing ETS and efforts to undermine U.S. regulatory agencies. The industry in the late 1980s began a major campaign to "produce scientific research and influence public opinion on the health consequences associated with ETS... the industry feared the ETS issue and any governmental regulation of smoking in public places... " In 1988, the industry founded the Center for Indoor Air Research (CIAR) to support the industry position that ETS was an insignificant health risk. The CIAR buffer "allowed industry-funded scientists to produce seemingly independent results aimed at contradicting ETS findings and disclaiming the EPA report [on passive smoking] while keeping such research under industry control... OSHA was also considered a threat to the industry's ETS efforts because if the EPA ruled that secondhand smoke was a Group A carcinogen, OSHA would then have the authority to regulate workplace smoking". The 1998 master settlement required CIAR to disband.

33. Using code names such as "Project Stealth" and "Project Ambrosia," cigarette companies have tested ingredients that hide ETS in a bid to make smoking more socially acceptable, but not necessarily safer.
                    Massachusetts Tobacco Control Program, September 13, 2000

34. In a tobacco industry statement to congress in the justice department lawsuit, all five tobacco companies still deny that environmental tobacco smoke causes disease in nonsmokers.
                    Report prepared for Rep. Henry Waxman, September 17, 2002

35. Secret poll for the U.S. Tobacco Institute: "What the smoker does to himself may be his business, but what the smoker does to the nonsmoker is quite a different matter. This we see as the most dangerous development yet to the viability of the tobacco industry that has yet occurred."      Roper Organization, 1978, *The Tobacco Atlas*, p. 34

# ETS and Lung Cancer

1. A landmark study in the British Medical Journal in 1981 by Japanese researcher Takeshi Hirayama concluded that lung cancer could be caused by passive as well as by active smoking. The tobacco industry responded by launching a public relations campaign to try to discredit Hirayama's work, despite the fact that several tobacco industry experts privately admitted that his conclusions were valid.

2. In a study from Moscow, nonsmoking women who lived with a smoking spouse had a 53% greater risk of lung cancer compared to nonsmoking women from homes where the husband does not smoke.
                    Reuters, February 10, 1998

3. Nonsmoking workers exposed to secondhand smoke on the job are 34% more likely to get lung cancer.
                    SCARC, February 26, 1993

4. In California, waitresses have the highest mortality of any female occupational group, with almost four times the expected lung cancer mortality and more than double the expected heart disease mortality. Nonsmoking waiters, waitresses, and bartenders have a 50% to 90% greater chance of developing lung cancer than other nonsmokers. Levels of environmental tobacco smoke in restaurants were 1.5 times higher than in homes with one or more smokers, and ETS levels in bars were 4.5 times higher than in residences with smokers. [Editor note: All California bars and restaurants were smoke-free after 1998.]                    JAMA, July 28, 1993, p. 491

5.  Waiters and waitresses have a 50% higher risk of lung cancer than other workers, mostly because of ETS exposure.
    Study by Dr. Michael Siegel, University of California Berkeley, reported in the Toronto Star, March 16, 1997

6.  A study from Greece concluded that nonsmoking women married to men who smoke more than a pack a day increase their risk of developing lung cancer by 3.4 times.                    JAMA, October 7, 1992, p. 1697

7.  The risk of developing lung cancer for nonsmoking women with spouses who smoke is about 30% higher than for those with nonsmoking spouses. For a spouse smoking 2 packs a day for 40 years, the increased risk is 80%, still far below the 30 to 40 times greater risk of lung cancer for active smokers.                    JAMA, June 8, 1994, p. 1752

8.  Autopsies from nonsmoking women married to smokers have a significantly higher number of precancerous lung abnormalities than samples from nonsmoking women not exposed to spouse's smoke.
    JAMA, October 7, 1992, p. 1697

9.  A smoker has a lifetime risk of 5 to 10% of developing lung cancer. The nonsmoking spouse of a smoker runs a risk of one in 500.                    New York Times, January 10, 1993, p. 22, and
    Journal of the National Cancer Institute, February 3, 1993, p. 179

10. The lifetime added risk of developing lung cancer from prolonged exposure to second hand smoke is roughly one in 1000. Although this is small, this is 1000 times greater than the one in a million lifetime cancer risk considered unacceptable for many other environmental contaminants.                    Consumer Reports, January 1995, p. 33

11. Never smokers married to smokers have a two-fold increased risk of lung cancer.
    American Journal of Public Health, May 1987, p. 598

12. Studies have shown that nonsmoking wives of smokers face four times the expected risk of lung cancer and die an average of four years earlier if their husbands are longtime smokers.                    AMA Fact Sheet on Passive Smoking

13. 17% of all lung cancer cases among nonsmokers are attributable to childhood exposure to second-hand smoke, and children who are exposed to heavy amounts of tobacco smoke at home are twice as likely to develop lung cancer as those who grew up in smoke-free households.                    NEJM, September 6, 1990, p. 632

14. There are 1700 lung cancer deaths in nonsmokers in the United States each year caused by exposure to parents' cigarette smoke during childhood and adolescence.                    NEJM, September 6, 1990, p. 632

15. Relative excess risk for nonsmokers living with smokers for developing lung cancer has been estimated to be 1.3 times (Journal of the American Medical Association, July 24, 1991, p. 471), two-fold increased risk (AJPH, May 1987, p. 598), or 3.3 times relative risk in a study from Sweden (American Journal of Epidemiology, January. 1987, p. 17).

16. Nonsmokers living with smokers in the household have a 26% increased risk of lung cancer, and a 23% increased risk of heart disease, compared to nonsmokers living in smoke-free households, in a study reported from London.
    CBS evening news, October 17, 1997

17. The lifetime risk of lung cancer from passive smoking is more than 100 times higher than the estimated effect of 20 years of exposure to chrysotile asbestos, the type normally found in asbestos-containing buildings.
    British Journal of Cancer 1986; 54:381-3

18. In a study from Moscow, non-smoking women who lived with a smoking spouse had a 53% greater risk of lung cancer compared with other non-smoking women.
    Reuters, February 10, 1998 from International Journal of Cancer

19. The estimated excess risk of lung cancer is 24% in female lifelong nonsmokers who live with spouses who smoke.
    British Medical Journal, February 12, 2000, p. 417

20. A ten-year study in Europe concluded that adults exposed to secondhand smoke at home and in the workplace have about a 20% increased risk of lung cancer. There was no increased risk of lung cancer found in children of smokers.                                                                    Reuters, October 6, 1998

21. Never-smoking women who are exposed to ETS and develop lung cancer are a genetically susceptible population. The more susceptible group (odds ratio 2.6) were more likely to be deficient in GSTM1 (glutathione S-transferase M1) activity.                        Journal of the National Cancer Institute, December 1, 1999, p. 2009

22. "It has been estimated that passive smoking in the workplace poses 200 times the acceptable risk for lung cancer, and 2000 times the acceptable risk for heart disease."        British Medical Association (www.tobaccofactfile.org)

23. In 1981, Japanese researcher Takeshi Hirayama published a landmark study showing that nonsmoking wives of heavy smokers had up to twice the risk of lung cancer as wives of nonsmokers. The tobacco industry decided to generate another study to refute Hirayama's work, and funded and published the study, all the while trying to hide its involvement.                                        British Medical Journal, December14, 2002, pp. 1413-1415

24. A new meta-analysis of the relationship between passive smoking and lung cancer was published in the Australia/New Zealand Journal of Public Health (June 2001, p. 203). The authors found that the pooled relative risk (RR) for never-smoking women exposed to environmental tobacco smoke (ETS) from spouses, compared with unexposed never-smoking women was 1.29.

25. "… secondhand or environmental tobacco smoke is carcinogenic to human beings. Meta-analyses show that there is a significant association between lung cancer and smoke exposure from a spouse (the excess risk is of the order of 20% for women and 30% for men) and also between lung cancer and exposure at work (excess risk 16-19%). Risks for other cancer types are inconclusive. There is at present insufficient evidence that children exposed to parental smoke have an altered risk of developing any cancer. In total, tobacco kills 4.2 million people annually, and is forecast by WHO 'to kill over ten million people per year by the late 2020s if robust steps to curb the epidemic are not taken immediately.'"                                        Quote from The Lancet, July 27, 2002, p. 267

26. Passive smoking is causally linked to lung cancer, with an increased risk of 20-30% among never smokers who are exposed to ETS.                                International Agency for Research on Cancer monograph, June 2002

# ETS and Cardiovascular Disease

1. Nonsmokers living with smokers have a 30% increase in the risk of death from myocardial infarction or ischemic heart disease.                                                            NEJM, March 31, 1994, p. 908

2. A relative risk estimate of 1.3 for heart disease mortality in nonsmokers exposed to ETS "corresponds to a lifetime risk of death of roughly 1 to 3% for exposed nonsmokers and approximately 4000 deaths annually in California."                                                            Tobacco Control, Winter 1997, p. 348

3. Nonsmoking Chinese women from Xi'an have a 24% increased incidence of coronary heart disease if their husbands smoke, and an 85% increase if they are exposed to passive smoke at work.
                                                            British Medical Journal, February 5, 1994, p. 380

4. Nonsmokers married to smokers have a 30% increase to as much as triple the risk for death from heart disease, compared to nonsmokers without household exposure to passive smoke.        JAMA, January 1, 1992, p. 94

5. Passive smoking is about half as risky in terms of developing heart disease as is smoking 20 cigarettes a day, despite the fact that the actual amount of smoke inhaled by a passive smoker is only about 1% of the smoke inhaled by an active smoker. Dr. Malcolm Law of the Wolfson Institute of Preventive Medicine in London says that this result "is likely to be due to the blood clotting system being very sensitive to small amounts of tobacco smoke."                                                            Times of London, October 17, 1997

6. About 47,000 people a year in the US die from heart disease caused by secondhand smoke, and 150,000 others suffer nonfatal heart attacks. Heart disease is by far the major mortality risk from passive smoking.

Associated Press, April 5, 1995

7. Nonsmokers who breathe passive smoke have a 30% increase in the risk of heart disease. The tobacco industry states that passive smokers inhale the equivalent of less than one cigarette per day, but this is a gross underestimation of the risk of passive smoking to the cardiovascular system, and ignores the complex chemistry of environmental tobacco smoke.

JAMA, April 5, 1995, p. 1051

8. Nonsmoking adolescents in homes where parents smoke have an 8.9% higher ratio of total cholesterol to high-density lipoprotein cholesterol, and 6.8% lower high-density lipoprotein cholesterol levels, suggesting that passive smoking, like active smoking, leads to "bad" alterations in lipid profiles predictive of an increased risk of atherosclerosis.

Pediatrics, August 1991, p. 259

9. Exposure to passive smoke increases the death rate from coronary heart disease by 20% to 70%, largely because of increased platelet aggregation as well as a decrease in the ability of the heart to receive and process oxygen. Longer term exposure results in plaque buildup and adverse effects on cholesterol. In 1985, there were an estimated 62,000 deaths in nonsmokers caused by their exposure to ETS.

Journal of the American College of Cardiology, August 1994, p. 546

10. A study has shown carotid artery thickening from exposure to passive smoke, evidence of a direct link between second-hand smoke and the progression of atherosclerosis.

USA Today, March 19, 1996

11. Marriage to a smoking spouse has been associated with a two-fold to three-fold increase in the risk of cardiac death.

Clinics in Chest Medicine, December 1991, p. 654

12. Researchers from the Harvard School of Public Health studied 26,000 nonsmoking nurses who had exposure to passive smoke over a ten-year period. The most consistently exposed nurses in the home or the workplace had a 91% higher risk of having a heart attack or heart-related death, almost a doubling of the risk. Those with only occasional exposure at work or home had an increased risk of 58%. Based on these figures, the annual number of U.S. heart disease deaths attributable to passive smoking may exceed 60,000, compared with the EPA estimate of about 3000 deaths from lung cancer in nonsmokers attributable to passive smoking.

San Francisco Chronicle, May 20, 1997, p. A9 (from Circulation, June 1997)

13. The excess risk of ischemic heart disease caused by exposure to environmental tobacco smoke is almost half that of smoking 20 cigarettes per day, even though the exposure is only about 1% that of active smoking. Platelet aggregation is a plausible mechanism for the low dose effect, and the overall risk of heart disease is increased by a quarter in nonsmokers exposed to environmental tobacco smoke.

British Medical Journal, October 18, 1997, pp. 973-980

14. In a study from New Zealand reported in the summer 1999 issue of Tobacco Control, researchers found that nonsmokers exposed to secondhand smoke at home or in the workplace were 82% more likely to suffer a stroke than were nonsmokers not regularly exposed to ETS. Active smokers were six times more likely to have a stroke than nonsmokers exposed to secondhand smoke.

Associated Press, August 18, 1999

15. Children with exposure to passive smoke have lower levels of "good" high-density lipoprotein cholesterol, a risk factor for premature coronary artery disease.     Archives of Pediatric and Adolescent Medicine, May 1999, p. 446

16. "A review of 12 epidemiologic studies has estimated that ETS accounts for as many as 62,000 annual deaths from coronary heart disease in the United States."     *Reducing Tobacco Use*, p. 195

17. In a study from Japan, passive smoke exposure caused vascular endothelial dysfunction of the coronary circulation in nonsmokers, an immediate compromise of the cardiovascular system. "Endothelial dysfunction may be at the heart of the development of atherosclerosis... Passive smoking increases the risk of cardiac death or morbidity about 30% compared with a doubling to quadrupling the risk associated with active smoking." Short term ETS

exposure also activates platelets, an effect which "probably acts synergistically with the effects on endothelial function."                                                                    JAMA, July 25, 2001, pp. 462-463 and 436-441

18. In a study from Greece, exposure to ETS in nonsmokers significantly increased the risk of developing non-fatal acute coronary syndrome (first acute myocardial infarction or unstable angina resulting in hospitalization). Exposure to tobacco smoke for more than 30 minutes a day at work was associated with a greater risk of acute coronary syndromes (increase of 97%) than was exposure in the home (an increase of 33%).
                                                                                    Tobacco Control, September 2002, p. 220

19. Exposure to ETS increases the risk of cardiovascular disease by 25% for a nonsmoker compared to a nonsmoker not exposed to ETS.                                                                Tobacco Control, September 2002, p. 223

20. Swedish researchers have confirmed an increased risk of myocardial infarction from exposure to environmental tobacco smoke, and suggest that the intensity of spousal exposure and exposure at work are important.
                                                                                                        Epidemiology 2001; 12:558

# ETS and Sudden Infant Death Syndrome (SIDS)

1. Maternal smoking is associated with an odds ratio for SIDS of 2.92. "If we could reduce smoking, we would have an opportunity to reduce SIDS by 30% to 60%."                                Respiratory Reviews, July 1999, p. 24

2. Smoking during pregnancy triples the risk of SIDS (Sudden Infant Death Syndrome). Maternal smoking is responsible for 35% of all SIDS deaths in the US, and 66% of SIDS deaths among the infants of women who smoked during their pregnancy. In all, an estimated 1900 SIDS deaths are caused by maternal smoking in the US each year.                                                                                 Tobacco-Free Youth Reporter, Fall 1995, p. 16

3. SIDS (Sudden Infant Death Syndrome) is the most common cause of death of infants between one month and one year of age, and accounts for about 50% of deaths of infants between two and four months of age. In a study from San Diego, breast-feeding was protective for SIDS among nonsmokers (overall adjusted odds ratio 0.37) but not smokers (odds ratio 1.38).                                                            JAMA, March 8, 1995, p. 795

4. Smoking is one of the most important preventable risk factors for SIDS; adjusted odds ratios range from 1.6 to 2.5 times increased risk for mothers who smoked 1 to 9 cigarettes per day during pregnancy (compared with nonsmokers) and from 2.3 to 3.8 for mothers who smoked 10 or more cigarettes per day during pregnancy.
                                                                        American Journal of Epidemiology, August 1, 1997, pp. 249 and 256

5. Infants of smoking smothers are three times more likely to die of sudden infant death syndrome (SIDS) than infants not exposed to smoke. SIDS is the number one cause of death in infants between one month and one year of age, and accounts for about 50% of deaths of infants between two and four months of age.
                                                                        JAMA, September 21, 1994, p. 841, and March 8, 1995, p. 795

6. In a study from Norway and Sweden, elimination of maternal smoking during pregnancy would have reduced the number of SIDS deaths by 46.7%.                                                      Pediatrics, October 1997, p. 616

7. British researchers concluded that nearly two-thirds of SIDS cases are linked to tobacco smoke. Even if a baby is merely in a room where smoking has occurred, the risk of dying from SIDS can increase eight-fold.
                                                                                                        Time, August 5, 1996, p. 16

8. Fetal exposure to maternal smoking before birth may have a greater impact on a baby's risk of dying from SIDS than does postnatal exposure to environmental tobacco smoke.                        Reuters Health, April 1, 1999,
                                                                                        (from the American Journal of Epidemiology, April 1999)

9. The odds ratio for SIDS is increased to 2.13 when the mother smokes.                            Thorax 1999; 54:357-366

10. 23.6 % of all SIDS deaths in the United States appear to be attributable to prenatal maternal smoking.

American Journal of Public Health, March 2001, p. 432

## ETS and Pets

1. Dogs such as bulldogs with short noses are 2.4 times more likely to develop lung cancer when they live in households with owners who smoke.          American Journal of Epidemiology, February 1, 1992, p. 234

2. In a study of 103 dogs with nasal cancer, long-nosed dogs with a smoker in the house had double the risk (odds ratio of 2.0) for developing nasal cancer, compared to control dogs from smoke-free households.

American Journal of Epidemiology 1998; 147:488-492

3. After a British woman's pet parakeet died of lung cancer caused by passive smoking, owner Eileen Wilson, 81, said, "I loved Peter, but I'm not going to give up smoking after all these years."

San Francisco Examiner, January 29, 1994

4. "Another reason not to smoke: secondhand smoke is dangerous not only for the people around you, but also for your pets. For instance, cats living with smokers are more than twice as likely to develop malignant lymphoma (a common feline cancer) as those living in smoke-free homes... Cats exposed to the most smoke have a quadrupled risk. Earlier studies have found that cigarette smoke increases the risk of lung cancer in dogs."

UC Berkeley Wellness Letter, February 2003, p. 8

5. Cats exposed to secondhand smoke are more than twice as likely to develop feline lymphoma, the most common form of cat cancer. It kills most victims within a year.          U.S. News and World Report, August 12, 2002, p. 13

6. Cats living in houses with people who smoke have a risk of feline lymphoma that is almost 2.5 times higher than that of cats living in nonsmoking households. Five or more years of exposure increased risk by 3.2 times, while having two or more smokers in the house increased the animal's risk by 4.1 times.

American Journal of Epidemiology 2002; 156:268

NEJM is New England Journal of Medicine
JAMA is Journal of the American Medical Association

# CHAPTER 6
# ASTHMA, ALLERGY, AND SMOKE EXPOSURE

1. Newborn infants of nonallergic parents have a fourfold higher risk of developing allergic disease before 18 months of age if the mother smokes.         Journal of Allergy and Clinical Immunology, November 1986, p. 898

2. Asthma is present in 4.8% of young children whose mothers smoke, but in only 2.3% of children of nonsmoking mothers.                                      Pediatrics, April 1990, p. 505

3. Parental smoking increases the risk of developing hay fever, or allergic rhinitis, by 360% before the age of five.
Journal of Allergy and Clinical Immunology, September 1990, p. 400

4. Current smokers without symptoms of allergy have higher levels of IgE immunoglobulin, the "allergic antibody", than do nonsmokers. The more pack years of smoking, the higher the average IgE level. The reason for this association is not known.         Journal of Allergy and Clinical Immunology, December 1994, p. 954

5. Maternal smoking causes a three-fold increase risk of an infant having abnormally high levels of IgE antibody in the umbilical cord blood at birth. Increased IgE is associated with an increased risk of allergy.     *Cigarettes*, p. 87

6. Having a mother who smokes doubles a child's risk of developing asthma. When asthma does develop, it is much more likely to begin in the first year of life, to be more severe, and to require full-time medication.
Pediatrics, April 1990, p. 505

7. Children of smokers have a much higher incidence and severity of asthma, bronchitis, colds, and ear infections. They also have impaired lung development and reduced lung function tests.
American Journal of Public Health, February 1989, p. 209

8. Babies born to mothers who smoke during pregnancy have lungs that are up to 10% smaller and do not function as well than lungs of babies whose mothers did not smoke. The damage is permanent, and these children are up to three times more likely to develop diseases such as asthma.         ABC news, June 20, 1994

9. Passive smoking in children is associated with an increase in the degree of the normal diurnal or circadian rhythm in diameter of the bronchi in the lungs, an early indicator of airway obstruction.
NEJM, December 1, 1988, p. 1452

10. In a study from England, having one parent (or both) who smoked quadrupled the risk for having an allergic disorder (asthma, eczema, food allergy) at age 12 months. Passive smoking is an important risk factor for the early development of allergy.         Archives of Diseases of Children, April 1992, p. 496

11. In a study of children with asthma in Washington DC and Baltimore, 56% lived with a household smoker.
Annals of Allergy, February 1994, p. 174

12. In a study of children with asthma and cockroach allergy living in the inner city, 58% lived in homes with at least one smoker.                                  NEJM, September 11, 1997, p. 791

13. In a study from West Virginia of 159 children less than two years old with infantile asthma, 59% had exposure to tobacco smoke in the home.         Journal of Allergy and Clinical Immunology, January 1998, p. S186

14. In a study from the University of Virginia, 75% of children who presented to an emergency department for acute wheezing had one or more smokers at home.         Pediatrics, October 1993, p. 535

15. Asthmatic children from homes with parents who smoke have a 63% increase in emergency room visits for wheezing as compared to asthmatic children from homes where there are no smokers. This suggests more severe asthma in the group with household smoke exposure.
American Review of Respiratory Disease, March 1987, p. 567

16. In a prospective study of 1200 children at the age of 2 years to determine environmental factors predisposing to allergies and asthma, maternal smoking was strongly correlated with both asthma and allergy in their children. 18 percent of children in homes where the mother smoked had diagnosed asthma, as opposed to 9 percent in homes where the mother did not smoke. Prevalence of any allergies was 28 percent in the maternal smoking versus 22 percent in the no smoking household group.                   Clinical and Experimental Allergy, June 1993, p. 506

17. One million asthmatic children in the United States are exposed to their parent's tobacco smoke.
                                                                                            Journal of Asthma, May 1993, p. 399

18. Children with asthma exposed to the most passive smoke (as identified by urine cotinine levels, a metabolite of nicotine) had 70% more asthma attacks than those with little or no exposure.   NEJM, June 10, 1993, pp. 1665-69

19. The 1993 EPA report *Respiratory Health Effects of Passive Smoking* concludes that levels of smoke present in homes are high enough to trigger as many as one million attacks of asthma in infants under 18 months of age, as well as 8,000 to 26,000 new cases of asthma in children each year in the United States.

20. The EPA report estimates that passive smoking induces additional attacks and increases the severity of symptoms in about 20% of this country's 2 to 5 million asthmatic children.
                                                                                    Journal of Respiratory Disease, August 1994, p. 723

21. Passive smoking worsens asthma symptoms in 207,000 children a year in Great Britain. It also causes 60,000 cases a year of bronchitis or pneumonia in babies, of whom 3,000 need hospitalization.
                                                                                                    Associated Press, October 18, 1997

22. In a study from France, severe asthmatic patients who required mechanical ventilation had an in-hospital mortality of 31% if they were smokers compared to 11% for nonsmokers who needed mechanical ventilation. The overall hospital readmission rate was also twice as high for smokers. 23% of this group of asthmatics were smokers.
                                                                                    American Review of Respiratory Disease, July 1992, p. 76

23. Smoking is an important risk factor for intubation for respiratory failure in hospitalized asthmatic teenagers, with an odds ratio of 21.3.                                                    Journal of Asthma 1995; 32:379

24. In a study from India, nonsmoking adults with asthma who had exposure to tobacco smoke at home or at work had more acute asthma episodes, more emergency visits, lower expiratory flow measurements, and more work missed than asthmatics not exposed to environmental tobacco smoke.          Chest, September 1994, p. 746

25. Courts in 11 states have ruled against parents who smoke in divorce custody suits, especially if the child has asthma or other respiratory problems.                                        Time, October 25, 1993, p. 56

26. A smoking mother lost custody of her 8 year old asthmatic daughter in Sacramento, California after the father found her repeatedly wheezing when he picked her up, and determined that the amount of nicotine in her blood was equivalent to smoking eight cigarettes a day.               New York Times, October 16, 1993, p. A8

27. In a study from Denmark, having a mother who smokes increased the risk of her baby having wheezy bronchitis by a factor of 2.4 times. 25 to 30% of babies whose mothers smoked had one or more episodes of wheezing.
                                                                        Journal of Allergy and Clinical Immunology, January 1994 (Abstract 368)

28. In a study from Tucson, babies whose mothers smoked a pack a day or more of cigarettes, and who were at home and not in a day care center, had a 2.8-fold greater risk of developing a lower respiratory tract illness such as pneumonia.                                                          Journal of Pediatrics, February 1991, p. 207

29. In a study of 1000 children in New Zealand, babies born to smokers had almost double the risk of developing asthma compared to those born to nonsmokers.        American Academy of Allergy News, February 1997, p. 10

30. "ETS is a risk factor for induction of new cases of asthma as well as for increasing the severity of disease among children with asthma." Asthma induction (relative risk 1.75 to 2.25) may occur in as many as 0.5 to 2% of ETS-exposed children.                                                                                    Tobacco Control, Winter 1997, pp. 349-350

31. In children with asthma, those with smoke exposure in the home have a 70% increased risk of wheezing with colds, a 60% increased risk of going to a hospital emergency room for wheezing, and a 40% increased risk of having persistent wheezing.     American Journal of Respiratory and Critical Care Medicine, January 1996, p. 218

32. In a group of San Diego seven-year-olds with atopic (allergic) parents, 42% of the group with no smoke exposure at home had positive aeroallergen skin tests, while 68% of the group with ETS at home had positive skin tests
.                                                                            Journal of Allergy and Clinical Immunology, June 1995, p. 1185

33. "Asthmatics who smoke suffer from increased mucus, decreased movement of cilia, increased susceptibility to infection, increased immediate allergic reaction and damage to small airway passages. In one study the rate of death due to asthma among current and former smokers was more than double the death rate due to asthma among nonsmokers. The death rate for people with asthma who had never smoked was 3.7 per 100,000; among current and former smokers it was 8.3 per 100,000."                                                *Cigarettes*, p. 10

34. People with medical conditions such as asthma are particularly vulnerable to environmental tobacco smoke. The Americans With Disabilities Act may provide such patients with a legal right to a smoke-free environment.
                                                                                                           JAMA, September 18, 1996, p. 909

35. Childhood asthma often goes into remission during adolescence and then recurs in adulthood. Maternal smoking during pregnancy and active smoking are significant risk factors for such recurrence.
                                                                                                           British Medical Journal, May 11, 1996, p. 1195

36. In a study from Munich, Germany, maternal smoking during pregnancy or lactation was associated with a 2.3-fold increase in the risk for atopic eczema in their babies.
                                                                                      Journal of the American Academy of Dermatology 1997; 36:550

37. A review of 36 studies showed no overall significant association of passive smoking with allergy skin test positivity, total serum IgE concentration, allergic rhinitis, or atopic eczema.            Thorax 1998; 53: 117-123

38. In a study from Munich, Germany, maternal smoking during pregnancy or lactation was associated with a 2.3 fold increased risk of atopic dermatitis in their babies.            Reuters Health e Line, April 15, 1997

39. Current smokers have an increased risk of sensitization and allergy to house dust mite, as well as higher total IgE levels on average.            Journal of Allergy and Clinical Immunology, November 1999, p. 934

40. In a study from California, asthmatic children who were exposed to ETS in the house required intubation for severe asthma exacerbations much more often than asthmatic children not exposed to passive smoke.
                                                                                                           Annals of Allergy, December 1999, p. 572

41. Allergy to tobacco leaf mediated by IgE manifest by urticaria and rhinoconjunctivitis has been reported as an occupational allergy in tobacco farmers and workers.            Annals of Allergy, February 1999, p. 194

42. In a study from San Francisco in the July 1998 American Journal of Respiratory and Critical Care Medicine, non-smoking asthmatics exposed to secondhand smoke had double the number of asthma-related emergency room visits compared to asthma patients not exposed to smoke. ETS was also associated with greater asthma severity.
                                                                                                           Reuters, July 17, 1998

43. In a study from San Francisco, high level ETS exposure was associated with a greater risk of emergency visits for asthma attacks (odds ratio 3.4) and hospitalization for asthma (odds ratio 12.2). Among adults with asthma, ETS was associated with a clear impairment in health status.
                                                                          2002 National Conference on Tobacco or Health Abstract EVAL – 344

44. ETS exposure is associated with increased asthma severity and worsened lung function in children with asthma
.                                                                                              Chest 2002; 122:409-415

45. Never smokers exposed to environmental tobacco smoke as children are more susceptible to developing asthma. In this group without a family history of asthma, the prevalence of asthma was 6.8%, compared to 3.80% among non-exposed.                     2002 AMA Annual Tobacco Report (from Chest, September 2001)

46. In utero exposure to tobacco smoke from the mother increases the risk of asthma and wheezing during childhood.
                                                                                              Respiratory Reviews, June 2001

47. In a study from Germany, smoking by mothers more than doubles the risk in children younger than age 3 years of developing allergic sensitization to foods.                                       Allergy 1999; 54:220-228

48. In a study from Finland, exposure to ETS in the workplace doubles the risk for a nonsmoker of developing adult asthma. Subjects exposed to smoke both at work and at home were almost five times more at risk compared to nonsmokers who had a smoke-free workplace and household.
    Findings presented at European Congress on Lung Disease and Respiratory Medicine in Berlin, September 25, 2001

49. In a nationally representative group of U.S. children with asthma, exposure to second hand smoke was associated with increased asthma severity and worsened lung function.                       Chest, August 2002, p. 409

50. In a study from Baltimore and Washington, D.C., exposure to higher levels of ETS in the home was associated with an increased frequency of nocturnal asthma symptoms among elementary school inner-city children with asthma. In this group, smoking in the home was reported by 29.4% of primary caregivers.
                                                                        Journal of Allergy and Clinical Immunology, July 2002, p. 147

51. Household ETS accounts for 8% to 13% of the prevalence of childhood asthma in the United States and 21% of all childhood asthma exacerbations.                                    Journal of Pediatrics, July 2002, p. 109

52. Maternal smoking during pregnancy almost doubles the baby's risk for developing asthma and wheeze. Passive smoke exposure in utero is a stronger risk factor than is postnasal ETS exposure in the home, although the latter is also a risk factor for asthma.             Journal of Allergy and Clinical Immunology, January 2000, p. 12

53. Maternal smoking during pregnancy is associated with increased prevalence of early onset of asthma in a genetically susceptible group of children.
                                                            American Journal of Respiratory and Critical Care Medicine, August 2002, p. 457

54. In a study from Pakistan, ETS exposure in the home was associated with a 60% to 70% increase in visits for acute exacerbations of asthma in children.               Journal of Allergy and Clinical Immunology, January 2002, p. 557

55. In a study from San Francisco of adult patients with asthma, 42% reported ever having smoked cigarettes, and 10% were current smokers.                              American Journal of Public Health, August 2000, p. 1307

56. In a study from San Francisco, asthmatic patients were found not to avoid smoking, as might be expected because they experience respiratory symptoms. The prevalence of both "ever smoking" as well as current smoking was the same in adults with asthma and those without asthma.        Public Health Reports, March-April 2001, p. 148

57. In a study from Los Angeles, children exposed to maternal smoking in utero are more likely to develop asthma than are children exposed to ETS only after birth.
                                                            American Journal of Respiratory and Critical Care Medicine 2001; 163:429-436

58. In a study from Sweden, childhood exposure to ETS is associated with an increased prevalence of asthma among adult never-smokers, especially in subjects without concomitant allergies. Children exposed to ETS were also more likely to become smokers themselves.                      Chest, September 2001, p. 711

59. In a study from Glasgow, Scotland, it was found that smoking by patients with asthma induces neutrophilic airway (lung) inflammation, in addition to the eosinophilic airway inflammation observed in nonsmoking asthma patients. In the smoking asthmatics, lung function was negatively related to sputum neutrophil proportion.

Chest, December 2001, p. 1917

60. In a study from Germany, cigarette smoking was a strong independent risk factor associated with severe asthma, and the greater the number of cigarettes smoked, the lower the lung function.    Journal of Asthma 2001; 38:41-49

# CHAPTER 7
# LUNG CANCER

1.  "Primary malignant neoplasms of the lung are among the rarest forms of disease."

    From *Primary Malignancies*, I. Adler, 1912 (reported by Richard Hurt, M.D.)

2.  Lung cancer was considered so rare that it was not listed as a cause of death in the International Classification of Disease system until 1930.                    Seminars in Oncology, August 1990, p. 407

3.  In 1921, Dr. Moses Barron of the University of Minnesota noted that there were eight cases of lung cancer treated at the university in the previous year, compared to a total of only four cases in the previous two decades since the turn of the century.                                               *They Satisfy*, p. 163

4.  "Before 1930 lung cancer was a rare disease not listed on the International Classification of Disease system in the United States; however, by the end of the 1930s a rapidly increasing lung cancer death rate among males had been noted by several scientists, including Dr. Harold Diehl and cancer surgeon Dr. Alton Ochsner of Tulane University. Dr. Ochsner recalled being aroused from his bed as a third-year medical student to witness a rare medical event that, according to his professors, he would probably not see again in his lifetime--an autopsy of a man who died of lung cancer. As a young cancer surgeon, he saw six lung cancer patients in a single year and concluded that an epidemic of lung cancer must be underway. All these patients were male, and all had a history of heavy cigarette smoking. This observation was among the first to link cigarette smoking and the new U.S. epidemic of lung cancer."                    *Changes in Cigarette-Related Disease Risks*, p. iii

5.  Drs. Alton Ochsner and Michael DeBakey in 1939 first reported the association of smoking and lung cancer.

    Surgery Gynecology Obstetrics 1939; 68:435

6.  A landmark article from the Journal of American Medical Association appeared on May 27, 1950: "Tobacco smoking as a possible etiologic factor in bronchogenic carcinoma" by E. L. Wynder and Evarts Graham. The same Journal of the American Medical Association issue featured a full page color ad for Chesterfields with the actress Gene Tierney and golfer Ben Hogan; the journal accepted tobacco ads until 1953. Another early article by Drs. Ochsner and DeBakey on lung cancer appeared in the March 1, 1952 issue of Journal of the American Medical Association, p. 691.

7.  If lung cancer deaths are excluded, total cancer mortality actually fell 13 percent from 1950 to 1982. Inclusion of lung cancer, however, results in an overall 8 percent increase in cancer deaths during this period.

    Executive Health Report, July 1990

8.  The amount of radiation as polonium-210 that a pack a day smoker absorbs into the lungs each year is equivalent to the radiation in 250 to 300 chest x-rays a year. This adds up to 80 REMS per decade, and is thought to be one of the main causes of lung and other smoking-induced cancers.

    Dean Edell, MD, ABC radio, September 14, 1993

9.  Lung cancer accounts for 22% of female cancer deaths, compared with 18% for breast cancer.

    American Journal of Public Health, September 1993, p. 1203

10. In 1986, lung cancer passed breast cancer as the number one cancer killer in females. In men, it had become the top cancer killer in 1952. Women's lung cancer death rates have risen dramatically; as late as the early 1970's, breast cancer killed twice as many women as lung cancer did.   Medical Clinics of North America, March 1992

11. Although the number of breast cancer cases in women each year exceeds lung cancer, the five year survival rate for lung cancer (13%) is much lower than for breast cancer (78%), accounting for the higher total death rate for lung cancer.                                                         JAMA, December 1, 1993, p. 2542

12. From 1950 to 1989, the overall cancer death rate for women dropped by 16%. But the death rate from lung cancer increased by 600%.                                                                  American Cancer Society

13. In the 20-year period from the mid-1960's through the early 1980's, the relative risk of fatal lung cancer approximately doubled in male cigarette smokers and increased nearly fivefold in female cigarette smokers.

*Changes in Cigarette-Related Disease Risks*, p. 305

14. There are 3800 lung cancer deaths each year in nonsmokers because of their exposure to second-hand smoke.

Journal of Respiratory Disease, May 1993, p. 635

15. Having a spouse who smokes doubles a nonsmoker's risk of developing lung cancer.

Seminars in Respiratory Medicine, October 1989, p. 387

16. "Q. Does cigarette smoking cause lung cancer?
"A. It's not been proven that cigarette smoking causes cancer.
"Q. If somebody is a two pack a day smoker for 20 years, and gets lung cancer, and every medical person is satisfied the reason that the person got lung cancer was because he smoked, you are saying it is not proven?
"A. That is correct. That is what I am saying." William I. Campbell, President, Philip Morris, in a deposition (Washington Monthly, February 1994, p. 6)

17. Asked under oath in testimony to Congress if he was aware that cigarettes caused cancer, Lorillard's president Andrew Tisch replied "I do not believe that." CSPAN, April 14, 1994

18. In men ages 35 to 44, the death rate from lung cancer in blacks is 2.3 times higher than for whites.

Thorax, August 1991, p. 565, and JAMA, January 30, 1991, p. 498

19. Lung cancer death rates in nonsmoking women from passive smoke are now higher than were total lung cancer death rates from active smoking in women 30 years ago. Associated Press, March 21, 1991

20. 1998 lung cancer estimates are 171,500 cases and 160,000 deaths. Lung cancer five year survival rates for 1986-1993 were 14% for whites and 11% for blacks, an improvement from 1960-63 survival rates of 8% and 5% in these two groups. CA--A Cancer Journal for Clinicians, January-February 1998

21. In the year 1930, 3,000 Americans died of lung cancer. By the early 1980s, the disease killed 3,000 Americans every nine days. Washington Monthly, March 1985, p. 48

22. In 1900, there were only 400 reported deaths from lung cancer, compared to 266,000 from tuberculosis. By 1930, lung cancer accounted for 2.3% of all cancer deaths (a total of about 2500); in 1940, 4.5% (7500 total); and in 1950, 15% of all cancer deaths (25,500 in the U.S.) *Tobacco in History*, pp. 123-125

23. U.S. lung cancer deaths in women increased from 5160 in 1960 to 50,200 in 1990, almost a ten-fold increase. Breast cancer deaths were 43,400 in 1990; since 1987, more women have died of lung cancer than breast cancer. Lung cancer death rates for males increased from 31,300 in 1960 to 91,100 in 1990. In 1996, estimated lung cancer deaths in males were 94,400, and in females, 64,300.

Cancer Facts and Figures 1994 (American Cancer Society)
and US News and World Report, February 5, 1996, p. 55

24. Cigarette smoking is responsible for 90% of lung cancer among men and 79% among women, about 87% overall. Cancer Facts and Figures 1994 (American Cancer Society)

25. In Japan, lung cancer in the early 1990's overtook stomach cancer as the most common cancer killer.

9th World Conference on Tobacco or Health, Paris, 1994 (T. Lam)

26. Of male deaths from smoking, lung cancer is responsible for 30 percent and other cancers an additional 8 percent, or 38 percent of the total deaths caused by cancer. In females, 24 percent of deaths are from lung cancer, and for all cancers combined, about 32 percent. *Deadly Choices*, p. 161

27. 51% of lung cancer cases being diagnosed are in former smokers, 41% in current smokers, and 8% in never-smokers. The former smokers with lung cancer had stopped smoking for an average of six years, and before quitting had averaged a pack and a half a day for 34 years. Overall deaths from lung cancer increased by 51 percent between 1980 and 1994 despite declines in smoking prevalence.          Associated Press, May 23, 1995

28. Almost half of all new cases of lung cancer are in former smokers. Those who quit 20 years ago still have double the risk of nonsmokers.          MSNBC, April 13, 1997

29. Lung cancer death rates among women who smoke increased six-fold from the 1960's to the 1980's. Among men, the rate nearly doubled.          Time, September 25, 1995, p. 24

30. The risk of lung cancer is 22 times higher among male smokers and 12 times higher among female smokers compared to nonsmokers.          *Tobacco and the Clinician*, p. 25

31. There is an increased risk of lung cancer associated with mentholated cigarette use in male but not female smokers.          Archives of Internal Medicine, April 10, 1995, p. 727

32. The risk of lung cancer is increased 10-fold for those who smoke 1-10 cigarettes per day, 40-fold in those who smoke 21-30 per day, and 70-fold in heavy smokers of 40 or more cigarettes a day.          Tobacco Control, Autumn 1995, p. 535

33. 20% of all lung cancers caused by factors other than actively smoking are due to passive environmental tobacco smoke exposure. This is a risk of about one in 1000, higher than almost any chemical whose exposure is regulated by the EPA. The risk of lung cancer in nonsmoking spouses of smokers rises to 2 in 1000.          New York Times, January 8, 1993, p. A9

34. The average relative risk ratio for passive smokers for lung cancer is 1.34. This risk, in comparison, is more than 100 times higher than the estimated effect of 20 years of exposure to asbestos while living or working in an asbestos-containing building.          Archives of Internal Medicine, January 11, 1993, p. 35

35. Asbestos workers who smoke are 53 times more likely to get lung cancer than nonsmokers not exposed to asbestos. (The risk rises to 87-fold in asbestos workers who smoke a pack a day or more.) For asbestos workers who do not smoke, the risk drops sharply; they are five times more likely to get lung cancer than nonsmokers not exposed to asbestos.          Washington Post National Weekly Edition, September 26, 1994, and It's Better Working Smoke Free, Europe Against Cancer 1992, p. 5

36. Nonsmoking asbestos workers have a 5.2-fold increased risk of developing lung cancer; smokers without asbestos exposure, a 10.8-fold increased risk. If an asbestos worker also smokes, the risk is increased by 53 times.          Clinics in Chest Medicine, December 1991, p. 660

37. "Workplace exposure to asbestos or alpha-radiation (the latter in uranium miners) synergistically increases the risk of lung cancer in cigarette smokers. Alcohol use interacts synergistically with tobacco in causing oral, laryngeal, and esophageal cancer."          Cecil Textbook of Medicine, 1996 edition, p. 34

38. A chemical found in cigarette smoke, benzopyrene, causes genetic damage in lung cells that is identical to the damage observed in many malignant tumors of the lung. This is the first specific scientific evidence linking smoking with lung cancer at the molecular and cell biology level.          Associated Press, October 19, 1996

39. A woman's magazine in 1996 warned that lung cancer may be caused by inhalation of dried bird droppings in bird owners, but did not mention smoking. The report was bracketed by ads for cigarettes.          The Osgood file, CBS radio, September 26, 1996

40. A former member of the Rolling Stones, Bill Wyman, was caught on camera in 1993 smoking a cigarette just before playing at a charity concert held to raise funds for the British Lung Foundation. A tabloid reported "Strike a Light! It's Bill at a Lung Cancer Charity Night."          *The Fight for Public Health*, Simon Chapman, BMJ Publishing Group, 1994, p. 88

41. A smoker's risk of dying from lung cancer by age 85 is one in four for men and one in nine for women.

Wall Street Journal, June 25, 1997, p. A23

42. After ten years of not smoking, the risk for lung cancer still remains at 30% to 50% of the rate for continuing smokers. *Smoke and Mirrors*, p. 10

43. There is a strong temporal relationship between lung cancer death rate and cigarette smoking prevalence, with a 30-year latency or lag period. The lung cancer death rate peaked in men in 1990 and is now declining; the male smoking prevalence rate was about 65% from 1940 to 1960 and has declined since to 28% in 1990. In women, smoking prevalence "did not rise above 2% until the 1930's, increased steadily to a peak of 38% in 1960, and then declined, more slowly than in men, to 23% in 1990. The lung cancer mortality rate began to rise substantially about 1965, approximately 30 years after the rise in smoking prevalence." The rate is still rising. Overall, the United States is approaching the height of the lung cancer epidemic, provided that smoking prevalence continues to fall. Chest, May 1997, pp. 1414-16

44. The lung cancer risk is higher in women smokers (27.9 times that of nonsmokers) than in men (9.6 times the risk). Richard Hurt, M.D., Mayo Clinic, May 12, 1997

45. Male smokers in China have a 3.8-fold increased risk for lung cancer, much lower than the average 20-fold increase in risk in male smokers in Western countries. This may reflect the relatively high background rate of lung cancer not related to smoking. The study did not address whether domestic air pollution from cooking, heating, and passive smoking, or exposure to industrial air pollution, was related to lung cancer in nonsmokers.

JAMA, November 12, 1997, p. 1503

46. In a study of 611 cancer-free survivors for more than two years after treatment of small-cell lung cancer, the risk for the development of second cancers (mostly non-small-cell cancers of the lung) was increased 3.5-fold relative to the general population. However, the risk was substantially increased in the group who continued to smoke; lung cancer survivors should stop smoking.

Journal of the National Cancer Institute, December 3, 1997, p. 1782

47. In a study from Italy, the odds ratio for lung cancer in current smokers was 13.4 for all lung cancer types, ranging from 34.3 for large cell carcinoma, 18.8 for squamous cell carcinoma, 14.3 for small cell carcinoma, and 7.9 for adenocarcinoma. The risk of lung cancer attributable to smoking was 88% for all types combined, including 95% for large cell, 91% for squamous cell, 89% for small cell, and 82% for adenocarcinoma. There is a higher prevalence of adenocarcinoma among nonsmokers, with a lower proportion of cases attributable to smoking. Chest, December 1997, p. 1474

48. Lung adenocarcinoma, a rare tumor type at the turn of the century, has replaced the squamous cell type as the most frequent histologic type of lung cancer. The odds ratios for major lung cancer types are consistently higher for women than men, likely because of higher susceptibility to tobacco carcinogens in women. In Connecticut, adenocarcinoma increased nearly 17-fold in women and 10-fold in men from 1959 through 1991. The increase might be from changes in cigarette design and smoking behavior. Cigarettes in the 1950's and before were unfiltered and had high nicotine content; the harshness meant less deep inhaling than is the case for more recent filtered low-nicotine brands. Another change is the increase in nitrate content of the tobacco blend in U.S. cigarettes, which raises the yield of nitrogen oxides and N-nitrosamines in the inhaled smoke. These factors result in increased exposure of the peripheral lung, the origin of most adenocarcinomas, to carcinogens in smoke. Journal of the National Cancer Institute, November 5, 1997, pp. 1563-64

49. The rise in the use of filter cigarettes with milder tobacco coincides with an increase in the incidence of adenocarcinoma, a type of cancer found at the periphery of the lungs. The reason might be that smokers now have to inhale more deeply to get the same nicotine dose. Adenocarcinoma was very rare in the 1950's, but it has now become the most common type of lung cancer, displacing squamous cell carcinoma found in the central bronchi of the lungs. Associated Press and Washington Post, November 4 and 5, 1997 (from a study in the Journal of the National Cancer Institute, November 5, 1997, p. 1563)

50. For each death from AIDS, there are $30,000 research dollars allocated. There are $7500 for breast cancer research for each death from the disease, but only $800 per death from lung cancer.

CBS evening news, February 20, 1998

51. A study from Santiago, Spain, concluded that "depending on the histologic type, between 1/5 and half of the lung cancer cases that occur among (those) exposed to both tobacco smoking and high concentration of domestic radon are due to the interaction between these two causes."

Abstract PO 59, 10th World Conference on Tobacco or Health, Beijing, 1997

52. Radon gas is the second leading cause of lung cancer after smoking. It is a colorless, odorless gas released when uranium decays in the ground. The gas can rise into homes through cracks in basements, and when inhaled, the radioactive alpha particles damage lung cells. A report by the National Research Council (Dr. Jonathan Samet, chairman) estimates that radon causes or contributes to between 15,000 and 21,800 of the 157,000 lung cancer deaths each year in the United States. Most of these deaths are in smokers, where the radon and smoking together were responsible for the lung cancer. Lung cancer deaths in nonsmokers attributable to radon total 2100 to 2900 each year. "Radon, particularly in combination with smoking, poses an important public health risk."

USA Today and Associated Press, February 20, 1998

53. 19,000 of the 160,000 annual lung cancer deaths in the United States result from a combination of smoking and exposure to radon gas.

Washington Post, September 16, 1998, p. A3

54. Radon gas was first recognized as a cause of lung cancer in miners in Germany before Hitler came to power, and the relationship between asbestos and lung cancer was similarly recognized there in 1943.

"German researchers were the first to establish – beyond clinical anecdote – the casual link between smoking and lung cancer. Two studies, one published in 1939, the other in 1943, compared the smoking habits of people with lung cancer and those without it. Although there are some methodological complaints about each, the studies nevertheless convincingly showed a strong and 'dose-dependent' link between the habit and the disease. American and British researchers didn't prove the same connection until after the war.

"Outside the academic world, smoking came under withering attack by Nazi officialdom. The hazards of smoking were taught in elementary schools. Posters and propaganda decried the economic drain of smoking… Starting in 1938, smoking was banned in many official offices and hospitals. Smoke-free restaurants opened. Sixty cities banned smoking on streetcars in 1941. That same year, regulations took hold banning tobacco advertisements 'that create the impression that smoking is a sign of masculinity,' as were all advertisements targeting women." Washington Post National Weekly Edition, August 9, 1999 p. 32

(from the book *The Nazi War on Cancer*, Robert N. Proctor, Princeton University Press, 1999)

55. In 1998 in the United States, there were 178,000 new lung cancer cases and 160,000 deaths from lung cancer.

Newsweek, July 19, 1999, p. 59

56. A decrease in the incidence of lung cancer in men began in the late 1980's, and between 1990 and 1996, incidence rates decreased by 2.6% per year. Rates in women are stabilizing, and have begun to decline in women ages 40 to 59. Estimated new lung cancer cases for the year 2000 are 164,100, with a total of 156,900 deaths. In 2000, lung cancer will account for 31% of all cancer deaths in men (compared to 11% for prostate and 10% for colon cancer), and 25% of all cancer deaths in women (ahead of 15% for breast cancer and 11% for colon cancer). The 5-year lung cancer survival rate was 14% for 1989-1995.

CA-A Cancer Journal for Clinicians, January-February 2000, pp. 9-16

57. The lung cancer death rate for men was 4.9 per 100,000 in 1930; in 1990 the rate had increased to 75.6 per 100,000.

Morbidity and Mortality Weekly Report, November 5, 1999, p. 986

58. Deaths from lung cancer in the United States increased from less than 400 cases recorded in 1900 to 4000 deaths in 1935, 11,000 in 1945, 36,000 in 1960, and 140,000 deaths a year by the mid-1980's.

Daedalus 1990; 119: 161

59. The proportion of widowhood attributable to lung cancer is 10%.

John Slade, M.D.

60. Lung cancer accounts for 14% of new cancer cases and 28% of the cancer deaths in the United States each year.                                          Journal of the National Cancer Institute, April 21, 1999, p. 687

61. Women are more susceptible than men to small cell lung cancer, the deadliest form of lung cancer, which is almost always caused by smoking.                                          Reuters, December 2, 1998

62. Prolonged ETS exposure in adults leads to about a 20% increased risk of lung cancer, a low excess risk compared to the 15- to 20-fold increased risk of lung cancer among current pack a day smokers. (See Chapter 5 for the association between ETS and lung cancer.)
                                          Journal of the National Cancer Institute, October 7, 1998, pp. 1416-1417

63. In the 1990s, lung cancer (90% attributed to smoking) accounted for 28% of all cancer deaths.
                                          JAMA, March 20, 2002, p. 1392

64. "We've got a vaccine for lung cancer. It's called tobacco control."                    Matthew Myers, President,
                                          Campaign for Tobacco-Free Kids (Tobacco Control, June 2002, p. 160)
                                          from Wall Street Journal, January 16, 2001

65. In a study from the Mayo Clinic and National Cancer Institute, screening for lung cancer using chest x-rays does not save lives or reduce lung cancer mortality rates. The chest films do detect a substantial number of tumors which do not result in illness or death, and such lesions are even more likely to be detected by spiral computed tomography (CT) scans. Critics have charged that spiral CT is being promoted for lung cancer screening without adequate proof that it will reduce lung cancer deaths.    JAMA, September 20, 2000, p. 1371

66. Lung cancer, the most lethal of all cancers, accounts for 28.5% of all cancer deaths. New lung cancer cases declined by 2.7% per year for men and 0.2% per year for women between 1992 and 1998, while during the same period, death rates for men declined by 1.9% per year, but increased among women by 0.8% per year.
                                          San Francisco Chronicle, June 6, 2001 (National Cancer Institute data)

67. The risk for developing lung cancer decreases by more than 90% for smokers who quit before age 35.
                                          Associated Press, August 3, 2000

68. An estimated 67,000 American women died from lung cancer in 2001.    New York Times, November 13, 2001

69. Although a former smoker's risk of lung cancer never drops to that of a lifelong nonsmoker, it does decline in 15 years to only twice that of a nonsmoker, instead of more than ten times.
                                          New York Times, November 13, 2000

70. In the United States in 1999, there were 171,000 newly diagnosed lung cancer cases, 92.6% of which were incurable.                                          *Clearing the Smoke*, p. 392

71. In 1950, lung cancer accounted for only 3% of female cancer deaths in the United States. In 2000, lung cancer accounted for about 25% of cancer deaths.                                          *Women and Smoking*, p. iii

72. Estimated U.S. lung cancer deaths in 2002 are 154,900 (89,200 men and 65,700 women). This is 25% of all female cancer deaths, compared to 39,600 for breast cancer.
                                          CA A Cancer Journal for Clinicians, January/February 2002, p. 25

73. Lung cancer deaths in the United States increased from 2,357 cases in 1933 to 7,121 in 1933, 7,121 in 1940, and 29,000 deaths in 1956.                                          *Tobacco* (Gately), p. 285

74. German scientists in 1943 published the first study demonstrating a strong link between smoking and lung cancer. Their work was previously ignored because it was seen as tainted by the Nazi connection.
                                          International Journal of Epidemiology, February 26, 2001

75. In the late 1990s, there were 1.2 million deaths from lung cancer worldwide (including 282,000 in women), making it the most frequent cause of death from cancer worldwide.     *Tobacco: The Growing Epidemic*, p. 14

76. A 60-year-old woman who smokes is almost ten times more likely to die of lung cancer, and nine times more likely to die from a heart attack or stroke, than from breast cancer.
ASH Smoking and Health Review, September-October 2002,
(from Journal of the National Cancer Institute, June 2000, pp. 799-804)

77. Over age 40, lung cancer kills more smokers than all other cancers combined.
Journal of the National Cancer Institute, June 2000, pp. 799-804

78. U.S. lung cancer deaths are 89,000 men and 66,000 women each year, more than deaths from breast, colon, and prostate cancer combined. The average survival after lung cancer diagnosis is 12 months. In 2001, cancer research funding was $464 million for breast cancer and $258 million for prostate cancer, compared to $189 million for lung cancer research.                NBC News (Tom Brokaw), November 25, 2002

79. About half of all lung cancer cases occur in people who have stopped smoking for a year or longer.
Contra Costa (CA) Times, May 19, 2002, p. A9 (from the New York Times)

80. In the United States in 2003, estimates are for 171,900 new cases of lung cancer, and 157,200 deaths. This is 31% of cancer deaths and 14% of new cancer cases in men, and 25% of deaths and 12% of new cancer cases in women.                CA A Cancer Journal for Clinicians, January-February 2003, pp. 7-9

81. A screening technique for detection of very early lung cancer, not visible on normal chest x-rays, using helical CT (computed tomography) is very expensive from both health policy and societal perspectives, and is unlikely to be a cost-effective method for early detection of lung cancer in smokers. There were an estimated 169,400 new cases of lung cancer and 154,900 lung cancer deaths in the United States in 2002.
JAMA, January 15, 2003, pp. 357 and 380

82. Several factors, including age, the number of cigarettes smoked, and years of smoking, determine whether a smoker or former smoker develops lung cancer. According to a study conducted at Memorial Sloan-Kettering Cancer Center in New York City, N.Y., smokers' risk of getting lung cancer varies considerably, from less than 1 percent to 15 percent. "Before this study, anyone who smoked for 25 or 30 years thought that they were at extra high risk of lung cancer when, in fact, there is lots of difference in risk," said Dr. Peter Bach, lead author. For instance, the study found that a 51-year-old woman who smoked a pack of cigarettes a day for 28 years and then quit has just a 0.8 percent chance of getting lung cancer in the next decade. On the other hand, a 68-year-old man who has smoked two packs a day for 50 years and continues to smoke has a 15-percent chance of getting lung cancer.     Quote from the Journal of the National Cancer Institute, March 19, 2003, pp. 470-478

# Kent Micronite Filters and Lung Cancer

1. Kent's micronite filter used from 1952 to 1956 contained crocidolite asbestos, a known cause of mesothelioma. The manufacturer admitted that it knew asbestos was a health hazard before it ever sold a Kent cigarette, and that it knew that asbestos was released from the filter more than two years before the filter design was changed. Advertisements at the time touted Kent's health protection and its "safe," "harmless," and "dust free" filter.
9th World Conference on Tobacco or Health, Paris, 1994 (p. 37 abstract book)

2. "Kent's micronite filter gives greater protection against nicotine and tars than any other cigarette on the market today. It is the greatest health protection in cigarette history." 1954 Kent ad (*Nicotine and Public Health*, p. 27)

3. Lorillard produced 13 billion Kent micronite filter cigarettes from 1952 to 1957 with the ad touting, "Just what the doctor ordered… maximum health protection." The filter was composed of 30% asbestos and 70% cotton and acetate. 20 out of the 36 workers of Specialties, Inc. which produced the filter subsequently died from lung

cancer and asbestos poisoning; one of the worker's wives also died from inhaling asbestos fibers from her husband's clothing.
Rep. Mike Synar, CSPAN, April 14, 1994

4.  "What can be labeled the greatest health fraud in cigarette history occurred in March 1952, when Lorillard Tobacco company introduced Kent cigarettes with its new 'Micronite filter' that was 'developed by researchers in atomic energy plants.' Lorillard ad copy stressed that the new filter removed seven times more tar and nicotine than any other brand. To bolster its claim, Lorillard cited none other than the Journal of the American Medical Association as its source. After strenuous objections from the AMA, Kent discontinued any direct reference to that organization but continued to picture health professionals and used the 'health protection' theme in both print and television ads for years, sometimes citing pseudoscientific test results in an effort to lend a degree of medical credibility to their claims. Ironically, the substance in the Kent micronite filter that allegedly provided 'health protection' turned out to be asbestos – one of the more dangerous occupational lung carcinogens known. Without any public disclosure whatsoever, the company quietly replaced the asbestos with cellulose in 1957. Millions of smokers who had switched to Kents were never informed either that the filter had contained asbestos or that the asbestos had been replaced."
*Tobacco and the Clinician*, p. viii

5.  Out of 33 workers at a Massachusetts Lorillard factory where asbestos "Micronite" filters were made for Kent cigarettes in the 1950s, 19 eventually died from cancer, including five from mesothelioma, the type associated with the inhalation of asbestos.
*Ashes to Ashes*, p. 186

6.  A 1954 Life magazine ad for the Kent Micronite filter (made with crocidolite asbestos fibers) stated that the filter is "... made of a pure, dust-free, completely harmless material that is... so safe that it actually is used to help filter the air in operating rooms of leading hospitals."
Tobacco Control, Spring 1994, p. 64

7.  The 1956 campaign for Kent cigarettes containing the asbestos Micronite filter implied that the filter solved the health problems of cigarettes and that it was endorsed by the AMA. Tobacco Control, Summer 1994, p. 136

8.  Kent cigarettes promised, "... the greatest health protection ever developed" by virtue of its new crocidolite asbestos filter. A lawsuit by a former Kent smoker who developed mesothelioma, an asbestos-related lung cancer, was dismissed in 1992 because he could not prove that he smoked Kents in the 1950s.
Journal of Psychoactive Drugs, July 1989, p. 281

9.  A jury ordered Lorillard, maker of Kent cigarettes, to pay former smoker Charles Connor $2.2 million after he discovered that he had mesothelioma, a cancer linked to asbestos. Kent cigarettes were manufactured with asbestos-containing micronite filters from 1952 to 1956. Connor was a Kent smoker in the 1950s before quitting in 1962. Kent ads at the time said that it was "the one cigarette that can show you proof of greater health protection."
Associated Press, April 20, 1999

# CHAPTER 8
# OTHER CANCERS

## Historical

1.  In 1775, Percival Pott described an epidemic of scrotal cancer in chimney sweeps in London, an early documentation of the carcinogenicity of chimney smoke.

    *Population and Development Review*, June 1990, p. 218

2.  In 1851, Sir James Paget saw a patient with leukoplakia of the tongue from pipe smoking, and "told him he certainly would have cancer of the tongue if he went on smoking." In 1859, Bouisson reported that of 68 cases of patients with mouth cancer at a French hospital, 66 smoked tobacco and one chewed tobacco. He also noted that cancer of the lip usually occurred at the spot where the pipe or cigar was held.

    *Population and Development Review*, June 1990, pp. 219-220

3.  In 1915, it was suggested that the relation of smoking to cancer of the mouth was "apparently so well established as not to admit even a question of doubt."                    *Cancer Wars*, p. 105

4.  The National Cancer Institute, formed in 1937, was slow to deal with the tobacco and cancer problem. "The NCI's annual plan for 1977-81 failed even to mention tobacco or cigarette smoking in its discussion of the origins and impact of cancer."                    *Cancer Wars*, p. 109

## General

1.  A panel of experts concluded that in types of cancer linked to smoking, the risk is higher than previously believed. Cancers of the bladder and kidney (renal pelvis) are five to six times more prevalent in smokers, and types newly declared to be caused by smoking are cancers of the liver, stomach, kidney, uterus, nasal sinus, and myeloid leukemia. Cancer types now thought not to be related to smoking are breast and prostate cancer, as well as cancer of the endometrium, or lining of the uterus. The panel also concluded that second hand smoke exposure increases the risk of lung cancer by 20%.                    Associated Press, June 20, 2002

2.  Since the 1950's, the tobacco industry has claimed that the evidence linking cancer with smoking is "merely statistical," and that it is "premature" to accept the "casual theory" that smoking may cause cancer. The point "is to insinuate doubt, to reassure smokers, and to stave off regulation through a combination of wishful thinking, nonsequiturs, and faulty logic."                    *Cancer Wars*, p. 106

3.  "To my knowledge, it's not been proven that cigarette smoking causes cancer." William Campbell, president and chief executive, Philip Morris USA.                    New York Times, December 7, 1993

4.  The common belief that there is an epidemic of death from cancer in developed countries is a myth. If the tobacco-caused cancer deaths are taken away, then the remaining cancer death rates are declining.

    9th World Conference on Tobacco or Health, Paris, 1994 (Richard Peto)

5.  Cancer death rates would have declined over the last three decades in the United States were it not for an increase in lung cancer and other cancers related to smoking.                    AMA Fact Sheet on Smoking

6.  Cigarette smoking contributed to 157,000 of the 514,000 total cancer deaths in the United States in 1991. Smoking directly contributes to 22% of all cancer deaths in women and 45% of all cancer deaths in men. Lung cancer has displaced coronary heart disease as the single leading cause of excess mortality among smokers.

    Journal of the National Cancer Institute, August 21, 1991, p. 1142

7.  Tobacco in 1990 was responsible for 28% of all cancer deaths in developed countries; 42% of cancer deaths in males and 10% in females.                    *Mortality from Smoking*, p. A23

8. More than 75% of the following cancers are attributable to smoking: lung, throat, mouth, vocal cords, and esophagus. 20% to 50% of bladder, kidney, pancreas, cervix and stomach cancers as well as leukemias are caused by smoking. *Medical Clinics of North America*, March 1992, p. 305

8. Women who smoke may have a decreased risk for thyroid cancer. *Tobacco: the Growing Epidemic*, p. 13

9. "Cancer is a communicable disease. You get it from tobacco companies."
Joe Tye, founder, STAT (Stop Teenage Addiction to Tobacco)

10. "The seven warning signs of cancer are (1) Philip Morris, (2) RJR Nabisco, (3) Brown and Williamson, (4) US Tobacco Company..." Alan Blum, MD, founder, DOC (Doctors Ought to Care)

11. "The cigarette company is to the lung cancer epidemic what the mosquito is to malaria. It is the vector of disease." John Slade, MD, New Jersey College of Medicine

12. "Q. Does cigarette smoking cause cancer?
"A. I don't believe so. There's been no conclusive scientific evidence that convinces me that cigarette smoking causes cancer.
"Q. This warning on the package which says that smoking causes lung cancer, heart disease and emphysema is inaccurate? You don't believe it's true?
"A. That's correct.
"Q. Because if you believed it were true, in good conscience you wouldn't sell this to Americans, would you, or foreigners, for that matter?
"A. That's correct." Andrew H. Tisch, chairman and CEO, Lorillard, in a deposition in a case brought by airline flight attendants exposed to tobacco smoke (Washington Monthly, February 1994, p. 6)

# Kidney, Bladder, and Prostate Cancer

1. Smoking doubles the risk for bladder cancer; 47% of bladder cancer deaths in men and 37% in women are caused by smoking. Bladder cancer is diagnosed in 47,000 Americans each year, with 10,200 deaths.
Cancer Facts and Figures 1994 (American Cancer Society), p.16 and Los Angeles Times, June 21, 1991

2. Year 2000 estimates for new cases of bladder cancer are 53,000, with 12,200 deaths.
CA-A Cancer Journal for Clinicians, January-February 2000, pp. 12-13

3. Women who smoke double the risk for bladder cancer, and mortality from kidney cancer is 30% higher.
*Women and Smoking*, p. 229

4. 70% of cancers of the renal pelvis and ureter in men, and 40% in women, are caused by smoking. Smokers have more than a threefold risk of developing these cancers. If all tobacco use were eliminated, kidney cancer would be reduced by 30 to 40%. Journal of the National Cancer Institute, March 18, 1992, p. 381
and Cancer Research 1992; 52:254

5. There is a twofold increased risk of kidney cancer among smokers compared with nonsmokers.
Cancer, June 1, 1997

6. Carcinogens in tobacco smoke are absorbed into the blood, and some are excreted unchanged or as active metabolites through the urinary tract. The urine of cigarette smokers is strongly mutagenic.
Clinics in Chest Medicine, December 1991, p. 636

7. Smoking is responsible for 30% to 40% of all bladder cancers; active smokers have as much as seven times the risk for bladder cancer and five times the risk for cancer of the renal pelvis as nonsmokers.
Clinics in Chest Medicine, December 1991, p. 645

8. "One study has estimated more than a doubling of penile cancer risk among men who smoke more than 10 cigarettes per day as compared with nonsmokers. Another study has estimated more than a tripling of risk for

9.  Smoking cigarettes is generally not thought to be associated with increased risk for developing prostate cancer. However, the subgroup of obese male cigarette smokers did have a higher risk (odds ratio of 2.31). As well, there is an association with cigar and pipe smoking. Epidemiology 2001; 12:546

10. Smoking has not been determined to increase risk for prostate cancer, but if men with prostate cancer smoke, the smoking appears to cause their cancer to become more invasive and aggressive. *Cigarettes*, p. 96

11. In a nine-year study of 450,000 men, those who developed prostate cancer and continued to smoke had a 34% greater likelihood of dying from the prostate cancer than men who had never smoked. American Journal of Epidemiology 1997; 145:466

12. Women who smoke and who are infected with genital warts have a much higher risk of genital and vulvar cancer than other women. Reuters and ABC News, October 14, 1997

# Cervical Cancer

1.  "The association of smoking with cervical cancer has been recognized only recently; the Centers for Disease Control and Prevention added cervical cancer to the categories of smoking-induced disease in 1988. While smokers as a group commonly have other risk factors associated with cervical cancer (including multiple sexual partners and the presence of sexually transmitted diseases), at least 12 studies have found that smoking increases the risk for cervical cancer after accounting for these other factors. Approximately 1,400 cervical cancer deaths each year (about 31 percent of the 4,514 total deaths) are estimated to be due to smoking." *Cigarettes*, p. 17

2.  Cigarette smoking accounted for about 30% of 13,500 new cases of cervical cancer reported in the US in 1993, and women who smoke double their risk for developing cervical cancer. NEJM, March 31, 1994, p. 910

3.  A study from London reported a link between smoking and early cancerous changes of the uterine cervix in women, and suggested that smoking cessation could have a beneficial effect on these cervical abnormalities. Lancet, April 6, 1996, p. 941

# Pancreatic Cancer

1.  A study from Harvard Medical School concluded that the proportion of pancreatic cancers attributable to cigarette smoking was 25%, accounting for a quarter of the 27,000 annual deaths from this cancer in the United States. Overall, a smoker has about twice the risk of a nonsmoker of developing pancreatic cancer; someone who smokes more than 40 cigarettes per day has about a five-fold increase in risk. Archives of Internal Medicine, October 28, 1996, p. 2255, and *Cigarettes*, p. 16

2.  About 27% of all pancreatic cancer deaths, 6750 each year in the US, are caused by smoking. The median survival period is only three months, and only 3% survive longer than five years. American Medical News, December 5, 1994, p. 33, and Journal of the National Cancer Institute, October 19, 1994, p.1510

3.  Cigarette smokers have a 70% increased risk of pancreatic cancer compared to nonsmokers. 29% of pancreatic cancer in blacks and 26% in whites is attributable to cigarette smoking. Journal of the National Cancer Institute, October 19, 1994, p. 1510

4.  There is a significant positive association between smoking and pancreatic cancer, with odds ratios for current smokers ranging from 1.3 to 5.5. CA-A Cancer Journal for Clinicians, July/August 2000, p. 243

5.  Smoking doubles the risk for pancreatic cancer, the fourth most common cause of death from cancer in the United States, and accounts for 25% to 30% of all pancreatic tumors. JAMA, July 11, 2001, pp. 169-170

# Leukemia and Childhood Cancers

1.  An estimated 6% of all childhood cancers and 18% of childhood acute lymphoblastic leukemia cases may result from smoking by the mother.                     American Journal of Epidemiology 1991; 133:123

2.  Children of women who smoked 10 or more cigarettes a day during their pregnancies have double the risk of developing acute lymphoblastic leukemia, Wilms' tumor, and non-Hodgkin lymphoma.
                                                                The Lancet, June 14, 1986, p. 1350

3.  There is a 30% excess risk of all types of leukemia in smokers, except for myeloid leukemia, where the excess risk is 40%. 14% of all leukemias are caused by cigarette smoking, or about 3600 of the 25,700 new cases of adult leukemia per year in the United States.
                                                    Journal of the National Cancer Institute, December 5, 1990, p. 1832

4.  The risk of myeloid leukemia is 50% greater in smokers. About 22% of all myeloid leukemias are caused by smoking.                     Archives of Internal Medicine, February 22, 1993, p. 469

5.  "Smoking may be associated with an increased risk for acute myeloid leukemia among women, but does not appear to be associated with other lymphoproliferative or hematologic cancers."
                                                    *Women and Smoking*, 2001 Surgeon General report, p. 231

6.  Up to 10% of cases of acute leukemia in adults could be smoking related.
                                                    Reuters, November 12, 1999 (from British Journal of Cancer)

7.  A study in the British Journal of Cancer found that children whose fathers smoked a pack a day or more had a 30% higher risk for developing cancer than did other children. "Damaged sperm is the likeliest culprit," said one of the study doctors, from the University of Birmingham, England.          Reuters, November 18, 1997

8.  Men who smoke father children who are far more likely to die of cancer. 15% of childhood cancers may be from this cause.                                     CBS News, December 11, 1996

9.  Men who smoke can damage their sperm and increase the risk of cancer in their children.
                                                                Reuters, December 16, 1996

10. In a study from Shanghai, China, "paternal smoking prior to conception may be associated with an increased risk for all childhood cancers combined and particularly for childhood acute lymphoblastic leukemia, lymphoma, and brain tumors. The elevated cancer risk was confined to children under age 5 years at diagnosis and associated with paternal smoking starting prior to conception, suggesting the possibility of prezygotic genetic damage." Children whose fathers smoked more than five pack-years prior to their conception had adjusted odds ratios of 3.8 for acute lymphoblastic leukemia, 4.5 for lymphoma, 2.7 for brain tumors, and 1.7 for all cancers combined. Other studies have found an increase in neuroblastoma and rhabdomyosarcoma in children whose fathers smoke. Cigarette smoking increases oxidative DNA damage in human sperm cells, and causes mutations in germ cells.
                                                    Journal of the National Cancer Institute, February 5, 1997, pp. 238-244

# Oral Cancer

1.  Tobacco causes about 70% of the 30,000 cases of oral cancer each year in the US, and is responsible for about 5600 of the 8000 yearly deaths from oral cancer. The five-year survival rate is 53%.
                                                                JAMA, April 27, 1994, p. 1232

2.  Tobacco use is the major risk factor for oral cancer. There were an estimated 29,600 new cases and 7925 deaths in 1994.                     Cancer Facts and Figures 1994 (American Cancer Society)

3.  The average smoker has a 14-fold higher risk of dying from cancer of the lung, throat, or mouth; a 4-fold higher risk of dying from cancer of the esophagus; and twice the risk of dying from bladder cancer.

    JAMA, September 1, 1999, p. 914

4.  Compared with the risk of nonsmoking nondrinkers, the relative risks for developing mouth and throat cancer are 7 times greater for those who use tobacco, 6 times greater for those who use alcohol, and 38 times greater for those who use both tobacco and alcohol.          Alcohol Alert newsletter, January 1998

5.  Year 2000 estimates for new cases of cancer of the larynx are 10,100, with 3900 deaths.

    CA-A Cancer Journal for Clinicians, January-February 2000, pp. 12-13

6.  About 80% of oral cancer patients are smokers, and the risk for developing oral cancer is five to nine times greater for smokers than for nonsmokers.     CA-A Cancer Journal for Clinicians, July/August 2002, p. 197

7.  About 70% of oral cancer cases are related to tobacco; the five-year survival rate is about 50%.

    Men's Journal, February 2002, p. 72

8.  Mouth and throat cancers constitute 33% of all cancers in India, compared to only 4% in the West.

    *Tobacco: the Growing Epidemic*, p. 41

9.  About 92% of oral cancers in men and 61% in women are caused by smoking; the risk for development of oral cancer compared to nonsmokers is 27-fold in men, and six times more likely in women who smoke.

    *Cigarettes*, p. 15

10. The five-year survival rate for oral cancer has improved little in the last four decades, holding steady at about 53%. Only 34% of blacks survived for five years after initial diagnosis, compared with 55% of whites.

    American Medical News, September 9, 1996, p. 10

11. Estimated new cases of cancer of the oral cavity and pharynx in the United States in 1998 are 30,300, with 8,000 deaths. For cancer of the larynx, estimates are 11,100 cases and 4300 deaths. Five-year cancer survival rates (1986-1993) for cancer of the oral cavity are 55% for whites and 34% for African Americans, and for laryngeal cancer, 69% and 54%, respectively.

    American Cancer Society data reported in CA-A Cancer Journal for Clinicians, January-February 1998

12. Non-drinking smokers have two to four times the risk of developing oral cancers as do abstainers of alcohol and tobacco. Heavy drinking smokers have a risk six to fifteen times greater than abstainers.

    CA-A Cancer Journal for Clinicians, November-December 1995, p. 329

13. In 1991, there were an estimated 12,500 new cases and 3640 deaths from laryngeal cancer; the prevalence has increased by 70% in the past 35 years. Cigarette smoking and alcohol use increases the risk by 75%, and 82% of cases of cancer of the larynx are attributable to cigarette smoking.

    Richard Hurt, M.D., lecture, Mayo Clinic, May 1997

14. The use of tobacco and alcohol, frequently in combination, is associated with an over 95% of the cases of squamous carcinoma of the head and neck.

    CA-A Cancer Journal for Clinicians, November-December 1995, p. 352

15. Patients with head and neck cancer who continue to smoke during radiation therapy have lower rates of response (45% vs 75%) and poorer two-year survival rates (39% vs 66%) than patients who do not smoke during radiation therapy.          NEJM, January 21, 1993, p. 159

# Esophageal, Stomach, and Small Intestinal Cancers

1.  Of the 10,200 deaths from cancer of the esophagus in 1993, about 80 percent were attributable to cigarette smoking.
    NEJM, March 31, 1994, p. 909

2.  The combination of smoking and drinking can boost the risk of esophageal cancer by more than 100 times.
    Reuters, August 9, 1999

3.  Smoking is a major risk factor for esophageal and gastric cardia (stomach) adenocarcinomas, accounting for about 40% of all cases. The risk of these cancers was increased 2.4-fold in current cigarette smokers, with little reduction in risk observed until 30 years after smoking cessation. The risk rose with increasing intensity and duration of smoking. The risks for developing squamous cell carcinoma of the esophagus were estimated to be more than five times higher among current smokers, 2.8 times higher among ex-smokers, and more than three times higher among liquor drinkers. The lag between smoking onset and the development of these cancers is extremely long; it may exceed 30 years.
    Journal of the National Cancer Institute, September 3, 1997, pp. 1248 and 1277-84

4.  The risk for mortality from stomach cancer is 40% higher for women smokers than nonsmokers.
    *Women and Smoking*, p. 226

5.  Male smokers in China have a 3.6-fold increased risk for esophageal cancer, and a 2-fold increase in liver cancer, the latter independent of alcohol consumption.
    JAMA, November 12, 1997, p. 1501

6.  In a study from the University of Southern California reported in the International Journal of Cancer, smoking tripled the risk of small intestinal cancer in men.
    Reuters Medical News, March 7, 1997

# Colon Cancer

1.  Cigarette smoking has been consistently associated with a higher risk of colorectal adenoma, a precursor of cancer. Recent studies indicate that an increased risk for colon and large bowel cancer emerges only after a very long induction period, about four decades after one begins smoking. New estimates are that 21% of colorectal cancer cases in men are attributable to smoking, or about 16,000 new cases and 6,000 deaths each year in U.S. men. This compares to about 7% of cases attributable to a family history in a first degree relative. "For women, the proportion of colorectal cancers attributable to smoking has not been appreciable to date, but may begin rising as the impact of women's smoking behavior in the 1950s and 1960s becomes manifest."
    Journal of the National Cancer Institute, December 4, 1996, pp. 1717-30

2.  Colorectal cancer ranks fourth in incidence and second in cause of death from cancer in the United States, and current smokers had almost double the risk (adjusted relative risk 1.81) for colorectal cancer compared with never smokers. For smokers of a pack a day or more, the relative risk was 2.14.
    Journal of the National Cancer Institute, July 19, 2000, pp. 1178-1179

3.  "People who smoke cigarettes for 20 years or more are about 40% more likely to die of colon cancer than are nonsmokers, according to a study that blames tobacco use for about 12% of U.S. colon cancer deaths."
    Associated Press, December 6, 2000

4.  A link exists between smoking and some types of colon cancer; there is a relative risk of about 2.0 for individuals who have smoked for 45 years or more.
    Journal of the National Cancer Institute, November 15, 2000, pp. 1831-36

5.  Long-term cigarette smoking is associated with an increased risk of colorectal cancer mortality in both men and women.
    Journal of the National Cancer Institute, December 6, 2000, p. 1888

6. For both men and women, smoking a pack a day for 10 to 14 years appears to double the risk of developing colon cancer decades later.                                                                    *Cigarettes*, p. xii

7. In a study of U.S. veterans, significant 20% and 40% excess risks of colon and rectal cancer mortality, respectively, were observed among cigarette smokers. However, a study of male construction workers in Sweden did not show an association between cigarette smoking and an increased risk of colorectal cancer.
                                                                    Journal of the National Cancer Institute, September 18, 1996, p. 1302

8. In a study from the Harvard School of Public Health, male heavy smokers had double the risk, and women 1.5 times the risk, of colon and rectal cancer compared to nonsmokers.                        USA Today, February 2, 1994

9. Adenomatous polyps are precursors of colon and rectal cancer. Current smokers increase their risk for developing these polyps by 2.6 fold. For smokers who drink as well, the excess risk is 4.2 times.
                                                                    Journal of the National Cancer Institute, February 15, 1995, p. 274

10. Cigarette smoking is a strong risk factor for anogenital cancer. American Journal of Epidemiology 1992; 135:180

11. The risk of anal cancer is high among premenopausal women who smoke (odds ratio 5.6), but not in men or older women. "We hypothesize an antiestrogenic mechanism of action for smoking in anal carcinogenesis."
                                                                    Journal of the National Cancer Institute, April 21, 1999, p. 708

12. In a study of patients with anal cancer, 55% were smokers compared to 21% of control subjects. The relative risk was 7- to 9-fold. A heavy smoker also has 77 times the risk of oral cancer compared to a nonsmoker.
                                                                    Journal of the American Academy of Dermatology, May 1996, p. 722

13. Smokers appear to have a modest increase in their risk of stomach cancer, about 50 percent over the risk of nonsmokers. If this association is casual, then at least one-fifth of stomach cancer would be attributable to smoking.                                                                    *Cigarettes*, p. 20

# Breast Cancer

1. In a study reported in the journal Epidemiology (Vol. 13, 2002, pp. 138-145), passive smoke exposure was not associated with an increased risk for developing breast cancer. There was a small increase in risk for breast cancer in women who began smoking before the age of 17.

2. Breast cancer patients who smoke have a much higher risk of the cancer spreading to their lungs, thus greatly decreasing their survival rates.                        ABC evening news (Peter Jennings), June 16, 2001

3. Breast cancer patients who smoke appear to be at increased risk for developing metastases to the lungs; the adjusted odds ratio was 1.96.                                                    Chest 2001; 119:1635-1640

4. In a study from New Jersey, no association was found between exposure to second hand smoke and female breast cancer mortality.                        Journal of the National Cancer Institute, October 18, 2000, p. 1666

5. Postmenopausal women who carry a defective or slow form of the acetylator enzyme N-acetyltransferase 2 (NAT2) and who smoke a pack a day or more appear to increase their risk for breast cancer four-fold. The prevalence of the slow form of NAT2 is about 55% in white women, 35% in blacks, 10-20% in Asians, and 65-90% in those of Middle Eastern descent. The enzyme is thought to help detoxify carcinogens in tobacco smoke.                                                                    JAMA, November 13, 1996

6. In a study from Switzerland, a three-fold increased risk of breast cancer was found among nonsmoking women who had been regularly exposed to tobacco smoke at home or at work. For active smokers of a pack a day or more, the risk for breast cancer was 4.6 times greater.
                        New York Times, May 5, 1996 (from May 1996 American Journal of Epidemiology)

7.  A Danish study found a 60% increase in the risk of breast cancer in women who had smoked cigarettes for more than 30 years. Smokers tended to develop cancer at a younger age, and those who had started to smoke before 16 and who smoked more than 25 cigarettes a day faced an 80% increase in breast cancer risk.

    New York Times, October 7, 1997

# Skin Cancer

1.  There is no known statistical association between smoking and the occurrence of malignant melanoma, but melanoma in a cigarette smoker is twice as likely to have metastasized at diagnosis: 23% vs. 11% in an Australian study. Smoking is also a predictor for poorer prognosis in people with basal cell carcinoma of the skin.

    Skin and Allergy News, July 1999, p. 38

2.  In a study from the Netherlands, smokers had a 1.9-fold increased risk for developing squamous cell carcinoma of the skin. There was no increase in the risk for basal cell carcinoma.

    Skin and Allergy News, August 1999, p. 3

3.  Smoking doubles the risk of developing squamous cell carcinoma of the skin, concludes a study from the Netherlands.

    Journal of Clinical Oncology 2001; 19:231-238

# CHAPTER 9
# CARDIOVASCULAR DISEASE

NOTE:    Please see Chapter 5 for section on ETS and cardiovascular disease.

1.  The Lancet in 1857 commented about tobacco: "The circulating organs are affected by irritable heart condition." *The Medical and Surgical History of the War of the Rebellion*, published in six volumes from 1875 to 1888, noted that abuse of tobacco may cause "irritable heart."
    Population and Development Review, June 1990, pp. 219-220

2.  Smoking causes about 40% of all the deaths from heart attacks in men and women less than 65 years old.
    Executive Health Report, July 1990

3.  More than 40% of all cardiovascular deaths are at least partly attributable to tobacco use. Compared with nonsmokers, cigarette smokers have double the risk for having a myocardial infarction (heart attack), and are 70% more likely to have a fatal complication from an infarct. Up to 80% of myocardial infarctions in smokers younger than age 49 may be related to smoking.        Postgraduate Medicine, February 1996, p. 102

4.  A 1958 study found a 70% increased risk of coronary artery disease in smokers compared to nonsmokers.
    Journal of the American Medical Association 1958; 166:1294

5.  The three major risk factors for premature coronary heart disease are smoking, elevated cholesterol, and high blood pressure. Any one of these factors doubles the risk of heart attack before age 60; two of three quadruples the risk, and if all three factors are present, the risk is increased eightfold.
    Archives of Internal Medicine, January 1992, p. 56

6.  Over 90% of patients with peripheral vascular disease are smokers. In those who fail to quit, there is a higher incidence of amputation needed.                                          The Lancet 1978; 2:234

7.  Smoking accounts for about 76% of all peripheral vascular disease, far overshadowing all other risk factors.
    *Cigarettes*, p. 36

8.  In one study, diabetic patients with gangrene were smokers in nearly all cases and, when compared with nonsmokers, had peripheral vascular disease rates of 33% versus 16%.
    Clinics in Chest Medicine, December 1991, p. 720

9.  Women who smoke and use oral contraceptives are up to 30 times more likely to have a heart attack and 22 times more likely to have a stroke than women who neither smoke nor use birth control pills.
    Journal of the American Medical Association, September 11, 1987, p. 1339

10. In women who smoke and use oral contraceptives, the risk of acute myocardial infarction is increased by 20.8 times. The risk of myocardial infarction is increased 41-fold in women who smoke and have a history of toxemia of pregnancy (compared to 4.5-fold in smoking women without a history of toxemia). There is no evidence that a smoker who chooses low tar and nicotine brands reduces the risk of myocardial infarction.
    Clinics in Chest Medicine, December 1991, p. 662

11. The use of oral contraceptive formulations with decreased estrogen content may lower the effects of the association of oral contraceptives and smoking on the risk for abnormal coagulation.
    Contemporary Ob/Gyn, March 1996, p. 126

12. In patients with heart attacks, nonsmokers had their first heart attack at a median age of 62. Heavy smokers had their first heart attack at a median age of 51, or 11 years earlier.        Associated Press, March 7, 1991

13. Cigarette smoking is equivalent to an additional two decades of aging in terms of the risk of damage to the carotid arteries in the neck. Smoking is the most significant risk factor for carotid artery atherosclerosis.
   Journal of the American Medical Association, February 24, 1989, p. 1178

14. A study from Wake Forest University of 10,900 people investigated risk factors for atherosclerosis. Smokers had a 50% increase in the rate of plaque accumulation in the carotid arteries, former smokers a 25% increase, and those exposed to environmental tobacco smoke a 20% increase. Each millimeter of increase in the intimal-medial thickness increases the risk of an acute coronary event by 2.14 times. The risk was even greater for people with hypertension or diabetes. The thickness of the carotid artery walls was measured with ultrasound. The fact that pack years of smoking, but not current versus past smoking, was associated with the progression of atherosclerosis suggested that some adverse cardiovascular effects of smoking may be cumulative and irreversible.
   Journal of the American Medical Association, January 14, 1998, pp. 119-124

15. In a study of carotid artery thickness, environmental tobacco smoke had about 34% of the impact on atherosclerotic progression that occurs with active smoking, a finding compatible with the relative risk of 1.3 found in epidemiologic studies.
   Journal of the American Medical Association, January 14, 1998, p. 158

16. A study from Greece showed that both active and passive smoking is associated with an acute deterioration, maintained for at least 20 minutes, of the elasticity of the aorta. This deterioration of aortic function and performance adversely influences coronary artery blood flow, and could also compromise left ventricular function.
   Annals of Internal Medicine, March 15, 1998, pp. 426-434

17. Both passive and active smoking is related to greater internal-medial wall thickness of the carotid arteries in the neck, a potent risk factor for carotid atherosclerosis.
   Archives of Internal Medicine, June 13, 1994, p. 1277

18. Smokers between the ages of 45 and 64 triple their risk of dying from heart disease compared to nonsmokers.
   Chest, September 1988, p. 449

19. Cigarette smoking is responsible for two-thirds of all heart attacks in women under age 50; a smoker in this age group runs a 5-fold increased risk of heart attack.
   *Your Good Health*, William Bennett, Harvard University Press, 1987, p. 95

20. Smoking leads to 7.7-fold increase in the risk of coronary artery spasm in women ages 36 to 41 who were evaluated for angina. 62% of patients were smokers compared to 17% of control subjects. Cigarette smoking accounts for 45% in men and 41% in women of the total risk for coronary heart disease for those under age 65.
   Circulation, March 1992, p. 905

21. Overall, smokers have a two- to fourfold greater incidence of coronary heart disease and about a 70 percent greater death rate from it.
   *Cigarettes*, p. 28

22. Smoking is associated with increases in the high density lipoprotein portion of cholesterol in the blood, the "bad" cholesterol, as well as increases in the triglyceride type of fat. Regular smokers are also more resistant to insulin.
   Chest, September 1988, p. 449

23. Smoking causes higher levels of free fatty acids in the bloodstream. In particular, this exposure causes higher levels of very low density lipoproteins. Smoking interferes with the normal metabolism of cholesterol and triglycerides.
   *Cigarettes*, p. 29

24. Cigarette smoking is responsible for more than 20% of all coronary heart disease deaths in men over age 65, but for about 45% of deaths in men under age 65. In women, smoking accounts for 10% of the deaths from coronary heart disease over age 65 and more than 40% of the deaths from this cause in women less than age 65. Overall, 30 to 40% of the nearly half million annual deaths related to coronary artery disease are attributable to smoking.
   Chest, September 1988, p. 449

25. Cigarette smoking increases the risk of sudden cardiac death, suggesting that it increases myocardial vulnerability to ventricular fibrillation, a fatal rhythm disturbance. The risk of sudden death in smokers is two-

fold higher in men without prior coronary heart disease, and six-fold higher in men with prior coronary heart disease.                                                  New England Journal of Medicine, January 30, 1986, p. 271

26. Smokers have a twofold to fourfold greater risk for sudden death from coronary artery disease than nonsmokers, two to eight times the mortality from ruptured aortic aneurysm, and a 3.7 to 4.9 times increased risk for stroke.

   Clinics in Chest Medicine, December 1991, p. 649

27. In ex-smokers, the excess risk for both stroke and coronary heart disease declines within 5 to 10 years to that of neversmokers.                           New England Journal of Medicine, September 18, 1986, p. 717

28. About 37,000 deaths from coronary heart disease in nonsmokers are due to passive smoke exposure in the household and workplace. This accounts for 70% of the estimated 53,000 yearly deaths from secondhand smoke.                                                                           Circulation, January 1991, p. 1

29. Exposure to secondhand smoke is estimated to increase the risk of heart disease in nonsmokers by 30%, causing an estimated 35,000 to 40,000 heart disease deaths a year in the US, or about ten times the number of lung cancer deaths attributed to secondhand smoke.             Consumer Reports, January 1995, p. 29

30. Among men and women under age 65, smoking causes more than 40% of deaths from coronary heart disease and more than 50% from cerebrovascular disease (stroke).                         *Nicotine Addiction*, p.339

31. In a study from Argentina, 55% of the myocardial infarctions in patients under age 55 were attributable to smoking.                                                                 *Tobacco Control* 1993; 2:127

32. In a study from Sweden, the excess risk of dying from cardiovascular disease was 1.4 times for smokeless tobacco users and 1.9 times for smokers of 15 or more cigarettes per day. Among men aged 35 to 55 years, the relative risk was 2.1 for smokeless tobacco users and 3.2 for smokers.

   American Journal of Public Health, March 1994, p. 399

33. Smokers have a threefold increase in frequency and a twelve-fold increase in duration of silent ischemic episodes. Smoking elevates "bad" low density and very low-density lipoproteins in the blood.
   *The Pharmacological Basis of Therapeutics*, Goodman and Gilman, 1990 edition, p. 547

34. Coronary bypass surgery is a strong motivator to quit smoking. Even without specific intervention, nearly one-half of smokers had quit 5 years after their surgery.             Annals of Internal Medicine 1994; 120:287

35. 35% of the 90,000 smoking-related deaths from coronary heart disease occur before age 65.
   Richard Hurt, M.D., Mayo Clinic, May 1997 lecture

36. 24 million Americans, or 10% of the population, will die prematurely of heart disease secondary to smoking.
   *Koop*, p. 165

37. In women 30 to 55 years old who smoke 25 or more cigarettes per day, the relative risk for fatal coronary heart disease is 5.5 times that of a nonsmoker. The relative risk for nonfatal myocardial infarction (heart attack) is 5.8, and for angina pectoris is 2.6.             New England Journal of Medicine, November 19, 1987, p. 1303

38. In a study of 120 men who had a myocardial infarction (heart attack) before age 36, 89% were smokers. There was a positive family history in 48%, hypertension in 21%, and lipid abnormalities in 20%.
   Western Journal of Medicine, April 1984, p. 201

39. In a study from Rochester, Minnesota, cigarette smoking accounted for 64% of all myocardial infarctions and sudden unexpected deaths in women 40 to 59 years of age.
   Mayo Clinic Proceedings, December 1989, p. 1471

40. Tobacco smoking accounts for about one half of coronary disease events in women. Smokers have double the incidence of coronary heart disease, a 70% greater death rate from coronary heart disease, an up to a fourfold

greater risk for sudden death than do nonsmokers.　　　Seminars in Respiratory Medicine, January 1990, p. 11

41. About 70% of smokers who survive a heart attack take up smoking again within a year.
British Journal of Addiction 1990; 85:295

42. Almost three in five smokers who have surgery for heart disease continue to smoke after their procedure.
Science Daily, November 12, 1998

43. After undergoing angioplasty for coronary artery disease, 63% of smokers in a study from the Mayo Clinic continued to smoke at least some of the time.　　　Reuters, March 5, 1998

44. A study from Great Britain showed that the risk for heart attacks for young adult smokers is about double what had been previously been believed, and that when cigarette smokers have a heart attack before age 50, there is an 80% chance that tobacco caused it.　　　New York Times, August 18, 1995, p. A9

45. In the above study, smokers in their thirties and forties have five times the chance of suffering a heart attack as nonsmokers of the same age, and switching to low-tar cigarettes does little to alter the risk. Among people in their thirties, the heart attack rate in smokers was 6.3 times that of nonsmokers. For those in their forties, the rate was 4.7 times higher, and for those in their fifties, it was 3.1 times higher. For smokers in their sixties and seventies, the risk was respectively 2.5 and 1.9 times that of nonsmokers. In the US yearly, there are about 40,000 heart attacks caused by smoking among people in their thirties or forties. A smoker's chance of having a heart attack falls precipitously after quitting, and in two years approximates that of someone who has never smoked.　　　British Medical Journal, August 19, 1995, p. 471

46. Thromboangiitis obliterans, or Buerger's disease, may be caused by nicotine poisoning. "In several cases, cessation of smoking without any further treatment whatsoever has resulted in complete disappearance of all symptoms."　　　Stop Smoking Before It Stops You, Emil Alban, Christopher Publ. 1949, p. 31

47. Smoking increases the risk for Buerger's disease, or thromboangiitis obliterans, an inflammatory condition of blood vessels leading to arterial occlusion and gangrene, first of the toes and then of the foot.　Cigarettes, p. 38

48. Most patients with thromboangiitis obliterans (Buerger's disease) are heavy cigarette smokers.
Mayo Clinic Proceedings, June 1998, p. 530

49. Passive smoking is associated in a dose-dependent manner with significant endothelial dysfunction, a key early event in atherogenesis and early arterial damage, in healthy teenagers and young adults.
New England Journal of Medicine, January 18, 1996, p. 154

50. Patients who smoke one year after heart bypass surgery had more than a nine-fold elevated risk of undergoing another bypass compared with patients who quit smoking at the time of surgery. And patients who smoked regularly five years after the procedure were 3.3 times more likely to need and undergo another bypass.
Associated Press, January 1, 1996

51. Smoking increases the heart rate by 10 to 25 beats per minute, or up to 36,000 extra beats a day. Smokers have a greater risk of irregular heartbeats (arrhythmias), which increases the risk of heart attack. Smoking also constricts blood vessels, triggering an increase in blood pressure, a key risk factor for both heart attack and stroke.　　　Mother Jones magazine, May-June 1996, p. 68

52. Both cigarette smoking and tobacco chewing increase the heart rate by an average of 7 to 12 beats per minute.
Seminars in Respiratory Medicine, January 1990

53. A transient elevation of blood pressure lasting for about 20 minutes follows every cigarette smoked.
The Tobacco Epidemic, p. 93

54. The heart rate may increase by as much as 30% during the first ten minutes of smoking, and there is also an acute increase in blood pressure. While some studies suggest that blood pressure returns to normal between episodes of smoking, repeated smoking does result in higher average pressure. *Cigarettes*, p. 27

55. Smoking reduces the effectiveness of medical treatment for hypertension, and reduces the effectiveness of the beta blocker class of drugs.

56. In a 1993 Gallup poll, 25% of respondents who smoked did not relate tobacco use to heart disease, 35% did not realize that smoking could lead to strokes, and 16% did not link smoking with lung cancer. *Tobacco*, p. 109

57. Each of the first four recipients of artificial hearts had smoked more than 250,000 cigarettes.
American Journal of Preventive Medicine, April 1985, p. 15

58. "Smoking directly reduces the life span of platelets and causes them to clump together abnormally. Independent of that, smoking causes the platelets to be stickier than normal, again causing them to be more likely to clump. That clumping in turn leads to blood-clot formation, which is compounded by smoking's effects on the blood's anti-clotting factors." *Cigarettes*, p. 28

59. Smoking increases blood viscosity, making the blood thicker, and makes red blood cells more rigid and less pliable. *Cigarettes*, p. 28

60. "Smokers have much higher rates than non-smokers of two potentially serious arrhythmias: the deadly arrhythmia called ventricular fibrillation, and ventricular premature beats. Arrhythmias are potentially dangerous when they occur in isolation, but they also increase the sufferer's chances of dying of a heart attack." *Cigarettes*, p. 31

61. In a study from Scotland, smokers had three times the risk of nonsmokers and ex-smokers of developing abdominal aortic aneurysm Reuters Medical News, April 21, 1997

62. In a study of 70,000 veterans aged 50-79, smokers had a five-fold increased risk for the development of abdominal aortic aneurysm. Annals of Internal Medicine, March 15, 1997

63. "Smokers have about eight times the risk of aortic aneurysms—and much higher death rates from ruptured aortic aneurysms—than do nonsmokers. Stopping smoking also slashes a person's risk of dying from a ruptured aortic aneurysm by approximately 50 percent. Accumulating evidence now indicates that the risk of developing cardiomyopathy is much greater in smokers." *Cigarettes*, pp. 30-31

64. Smokers who continue to puff away after having balloon angioplasty double their odds of a heart attack or early death. Time, March 24, 1997, p. 40

65. In an American Cancer Society study of 121,000 men, smoking one cigar a day appeared to increase the risk of death from coronary heart disease by 30% in men ages 75 and younger. Washington Post, November 16, 1999

66. In a meta-analysis of studies of the risk of coronary heart disease associated with passive smoking among nonsmokers, the authors concluded that the relative risk of coronary heart disease in nonsmokers exposed to environmental tobacco smoke was 1.25. New England Journal of Medicine, March 25, 1999, p. 920

67. Only 29% of current smokers in a large telephone survey believed that they were at higher risk than average risk for having a heart attack, and only 40% of the group acknowledged that they were at a higher risk for cancer. Journal of the American Medical Association, March 17, 1999, p. 1019

68. In apparently healthy long-term smokers, myocardial blood flow averages 14% less than in non-smokers. Smoking is associated with significant vascular dysfunction even before evidence of atheroma is present.
The Lancet, July 18, 1998, p. 205 (from Circulation 1998; 119-125)

69. "Healthy" smokers average about 14% less blood flow to the heart than nonsmokers, according to a UCLA study reported in the July 1998 issue of Circulation.                    Reuters, July 13, 198

70. Smoking elevates heart rate by 15 to 20 beats per minute and systolic and diastolic blood pressure by about 12 mm of mercury. The peak effect is after about 10 minutes of smoking, and the heart rate and blood pressure gradually drop toward the pre-smoking level, which is reached after about 30 minutes. The heart rate and blood pressure increases are paralleled by about 20% elevations in myocardial oxygen uptake and increased coronary artery blood flow.                    *Nicotine Safety and Toxicity,* pp. 42 and 43

71. In Korea, smoking is a major independent risk factor for atherosclerotic cardiovascular disease, and a low cholesterol level confers no protective benefit against this smoking-related vascular disease.
                    Journal of the American Medical Association, December 8, 1999, p. 2149

72. Female nurses who smoke just one to four cigarettes a day have a 2.5-fold increased risk of fatal coronary heart disease.                    *Cigarettes,* p. 26

73. Smoking increases mortality from coronary artery disease by 70%, and smokers began to have angina about 10 years earlier than nonsmokers or former smokers.
                    New England Journal of Medicine, March 13, 1997, pp. 759-760

74. In a study from Sweden, smokers who are physically active have a 40% lower risk of dying from heart problems than smokers who do not exercise. Sedentary smokers have a risk of cardiac death four times higher than that of active nonsmokers.
                    American Medical News, May 5, 1997 (from Archives of Internal Medicine, April 28, 1997)

75. The risk for sudden coronary death is nearly double in current smokers without a history of heart disease.
                    Reuters, February 20, 1997

76. Smoking stiffens the aorta within one minute after lighting up, and the effect lasts 20 minutes or more.
                    Reuters Health eLine, January 7, 1997

77. Women who smoke 25 to 34 cigarettes a day are 1.8 times more likely to develop a pulmonary embolism than their nonsmoking counterparts, and smoking more than 34 cigarettes a day increased the risk by 3.4 times.
                    Reuters Medical News, February 25, 1997

78. Smokers with no history of heart disease are 20 times more likely than nonsmokers to suffer from myocardial ischemia, or inadequate oxygen supply to the heart, if they smoke in the 24 hours before surgery.
                    Reuters, October 22, 1997

79. The so-called "smokers' paradox" is the fact that a smoker is much more likely to suffer a heart attack than a nonsmoker, but also more likely to survive it. The reason for this, a study in the February 2002 issue of Nicotine and Tobacco Research suggests, is mainly that the smoker tends to be much younger at the time of the heart attack. The smokers were, on average, 14 years younger at the time of the heart attack, and were only half as likely as nonsmokers to die while hospitalized. The age difference between the groups accounted for almost all the observed difference in mortality rates.                    2002 AMA Annual Tobacco Report

80. In a study from the Journal of Nicotine and Tobacco Research in August 2001, 8 weeks of smoking reduction resulted in clinically significant improvements in established cardiovascular risk factors, including improvements in the high-density/low-density lipoprotein (HDL/LDL) ratio, fibrinogen, and white blood cell count. (Following a year of abstinence from smoking, heart disease risk is decreased by half.)

81. Cigarette smoking is strongly associated with an increased risk of coronary heart disease among women with Type 2 diabetes; the relative risk is 2.68 for current smokers of 15 or more cigarettes per day.
                    Archives of Internal Medicine, February 11, 2002, p. 273

82. Smokers are twice as likely as nonsmokers to have heart disease, and three times more likely to have a heart attack.
*Tobacco: The Growing Epidemic*, pp. 41-42

83. Smokers of cigarettes with higher tar yields is associated with an increased risk for acute myocardial infarction (heart attack), and there is a dose-response relationship between total tar consumption per day and heart attack.
Archives of Internal Medicine 2002; 162:300

84. During the 1980s and early 1990s, the rate of heart attacks in women increased by 36%, at a time when heart attacks in men declined by 8%. The increase in smoking in women was one of the major factors cited in the study from the Mayo Clinic.
2002 AMA Annual Tobacco Report

85. Cigarette smoking affects endothelial (blood vessel) nitric oxide biosynthesis and, in a study from the June 2002 issue of the Journal of the American College of Cardiology, light smokers had similar detrimental effects on the nitric oxide biosynthetic pathway as did heavy smokers. These data may have important implications concerning the amount of active cigarette exposure that impacts cardiovascular risk.
2003 AMA Annual Tobacco Report

86. 55% of deaths from cerebrovascular disease among women younger than 65 years, and 6% of deaths from CVD in older women, are attributable to smoking. *Women and Smoking*, 2001 Surgeon General report, p. 239

87. The excess risk for coronary heart disease associated with smoking is reduced by 25 to 50% after one year of abstinence; after 10 to 15 years, the risk declines to that of never smokers.
*Women and Smoking*, 2001 Surgeon General report, p. 233

88. "Smoking is a strong, independent risk factor for arteriosclerotic peripheral vascular disease among women."
*Women and Smoking*, 2001 Surgeon General report, p. 244

89. In studies from the 1980's, women who smoked and used oral contraceptives (with higher doses than those used at present) had a risk of heart attack about 10 times that of women without these two risk factors.
*Women and Smoking*, 2001 Surgeon General report, p. 237

90. The relative risk for death from abdominal aortic aneurysm is 3.9 among current women smokers compared with never smokers. *Women and Smoking*, 2001 Surgeon General report, p. 247

91. "You're a social smoker, no more than one or two a day, or at night at a bar. No harm in that, right? Wrong." A study from the Journal of the American College of Cardiology suggests that even light smoking has dangers. One or two cigarettes a day limits the ability of blood vessels to dilate, the same limitation as in heavy smokers, and this can be the first step toward arterial plaque buildup.
U.S. News and World Report, June 17, 2002, p. 57

92. Cigarette smoking may account for as much as two thirds of the incidence of coronary heart disease among women younger than age 50. About 41% of deaths from coronary heart disease among U.S. women younger than age 65 years of age, and 12% among women older than age 65, are attributable to cigarette smoking.
*Women and Smoking*, 2001 Surgeon General report, p. 232

93. Smoking cigarettes with higher tar yields is associated in a dose-response relationship with an increased risk for myocardial infarction. Archives of Internal Medicine, February 11, 2002, p. 300

94. Smoking cessation reduces blood pressure and heart rate; in smokers who quit for at least six weeks, the blood pressure decreased an average of 5.3 mm of mercury, and the heart rate decreased an average of 7 beats per minute. Journal of the American Society of Hypertension, September 2001

95. Smoking a cigarette typically increases blood pressure by 5 to 10 mm Hg for 15 to 30 minutes and increases heart rate for up to an hour, with average increases of 10 to 20 beats/minute; however, hypertension is not more

prevalent in cigarette smokers compared with nonsmokers. This is probably because blood pressure is typically measured in most studies at a time when the subject has not recently been smoking.

Quote from Nicotine and Public Health, p. 67

96. Successful smoking cessation reduces systolic blood pressure and heart rate during the daytime (when patients typically smoke). American Journal of Hypertension 2001; 14:942-949

97. The first cigarette of the day increases the heart rate by 10 to 20 beats per minute.

Cigarettes (Parker-Pope), p. 68

98. The relative risk of heart attack associated with high blood pressure is far greater in women who smoke than in male smokers. "… female smokers in the highest tertile had an adjusted risk of acute MI that was 4.8-fold greater than those whose systolic blood pressure was less than 140 mmHg. Women smokers in the intermediate blood pressure category had twice the MI risk of smokers in the lowest tertile."

Internal Medicine News, August 15, 2000, p. 21

# Facial Wrinkling and "Smoker's Face"

1. .Smoking is associated with prominent and premature facial wrinkling and aging, particularly in the periorbital ("crow's foot") and perioral areas of the face. Chest, May 1986, p. 622

2. Smokers in their forties have facial wrinkles similar to those of nonsmokers in their sixties. Skin damage occurs because of smoking-induced constriction of blood vessels, leading to skin atrophy, leathery-looking skin, and the wrinkling. Smoker's skin also has less elastin, which allows the skin to stretch. *Cigarettes*, pp. 30-31

3. "Smokers in the age group from 40 to 49 years frequently have facial wrinkles that are similar to those of nonsmokers who are 20 years older."

Mayo Clinic Family Health Guide, David Lasson, William Morrow & Company, 1996, p. 318

4. Because of premature wrinkling of the facial skin caused by circulatory problems, smokers look 5 years older on average than their actual chronological age. Dean Edell, M.D., ABC radio, March 21, 1994

5. In a study from London of sets of twins, one of whom smoked and the other did not, the smoking twin had skin an average of 25% thinner than the nonsmoker; in several cases, the difference was 40%. Thinning accounts for the premature wrinkling and aging of the skin seen in smokers. Associated Press, January 13, 1997

6. Smokers have significantly more elastosis in their facial skin than nonsmokers; this increased elastotic material may cause the gray hue and prominent wrinkling associated with "smoker's face."

Skin and Allergy News, December 1999

7. Characteristics of "smoker's face" include increased wrinkling, gauntness, and discoloration. An increase in elastotic material, or elastosis, may contribute to the clinical features of "smoker's face."

Journal of the American Academy of Dermatology 1999; 41:23

8. "Scientists say they have discovered why smokers look older than nonsmokers: smokers' skins lose elasticity and wrinkle. Dermatologists claim that simply looking at a person's face can show whether he or she is a smoker. The underlying reason is that smoking activates the genes responsible for a skin enzyme that breaks down collagen in the skin. Thus, smokers look much older."

ASH Smoking and Health Review, May-June 2001, p. 6

# Stroke

1. The risk of stroke is increased by four times for smokers less than 65 years old, and smoking is the cause for about half of all strokes in this population. Executive Health Report, July 1990

2.  Smokers have almost twice the risk of dying of stroke. About 400,000 Americans suffer strokes each year, and 50 to 55 percent are directly related to cigarette smoking.
    *Journal of Respiratory Disease*, May 1993, p. 628, and *New York Times*, November 2, 1993, p. A13

3.  Smokers of more than one pack a day have an 11-fold increased risk of subarachnoid brain hemorrhage, or one variety of stroke. 38% of subarachnoid hemorrhages are attributable to current smoking. The excess risk for stroke largely disappears between two and four years after cessation in former smokers.
    *Stroke* 1992; 23:1242 and *American College of Physicians Journal Club*, July 1993, p. 27

4.  The risk for subarachnoid hemorrhage is increased 5.7-fold in smokers.
    *Clinics in Chest Medicine*, December 1991, p. 664

5.  In young adults age 15 to 45 years, a smoker was 1.6 times more likely to have an ischemic stroke, or cerebral infarction, than a nonsmoker.
    *Archives of Neurology* 1990; 47:693

6.  Cigarette smoking accounts for 51% in men and 55% in women of the total risk for cerebrovascular disease (stroke) for those under age 65. Women who smoke have a 5.7-fold increased risk for stroke.
    *Journal of the American Medical Association*, February 19, 1988, p. 1026

7.  Women under age 45 with migraine headaches and who smoke have an 11.7 times greater risk of stroke.
    *USA Today*, February 15, 1993

8.  Smokers under age 65 have a threefold increased risk of coronary heart disease and more than a fourfold risk of having a stroke.
    *Journal of the National Cancer Institute*, August 21, 1991, p. 1145

9.  Current smokers have 3.7-fold increased risk of stroke compared with never smokers.
    *Journal of the American Medical Association*, July 12, 1995, p. 155

10. Tobacco is responsible for 26,500 stroke deaths a year in the US.
    *US News and World Report*, January 23, 1989, p. 9

11. Over a quarter of strokes, at least 61,500 each year, could be prevented if people stopped smoking. The total yearly savings could be about $3 billion.
    *Cigarettes*, p. 102

12. Smoking increases the risk for carotid artery disease and transient ischemic attacks, or "warning" strokes.
    *Cigarettes*, p. 103

13. Smoking increases the risk for both the hemorrhagic and occlusive/ischemic type of stroke.  *Cigarettes*, p. 103

14. "Cigarette smoking accelerates atherosclerosis and promotes acute ischemic events. The mechanisms of effects of smoking are not fully elucidated but are believed to include (1) hemodynamic stress: nicotine increases heart rate and transiently increases blood pressure; (2) endothelial injury; (3) development of an atherogenic lipid profile: smokers have on average higher LDL, more oxidized LDL, and lower HDL cholesterol than nonsmokers; (4) enhanced coagulability; (5) arrhythmogenesis; and (6) relative hypoxemia due to effects of carbon monoxide. Carbon monoxide reduces the capacity of hemoglobin to carry oxygen and impairs the release of oxygen from hemoglobin to body tissues, resulting in a state of relative hypoxemia. To compensate for this hypoxemic state, smokers develop polycythemia, with hematocrits often 50% or more. The polycythemia also increases blood viscosity, which adds to the risk of thrombotic events."
    *Cecil Textbook of Medicine*, 1996 edition, p. 34

15. In a study from Australia, the risk for ischemic stroke was twice as high for nonsmokers whose spouses smoked as for those whose spouses did not smoke.    *American Journal of Public Health*, April 1999, p. 572

16. The relative risk of stroke among hypertensive smokers is five times that of smokers without hypertension, and 20 times that of normotensive nonsmokers. The British Regional Heart Study showed a relative risk for stroke of 3.7 in all current smokers.    *British Medical Journal*, October 10, 1998, p. 962

17. Smokers have more than a five-fold increased risk for subarachnoid hemorrhage of the brain; the risk persists even after smoking cessation.                                                     Neurosurgery 2001; 49:607-613

18. In a study from Johns Hopkins, current smoking increased the risk for subarachnoid hemorrhage by a factor of 5.2 times. The increased risk in former smokers remained high at 4.5 odds ratio. Hypertension is the other major risk factor for this type of brain hemorrhage.                          Neurosurgery, August 2001, pp. 607-613

19. There is a two to threefold excess risk for ischemic stroke and subarachnoid hemorrhage among women who smoke compared to nonsmokers.                          *Women and Smoking*, 2001 Surgeon General report, p. 240

# CHAPTER 10
# CHRONIC OBSTRUCTIVE PULMONARY DISEASE (COPD), EMPHYSEMA, AND OTHER LUNG DISEASE

1. About 15% of one pack per day and 25% of two pack per day cigarette smokers will eventually develop COPD if they continue their habit.                                                   *The Tobacco Epidemic*, p. 85

2. Chronic obstructive pulmonary disease (COPD) is the fourth leading cause of death in the US, with a mortality of more than 90,000 in 1991. Almost 13 million Americans are diagnosed with COPD, probably an underestimate, and the annual cost in direct and indirect medical expenses for the disease is more than $12 billion.                                        Journal of the American Medical Association, November 16, 1994, p. 1539

3. There are 14 million patients with COPD (chronic obstructive pulmonary disease) in the United States, an increase of 40% since 1982. 1.5 million of these have emphysema; the rest have the chronic bronchitis type of COPD. It is the fourth leading cause of death by diagnosis in this country, and mortality from COPD has increased by 71% since 1982. 80 to 90% of cases are caused by smoking, and the increased risk is thirty-fold for heavy smokers compared to nonsmokers. Only about 15% of smokers develop overt COPD. However, all smokers have an accelerated loss of pulmonary function with increasing age, and more than half of one pack per day middle age smokers complain of chronic cough.
                                    Michael S. Stulbarg, M.D. Audio Digest Internal Medicine, November 6, 1996

4. Mean lung function measured by FEVI (forced expiratory volume in one second) averages 23% lower in male smokers and 18% lower in female smokers compared with never smokers of the same age and height. Measurement of lung function identifies smokers at increased risk of disease and death, and the concept of "lung age" (telling a smoker "you have the lung capacity of nonsmoking 70-year-old") may have a powerful effect in motivating smoking cessation.
                                    Journal of the American Medical Association, June 2, 1993, pp. 2741 and 2785

5. In COPD, patients who are successful in smoking cessation experience an actual improvement in lung function over the first 2 to 3 years after quitting, as well as a decrease in the rate of age-related decline of lung function thereafter.                    Journal of the American Medical Association, November 16, 1994, p. 1540

6. If Americans did not smoke, there would be 85% less emphysema and chronic bronchitis, 90% less lung cancer, and 33% less heart disease.

7. Chronic obstructive pulmonary disease was the fourth leading cause of death in 1997, with 109,029 deaths, or 4.7% of the total. The top three were heart disease, cancer, and cerebrovascular disease.
                                    CA-A Cancer Journal for Clinicians, January-February 2000, p. 22

8. There are 15 million Americans with COPD. This is now the fifth leading cause of death in the United States, deaths from COPD have increased by 22% in the last decade, and there is a 50% total mortality in the 10 years after diagnosis, the same mortality as breast cancer.
                                    Allan Siefkin, M.D., lecture in San Francisco, April 14, 1999

9. Chronic obstructive pulmonary disease – emphysema and chronic bronchitis – is the leading cause of death in China, with a mortality rate five times that of the United States. Air pollution, much from coal smoke, kills at least 1.9 million people a year in the country, and cigarettes account for only 50% of the lung cancer risk (compared to 90% in Western countries); the greater air pollution accounts for the rest.
                                    World Bank data reported in *Earth Odyssey*, Mark Hertsgaard, Broadway Books, 1998, pp. 162 and 177

10. The total cost for COPD in the United States in 1993 was $25 billion, including $15 billion in direct medical costs.                    Bartolome Celli, M.D., American Academy of Allergy lecture, San Diego, March 2000

11. In the United States, an estimated 16 million persons had COPD in 1994, a 60% increase from 1982. In 1993, COPD was the fourth most common cause of death, causing 95,910 deaths, more than twice the 47,335 deaths

in 1979. For unknown reasons, only about 15% of cigarette smokers develop clinically significant COPD. In COPD patients with FEV1, less than 0.75 liters (about 20% of predicted), the mortality rate is 30% at one year and 95% at ten years. *The Merck Manual*, Mark Beers and Robert Berkow, Editors, 1999 edition, pp. 569-575

12. More than 90% of patients with the diagnosis of pulmonary eosinophilic granuloma are current or past cigarette smokers. *Textbook of Respiratory Medicine*, John Murray and Jay Nadel, editors, W.B. Saunders, 1994, p. 1927

13. A study from Northern California showed a strong association between smoking and adult respiratory distress syndrome (ARDS), a rapidly progressive syndrome of lung injury with an overall fatality rate of 40 to 60%. The authors concluded that approximately 50% of ARDS cases were attributable to cigarette smoking. Chest, January 2000, p. 163

14. Smoking is a risk factor for active tuberculosis in British, but not American, studies. John Slade, M.D.

15. "Smokers suffer more – and more severe – respiratory infections than do nonsmokers. In one study, college students who smoked had more coughs, more acute and chronic phlegm production, more wheezing and more lower respiratory tract symptoms with their colds. Pneumonia is not only more common, but much more likely to be fatal among smokers of any age. Among high-risk or medically compromised adults, the risk of pneumococcal infection is approximately four times as high among those who smoke. Among pregnant women who contract pneumonia, those who smoke more than 10 cigarettes per day are more likely to have an adverse outcome (defined as maternal-fetal death, preterm delivery, fetal death and early miscarriage)." *Cigarettes*, p. 10

16. A September 2001 study from Finland in the journal Thorax found that the natural decline in forced expiratory volume in 0.75 seconds, a measure of lung function, was 46.4 ml/year in never smokers, and 66 ml per year in current (continuous) smokers.

17. In a study from Finland, the decline in lung function measured by forced expiratory volume in 0.75 seconds was 46 milliliters a year in never smokers compared to 66ml in current smokers. Former smokers had intermediate values. (All adults lose lung function as they age.) Thorax, September 2001 (from 2002 AMA Annual Tobacco Report)

18. About 90% of mortality from COPD among American women is attributable to cigarette smoking. *Women and Smoking*, 2001 Surgeon General report, p. 261

19. 10 million Americans are diagnosed with COPD, which includes emphysema and chronic bronchitis, and another 14 million have it but are not yet diagnosed. In 1980, 37,000 men and 16,000 women died from COPD; in 2000, deaths had increased to 59,000 men and 60,000 women. NBC evening news, August 2, 2002 (data from Centers for Disease Control)

20. By the year 2020, COPD will be the third leading cause of death in the world. Bartolome Celli, M.D., 2000 meeting of the American College of Chest Physicians

21. There are 100,000 yearly deaths from COPD in the United States, the third leading cause of death, and 17 to 18 million people with COPD in the country. In 2020, it is expected to be the third leading cause of death worldwide. Nonsmokers lose 15 to 20 milliliters of lung capacity each year with aging; smokers may lose 60 to 100 milliliters. COPD patients requiring oxygen therapy have a two year mortality of 50%. Samuel Louie, M.D., lecture, University of California, Davis, October 24, 2002

22. 600 million people worldwide have COPD or "smoker's lung," and it causes 3 million deaths each year. Associated Press, September 3, 2000

23. Pipe and cigar smokers have mortality rates from COPD that are intermediate between those of cigarette smokers and nonsmokers. *Nicotine and Public Health*, p. 191

24. The number of Americans who have diagnosed COPD increased from 7.1 million in 1980 to 10.5 million in 2000, and deaths more than doubled, rising from 52,000 to more than 119,000. 2000 was also the first year where more women than men died of COPD.  Respiratory Reviews, October 2002, p. 17

25. COPD is the fourth leading cause of mortality in the United States (112,009 deaths in 2000), yet it ranks only 27th in research funding. The other top causes are heart disease (711,000), cancer (553,000), stroke (168,000), accidents (98,000), diabetes (69,000), influenza and pneumonia (65,000), and Alzheimer's disease (49,600). More women than men now die from COPD, and both COPD prevalence and mortality are greatly under reported.  Advanced Studies in Medicine
(Johns Hopkins University), February 2003, pp. 587-90

# CHAPTER 11
# OTHER HEALTH PROBLEMS

**Includes cataracts and eye problems, depression, AIDS risk, thyroid disease, diabetes, ulcers, osteoporosis and fractures, and surgical complications**

1.  "For more than 300 years tobacco has given solace, relaxation, and enjoyment to mankind. At one time or another during those years, critics have held it responsible for practically every disease of the human body. One by one these charges have been abandoned for lack of evidence."
    From 1954 full page ad "Frank Statement to Cigarette Smokers" (Washington Post, May 11, 1997, p. C2)

2.  There are over 70,000 medical articles detailing the dangers of smoking.                *Cigarettes*, p. xiii

## Influenza, Snoring, and Infections

1.  24% of pneumonia and influenza deaths are attributable to smoking..        JAMA, November 10, 1993, p. 2208

2.  Smoking more than doubles the risk for an elderly woman of dying from pneumonia.
    Journal of the National Cancer Institute, June 2000, pp. 799-804

3.  Smoking increases vulnerability to influenza. In one outbreak of influenza among 336 men in a military unit, 68.5 percent of current and occasional smokers suffered influenza, as compared with 47.2 percent of never and former smokers. Overall, smoking is thought to play a significant role in 31 percent of all influenza cases and 41 percent of severe cases. Vaccination against influenza is less effective in smokers, and the death rate among smokers who suffer influenza is much higher than among nonsmokers.                *Cigarettes*, p. 10

4.  Invasive pneumococcal infection is strongly associated with cigarette smoking (odds ratio 4.1); 51% of the disease burden in smokers is attributable to their smoking.
    New England Journal of Medicine, March 9, 2000, pp. 681-9

5.  Smokers are four times more likely than nonsmokers to develop pneumococcal (caused by the bacteria streptococcus pneumoniae) sepsis or meningitis. Nonsmokers exposed to passive smoke on a frequent basis had a 2.5-fold increased risk, and heavy smokers (at least 25 cigarettes a day) had a 5.5-fold increased risk.
    San Francisco Chronicle, March 9, 2000 (from the NEJM, same date)

6.  Although cigarette smoking is known to have detrimental effect on the immune system, the nature of the immunosuppression is poorly understood. In a joint study from Denver and Boston, it was found that cigarette smoke contains potent inhibitors of cytokine production. Cytokines play important roles in the host defense against infection and cancer.        Journal of Allergy and Clinical Immunology, August 2000, pp. 280-287

7.  One alteration in the immune system of babies with passive smoke exposure is a significant reduction in natural killer-cell activity. The clinical significance of this alteration is not known, but could be involved in the increased incidence of lower respiratory tract viral infection and childhood cancer observed in infants exposed to passive smoke.                Journal of Allergy and Clinical Immunology, January 1999, p. 172,
    and Respiratory Reviews, April 1999

8.  Smokers have an increased risk of acquiring epidemic influenza, a decreased immune response to influenza vaccination, a decreased response to hepatitis B vaccine, and an apparent increased risk of varicella pneumonia.        *Cigarettes*, p. 160, and Clinics in Chest Medicine, December 1991, p. 649

9.  Cigarettes (both tobacco and marijuana) are commonly contaminated with fungi, especially Aspergillus fumigatus, and invasive aspergillosis remains a significant cause of illness and death in patients who are immunocompromised. There have not been fungal spores isolated in the tobacco smoke itself.
    JAMA, December 13, 2000, p. 2875

10. In a study of teenagers with primary pulmonary tuberculosis, 42% admitted to being smokers.

Chest 1974; 65:100

11. Persistent smoking increases the risk for snoring in men, with an odds ratio of 1.4 (40% increased incidence).

Chest 1998; 114:1048-1055

12. Smokers of more than 15 cigarettes a day are 6.5 times more likely to be frequent snorers. *Cigarettes*, p. 118

13. Current smokers have a 2.3-fold greater risk of snoring and 4.44-fold increased risk of moderate or severe sleep-disordered breathing as compared to never-smokers. Heavy smokers of two packs a day or more increase their risk for moderate or severe sleep-disordered breathing by a factor of 40.47 times.

Archives of Internal Medicine, October 10, 1994, p. 2219

14. Smoking may represent a risk factor for immunoglobulin G deficiency, and an increased risk for respiratory bacterial infections. Annals of Allergy, May 1993, p. 418

15. Smokers have about 30% higher white blood cell counts, perhaps reflecting the increase in number of infections they have. They also have impaired neutrophil function, fewer natural killer cells, an increased number of eosinophils, and decreased amounts of the immunoglobulins IgA and IgG in saliva.

*Cigarettes*, pp. 158-159

# Cataracts and Eye Problems

1. Smoking triggers 200,000 of the one million yearly cases in the United States of cataracts, the leading cause of blindness. This costs the nation $800 million in extra Medicare services. But Philip Morris funds Helen Keller Services for the Blind and Entertainment for the Blind. World Smoking and Health No. 1, 1993, p. 2

2. Cataracts cause visual impairment in 3 million Americans, a million of whom have operations each year to have clouded lenses removed from their eyes. Smoking causes 20% of these cases; male smokers of a pack a day or more double their risk of cataract, and women smokers have a 60% greater risk.

JAMA, August 26, 1992, p. 989 and Time, September 7, 1992, p. 22

3. Age-related macular degeneration involves a deterioration of the center of the visual field, causing a roughly circular area of blindness that gradually grows larger. It is responsible for at least 1.7 million cases of impaired vision in Americans over 65, and is the leading cause of new cases of blindness in that age group. Smoking increases the risk of this condition by two to three times; almost one third of cases are attributable to smoking.

Associated Press, October 9, 1996 (from JAMA issue same date)

4. As compared to nonsmokers, smokers are 2.5 times more likely to develop age-related macular degeneration, which is untreatable and blinding in most cases, and up to 3 times more likely to develop cataract. The increased risk of blindness should be added to the better-known arguments against smoking.

Survey of Ophthalmology 1998; 42:535-547

5. Current smokers of a pack a day or more had double the risk of cataract compared with never smokers. While some smoking-related damage to the lens may be reversible in smokers who quit, smoking cessation reduces the risk of cataract primarily by limiting the total dose-related damage to the lens.

JAMA, August 9, 2000, p. 713

# Depression and Psychiatric Problems

1. There is a strong positive correlation between smoking and depression, and a study from the Harvard School of Public Health found that in a population of nurses, those smoking 1 to 25 cigarettes per day had twice the risk of committing suicide. The group smoking 25 or more cigarettes had four times the risk of suicide when compared to the nonsmokers. JAMA, September 1990, p. 1541

2.	In a study of 6863 adolescents ages 12 to 18 in the United States, smoking status was a significant predictor for developing symptoms of depression. Overall, 18.8% of "current established smokers" developed depressive symptoms, compared to 9.8% of nonsmokers. The odds ratio for depression was 1.86 for male and 2.05 for female smokers (1.00 for never smokers).	*Annals of Behavioral Medicine* 1997; 19(1):42-50

3.	In a study from Australia, subjects reporting high levels of depression and anxiety were twice as likely to be smokers.	*Archives of General Psychiatry* 1998; 55:161

4.	Among patients seeking smoking cessation treatment, as many as 25 to 40% have a past history of major depression. This is triple the rate for nonsmoking adults.
	*American Journal of Psychiatry*, October 1996 supplement, p. 21

5.	Dr. Cynthia Pomerleau from the University of Michigan Substance Research Center has evidence that many longtime smokers have an underlying psychiatric problem that nicotine may help to ameliorate. Nicotine can either sedate or stimulate, helping a person with anxiety to relax, but stimulate a depressed patient. The psychiatric disorder can be unmasked or worsened by nicotine withdrawal, which leads to higher relapse and lower successful quit rates. Different studies have shown (compared with people with no psychiatric disorder) rates of nicotine dependence twice as high among those with anxiety disorder as well as the diagnosis of attention deficit hyperactivity disorder, and smoking rates three times as high among those with major depression.	*New York Times*, August 27, 1997, p. C8

6.	History of daily smoking increases significantly (odds ratio 1.9) the risk for major depression.
	*Archives of General Psychiatry* 1998; 55:161

7.	Major depression is more common among smokers (6.6% versus 2.9%), and smokers with a history of depression are less likely to have succeeded in smoking cessation than were smokers without such a history (14% versus 28%). Depressed smokers are 40% less likely to quit than non-depressed ones and they are more likely to relapse. The overwhelming majority of alcoholics are smokers, and co-morbidity with major depression is high.	*American Journal of Psychiatry*, April 1993, p. 547, and October 1993, p. 1547

8.	Smokers who have histories of major depression are only half as likely to be successful long-term quitters as smokers without depression. Also, major depression is much more common among smokers than nonsmokers.
	*Journal of the American Medical Women's Association*, January 1996, p. 39

9.	Seriously depressed young people are more likely than others to become daily smokers, and the tobacco habit itself can also raise the risk of depression. A study from Case Western Reserve University in Cleveland published in the February 1998 issue of the Archives of General Psychiatry concluded that the link between smoking and depression is a "two way street."	*San Francisco Chronicle*, February 12, 1998, p. A3

10.	An estimated 30-40% of people who begin smoking cessation programs are depressed, or about three times the rate of depression in nonsmokers. In another study, 74% of patients with schizophrenia smoked.
	*Cigarettes*, p. 114

11.	About a third of smokers have a history of major depression, compared with a lifetime prevalence of 10% to 15% in the general population. They tend to have only about half the success rate in smoking cessation as do smokers without a history of depression. 75% of smokers with a history of major depression developed depressive symptoms during withdrawal, which quickly disappeared when the patient returned to smoking. 30% of smokers without a positive history of depression developed these symptoms during withdrawal. In a St. Louis epidemiologic study, major depression was more than twice as common in smokers, and 76% of subjects with a history of depression had ever smoked, compared to 52% without a history of depression.
	Mayo Clinic Nicotine Dependence Conference (Paul Frederickson, M.D.),
	May 13, 1997, and *Journal of Clinical Psychiatry*, October 1996, p. 468

12.	Research suggest that cigarette smoke inhibits the activity of monoamine oxidase B (MAOB); this inhibition may lead to a rise in the brain levels of phenylethylamine, a neuroactive compound linked to schizophrenia as well as other psychiatric disorders.	*Reuters Medical News*, October 7, 1997

13. Nicotine may improve cognitive functioning in schizophrenia; 75 to 90% of schizophrenics are smokers.
    Paul Newhouse, M.D., Tenth National Conference on Nicotine Dependence, Minneapolis, October 17, 1997

14. As many as three quarters of all schizophrenics are smokers; other data report that between 80% and 90% of all hospitalized schizophrenics are smokers. *Tobacco*, pp. 85-86

15. The prevalence of cigarette smoking can be as high as 90% among persons with schizophrenia.
    Epidemiologic Reviews 1995; 17:56

16. Smokers have more sleep difficulties than do nonsmokers and tend to exhibit more depression, irritability, and anxiety.          Goodman and Gilman's *The Pharmacological Basis of Therapeutics*, 1990 edition, p. 547

17. Smoking quadruples the risk of panic attacks – sudden onset of overwhelming feelings of anxiety, heart palpitations, and shortness of breath.
    Time, December 27, 1999, p. 180 (from December 1999 Archives of General Psychiatry)

18. Persons with mental illness are about twice as likely to smoke as other persons, but have substantial quit rates.
    JAMA, November 22/28, 2000, p. 2606

19. The association between depression and smoking is unresolved, with different conclusions whether smoking may be a causal factor in depression, or whether depressed people smoke to "self-medicate" with nicotine. A study in the Australia New Zealand Journal of Psychiatry (June 2001, p. 329) concluded that cigarette smoking and depression may be linked by shared early deprivational variables, rather than cigarette smoking causing depression or vice-versa.          2002 AMA Annual Tobacco Report

20. Cigarette smoking may increase the risk of certain anxiety disorders during late adolescence and early adulthood. These include generalized anxiety disorder, panic disorder and agoraphobia.
    JAMA, November 8, 2000, p. 2348

21. About two-thirds of gamblers seeking treatment are daily cigarette smokers, and smoking status is associated with more severe gambling and psychiatric symptoms.          Addiction 2002; 97:745-753

22. 44% of cigarettes sold in the U.S. are smoked by people with a diagnosable mental illness such as depression or alcohol abuse.          Time, December 4, 2000, p. 29

23. People with diagnosable mental illness account for nearly 45% of the total cigarette market in the United States, estimated a report from the Harvard Medical School          Reuters, November 21, 2000

# HIV

1. HIV-seropositive patients who smoke have a substantially increased risk for developing bacterial pneumonia compared with nonsmokers with HIV infection.          JAMA, August 17, 1994, p. 564

2. Smoking is an independent risk factor for invasive pneumococcal infection in patients with HIV, who already have an extremely high incidence of pneumococcal disease.
    New England Journal of Medicine, July 20, 2000, p. 220

3. In HIV positive patients, progression time to full-blown AIDS is significantly reduced in smokers (mean 8.2 months) compared to nonsmokers (mean 14.5 months). Smokers also developed pneumocystis pneumonia more rapidly (9 months) compared to 16 months for nonsmokers.
    Tobacco Control, Spring 1993, p. 157

4. HIV-infected patients who smoke develop full-blown AIDS twice as quickly as nonsmokers infected with HIV. In a four year study period, smokers with the virus were nearly twice as likely to die of AIDS.
    American Medical News, June 14, 1993

# Thyroid Disease

1. Smoking decreases both thyroid secretion and thyroid hormone action in women with hypothyroidism. Smoking does not cause hypothyroidism, but increases its severity. The most dramatic effect of smoking on the thyroid is its association with Graves' hyperthyroidism. The odds ratio for smoking among patients with Graves' hyperthyroidism with and without opthalmopathy were 7.7 and 1.9, respectively, and smokers had more severe eye disease.                                                  NEJM, October 12, 1995, p. 1001

2. Graves' disease is associated with an overactive thyroid gland and often a swelling of muscles behind the eyes that makes them bulge out (as with the actor, the late Marty Feldman). 81% of a survey population with Graves' disease were smokers, and the incidence of the disease was 7.7 times higher in smokers. Of the 27 people with the worst form of the disease, 26 were smokers.          American Medical News, February 1, 1993

3. Smoking and goiter (thyroid gland enlargement) are strongly associated in countries with iodine deficiency. In a study from Denmark, the prevalence of thyroid enlargement and palpable, visible goiter was 10.8% and 1.1% among nonsmokers and 28.4% and 4% among heavy smokers, respectively. Thiocyanate, which inhibits iodine transport and is present in cigarette smoke, is thought to be a contributor to thyroid enlargement caused by iodine deficiency.
   Respiratory Reviews, May 2002, p. 2 (from February 25, 2002 Archives of Internal Medicine)

# Diabetes

1. In a study from Japan, men who smoked had a 3.27 times higher risk of developing non-insulin-dependent diabetes.                                              American Journal of Epidemiology, January 15, 1997

2. A study of adult onset (Type 2) diabetics in Italy found that smokers had double the risk of premature death (1.3% annual death rate) compared to nonsmoking adult onset diabetics (0.6% annual death rate).
   San Antonio Express, November 6, 1997 from American Society of Nephrology annual meeting

3. Smoking appears to increase the risk for developing diabetes, and is also an important risk factor for insulin resistance.                                                                             *Cigarettes*, pp. 138-139

4. In a study from the Harvard School of Public Health, the relative risk of diabetes was 1.42 among women who smoked 25 or more cigarettes per day compared with nonsmokers. In another study of middle-aged Dutch men, the relative risk of diabetes was 3.3 times the risk in nonsmokers.
   American Journal of Public Health, February 1993, p. 211

5. Young diabetics who smoke are two to three times more likely to develop kidney damage and renal failure than nonsmoking diabetics.                                                      JAMA, February 6, 1991, p. 614

6. Diabetic smokers have significantly higher blood pressure and heart rates compared to nonsmokers with diabetes. This suggests that smoking acts as one of the risk factors for development of kidney disease through elevated blood pressure.
   Reuters, November 3, 1998, from the September 1998 American Journal of Hypertension

7. Children of mothers who smoked after the fourth month of pregnancy are much more likely to develop early onset (before age 33) type 2 diabetes than were the children of nonsmokers. The offspring of moderate and heavy smokers had more than a fourfold increased risk of type 2 diabetes.
   Respiratory Reviews, March 2002, p. 1

8. In a study from Boston on smoking and diabetes (American Journal of Medicine 2000; 109:538), the risk of type 2 diabetes in men was 70% and 50% higher among current smokers of 20 or more cigarettes a day, and less than 20 cigarettes, respectively, compared with nonsmokers.

9. In a study from Japan, men who smoked more than 31 cigarettes a day were four times as likely as nonsmokers to develop diabetes.                    Time, August 14, 2000, p. 86 (from Annals of Internal Medicine, August 2000)

10. Smoking is an independent risk factor for the development of type 2 diabetes mellitus; the adjusted relative risk is 1.7 for current smokers of a pack a day or more, and 1.5 for lighter smokers.
                        American Journal of Medicine 2000; 109: 538-542

11. Smoking induces albuminuria (protein in the urine) and accelerates progression to renal (kidney) failure in persons with diabetes. In a study from the Netherlands, smoking was also associated with albuminuria and abnormal renal function in nondiabetics.                    Annals of Internal Medicine 2000; 133: 585-591

# Parkinson's, Alzheimer's, Hearing Loss

1. 25 different diseases and causes of death are significantly associated with cigarette smoking, 24 positively and one negatively.                    British Medical Journal, October 8, 1994, p. 909

2. Smoking is a major risk factor for 7 of the top 14 causes of death for people older than age 65.
                        *Nicotine Addiction* p. 385

3. Nicotine is of therapeutic benefit in ulcerative colitis and perhaps also in Parkinson's disease.
                North Carolina Medical Journal, January 1995, p. 48 and NEJM, March 24, 1994, p. 811

4. Smokers have only half the risk of nonsmokers of developing Parkinson's disease.
                        JAMA, April 24, 1996, p. 1217

5. Nicotine can improve some aspects of memory in patients with Alzheimer's disease.
                        *Nicotine Safety and Toxicity*, p. 141

6. In a study from the Netherlands, smokers were more than twice as likely (relative risk 2.3) to develop Alzheimer's disease as are nonsmokers.                    The Lancet, June 20, 1998, pp. 1840-43

7. In a study from the Netherlands of people age 65 and older who did not have dementia, those who smoked were more likely to have impairment in short term memory, time and place orientation, attention and calculation compared to people who had never smoked.            San Diego Union-Tribune, October 5, 1998

8. A medical research organization in the United Kingdom has accepted a donation of $220,000 from British American Tobacco. The money is being used to examine effects of nicotine on the brain and to compare brains of smokers and non-smokers, after several epidemiological studies suggested that smokers may have a lower incidence of Alzheimer's dementia and Parkinson's disease.
                        British Medical Journal, September 7, 1996, p. 577

9. There is an inverse dose-response relationship between Parkinson's disease and smoking, providing indirect evidence that smoking is biologically protective.                    JAMA, April 7, 1999, p. 1154

10. Smoking is protective against Parkinson's disease; 34 of 35 studies show this effect, and it appears not to be an artifact, although the mechanism for the protection is unclear. Current smokers have only 50% of the risk compared to nonsmokers, and former smokers show intermediate protection.            Paul Newhouse, M.D.,
                Tenth National Conference on Nicotine Dependence, Minneapolis, October 17, 1997

11. Nicotine patch therapy shows promise in the treatment of children with Tourette's syndrome, a condition affecting 100,000 people in the United States and marked by facial tics and often uncontrollable movements and vocalizations.                    San Francisco Chronicle, February 22, 2000, p. A2

12. Cigarette smoking may play a role in age-related hearing loss. In a study from Wisconsin of 3700 adults ages 48 and older, current cigarette smokers were 1.7 times as likely to have hearing loss as nonsmokers.

JAMA, June 3, 1998, p. 1715

13. In a study of Japanese men, smokers were much more likely to have hearing impairment, particularly high frequency hearing loss. Journal of Occupational and Environmental Medicine 2000; 42:1045-1049

14. Smoking causes long-term but reversible adverse effects on the ability to smell.

JAMA, March 2, 1990, p. 1233

# Dental Problems

1. Smokers are up to four times more likely than nonsmokers to develop gum disease. 46% of smokers ages 19 to 30 compared to 12% of nonsmokers had gum disease. Between ages 31 and 41, 86% of smokers had gum disease compared to 33% of nonsmokers. San Francisco Chronicle, February 1, 1993, p. A4

2. Tobacco use plays a significant role in refractory periodontitis, with tobacco users having a 90% refractory rate, compared to only 30% in non tobacco users. Smokers also have poorer success rates for soft tissue and bone graft procedures and implants. Larry Williams, D.D.S., Norfolk, Virginia

3. In a study from the University of Buffalo, 80% of patients with periodontitis, a gum disease that can lead to the loss of teeth, were smokers of 10 cigarettes a day or more.

Minneapolis-St. Paul Star Tribune, October 12, 1997

4. Tobacco use is a significant risk factor for poor dental health among older adults, including tooth loss, periodontal disease, and cavities or caries. American Journal of Public Health, September 1993, p. 1271

5. Smoking is a strong risk factor for periodontal disease; nicotine is a potent vasoconstrictor, and reduces blood flow to the gingiva, or gums. Independent of oral hygiene, smokers' teeth have more brown staining, plaque accumulation (soft bacterial deposits), and calculus, or calcified deposits on the teeth. *Cigarettes*, p. 130

6. Researchers at Tufts University in Boston have concluded that smoking could double a person's risk of losing teeth; they suspect that cigarette use influences the loss of bone around the teeth.

JAMA, October 23-30, 1996, p. 1292, and Time, November 11, 1996, p. 26

7. Exposure to secondhand smoke can nearly double the risk that children ages 4 through 11 will develop cavities. The nicotine metabolite cotinine is thought to encourage tooth-destroying bacteria to grow and multiply.

Time, May 14, 2001, p. 76 (source cited: Pediatric Academic Society meeting)

8. ETS exposure at home is a risk factor for periodontal disease in nonsmokers; in a study from North Carolina, the adjusted odds ratio was 1.6. American Journal of Public Health, February 2001, p. 253

9. Smokers are four times as likely as nonsmokers to develop gum disease, which is the major risk factor for tooth loss. CBS news, May 30, 2000

10. Smoking is a major risk factor for periodontal disease, with 30 to 75% of cases liked to cigarette smoking.
*Clearing the Smoke*, p. 563

11. 52.8% of periodontitis, or severe gum disease that is one of the main causes of tooth loss, is attributable to current and former smoking. In a study from the Centers of Disease Control, current smokers were about four times more likely than people who have never smoked to have periodontitis. The gum disease destroys the tissue and bone surrounding the teeth, and is usually caused by bacteria contained in plaque buildup. Smoking can suppress the body's immune system, and it also reduces blood flow to the gums. 55% of the study subjects with gum disease were smokers, and 21.8% were former smokers. Associated Press, May 30, 2000
and Reuters, March 6, 2003

# Ulcers

1. In a 1991 study from Sweden, one quarter of peptic ulcers diagnosed for the first time in people ages 35 to 84 were estimated to be caused by smoking. Smokers are more prone to becoming infected with the bacterium Helicobacter pylori that is associated with a greatly increased risk of developing ulcers.

   *Cigarettes*, pp. 146-147

2. Cigarette smoking is associated with an increased risk of developing duodenal ulcer and ulcer-related complications, including delayed ulcer healing and death.

   Annals of Internal Medicine, November 1, 1993, p. 882

3. 20% of peptic ulcer cases in women in the U.S. are attributable to cigarette smoking. Regular smokers were 1.8 times more likely to develop ulcers than never smokers.     Archives of Internal Medicine, July 1990, p. 1437

4. A significant number of former smokers have stopped suffering from heartburn after quitting smoking.

   San Francisco Chronicle, May 9, 1999, p. 8

5. Women who smoke have an increased risk for peptic ulcers and Crohn's disease, and smokers with Crohn's disease have a worse prognosis than do nonsmokers.

   *Women and Smoking*, 2001 Surgeon General report, p. 325

# Osteoporosis

1. Smoking is a moderate risk factor for osteoporosis for both men and women, with a risk nearly 2.5 times that of their nonsmoking counterparts. One of the mechanisms of osteoporosis is smoking-related decrease of estrogen, a mechanism which applies to men as well as women.     *Cigarettes*, p. 63

2. "Cigarette smoking is a risk factor for osteoporosis, reducing the peak bone mass attained in early adulthood and increasing the rate of bone loss in later adulthood. Smoking antagonizes the protective effect of estrogen replacement therapy on the risk of osteoporosis in postmenopausal women."

   Cecil Textbook of Medicine, 1996 edition, p. 35

3. Smoking accelerates bone loss in older women and increases the risk of osteoporosis. It also reduces the protective effect of oral estrogens on osteoporosis.

   9th World Conference on Tobacco or Health, Paris, 1994 (T. Hirayama)

4. Smoking is positively and significantly associated with decreased hip bone mineral density in old age. Bone loss associated with smoking would be expected to increase the risk of hip fracture in those who do not die earlier from another complication of tobacco use.

   American Journal of Public Health, September 1993, p. 1265

5. Although estrogen replacement therapy helps to protect nonsmoking post-menopausal women from hip fracture, smoking may negate the protective effect of estrogen replacement.

   Annals of Internal Medicine, May 1, 1992, p. 716

6. Smokers suffer more fractures because they have higher rates of osteoporosis, or decreased bone density. Back pain is more common in smokers, and surgery to treat back problems, especially spinal fusion, is less successful.     *Cigarettes*, pp. 56-57

7. A nonsmoker's broken leg heals an average 80% faster than a smoker's broken leg. Experts theorize that reduced blood flow in smokers interferes with bone healing.     *Cigarettes*, p. 58

8. Women who smoke have levels of osteoporosis equivalent to about five years of aging, and double their risk for fractures.                               Mayo Clinic Nicotine Dependence Seminar, May 13, 1997

9. Regular exercise and not smoking is important in achieving maximal peak bone mass in adolescents and young adults. In men, smoking had a deleterious effect on bone mineral density, reducing average femoral neck bone mineral density by 9.7% as compared with nonsmokers.         British Medical Journal, July 23, 1994, p. 234

# Fractures

1. Smoking is a major cause of hip fracture, and the effect of smoking on bone mineral density increases cumulatively with age. Smoking has no effect on bone density in women until after the menopause, when smokers lose an additional 0.2% of bone mass each year, or a difference of 6% at age 80. The cumulative risk of hip fracture to age 85 in women is 19% in smokers and 12% in nonsmokers; to age 90 it is 37% and 22%. Among all women, one hip fracture in eight is attributable to smoking. The study from the Royal London School of Medicine concludes as follows. "Smoking in women from the time of the menopause onwards increases the risk of hip fracture in old age by about half. This is an insufficiently recognized major adverse effect of smoking, and it has substantial implications on health care costs. The lower risk in former smokers indicates that stopping smoking prevents further excess bone loss, and stopping at the time of the menopause should avoid the excess risk."                               British Medical Journal, October 4, 1997, pp. 841-845

2. The age-adjusted relative risk for hip fracture among women who smoke appears to be between 1.5 and 2.0.
                               *Women and Smoking*, 2001 Surgeon General report, p. 318

3. In a study from Japan, smoking increased the risk for hip fracture by more than two times for both men and women over age 40.                               *Tobacco and Health*, p. 521

4. One in eight hip fractures, particularly common in elderly women, is attributable to smoking.
                               Reuters, October 3, 1997

5. A speaker at a meeting of the American Academy of Orthopaedic Surgeons reported that nonsmokers' long bone leg fractures healed 80 percent faster than similar fractures in smokers. Nicotine impairs circulation, and poor circulation is the apparent reason for the delayed healing.     San Francisco Examiner, February 26, 1995

4. Giving up cigarettes for seven to ten days after an operation can significantly reduce post-surgical complications.                               U.S. News and World Report, April 24, 1995, p. 70

5. It takes an average of 39 weeks for a bone fracture to heal in a smoker, compared to 21 weeks in a nonsmoker.
                               Health, September 1995, p. 16

6. Smoking is consistently associated with increased risk of vertebral fractures.
                               JAMA, December 20, 1995, p. 1834

7. Smokers are four times more likely than nonsmokers to require surgery to fuse the spine, particularly for problems of the lower back. The time for healing after spinal fusion surgery was much slower for smokers, and the surgery complication rate was higher. Tobacco use leads to bone weakening and a diminution of the production of new, healthy bone cells.                               Reuters Health eLine, July 1997

# Wound Healing and Surgery

1. Smokers have more than double the rate of complications after skin flap surgery to repair facial defects, 37% versus 17%.                               Skin and Allergy News, November 1995, p. 11

2. Smoking delays wound healing, a problem that is especially true for smokers undergoing plastic or reconstructive surgery. Skin flaps have a significantly reduced chance of survival because of impaired blood flow, and in one study, smokers undergoing plastic surgery had a 12.5 times greater risk of unsuccessful

3. Smoking delays wound healing by at least six mechanisms: (1) a decrease of blood flow, (2) carbon monoxide limits oxygen transport to the wound, (3) smoking-induced catecholamines stimulate the formation of chalones, which slow the rate of epithelialization, or the formation of new skin cells, (4) hydrogen cyanide in smoke inhibits body chemicals from working normally to transport oxygen from cell to cell, (5) nicotine reduces the formation of red blood cells, fibroblasts and macrophages, and (6) smoking causes increased platelet stickiness, which increases the chance that an abnormal number of clots will form at the wound site.
   *Cigarettes*, pp.50-51

4. Smoking significantly increases a person's chances of suffering complications when undergoing surgery. The risks are multiple: Smokers who require anesthesia are much more likely to suffer anesthesia-associated complications, and their surgical wounds don't heal well. Smokers require a significantly longer time in the recovery room to stabilize than do nonsmokers, and they need supplemental oxygen for a longer time after surgery. The inability to clear secretions is magnified in smokers and is associated with their much greater risk of developing respiratory infections such as pneumonia and bronchitis. Smokers also have a greater chance of suffering a collapsed lung after undergoing anesthesia and surgery. *Cigarettes*, pp. 48-49

5. In a study of 410 patients in Syracuse, New York undergoing elective non-cardiac surgery, postoperative pulmonary complications occurred in 22% of current smokers compared to 4.9% of never smokers. Because of this nearly six-fold increased risk for complications, the authors advise all smokers to stop smoking for at least four weeks prior to elective surgery. If this is not possible, all current smokers should become abstinent for the 24 hours immediately before surgery to lower their carboxyhemoglobin level. Reducing rather than stopping smoking before surgery did not decrease the risk Chest, April 1998, pp. 857 and 883

6. Smoking a single cigarette can reduce blood flow to the fingers by more than 40% for up to an hour, posing a significant problem for surgery involving the hands. *Cigarettes*, p.52

7. In a study of 1186 patients undergoing face lifts, 10.2% were complicated by skin sloughing, and 80% of the group with this complication were current smokers. A patient undergoing a face lift who smoked had a 12.46 times greater chance of skin slough than a nonsmoker.
   Journal of the American Academy of Dermatology, May 1996, p. 718

8. In a study of 500 outpatient surgery patients at the Medical College of Wisconsin in Milwaukee, patients who smoked in the 24 hours before surgery had 20 times the risk for myocardial ischemia, or inadequate oxygen supply to the heart. Reuters, October 22, 1997

9. In a study from Denmark of postoperative complications in patients undergoing hip and knee replacement surgery, the overall complication rate was 52% in continuing smokers compared with 18% in a smoking intervention group. The complications included wound-related, cardiovascular, and secondary surgery. The authors concluded that an effective smoking program 6 to 8 weeks before surgery markedly reduced postoperative morbidity. The Lancet, January 12, 2002, p. 114

10. Postoperative pulmonary complications are about double in current smokers and recent smokers undergoing pulmonary surgery, compared to nonsmokers. Preoperative smoking abstinence of at least four weeks is necessary to reduce these complications. Chest, September 2001, p. 705

## Skin and Throat Disorders

1. Patients with peritonsillar abscess, or quinsy, are 70% more likely to be smokers than the general population.
   The Lancet, June 20, 1992, p. 1552

2. Oral ulcers associated with Behcet's syndrome may be related in some cases to stopping smoking, and nicotine replacement therapy may be useful for treatment. Recurrent aphthous ulcers are also less common among tobacco users. New England Journal of Medicine, December 14, 2000, pp. 1816-17

3.  Acute necrotizing ulcerative gingivitis, also known as "trench mouth" or Vincent's disease, occurs almost exclusively in smokers and is strongly dose related.

    *Journal of the American Academy of Dermatology, May 1996, p. 723*

4.  The relative risk of palmoplantar pustulosis, a skin condition resembling psoriasis, is 7.2 times greater in smokers.

    *Journal of The American Academy of Dermatology, May 1996, p. 719*

5.  Smokers have at least a two- to threefold increased risk of developing psoriasis. Smoking may precipitate as many as one quarter of all psoriasis cases, and may possible contribute to as many as half the cases of palmoplantar pustulosis.

    *Cigarettes*, p. 43

6.  Most studies suggest a two to threefold increase in risk of psoriasis in smokers.

    *South China Morning Post, June 17, 1998 (Tobacco and Health News website)*

7.  Women who smoke more than 15 cigarettes a day are 3.9 fold more likely to have psoriasis, compared to a 1.4 fold increased risk for men who smoked this often. Overall, people who smoked 25 or more cigarettes a day are 2.1 fold more likely to have psoriasis. For pustular psoriasis, the increased risk was 10.5 fold for smokers of 15 or more cigarettes a day. The study authors from Milan, Italy pointed to the possible role of hormonal factors, since smoking has well-defined antiestrogenic effects.

    *Archives of Dermatology, December 1999, pp. 1479-1484*

8.  Smoking more than 24 cigarettes a day increases by 2.2 fold the risk for developing psoriasis, in a report from Italy.

    *Skin and Allergy News, December 1998, p. 20*

9.  Smoking may increase the risk of systemic lupus erthematosus; the odds ratio is 2.3.

    *International Journal of Dermatology 1995; 34:333*

10. Cigarette smoking appears to be a major risk factor for development of systemic lupus erythematosus. It has also been associated with rheumatoid arthritis, Raynaud phenomenon, Goodpasture syndrome, Graves disease, and increased severity of autoimmune disease.

    *Journal of Respiratory Diseases, September 2002, p. 448*

11. Patients with cutaneous lupus erythematosus who smoke are much less likely than nonsmokers to respond to hydroxychloroquine, the antimalarial drug used as first-line therapy. In a study from the University of North Carolina, Chapel Hill, there was a 90% response rate for nonsmokers, but a response rate to hydroxychloroquine of only 40% in smokers. The mechanism for this effect is not known.

    *Skin and Allergy News, September 2000, p. 24*

12. In a study from North Dakota, there was a strong association between smoking and discoid lupus erythematosus, with an odds ratio of 12.2, significantly higher than that reported for systemic lupus erythematosus, odds ratio 2.3.

    *Cutis, April 1999, p. 234*

## Miscellaneous Health Problems

1.  Smokers have an increased risk of infertility in both sexes, osteoporosis, upper and lower respiratory tract infections, sensorineural hearing loss, and two major causes of blindness, cataracts and macular degeneration.

    *JAMA, August 9, 2000, p. 743*

2.  Two cases of acute eosinophilic pneumonia in young people 10 days and 3 days after smoking initiation have been reported from Japan.

    *Tobacco Control, Winter 1995, p. 400*

3.  Disseminated cryptococcus neoformans infection (DCI) is the most common invasive fungal disease and the third most common central nervous system disorder in patients with HIV infection. In a study from San Diego, the risk for developing the opportunistic infection DCI increased by 4.75 times in smokers compared with

nonsmokers, and 74% of cases were in smokers. JAMA, February 26, 1997, p. 629

4. Women who smoke have less endometrial cancer, fewer uterine fibroids, less endometriosis, and less hyperemesis gravidarum, or severe nausea during pregnancy. *Cigarettes*, p. 90

5. Smoking has a protective effect for ulcerative colitis, with odds ratios between 0.34 and 0.48, and smokers with the disease exhibit a better clinical course. *Clearing the Smoke*, p. 562

6. Anecdotal evidence suggests that nicotine may ameliorate symptoms of ulcerative colitis. Chewing tobacco users have double the risk of developing ulcerative colitis, but smokers may have a lower risk. *Cigarettes*, p. 150-151

7. Transdermal nicotine provokes gastroesophageal reflux and heartburn. Crohn's disease is primarily a disease of smokers, and smoking exacerbates symptoms. In contrast, nicotine promotes healing in ulcerative colitis, which is primarily a disease of nonsmokers. *Nicotine Safety and Toxicity*, p. 165

8. In a study from the Mayo Clinic, transdermal nicotine was associated with improvement of 39% of nonsmoking patients with ulcerative colitis, compared to 9% of patients on placebo patches. Annals of Internal Medicine, March 1, 1997, p. 364

9. In a report from Norway, 90% of nonsmoking mothers were breast feeding at three months, compared to 65% of smokers. Many of the latter had stopped early because of "too little milk." 40% of infants breast fed by smokers had infantile colic, compared to 26% of the babies of nonsmokers. JAMA, January 6, 1989, p. 42

10. Smoking is a risk factor for low back pain. Industrial workers who smoked at baseline had a 40% higher incidence of back pain during a four-year follow-up period. Spine, February 1989, p. 141

11. In an Army infantry training unit, there was a threefold higher rate of lower back and lower extremity injury among smokers compared to nonsmokers. American Journal of Preventive Medicine 1994; 10:145

12. In a study from France of patients with asthma who required mechanical ventilation in an intensive care unit, 23 percent were smokers. Smoking was associated with a higher mortality from asthma both during hospitalization and after discharge. American Review of Respiratory Disease, July 1992, p. 76

13. Elderly women who smoke have poorer muscle strength, agility and balance, and generally feel older than their nonsmoking contemporaries. For these women, smoking may have the same effect as adding five years to her age. ASH Review, January-February 1995 p. 4

14. In kidney transplant recipients, smoking is significantly associated with reduced graft survival, with a relative risk of 2.3 for graft loss. Smokers had kidney graft survival of 84% at one year, 65% at five years, and 48% at ten years, compared with 88%, 78%, and 62% at comparable times for nonsmokers. Transplantation 2001; 71:1752-57

15. Long-time smokers face an increased risk of multiple sclerosis, according to researchers from Harvard University. They found that women who smoked a pack a day for 25 years of more were more likely than nonsmokers to develop the disease. Compared with nonsmokers, the risk that current smokers would develop MS was increased by 60%. Smoking has also been linked to other immune system-related diseases such as rheumatoid arthritis and lupus. American Journal of Epidemiology 2001; 154:69-74

16. Smoking has been associated with a worsening of upper body motor functioning in multiple sclerosis. *Cigarettes*, p. 104

17. In a study from Norway, decline in physical fitness and lung functions among healthy middle aged men was considerably greater among smokers than among nonsmokers, and could not be explained by differences in age and physical activity. British Medical Journal, August 16, 1995, p. 715

18. Tobacco use, specifically nicotine and polycyclic aromatic hydrocarbons, may suppress the body's immune function by mechanisms that have not been established. Cigarette smoking is associated with reductions in serum immunoglobulins, helper/suppressor T-cell ratios, mitogen-induced lymphocyte transformation, and natural killer cytotoxic activity.                    Journal of Allergy and Clinical Immunology, April 1995, p. 901

19. Green tobacco sickness, a type of nicotine poisoning, can occur in tobacco harvesters when nicotine contained in the sap of tobacco leaves is absorbed through the skin. Symptoms are weakness, nausea, vomiting, headache, and difficulty breathing. In Kentucky, about 600 workers during the late summer harvest each season seek emergency care for this condition.          Southern Medical Journal, September 1993, p. 989 and
Morbidity and Mortality Weekly Report, April 9, 1993, p. 237

20. In a study of Hispanic migrant workers involved in tobacco harvesting in North Carolina, 41% of the workers had at least one episode of green tobacco sickness caused by transdermal absorption of nicotine from green tobacco leaves.                    JAMA, March 22/29, 2000, p. 1557

21. In a study from the Wake Forest University School of Medicine published in the March 2000 issue of the American Journal of Industrial Medicine, 41% of tobacco farm workers contracted "green tobacco sickness," a form of acute nicotine poisoning from nicotine absorption from tobacco leaves through the skin, at least once during a summer harvest season.                    American Medical News, March 6, 2000, p. 4

22. Cigarette smoking decreases exhaled nitrogen dioxide. Since nitric oxide is important in defending the respiratory tract against infection, in counteracting bronchoconstriction and vasoconstriction, and in inhibiting platelet aggregation, this effect may contribute to increased risks of chronic respiratory and cardiovascular diseases in cigarette smokers.
American Journal of Respiratory and Critical Care Medicine, August 1995, p. 609

23. "Smoking is considered the major risk factor in causing carpal tunnel syndrome according to a study by the Mayo clinic. This is because the nerves around the carpal tunnels are being deprived of oxygen by the vessel-constricting effects of nicotine."          ASH Smoking and Health Review, July-August 2001, p. 6

24. Alcohol use and cigarette smoking may exacerbate liver dysfunction in individuals with hepatitis C virus infection.                    Archives Of Internal Medicine 2002; 162:811

25. Smoking increases the risk for pulmonary embolism in women, with a relative risk of 1.8 in smokers of 25 to 34 cigarettes a day, and 3.4 for those smoking 35 or more cigarettes a day.    JAMA, February 26, 1997, p. 643

26. Among adult non-diabetic offspring, the risk of obesity correlates significantly with the degree of maternal smoking, with an odds ratio of 1.34 to 1.38.                    Respiratory Reviews, March 2002, p. 1

27. In a study from the Netherlands, colic was twice as likely in babies up to six months old whose mothers smoked 15 to 30 cigarettes a day, either during or after pregnancy.          Time, October 16, 2000

28. Women who smoke may have a modestly elevated risk for rheumatoid arthritis.
*Women and Smoking*, 2001 Surgeon General report, p. 330

29. A study from the University of Alabama found that women who smoke double their risk of developing rheumatoid arthritis later in life.          ASH Smoking and Health Review, November-December 2000, p. 6

30. There is a striking association between heavy cigarette smoking and rheumatoid arthritis; a history of 41 to 50 pack years smoked had an odds ratio of 13.54.          Annals of the Rheumatic Diseases 2001: 223-227

31. In a study from Yale, the prevalence of both acute and recurrent or chronic sinusitis was increased in smokers, but did not rise with passive exposure to cigarette smoke. In the United States, 66 million adults, or 35% of the adult population, reported having sinus problems or sinusitis at least once during the previous year.
Abstract reported in JAMA, November 1, 2000, p. 2170

32. Sinus infections (sinusitis) affects 14.1% of the U.S. population, but the relationship to smoking or ETS exposure is poorly documented in the medical literature. In a study from Yale, the direct use of tobacco, but not household passive tobacco smoke exposure, was linked to an increased prevalence of sinusitis.

Archives of Otolaryngology Head and Neck Surgery, August 2000, pp. 940-946

33. Smoking is a major triggering factor for the development of acne inversa, formerly known as hidradenitis suppurativa, a severe painful skin disease associated with abscesses, fistulas, scarring, and unpleasant odor.

Skin and Allergy News, February 2003

34. "It is an admitted fact that a disease of vision – tobacco amblyopia – is contracted by smokers... Allowing that such incidental evils may arise from even comparatively moderate indulgence in tobacco, they are after all as nothing compared to the vast aggregate of gentle exhilaration, soothing, and social comfort extracted from Virginia weed."

Encyclopedia Britannica, 10th edition, New American supplement, 1902, page 427 (Tobacco Control, December 2000, p. 432)

35. In a study from the Netherlands, smoking more than tripled the risk of a common type of skin cancer, squamous cell carcinoma.

US News and World Report, January 8, 2001, p. 55

36. Postmenopausal women who smoke have lower bone densities than nonsmoking women.

British Medical Association (www.tobaccofactfile.org)

37. The odds of developing both ulcerative colitis and primary sclerosing cholangitis are significantly decreased among both current and former smokers; nicotine has a protective effect.

Gut 2002;51:567-573

38. Smokers are 50 to 60% less likely to exercise than are nonsmokers, and smokers are 15 to 20% more likely to suffer from back injuries than are nonsmokers.     From *Kicking the Habit, Why Golf and Smoking Don't Mix*, Glaxo Smith Kline (Golf Digest, March 2003, p. 126)

39. Smoking could dull the body's protective cough reflex, making smokers more susceptible to respiratory infections, reported a study from Albert Einstein Hospital in New York City. "Cough reflex sensitivity is significantly diminished in young, healthy, male current-smokers compared to a similar population of nonsmokers. The mechanism of cough suppression in smokers remains speculative but may involve long-term tobacco smoke-induced desensitization of the cough receptors within the airway epithelium."

Chest 2003; 123:685-688

40. Heavy smoking can lead to bladder control problems and urinary incontinence among women.

British Journal of Obstetrics and Gynecology, March 2003
(Reuters, March 6, 2003)

# CHAPTER 12
# IMPOTENCE

1. Up to 10 million US men are impotent, and half of these cases are caused by diabetes, alcohol, smoking, aging, and medication. In a study of 4500 US Army Vietnam veterans ages 31 to 49, 2.2 percent of nonsmokers and 2 percent of former smokers were impotent, compared with 3.7 percent of current smokers. An Associated Press headline of December 2, 1994 read: "Joe Camel and Marlboro Man Are Probably Not Studs."

2. In men with treated heart disease, the age-adjusted probability of complete impotence was 56% for current smokers, compared to 21% for nonsmokers. Among men treated for hypertension, 20% of smokers were impotent compared to 8.5% of nonsmokers.               Journal of Urology, January 1994, p. 57

3. Smoking is much more common in impotent men than in the general population. 58 to 64% of impotent men in several studies were smokers.               Journal of Urology, July 1991, p. 761

4. In a study of sedentary men ages 40 to 55, 21% of smokers reported sexual dysfunction and erectile failure, compared to only 4% of nonsmokers.      9th World Conference on Tobacco or Health, Paris, 1994 (J. White)

5. Smoking's adverse effects on erections and resulting 50% higher risk of impotence is apparent at about age 40. Smokers also tend to be physiologically about 8 years older that their chronological age.
               Reported in USA Today from American Journal of Epidemiology, December 1994

6. The risk of impotence is increased by 60% in twenty "pack-year" smokers between the ages of 30 and 50 (one pack per day for twenty years is twenty "pack years"; two packs per day for ten years also equals twenty "pack years").      Michael Eriksen, American Society of Addiction Medicine, Atlanta, November 12, 1993

7. Smoking increases impotence by at least 50% among healthy young men aged 31 to 49. The problem is even worse in older men, and 70% of the men attending impotence clinics were smokers in one study. Ann Landers published a suggestion for a new health warning label: **WARNING: SMOKING IS A CONTRIBUTING FACTOR TO SEXUAL IMPOTENCE.**               ASH Review, January 1995, p. 4

8. In a clinic for men with impotence, 58.4 percent were current smokers, and another 23 percent were former smokers. 81 percent of the total were current or former smokers.               Urology, June 1986, p. 495

9. "Smoking plays a role in male impotence, delayed conception in women, and a predisposition for male smokers' offspring to develop brain tumors because of smoking-induced defective genes in the parent's sperm: the sins of the fathers."               *No Stranger to Tears*, p. 336

10. A group of Israeli doctors believes that the fear of impotence is stronger incentive for their patients to give up smoking than is the fear of death. In a study of 886 smokers suffering from impotence, 80% quit after they were encouraged to do so.               Tobacco Free Youth Reporter, Fall 1995, p. 23

11. Smoking seriously reduces blood flow to the penis, in some instances causing impotence.      *Cigarettes*, p. 96

12. Smoking just two cigarettes causes acute vasospasm of the penile arteries, and smoking appears to at least double the risk of becoming impotent. In one study of patients at an impotence clinic, 39% were diagnosed as having vascular impotence; 97% of those men smoked. In another study, 82% of men with vascular impotence were smokers.               *Cigarettes*, p. 90

13. Male smokers are about twice as likely as nonsmokers to suffer from impotence.      Reuters, November 5, 1998

14. In a study of men ages 24 to 36 seeking treatment for infertility, Panayiotis Zavos, Ph.D., "confirmed the results of earlier studies demonstrating that smoking harms sperm quality in every way, from longevity to motility. But Zavos also found that smoking affected sexual behavior. The smokers had sex an average of 5.7

times per month, while the nonsmokers reported an average of 11.6 encounters. And on a scale of 1 to 10, the smokers rated the quality of sex at a lackluster 5.2, compared to 8.7 for nonsmokers."

Men's Journal, March 2000, p. 69

15. In a study from Boston University School of Medicine, smokers had significantly shorter erect penises than nonsmokers.　　　　　　　　The Observer, July 27, 1998 (Tobacco and Health News website)

16. In April 1999, the 60-foot Marlboro Man on Sunset Boulevard in Hollywood was replaced by a new giant cowboy. "But this one has a limp cigarette dangling from his lips. Behind him is the word 'Impotent' in big red letters."　　　　　　　　Contra Costa (California) Times, April 24, 1999, p. A12

17. The government of Canada has proposed that cigarette packs carry photographs of diseased hearts and cancerous lips and lungs. Another warning would attempt to dispel the perception that smoking has sex appeal: "Cigarettes may cause sexual impotence due to decreased blood flow to the penis. This can prevent you from having an erection."　　　　　　　　New York Times, January 20, 2000

18. Smoking is a major cause of male impotence. Males who smoke have sperm with decreased density, decreased mobility and increased morphologic abnormalities.　　*Reducing the Health Consequences of Smoking*, p. 75

19. A new suggested warning label for cigarette packs: Smoking just two cigarettes constricts blood flow to the penis enough to cause at least temporary impotence.　　　　　　　　Associated Press, October 30, 1996

20. Two decades of evidence – including 19 different studies involving more than 3,800 men – shows conclusively that smoking can lead to impotence, according to a new article in Preventive Medicine. 40% of impotent men studied were smokers, compared with only 28% of men overall. "Our review shows a clear relationship," the authors wrote.　　　　　　　　Preventive Medicine, June 2001

21. Hypertensive men who smoke are 26 times more likely to have erectile dysfunction than men without these risk factors.　　　　　　　　Dean Edell, M.D. ABC radio, May 22, 2001

22. Middle age men who smoke have about a 24% rate of impotence, about twice that of nonsmokers. Heavy exposure to passive smoke also doubles the risk of erectile dysfunction.

ASH Smoking and Health Review, November – December 2000, p. 6

23. In a study of 5,400 men in Hong Kong who were taking Viagra, 926 failed to respond to the drug. Of the non-responders, 90% were smokers, suggesting that male smokers do not respond as well to Viagra.

2002 AMA Annual Tobacco Report

24. In a study from Tulane in New Orleans, researchers determined that men who smoked more than 20 cigarettes a day were 60 percent more likely to have erectile dysfunction than men who never smoked. Men who smoked between 11 and 20 cigarettes a day had a 36 percent higher risk, while men who smoked fewer than 10 cigarettes daily had a 16 percent higher risk.　　　Tobaccofreekids.org Tobacco News, March 12, 2003, from American Heart Association meeting

# CHAPTER 13
# PHYSICAL FITNESS AND CARBON MONOXIDE

1. A 1929 American Tobacco Company ad claimed that cigarettes were actually health-giving. "For years this has been no secret to those who keep fit and trim. They know that Luckies steady their nerves and do not hurt their physical condition. They know that Lucky Strikes are the favorite cigarettes of many prominent athletes who must keep in good shape. They respect the opinions of 20,679 physicians who maintain that Luckies are less irritating to the throat than other cigarettes."
*They Satisfy*, p. 101

2. Ads for Camels in 1935 featuring Lou Gehrig claimed "They Don't Get Your Wind... So mild, you can smoke all you want." And tennis star Bill Tilden was quoted, "Playing competitive tennis day after day, I've got to keep in top physical condition. I smoke Camels, the mild cigarette. They don't get my wind or upset my nerves."
*Ashes to Ashes*, p. 88

3. The average young nonsmoking Navy man runs a mile and a half on the physical fitness test in 11 minutes 20 seconds. The average smoker of a pack a day or more takes a minute and half longer to run the same distance. For men over age 30, the averages are 12 minutes 20 seconds for nonsmokers and 15 minutes 15 seconds for the smoking group.
Military Medicine, November 1988, p. 489

4. In a study of physical fitness in 19 year olds, the average nonsmoker was able to run 2613 meters in 12 minutes. The average 19 year old smoker of a pack a day or more, however, was able to run only 2253 meters in the same time, or 360 meters behind the nonsmoking group.
B Marti et al, Preventive Medicine 17, 1988

5. Women over age 65 who smoke are weaker and have poorer balance and poorer performance on measures of integrated physical function than nonsmokers. This decline in physical function was 50% to 100% as great as that associated with a five year increase in age, and most measures worsened with increasing number of pack-years of smoking.
JAMA, December 21, 1994, p. 1825

6. "I'm going to focus on staying as healthy as possible. That means doing regular exercises – but hiking, not running . . . . I don't feel any desire to drink or do coke. Especially coke. I see people drinking wine when I'm out to dinner, and I think, Oh, one glass. But it's better that I don't." Actress Melanie Griffith, early in her third pregnancy, at about the time she was photographed smoking cigarettes.
In Style magazine, March 1996

7. Well known climber Jim Bridwell was the first to climb El Capitan in Yosemite in one day. "A notorious tobacco fiend, Bridwell has defended his habit by saying it trains his lungs for altitude because it makes his every breath feel as if he's at 8000 meters."
Climbing magazine, September 15, 1998, p. 76

8. The "record highest altitude for smoking" appears to be held by a Sherpa in Nepal who continued to smoke on three visits to the South Col on Mt. Everest, elevation 8000 meters (over 26,000 feet).
from *Filming the Impossible*, Leo Dickinson, 1982

9. Smoking may impair acclimatization to high altitudes and cause a decreased capacity for oxygen delivery to the lungs. In a study of 109 men working on a project in Peru at an altitude of 10,500 feet (3200 meters), ten had to return to lower altitude for nonmedical reason, all of whom were smokers.
*High Altitude Medicine*, Herbert Hultgren, Hultgren Publications, 1997, pp. 178 and 470

# Carbon Monoxide

1. "Mainstream cigarette smoke has carbon monoxide present at concentrations similar to that found in automobile exhaust. It is the dilution of the smoke with room air and the intermittent nature of smoke inhalation that prevents cigarette smoke from being immediately lethal."
Clinics in Chest Medicine, December 1991, p. 633 (David Burns, M.D.)

2.  The average smoker has exhaled carbon monoxide of 33 parts per million, which equates to a 5.5% percentage of carboxyhemoglobin. Heavy smokers have carboxyhemoglobin levels of 8% and exhaled CO of 48 ppm.
    Smokerlyzer brochure, Bedford Scientific, UK and Journal of Family Practice, June 1992, p. 690

3.  Red blood cells have a 210 to 250 times greater affinity for carbon monoxide (CO) than for oxygen, and fetal hemoglobin binds to CO with an even greater affinity. Exhaled CO correlates with carboxyhemoglobin (COHb) blood levels, and a one pack per day smoker has a reading of 25 to 35 parts per million. A 59ppm CO level equals a 10% COHb, or a 10% loss of oxygen-carrying capacity, which may reduce mental awareness and slow reaction time.
    American Society of Addiction Medicine, Atlanta, November 12, 1993 (L. Nett) and Reader's Digest, March 1995, p. 129

4.  When people smoke normally, their carbon monoxide levels are lowest in the morning and level off at their highest values by midday. The typical one-pack-per-day smoker achieves levels in expired air averaging between 25 and 35 parts per million. However, even these "average" smokers may hit short-term levels of greater than 100 parts per million. Firefighters are now routinely checked with portable CO analyzing machines while combating fires. If their levels exceed 150 parts per million they may be relieved and given oxygen, since even these generally healthy people run a risk of heart attacks.
    Quote from *Nicotine*, p. 34

5.  Carbon monoxide in tobacco smoke decreases the threshold for ventricular fibrillation.
    Clinics in Chest Medicine, December 1991, p. 635

6.  Expired air carbon monoxide levels correlate with carboxyhemoglobin 5 to 1; the average pack-a-day smoker has about 8% carboxyhemoglobin in the afternoon, which corresponds to 40 parts per million carbon monoxide in expired air.
    Psychiatric Clinics of North America, March 1993, p. 53

7.  The carbon monoxide in cigarette smoke (it makes up from 2.7 to 6 percent of the smoke) reduces the oxygen-carrying capacity of the blood. Cigarette smoke averages about 400 parts per million of carbon monoxide, or eight times greater than the maximum level of carbon monoxide permitted in industry.
    *Cigarettes*, p. 30

8.  Carbon monoxide emissions from one cigar are 30 times higher than for one cigarette, and secondhand smoke from one cigar equals the smoke of three cigarettes.
    American Lung Association data reported in Ann Landers column, March 1997

# CHAPTER 14
# PREGNANCY AND FERTILITY

1.  About 15% of U.S. women still smoke during pregnancy. Newborns of these mothers have the same nicotine levels as adult smokers, and almost certainly spend their first days of life going through withdrawal.
    Associated Press, February 9, 1997

2.  Maternal smoking is responsible for 14% of all premature births in the United States; the risk for early labor and delivery is increased by one-third to one-half if the mother is a smoker.
    American Journal of Diseases of Children, June 1981, p. 501

3.  Infant mortality increases from 15 per 1000 live births in white nonsmokers to 23 per 1000 for white women who smoke more than one pack of cigarettes per day. The comparable rates for black women are 26.0 for nonsmokers and 39.9 for the second group. The odds for a spontaneous abortion in one study were 46% higher for the first 10 cigarettes smoked per day and 61% greater for the first 20 cigarettes smoked per day compared with no cigarettes during pregnancy. Smoking also accounts for 21% to 39% of the incidence of low-birth-weight-babies. In terms of fertility, smokers have 3.4 times the risk of taking more than a year to conceive, and twice the risk of infertility (not pregnant 5 years after ceasing contraceptive use).
    Clinics in Chest Medicine, December 1991, p. 652

4.  Complications during pregnancy and labor in smokers include an increased risk of bleeding and premature rupture of membranes. As well, the likelihood of spontaneous abortion is almost double for women who smoke.
    *Nicotine*, p. 56

5.  Babies of mothers who smoke during pregnancy are twice as likely to be aborted, to be stillborn, or to die soon after birth as the babies of non-smoking mothers. One in five of babies who dies would have been saved if their mothers had not smoked.
    *Licit and Illicit Drugs*, p. 233

6.  Smoking during pregnancy increases the risk of spontaneous abortion (miscarriage), preterm delivery, premature rupture of placental membranes, placenta previa, abruptio placenta, and bleeding during pregnancy.
    *Preventing Tobacco Use Among Young People*, 1994 Surgeon General report, p. 28

7.  A dose-response pattern has been found for smoking and abruptio placenta, placenta previa, bleeding during pregnancy, prolonged premature rupture of membranes, and impaired physical and intellectual development of the infant.
    Clinics in Chest Medicine, December 1991, p. 652

8.  Pregnant women who smoke are 46% more likely to have a baby who dies before its first birthday.
    American Medical News, December 28, 1992

9.  Smoking by pregnant women in Spain increased from 18% in 1980 to 29% in 1990.
    The Lancet, May 22, 1993, p. 1350

10. Of the 4 million American women who give birth each year, some 820,000 smoke cigarettes.
    American Journal of Public Health, January 1998, p. 9

11. 40% of US women smokers quit when they become pregnant. Of these, 70% relapse in the first year postpartum. 5% to 6% of perinatal deaths, 17-26% of low birth weight births, and 7-10% of premature deliveries are attributable to smoking during pregnancy.
    *Nicotine Addiction*, p. 282

12. About 35 to 40% of smokers quit during pregnancy, and another 25 to 30% reduce their intake, but less than a third maintain the change postpartum.
    Obstetrics and Gynecology, November 1992, p. 743

13. Nursing mothers who smoke produce 46% less milk than non-smokers. The milk also contains 19% less fat and, ounce for ounce, 10% fewer calories.
    San Francisco Chronicle, May 9, 1994, p. E9,
    and Pediatrics, December 1992, p. 934

14. In a study from Norway, smoking adversely affected lactation and breast feeding. 90% of non-smoking mothers continued breast feeding for at least three months compared to 65% of the smoking mothers; more of the latter group said that they stopped breast feeding early because of "too little milk." Also, 40% of the babies with smoking mothers had infantile colic, compared with 26% of babies of the non-smoking mothers.

JAMA, January 6, 1989, p. 42

15. Smoking during pregnancy accounts for 14% of preterm deliveries and up to 30% of low-birth weight babies. It is also responsible for 4600 infant deaths each year.　　　　　American Medical News, July 4, 1994, p. 14

16. Cigarettes may actually be worse for a fetus than cocaine; both decrease blood flow to the fetus and deprive it of oxygen and nutrition. Many of the bad things attributed to cocaine, like low birth weight, behavior problems, and learning difficulties, are exactly the same things associated with cigarette smoking, a habit that is acknowledged by up to 85% of crack cocaine users.　　　　　JAMA, February 23, 1994, p. 576

17. In 1991, North Carolina began a new campaign to reduce infant mortality. Brochures and posters warned pregnant women about alcohol and illicit drugs, but warnings about the hazards of smoking were conspicuously absent. State funding for the educational materials was granted only with the provision that not one word about smoking be included. The health authorities ultimately had to choose between publishing the censored materials or not publishing anything at all. The state has the second highest infant mortality rate in the country, and is also the number one tobacco producing state, growing 40% of the nation's crop.

JAMA, December 25, 1991, p. 3399

18. In surveys of smoking during pregnancy in 1967 and again in 1980, the percentage of smokers in married pregnant women with more than 16 years of education (college graduate) dropped from 34 to 11 percent. In the group with less than a high school education, smoking rates decreased from 48 to only 43 percent.

American Journal of Public Health, July 1987, p. 823

19. In 1989, the prevalence of smoking among college educated pregnant women was 5%, while that among pregnant women without a high school diploma was 42%. There is a 25 to 50 percent higher fetal and infant death rate among women who continue to smoke.　　　　　*Tobacco Use*, p. 27

20. In 1989, 19% of all women who gave birth reported tobacco use during pregnancy. Mothers whose prenatal care was poor or inadequate were twice as likely to be smokers (32% versus 16%). Among mothers with less than a high school education, 41 to 46% were smokers (even higher among white women, 44 to 48%). Only 5% of mothers who were college graduates were smokers during pregnancy.

Morbidity and Mortality Weekly Report, 1990

21. Unmarried pregnant white women are 40% more likely to smoke than their married pregnant counterparts.

JAMA, January 6, 1989, p. 70

22. In Missouri, 23% of married pregnant women but 41% of unmarried pregnant women were smokers in a 1990 survey.　　　　　Public Health Reports, January 1991, p. 52

23. In Washington State from 1984 through 1988, 31.7% of married pregnant teenagers and 42.8% of unmarried pregnant teenagers smoked during their pregnancies. The overall smoking prevalence for pregnant teens increased from 32% in 1984 to 37% in 1988.

American Journal of Diseases of Children, December 1990, p. 1297

24. Women in the lowest age and socioeconomic categories have the highest likelihood of smoking during pregnancy. Between 1974 and 1985, smoking declined five times faster among college graduates compared with those with less than a high school education.　　　　　American Journal of Public Health, May 1990, p. 544

25. Tobacco's toxic elements accumulate in the fetuses of non-smoking pregnant women who live with smokers. One baby in a study was exposed to so much secondhand smoke that it was equivalent to the mother herself smoking five cigarettes a day.　　　　　San Francisco Chronicle, February 23, 1994, p. A5

26. Perinatal mortality was 270 per 1000 (27%) for children of smoking women in Dacca, Bangladesh. This was twice as high as for children of nonsmokers. The Lancet, May 16, 1981, p. 1092

27. Mothers who smoke have a significantly increased risk for episodes of uterine bleeding during pregnancy. After birth, infants of smokers also had more frequent (relative risk 2.76) and longer episodes of obstructive sleep apnea, or periods of not breathing during sleep. Pediatrics, May 1994, p. 788

28. Exposure to maternal smoking during pregnancy, even if only in the first trimester, is associated with long term and potentially irreversible reduction in lung function. American Journal of Epidemiology, June 1994, p. 1139

29. In a study from New York, maternal smoking during pregnancy selectively increased by four times the probability that their female children would eventually smoke. Maternal smoking during pregnancy thus may create a serious risk for smoking in their female but not male children.
American Journal of Public Health, September 1994, p. 1407

30. There is a five-fold increased risk of etopic (tubal) pregnancy in heavy smokers and an excess risk 2.5 times normal of ectopic pregnancy in all smokers. American Journal of Public Health, September 1989, p. 1239

31. A pack a day pregnant smoker increases her chance of premature delivery by 20%. *Cigarettes*, p. 85

32. Tobacco use by pregnant women is responsible for an estimated 14,000 to 26,000 infants being admitted to neonatal intensive care units each year. *Cigarettes*, p. 85

33. About 15,000 admissions each year to neonatal intensive care units, or 7% of the total, are the consequence of maternal smoking. This accounts for about 9% of total national expenditures for neonatal intensive care services, or $272 million in 1983. The average cost for neonatal care was $288 higher for infants born to smokers than for those born to nonsmokers. American Journal of Preventive Medicine, April 1988, p. 216

34. In 1987, the estimated direct medical cost of a complicated birth for a smoker was 66% higher than for a nonsmoker, and represented 11% of the total medical expenditures for all complicated births. The total smoking-attributable costs were an estimated $2.0 billion in 1995 dollars, based on a smoking prevalence of 27%. Morbidity and Mortality Weekly Report, November 7, 1997, p. 1049

35. The elimination of smoking would reduce infant deaths by 10% and decrease the incidence of low birth weight babies born by 25%. Pediatrics, May 1994, p. 866

36. If all pregnant women stopped smoking, the number of fetal and infant deaths would be reduced by 10%. Compared with nonsmoking primagravidas, women smokers or one of one or more packs per day had a 56% greater risk of fetal or perinatal death. American Journal of Epidemiology 127:274, 1988

37. In a survey of Native American women in the state of Washington, 39.8% smoked during pregnancy.
American Journal of Public Health, December 1990, p.1297

38. In a study of women who gave birth in Inuvik in arctic Canada, 64% smoked during their pregnancies. Most were Inuit Eskimos and Native American Indians.
Canadian Medical Association Journal, July 15, 1992, p. 181

39. The incidence of placenta previa during pregnancy is increased 2.6-fold in smokers.
American Journal of Obstetrics & Gynecology, July 1991, p. 28

40. About 10% of the 38,351 infant deaths that occurred in 1990 may be attributable to smoking.
JAMA, September 22, 1994, p. 1443

41. In an American study, the infant mortality rate was 12.1 deaths per 1000 births among infants of mothers who had smoked during pregnancy compared with 7.6 among infants of nonsmokers, an increased risk of 60% or odds ratio of 1.6. The odds ratios for smoking were particularly high for deaths from respiratory disease (3.4

times) and SIDS (1.9). If no mother had smoked, infant mortality would have been reduced by 10%, and deaths from SIDS and respiratory illness by 28% and 46%, respectively. *Thorax*, August 1994, p. 731

42. Smoking during pregnancy increases the risk of perinatal death by 26%, and an estimated 3,700 infant deaths in the perinatal period are caused by maternal smoking each year in the US. This represents 7% of all perinatal deaths, and 21% of perinatal deaths among the offspring of women who smoke during pregnancy. These deaths are caused primarily by complications from low birth weight and premature separation of the placenta.
*Journal of Family Practice*, April 1995, p. 385

43. In preterm infants born to mothers who smoked more 10 cigarettes a day during the latter half of pregnancy, the risk of mild intracranial hemorrhage (bleeding into the brain) was increased threefold.
*Journal of Pediatrics*, September 1995, p. 472

44. Maternal smoking during pregnancy is associated in a dose-dependent manner with increased blood pressure in their babies which does not return to normal until the second year of life. Whether this early increase in blood pressure is related to the development of essential hypertension later in life is not known.
*Journal of Pediatrics*, June 1996, p. 806

45. Pregnant women who smoke are on average 40% more likely than nonsmokers to give birth prematurely, and about 30% more likely to have their babies die in the newborn period. *Ashes to Ashes*, p. 462

46. Eliminating smoking during pregnancy could prevent about 17% to 26% of low birth weight births, 7% to 10% of preterm deliveries, 1200 to 2200 yearly deaths from SIDS, and 5% to 6% of perinatal deaths.
*Journal of the American Women's Association (JAMWA)*, January 1996, p. 11

47. Smoking during pregnancy doubles the risking for having a low birth weight baby, and increases the risk for spontaneous abortion (miscarriage) by 70%, premature birth by 36%, and having a baby who dies during the newborn period by 25%. *The Health Consequences of Smoking for Women*, 1980 Surgeon General report

55. Children whose mothers smoked during pregnancy had significantly lower IQ scores (4 to 9 points) than the children of non-smokers in a study from Pediatrics in February 1994. This difference is comparable to the effects that moderate levels of lead exposure have on children's IQ scores. *Associated Press*, February 11, 1994

56. There is an association between prenatal cigarette smoking and childhood intellectual development, with a decrement of almost 7 IQ points in children born to smokers. This difference is comparable to deficits observed in children with low level environmental lead exposure. *JAMA*, June 7, 1995, p. 1709

57. Women who smoke while pregnant could be dooming their babies to lower IQs. Children ages 3 and 4 whose mothers smoked 10 or more cigarettes a day during pregnancy scored about nine points lower on intelligence tests than the offspring of nonsmokers. Tobacco smoke could influence the developing fetal nervous system by reducing oxygen and nutrient flow to the fetus. *Pediatrics*, February 1994, p. 221

58. Children of mothers who smoke are shorter and have poorer school performance compared to children of nonsmoking mothers. *British Medical Journal*, November 12, 1988, p. 1233

59. Children born to women who smoke have an average delay of three to five months in reading and math ability compared to their peers. *Newsweek*, November 12, 1985, p. 77

60. In a study from Pennsylvania, children of mothers who smoked during pregnancy had increased frequency of hyperactivity and short attention span, as well as lower scores on spelling and reading tests.
*Obstetrics and Gynecology*, November 1984, p. 60

61. Pregnant women who smoke more than 10 cigarettes a day have a 4.4-fold increased risk of having boys with "conduct disorder", defined as serious antisocial problem or destructive behavior (lying, stealing, vandalism, aggression) for six months or more.
*Associated Press*, July 15, 1997 (from July 1997 *Archives of General Psychiatry*)

62. A study from Archives of General Psychiatry reported that boys whose mothers smoked during pregnancy were 4.4 times more likely to engage in aggressive, destructive or other problem behaviors, or what psychiatrists call "conduct disorder" that begins much earlier and is much more severe than typical juvenile delinquency. Nicotine may disrupt fetal brain development. Time, July 28, 1997, p. 23, and Associated Press, July 15, 1997

63. In a study from Denmark in the March 1999 issue of Archives of General Psychiatry, men whose mothers smoked a pack a day or more during the third trimester were twice as likely as others to have been arrested for a violent crime, and nearly that likely to be chronic criminals. Newsweek, March 29, 1999, p. 81

64. "As if there weren't enough reasons to quit, a new study links smoking during pregnancy to serious psychological problems in children. Prepubescent boys whose moms smoked are four times as likely to steal, set fires, lie or exhibit other aggressive behavior. Adolescent girls, meanwhile, are five times as likely to abuse drugs." Reported in Time, July 12 1999, p. 82, from an article from the July 1999 issue of the Journal of the American Academy of Child and Adolescent Psychiatry

65. Women who smoke while pregnant are far more likely to have children who develop behavior problems as toddlers, a study has found. Nearly all 2-year-olds exhibit some rebelliousness, risk-taking and impulsiveness, but such behavior was four times more likely in toddlers whose mothers smoked during pregnancy, according to the study published in the Archives of Pediatrics & Adolescent Medicine. The findings suggest a chemical root for the problem behavior, since the researchers took into account sociological factors that might have affected the children, such as a mother's stress, personality and income level. Previous studies have linked smoking during pregnancy to low birth weight, retardation and even adult criminal behavior. Quote from Contra Costa (California) Times, April 18, 2000, p. D1

66. The more a woman smokes during her pregnancy, the greater the risk for serious behavior problems in her child. A possible explanation for the link is that low levels of serotonin in the brain are associated with increased levels of aggression. American Health, January-February 1996, p. 30

67. Stillbirths and early neonatal deaths are increased by about 33% in the babies of smokers as compared with those of nonsmokers. The effects of smoking in pregnancy extend well beyond infancy, with a reduction in growth and educational achievement. NEJM, March 31, 1994, p. 910

68. A study published in the April 1996 issue of Pediatrics presented data that women who smoked while pregnant were 50 percent more likely to have mentally retarded children. About 35% of women who gave birth to retarded children reported smoking as few as five cigarettes a week during pregnancy. Women who smoked during the last six months of pregnancy, when a fetus develops many organs, were 60% more likely to have retarded children than women who did not smoke then. Pregnant women who smoked at least a pack of cigarettes a day were 85 percent more likely to give birth to a retarded child. The researchers considered children retarded if their I.Q. was lower than 70 when they were 10 years old. Overall, 35% of mothers of retarded children were smokers, compared with 23% of mothers of non-retarded children. Associated Press, April 9, 1996

69. Smoking is associated with a higher risk of menstrual problems. Current smokers report heavier, more changeable, and irregular periods as well as severe period pain, when compared to never smokers or former smokers. Abstract PO 122, 10th World Conference on Tobacco or Health, Beijing, 1997

72. In one study, HIV-positive mothers who smoked were 3.3 times more likely to transmit the infection to their fetuses before birth, compared to nonsmoking HIV-positive mothers. *Cigarettes*, p. 86

73. Among pregnant women infected with HIV who smoked, about a third had HIV-seropositive babies, compared to 22% of HIV-positive mothers who did not smoke. The increased risk is thought to be due to the adverse effects of smoking on the placenta. Reuters Health eline, May 2, 1997

74. In a study from Sweden, pregnant women who smoke have an increased risk of having a very premature infant.
Reuters, November 26, 1998 (from the Journal of Obstetrics and Gynecology 1998; 179:1051-1055)

75. The odds ratio for a very preterm (premature) delivery among pregnant women who smoked 10 or more cigarettes a day was 1.6, or a 60% increased risk.                                    NEJM 1999; 341: 943

76. In a 1987 survey, 26% of non-pregnant women and 16.3% of pregnant women reported being smokers. By 1996, only 11.8% of pregnant and 23.6% of non-pregnant women were smokers. In the ten years of the survey, pregnant women were about half as likely to be current smokers compared to women who were not pregnant.
JAMA, January 19, 2000, pp. 361-366

77. About 60% of women who smoke before pregnancy continue to smoke during pregnancy.
*Nicotine Safety and Toxicity*, p. 99

78. Only one in six British women who smoke give up the habit when they become pregnant.
British Medical Journal, September 10, 1998

79. There is "strong evidence that the reduced lung function in infants born to smoking mothers is in large measure due to an in-utero alteration in lung development that occurs prior to the middle of the third trimester."
American Journal of Respiratory and Critical Care Medicine, Vol. 158, 1998, p. 690 (Fernando Martinez)

80. "...the direct additional health care costs in the United States associated just with the birth complications caused by pregnant women smoking or being exposed to secondhand smoke could be as high as $2 billion per year or more, with the costs linked to each smoking-affected birth averaging $1142 to $1358."
1995 CDC data published by Campaign for Tobacco-Free Kids

81. The percentage of pregnant women who smoked at some point during their pregnancies dropped from 18.4% in 1990 to just over 12% in 1999. This 12%, however, translates into half a million mothers who continue to smoke during their pregnancy. The highest rate was in white teenagers, 30% of whom smoked during pregnancy. There was a huge disparity in different states, with West Virginia "leading" at 26.1%, and Texas the lowest at 6.9%. American Indian women had the highest rate of all ethnic groups, 20%, and women of Chinese descent the lowest, only 0.5%. There were also major differences in rates depending upon educational status in the CDC study. Only 2% of college graduates smoked during pregnancy in 1999, compared with 29% of pregnant women who had not finished high school.
Los Angeles Times, August 29, 2001 (from Centers for Disease Control report)

82. The rate of smoking during pregnancy dropped 33% between 1990 and 1999, so that in 1999 just over 12% of all women reported smoking during their pregnancies. The greatest success in reducing smoking was for women in their late twenties and early thirties, where there was over a 40% drop since 1990. Teenagers were more likely than women of any other age to smoke while pregnant. After experiencing a dramatic 20% decline in the first part of the decade, smoking rates among pregnant teenagers--unlike women of all other ages-- increased by 5% from 1994 to 1999. The highest rate in 1999 (19%) was for women 18-19 years of age. About 2% of mothers with four or more years of college smoked during pregnancy, in contrast with 29% for those not completing high school. Of all groups, American Indian women still have the highest rate of smoking during pregnancy (20%) and had the smallest percent reduction.                    2002 AMA Annual Tobacco Report

83. In 1998, the prevalence of smoking during pregnancy was only 2.2% among mothers with 16 years or more of education (college degree), compared to 25.5% smoking rates in pregnancy for women with only 9 to 11 years of education (less than high school degree).          *Women and Smoking*, 2001 Surgeon General report, p. 73

84. In 1998, 13% of American women continued to smoke while pregnant. About 25% of smoking women quit on their own when they became pregnant; about half of this group restarts within six months of giving birth. 5% of all perinatal deaths can be linked to smoking during pregnancy.   American Medical News, January 15, 2001

85. About 30% of women smokers quit spontaneously early in their pregnancies.
American Journal of Public Health, September 2001, p. 1393

86. Postpartum relapse in women who stop smoking during pregnancy has been reported at 32 to 54% six weeks after delivery, 56 to 65% at six months, and a 67% relapse rate one year after delivery.

*Women and Smoking*, 2001 Surgeon General report, p. 564

87. In a study from the United Kingdom, a self help approach to smoking cessation during pregnancy was ineffective when implemented during routine antenatal care. The authors concluded that more intensive interventions needed to be developed.

British Medical Journal, December 14, 2002, p. 1383

88. For every dollar invested in stop smoking interventions for pregnant women, an estimated six dollars is saved in averting the costs associated with the delivery of babies with low birth weight. Brief cessation counseling in pregnancy is likely for smokers to be more cost effective than all the rest of their prenatal care.

Western Journal of Medicine, April 2001, p. 277

89. Women who stop smoking during pregnancy appear to be less likely to relapse if they breast feed their babies.

*Women and Smoking*, 2001 Surgeon General report, p. 488

90. A 55-cent per pack tax increase would cut smoking rates among pregnant women by about 22% nationwide, and by about 16% in pregnant teens.

American Journal of Public Health, November 2001

91. Elimination of maternal smoking might lead to a 10% reduction in all infant deaths and a 12% reduction in death from perinatal conditions.

*Women and Smoking*, 2001 Surgeon General report, p. 296

92. Smoking during pregnancy results in the death of an estimated 599 male and 408 female babies annually in the United States.

JAMA, May 8, 2002, p. 2355

93. Smoking during pregnancy causes about 1000 infant deaths each year.

Morbidity and Mortality Weekly Report, April 12, 2002

94. In a study from the Mayo Clinic, there was an alarming incidence (19%) of cigarette smoking among pregnant women with asthma, and the incidence of prematurity and birth abnormalities were twice as common in women who smoked and had asthma compared to nonsmokers. Other adverse perinatal outcomes were also significantly greater in pregnant asthmatics who smoked.

Journal of Asthma and Clinical Immunology, February 2001, p. 569

95. In the United States, 23.6% of all SIDS deaths appear to be attributable to prenatal maternal smoking.

American Journal of Public Health, March 2001, p. 432

96. 11% to 14% of preterm births are attributable to smoking during pregnancy.

Women and Smoking, 2001 Surgeon General report, p. 290

97. Women who smoke may have an increased risk for ectopic pregnancy, preterm premature rupture of membranes, abruptio placentae, and placenta previa.

*Women and Smoking*, 2001 Surgeon General report, pp. 278 and 281

98. Maternal parental smoking is related to criminal and substance abuse outcomes in both male and female offspring.

American Journal of Psychiatry 2002; 159:48

99. In a study from Sweden, children of mothers who smoke were more likely to develop both type 2 diabetes and obesity later in life.

JAMA, February 13, 2002, p. 706

100. In a study from Denmark, maternal smoking was associated with an increase risk (adjusted odds ratio 2.0) of infantile hypertrophic pyloric stenosis.

British Medial Journal, November 2, 2002, p. 1011

101. Pregnant women who smoke regularly are 40% more likely to have autistic children.

ASH Smoking and Health Review, July-August 2002, p. 6

102. Pregnant women who smoke increase by 5.5 times their risk of developing varicella zoster (chicken pox) virus pneumonia, a complication of natural chicken pox infection.        Skin and Allergy News, May 2002, p. 38

103. There tends to be a decreased head circumference in babies born to mother who smoke.
Dean Edell, M.D., ABC radio, June 12, 2001

104. In the August 2001 edition of the American Journal of Epidemiology, a Danish study reports that women who smoke while pregnant nearly double the risk of stillbirth. Exposure to tobacco smoke in utero was associated with an increased risk of stillbirth (odds ratio =2.0), and infant mortality was almost doubled in children born to women who had smoked during pregnancy compared with children of nonsmokers (odds ratio=1.8). Among children of women who stopped smoking during the first trimester, stillbirth and infant mortality was comparable with that in children of women who had been nonsmokers from the beginning of pregnancy. Approximately 25% of all stillbirth and 20% of all infant deaths in a population with 30% pregnant smokers could be avoided if all pregnant women stopped smoking by the sixteenth week of gestation.

# Smoking and Low Birth Weight

1. Maternal smoking is the most important cause of intrauterine growth retardation. The average baby born to a smoker is 8 ounces lighter because of this oxygen deprivation during pregnancy.  AMA, January 3, 1986,  p. 22

2. Cigarette smoking during pregnancy reduces by as much as 25% the amount of oxygen that reaches the fetus.
American Lung Association Fact Sheet, Women and Smoking (August 1997 Update)

3. A smoking cessation program offered to all pregnant smokers could save five dollars for every dollar spent by preventing low birth weight-associated neonatal intensive care and long term care.
Morbidity and Mortality Weekly Report, October 5, 1990, p. vii

4. Maternal smoking during the third trimester of pregnancy increases by 2.2 times the risk for the birth of a small for gestational age, or low birth weight, baby.        American Journal of Public Health, July 1994, p. 1127

5. Maternal smoking is the reason that 53,000 babies a year in the United States are born with low birth weight, and an additional 22,000 need expensive intensive care in the newborn period.
Action on Smoking and Health letter, August 1996

6. If smoking were eliminated, there would be 25% fewer babies born with low birth weight and 41% fewer childhood deaths between one month and five years of age.
Pediatric Clinics of North America, April 1987, p. 363

7. In a review of five clinical studies, 21% to 39% of the incidence of low birth weight babies was attributable to maternal cigarette smoking. Compared with non-smokers, light and heavy smokers have 54% and 130% increases in the prevalence of low birth weight babies under 2500 grams, or about 5 1/2 pounds. In other studies, children of smokers have shown deficits in growth, intellectual and emotional development, and behavior.                                                                              JAMA, May 24, 1985, p. 2998

8. Fetal growth may be adversely affected when the mother is passively exposed to tobacco smoke during pregnancy. A mean birth weight deficit of 88 grams, about 3 ounces, was found in newborns of nonsmoking mothers whose fathers smoked more than 20 cigarettes a day.
American Journal of Public Health, September 1994, p. 1489

9. In the 1980's, maternal smoking contributed to 17% to 26% of low birth weight babies born in the United States. The mean average excess medical cost per live birth for each pregnant smoker was $511 (in 1995 dollars); direct medical expenditures on low birth weight babies from maternal smoking are $263 million per year. An annual drop of one percentage point in smoking prevalence in pregnant women over seven years would prevent 57,200 low birth weight infants and save $572 million in direct medical costs.
Pediatrics, December 1999, pp. 1312-1320

10. Passive smoke exposure in nonsmoking pregnant women doubles the risk for a mother delivering a small for gestational age baby. American Journal of Public Health, October 1998, p. 1523

11. In 1997, 13.2% of women giving birth said that they had smoked during their pregnancy. 20 to 30% of low birth weight cases in babies are attributable to smoking during pregnancy. Reuters, May 27, 1999

12. In 1999, 12.1% of women who smoked during pregnancy had low birth weight babies, compared with 7.2% of women who did not smoke. Los Angeles Time, August 29, 2001 (CDC data)

13. "Some women would prefer having smaller babies."
Joseph Cullman, president of Philip Morris on CBS's "Face the Nation", January 1971, commenting on a study which showed that mothers who smoked gave birth to smaller babies

## Congenital Anomalies

1. One study found an increased risk of 1.6 for congenital malformations among babies born to heavy smokers; another reported a 2.3 fold higher risk of birth defects. However, other studies have not demonstrated an increased risk, and the overall evidence that cigarette smoking is related to congenital malformations is unclear.
*Reducing the Health Consequences of Smoking*, p. 73

2. In a study from Budapest, Hungary, maternal smoking during pregnancy raised the risk by 48% (relative odds 1.48) of delivering a baby with congenital limb deficiency (isolated absence of a single arm or leg).
British Medical Journal, June 4, 1994, p. 1473

3. In a study from Seattle, maternal smoking during pregnancy was associated with a 2.3-fold increased risk of congenital urinary tract anomalies in offspring. American Journal of Public Health, February 1996, p. 249

4. Babies of mothers who smoke during pregnancy run twice the risk of cleft lips and palates. If there were no smoking during pregnancy, it would reduce from 7000 to 5000 the total yearly number of US babies with oral clefts. Corrective surgeries and treatment cost up to $100,000 per child.
American Medical News, April 8, 1996 (from March 1996 American Journal of Human Genetics)

5. Fetuses whose mothers smoke are 50 to 70% more likely to develop a cleft lip or palate. 13% of pregnant American women still smoke. Newsweek, April 24, 2000, p. 78

6. "To date, most studies have found no association between cigarette smoking during pregnancy and the overall risk for birth defects." *Women and Smoking*, 2001 Surgeon General report, p. 303

7. Maternal smoking is associated with an increased risk of birth defects, including hydrocephaly, microcephaly, omphalocele/gastroschisis, cleft lip and palate, clubfoot, and polydactyly/syndactyly. [This is in contrast with the previous entry – editor] Public Health Reports, July-August 2001, p. 327

8. Maternal smoking is not generally associated with an increased risk for cleft lip or cleft palate in babies. However, the subset of mothers who smoke and carry a genotype called GSTT1 had a much increased risk (odds ratio 3.2) of delivery babies with oral clefting. Epidemiology 2001; 12:502-507

## Miscarriage

1. Smoking may account for as many as 7.5% of all miscarriages, or 115,000 in the US each year, and the deaths of 5600 babies, including an estimated 1900 from Sudden Infant Death Syndrome (SIDS). It also contributes to 53,000 low birth weight babies a year, and 22,000 babies who require intensive care at birth.
Associated Press, April 13, 1995, and Journal of Family Practice, April 1995, p. 385

2. "It's very clear that you cannot be pro-life and be pro-tobacco. Tobacco is a major cause of abortions in America." Joe DiFranza MD, tobacco control researcher, CNN Headline News, April 11, 1995

3. An estimated 15,000 abortions, or miscarriages, each year are caused by tobacco. This represents 19% of all miscarriages experienced by smoking women. Smoking during pregnancy increases a woman's risk of miscarrying by 24%. Tobacco-Free Youth Reporter, Fall 1995, p. 16

4. In a study of 1000 black inner-city women, smoking cigarettes was responsible for 16% of miscarriages, and cocaine caused 8%. 80% more miscarriages occur among women who smoke cigarettes. Reuters, February 3, 1998 (from NEJM)

5. Cigarette smoking in pregnancy is associated with an 80% increased risk of spontaneous abortion, or miscarriage (odds ratio of 1.8). NEJM, February 4, 1999, p. 333

6. 50% of female smokers in a survey were unaware that smoking during pregnancy increases the risk for stillbirth and miscarriage.

7. About 11% of all spontaneous abortions are attributable to smoking. Among women who smoke a pack a day or more, smoking causes 40% of all spontaneous abortions. American Journal of Public Health, January 1992, p. 85

8. Maternal smoking increases the risk of miscarriage, stillbirth, and neonatal death by 25 to 35%. This represents an annual loss of almost 5000 fetuses and newborn infants in England. Thorax, August 1994, p. 731

9. In a study from Australia, three or more miscarriages were reported by 7.4% of current smokers, 5.3% of former smokers, and 3.7% of never smokers in a survey of 14,000 women ages 45 to 49. Among the same number of women ages 18 to 22, one or two miscarriages were reported by 6.2% of current smokers, 4.7% of former smokers, and only 1.4% of never smokers. Abstract OS 79, 10th World Conference on Tobacco or Health, Beijing, 1997

10. In 1980, about a quarter of women smoked regularly during pregnancies. This means that of the 3.6 million women who delivered in 1980, approximately 900,000 women smoked during pregnancy. Because maternal smoking during pregnancy increases the number of "spontaneous" abortions by approximately five abortions per hundred pregnancies, such smoking by nearly one million women in the United States may have caused approximately 50,000 abortions in 1980. American Journal of Preventive Medicine, April 1985, p. 13

11. A 1992 study estimated that smoking accounted for 11% of all spontaneous abortions "and could have explained 40% of spontaneous abortions among women smoking 20 or more cigarettes per day." In a small case-control study of habitual abortion (two or more spontaneous abortions), current smokers had a relative risk of 1.4. *Women and Smoking*, 2001 Surgeon General report, p. 283

# Fertility and Menopause

1. Nicotine is toxic to sperm, and reduces its ability to penetrate eggs by 12 to 16 percent. Nicotine lowers the sperm count, causes sperm to clump together, reduces sperm swimming ability and causes it to grow in abnormal shapes. San Francisco Chronicle, February 4, 1991, p. A4

2. Two studies reported in the March 1998 issue of the journal Fertility and Sterility showed that men who smoke had poorer quality and more structurally abnormal sperm, and that smoking might impair fertility. American Medical News, April 27, 1998

3. Male smokers have lower levels of testosterone, a reduced volume of semen ejaculated with decreased sperm production and lower sperm count, an impairment of sperm motility and movement, a higher percentage of sperm with abnormal morphology or shape, and an increase in the number of white blood cells in the sperm, or pyospermia. *Cigarettes*, pp. 96-97

4.  In men in fertility clinics, cigarette smoking is associated with significant decreases in sperm penetration assay scores and with increased numbers of seminal fluid white blood cells.

    Journal of Urology, October 1990, p. 900

5.  In a study from the Czech Republic, male teenage smokers had sperm damage and significant evidence of chromosomal damage that could cause genetic abnormalities in their children.

    San Francisco Chronicle, October 2, 1998, p. A2

6.  Smoking men are at nearly double the risk for cancer-linked sperm mutations than non-smoking men.

    ASH Smoking and Health Review, July-August 1999 (from Fertility and Sterility, August 1999)

7.  Smoking more than 10 cigarettes daily has been linked to 10% to 15% lower sperm counts compared to nonsmoking men.

    Reuters, March 23, 1998

8.  Women who smoke more than 10 cigarettes a day are 40% more likely to enter menopause earlier than nonsmokers.

    Journal of Clinical Epidemiology 1998; 51:1271

9.  Females who smoke have a 28% reduction in fertility, and are 3.4 times more likely to take longer than a year to become pregnant. Heavy smokers have only 57% of the pregnancy rate of non-smokers.

    JAMA, May 24, 1985, p. 2979

10. In vitro fertilization rates of eggs (oocytes) is much reduced in women who smoke. The mechanism is unknown, but there is a strong association between smoking and reduced fertility.

    The Lancet, December 5, 1992, p. 1409

11. Smoking causes women to have their natural menopause one to two years early.

    Morbidity and Mortality Weekly Report October 5, 1990, p. 8,
    and Archives of Internal Medicine, January 1988, p. 143

12. Premenopausal women who give up smoking tend to go through menopause at the normal time.

    The Harvard Guide to Women's Health, Karen Carlson, Harvard University Press, 1996, p. 583

13. Women who smoke may experience menopause up to eight years earlier than nonsmokers.

    from What Every Woman Should Know:
    Staying Healthy after 40, Lila Nachtigall, Warner Books, 1995

14. Women who smoke are 3 to 4 times more likely than nonsmokers to take more than one year to become pregnant, and are 3 times as likely to be infertile. This is because smoking lowers levels of the hormone necessary for ovulation and the implantation of a fertilized egg in the uterus.

    Reducing the Health Consequences of Smoking, p. 75

15. Smoking probably reduces a woman's probability of conceiving by one-third per cycle.

    Journal of the American Medical Women's Association, January 1996, p. 29

16. Infertility is two to three times more prevalent in women who smoke.      The Tobacco Epidemic, p. 95

17. Ovulation does not occur normally in smokers, impairing a woman's ability to conceive.      Cigarettes, p. 83

18. The fertility rates of women who smoke are about 30% lower than those of nonsmokers, and smokers are about 3.4 times more likely to take more than a year to conceive than are nonsmokers.

    New York Times, October 25, 1996, p. A39

19. "Cigarette smoking...seems to alter fallopian tube function, which in turn seems to destroy eggs and impair the density, movement, and shape of sperm."      The Harvard Guide to Women's Health, Karen Carlson,
    Harvard University Press, 1996, p. 322

20. Nonsmoking women living with a smoker are 34% less likely to become pregnant than women from smoke-free homes, concludes a study from Bristol University.
Time, December 18, 2000

21. In a study from France of women undergoing in vitro fertilization, smokers of more than 10 cigarettes a day had only a 15% chance of successful implantation, compared with about 23% for nonsmokers.
2002 AMA Annual Tobacco Report

22. "Women who smoke have increased risks for conception delay and for both primary and secondary infertility."
*Women and Smoking*, 2001 Surgeon General report, p. 307

23. Men who have difficulty fathering children reduce their chances of success by about two thirds if they smoke. Smoking alters the DNA of sperm.
ASH Smoking and Health Review, July-August 2002, p. 6

24. The polycyclic aromatic hydrocarbons (PAHs) in tobacco smoke accelerate the death of egg cells, or oocytes, in the ovaries, and egg cell death may explain why women who smoke reach menopause two to three years earlier than nonsmokers, as well as why women who smoke have a higher incidence of infertility.
2002 AMA Annual Tobacco Report

# CHAPTER 15
# CHILDREN AND TEEN SMOKING

1.  "The early use of tobacco is one of the most lamentable evils which afflict the rising generation. Cigarettes have done more to demoralize and vitiate youth than all the liquor-shops in the land."   New York Times editorial, 1909

2.  "A vigorous effort to prevent initiation of tobacco use by children and youths must be the centerpiece of the nation's tobacco control policy, and should be among its highest public health priorities."
    *Growing Up Tobacco Free*, p.11

3.  Adolescents who smoke greatly overestimate smoking prevalence in both their peer group and with adults. Ninth graders who smoke estimate that 55% of their peers are also regular smokers (actual figure 12%), and also estimate that 66% of adults smoke (actual figure is 25%).   *Growing Up Tobacco Free*, p. 79

4.  There are 6 million teenagers in the United States who smoke, and another 100,000 children age 12 or younger who smoke.   NEJM, March 31, 1994, p. 910

5.  7% of high school seniors with an A average are smokers. 47% of students with a D average or less are smokers.
    Internal Medicine World Report, June 1991

6.  Cigarette smoking increases with decreasing academic performance, particularly for girls.
    Pediatric Clinics of North America, April 1987, p. 370

7.  Of the four million adolescents who smoke, more than three-quarters come from homes where one or both parents also smoke.   American Medical News, January 24, 1994, p. 11

8.  In a study from Minnesota, 73% of adolescent smokers had other smokers in their households, and only 46% were living with both biological parents. 52% had parents who were divorced. In another survey of adolescents who smoked, 75% came from families where one or both parents also smoked.   Pediatrics, October 1996, p. 666

9.  Another study estimates that if both parents smoke, there is a 63% chance that their child will become a smoker. If neither parent smokes, this chance drops to 6%.   Postgraduate Medicine, July 1988, p. 21

10. The most effective means to have children not begin to smoke is to have nonsmoking parents. Adolescents with one or both parents who smoke are almost twice as likely to become smokers themselves.
    1994 Surgeon General report, *Preventing Tobacco Use Among Young People*, p. 129

11. Candy cigarettes send a message to children that smoking is accepted and "normal" behavior.
    Pediatrics, January 1992, p. 27

12. Children and teens are generally not interested in the long-term health hazards of smoking. Instead, reasons not to start should emphasize short-term effects such as impairment of physical fitness, bad breath, and yellow teeth. Adolescents should also be made aware of the "con job" of the cigarette companies, who are manipulating them through their advertising into an addictive and very expensive behavior.
    Journal of School Health, May 1989, p. 184

13. The three most heavily advertised brands, Marlboro, Camel, and Newport, are the choice of 86% of teenagers who smoke. By contrast, these three brands have only 32.7% of the adult market.
    1993 data from the Centers for Disease Control and Prevention

14. 85 to 90% of children and teenagers who smoke choose one of these brands: Marlboro (43% market share), Camel (30%), or Newport (20%, and the most popular brand among blacks). These are also among the most heavily advertised brands in the United States, suggesting that advertising influences teens in their choice of brands.
    Mortality and Morbidity Weekly Report, 1992

15. Cigarette brands popular with young adolescents are more likely than adult brands to advertise in magazines with a higher percentage of young (ages 12-17 years) readers. "Youths are more heavily exposed to magazine cigarette advertisements for brands that are popular among youth smokers than for brands smoked almost exclusively by adults."                                                                            JAMA, February 18, 1998, pp. 516-520

16. 68.7% of current smokers ages 12 to 18 choose Marlboro as their brand. But black adolescents most frequently chose Newport (70%).                                                                            JAMA, September 21, 1994, p. 843
                                                            and Morbidity and Mortality Weekly Report, March 13, 1992, p. 170

17. In a 1989 study, 71% of white adolescents who smoked preferred Marlboro, while 82% of black adolescent smokers chose a mentholated brand (Newport 61%, Kool 11%, and Salem 10%). Only 8% of black adolescent smokers chose Marlboro.                                                                            JAMA, April 8, 1992, p. 1893

18. In a 1992 study of ninth grade smokers, 91.2% chose one of the three most heavily advertised brands, Marlboro (45.1%), Newport (23.7%), and Camel (22.4%).                                                                            Tobacco Control, Winter 1997, p. 534

19. At present smoking rates, 20 million of the 250 million children in Europe who do not yet smoke will eventually die from tobacco-induced disease.                                                                            The Lancet, September 21, 1991, p. 748/

20. Each day, about 6000 American children and teenagers try a cigarette for the first time, and about half of them eventually become daily smokers.                                                                            Public Health Reports, July/August 1997, p. 292

21. An estimated 4.5 million U.S. children ages 12 to 17 now use tobacco products.
                                                                            New York Times, September 18, 1997, p. A18

22. About 3000 young people, 80% to 90% younger than age 18, become new smokers each day. These 1 million new smokers each year partially replace the 2 million smokers who either quit or die each year.
                                                                            JAMA, February 23, 1994, p. 628

23. Because of the 1200 Americans who die each day from smoking, and the 3600 each day (1.3 million per year) who successfully quit, the tobacco companies must attract almost 5000 new smokers each day to keep the "status quo" and their sales steady. About 3000 children and adolescents each day begin to smoke.
                                                                            Disease-a-Month, April 1990, p. 205

24. 3000 adolescents become regular smokers each day. The average age to begin smoking is 13, and the average age to begin using smokeless tobacco is 10.                                                                            American Medical News, July 19, 1993

25. 80 to 90% of regular smokers begin the habit before high school graduation, and 60% began before age 14.
                                                            NEJM, April 7, 1994, p. 979 and American Medical News, January 24 1994, p. 11

26. 90% of smokers begin to smoke before age 20, and 50% begin before age 13. Each 10% price increase of cigarettes reduces smoking by 4% overall, but teenagers are much more price-sensitive, and a 10% price hike results in a 14% decline in consumption in this group, the vast majority representing a decision not to begin to smoke.        Los Angeles Times, February 7, 1987 and Journal of Public Health Policy, September 1984, p. 312

27. In a more recent study, health economists estimate that each 10% cigarette price increase would result in 7% fewer teen smokers, and that teens who continue to smoke will smoke 6% fewer cigarettes.
                                                                            Associated Press, August 4, 1997

28. "It is no coincidence that in 1993--the year that saw a sharp increase in the number of teenagers who started smoking--tobacco companies lowered the price by 40 cents on the three brands that young people predominately smoke . . . "                                                                            British Medical Journal, August 23, 1997

29. In Canada, tax increases reduced adolescent smoking by 62% and adult smoking by 35% between 1982 and 1992.
                                                                            American Journal of Public Health, April 1994, p. 546

30. In Canada from 1979 to 1991, the real price of cigarettes increased by 158%, and teenage cigarette use fell by two
thirds. World Smoking and Health No. 3, 1992, p. 10

31. A 10% increase in the price of cigarettes, about 18 cents a pack, cuts adult smoking by 4% and teen smoking by
12%. Estimates are that a 50-cent increase would cut the number of teen smokers by a million and save 250,000
from a premature death. USA Today, April 3, 1997, p. 14A

32. An increase of only 20 cents a pack would reduce teenage smoking by 18%, cut the total number of smokers by
half a million, and would eventually result in 125,000 fewer premature deaths yearly.
Hospital Practice, June 15, 1993, p. 8

33. A study from the National Bureau of Economic Research showed that a 75-cent increase in the cost of a pack of
cigarettes in 1992 – 1994 would have cut overall youth smoking in half and reduced the number of underage
smokers by 1.6 million and future smoking-related premature deaths by 400,000.
ASH Smoking and Health Review, July-August 1996, p. 4

34. When high school dropouts are included (as many as 70% of dropouts smoke), the adolescent smoking rate is
about 25%, the same as the adult rate. American Medical News, January 24, 1994, p. 11, and
American Journal of Public Health, February 1988, p. 176

35. Of the 434,000 US tobacco-related deaths in 1988, one half occurred in people who began smoking by age 13, and
one quarter in people who began smoking by age 11. American Journal of Public Health, March 1993, p. 468

36. Nearly all first use of tobacco occurs before high school graduation; if adolescents can be kept tobacco-free until
this time, most will never start using tobacco. Over three million children and adolescents smoke cigarettes, and
over one million adolescent males currently use smokeless tobacco. Smoking appears to reduce the rate of lung
growth and the level of maximum lung function that can be achieved.
*Preventing Tobacco Use*, 1994 Surgeon General report, p. 5

37. One out of three adolescents in the United States is using tobacco by age 18, and almost all first use has occurred
by high school graduation. 28% of the nation's high school seniors are currently cigarette smokers.
*Preventing Tobacco Use Among Young People*, 1994 Surgeon General report introduction

38. Each day in the United States, 3000 children begin to use tobacco. Of these, about 40% begin experimentation in
grade school, and initiation of regular daily smoking is highest among children 12 to 14 years of age.
Pediatrics, May 1994, p. 866

39. In adolescents, smoking increases levels of very low density lipoprotein cholesterol (the "bad cholesterol") by 12%
and of triglycerides also by 12%. It decreases levels of high-density lipoprotein cholesterol (the "good
cholesterol") by 9%. 1994 Surgeon General report, p. 28

40. Only 14% of teen smokeless tobacco users report that their father disapproved of the habit; 60% said that their
mother disapproved. 1994 Surgeon General report, p. 142

41. 61% of smokers began the habit by the eighth grade, and one quarter of high school senior smokers reported
starting before sixth grade. *Nicotine Addiction*, p. 365, and 1994 Surgeon General report, p. 88

42. If current smoking prevalence rates remain the same, 20 million of the 70 million children in the US today will
become smokers, and at least 5 million will eventually die from smoking-related diseases.
*Nicotine Addiction*, p. 367

43. Of every 100 high school smokers, 95% plan to quit within five years of graduation, but only 25% actually
succeed. American Medical News, January 24, 1994, p. 11

44. "Children tend to vastly underestimate the likelihood that they will become addicted to these products. Although
only 5 percent of daily smokers surveyed in high school said they would definitely be smoking five years later,

close to 75 percent were smoking 7 to 9 years later. A survey conducted in 1992 found that approximately two-thirds of adolescents who smoked said they wanted to quit and 70 percent said they would not start smoking if they could make that choice again."
*Stop the Sale, Prevent the Addiction*

45. "Empirical data, moreover, support the position that minors do not make well-informed choices about smoking. Among high school seniors who were surveyed between 1976 and 1986, 45% of daily smokers believed that they would not be smoking within 5 years; yet in follow-up studies 5 to 6 years later, 73% remained daily smokers. In 1992, approximately two thirds of adolescent smokers reported that they wanted to quit smoking, and 70% indicated that they would not have started if they could choose again."  JAMA, February 5, 1997, p. 414

46. 92% of female teens who smoke do not expect to be smoking in one year, revealing a dangerous naiveté about the addictiveness of tobacco.  JAMA, February 23, 1994, p. 630

47. Only 5% of adolescents who smoke believe that they will still be smoking 5 years later. In fact, 75% of them are still smoking 8 years later.  *Nicotine Addiction*, p. 376

48. A 1992 document from Imperial Tobacco Limited details a project called "Project 16," noting that many young people who begin smoking "in the 14-16 age range" doubt that they will become addicted to cigarettes. "Once addiction does take place, it becomes necessary for the smoker to make peace with the accepted hazards. This is done by a wide range of rationalizations."  Washington Post, February 5, 1998, p. A3

49. About 3000 children start smoking every day in the US. During their lifetime, of these 3000, about 30 will die in traffic accidents, and about 22 will be murdered, but 750 will die from smoking-related causes, with an average of 21 years of life lost. (*Nicotine Addiction*, p. 379) Subsequent estimates (1994 World Conference on Tobacco or Health in Paris) are even worse; 50% of all regular smokers who began as teenagers will be expected to eventually die from smoking-induced illness.

50. According to the World Health Organization, 800 million of the world's two billion children are destined to become smokers, and tobacco will eventually kill at least one third of the smoking group.
World Watch magazine, July-August 1997, p. 25

51. Number of adult smokers who successfully quit smoking each year: 1.3 million. Teenagers who start smoking each year: 1.1 million.  US News and World Report, November 29, 1993, p. 11

52. High school student smoking rates rose by nearly a third between 1991 and 1997, rising from 27.5% to 36.4%. The sharpest rise was an increase of 80%, from 12.6% to 22.7%, in African American students. The highest youth smoking rates are in white male high school students, with 51.5% saying that they smoked a cigarette in the previous month in 1997, and in white female students, with a 40.8% smoking rate.
New York Times, April 3, 1998, p. A20 (from Centers for Disease Control and Prevention)

53. "When the tobacco use rates of high school seniors, high school dropouts, and adolescent smokeless tobacco users are considered together, the daily tobacco use prevalence rate of US adolescents is approximately that of adults--about 25%--thus providing the necessary replacement smokers for those adults who quit or die from their tobacco use." About 70% of high school dropouts are smokers.  Preventive Medicine 1993; 22:514

54. Of California teenagers who have nonsmoking parents and best friends who do not smoke, only 6% are smokers. In the group with best friends who smoke and one or both smoking parents, 40% are current smokers.
*Tobacco Use in California*, p. 111

55. Among teenage high school dropouts, from 43% to 70% are current smokers.
Morbidity and Mortality Weekly Report, February 25, 1994, p. 4

56. The US has 374,000 cigarette vending machines.  *Strategies to Control Tobacco Use*, p. 239

57. All 50 states and the District of Columbia have adopted a minimum age of 18 for the sale of tobacco. In 1993, 21 states had laws restricting vending machine sales, and at least 30 cities had totally banned vending machines.

*1994 Surgeon General report*, p. 249

58. The prevalence of smokeless tobacco use among teens ages 16 to 19 increased nearly 10-fold between 1970 and 1985. In 1993, 10.7% of high school seniors used smokeless tobacco. *Growing Up Tobacco Free*, p. 8

59. Adolescent smokers tend to discount long-term health risks. Only half of high school seniors who smoked reported believing that smoking a pack a more per day is a serious health risk. *Growing Up Tobacco Free*, p. 14

60. Adolescents underestimate the magnitude of the risks of smoking. Nearly half (47%) of eighth graders in 1993 denied that there is "great risk" associated with smoking a pack a day of cigarettes. Even among high school seniors, more than 30% denied that there was "great risk" associated with pack-a-day smoking.

*Growing Up Tobacco Free*, p. 240

61. In young American Indians and Alaskan Natives, weekly use of smokeless tobacco by boys was 43% and by girls 34%. *Growing Up Tobacco Free*, p. 75

62. The fifth grade edition of Weekly Reader, the free magazine circulated to grade school students nationwide, recently featured an article on smokers' rights and how tobacco industry profits and jobs would be hurt by increased excise taxes. The magazine is published by a unit of Kohlberg Kravis Roberts and Co., the majority shareholders in RJR Nabisco. *Tobacco Industry Strategies*, p. 12

63. Before RJR Nabisco purchased the Weekly Reader, which now reaches more than 8 million school children, 62% of its tobacco articles were anti-smoking. After the purchase, the figure dropped to 24%.

Washington Monthly, December 1995, p. 5

64. The more than one million young people who start to smoke each year will add an estimated $10 billion to the cost of health care in the US during their lifetimes. *Tobacco Use: An American Crisis*, p. 34

65. In response to the question "Do you think that you will be smoking cigarettes five years from now?" nearly 9 of every 10 high school seniors who smoked predicted they would be off the habit. But in follow-ups of those who smoked a pack a day, 70% were still smoking a pack or more five or six years later.

US News and World Report, September 26, 1994, p. 24

66. One third to one half of children who experiment with even a few cigarettes go on to become regular smokers, a process that takes an average of two to three years. American Journal of Public Health, April 1994, p. 544

67. About 30% of cigarette experimenters eventually become established smokers; in California, over half (50.7%) of 17 year-olds had experimented with cigarettes. A University of California, San Diego study estimated that tobacco promotional activities influenced 34% of these adolescents, or 17% of the total population of this age, to experiment with cigarettes before they reached age 18. Nationally, this would be over 700,000 adolescents each year. This is the first longitudinal evidence that tobacco promotional activities are causally related to the onset of smoking. JAMA, February 18, 1998, pp. 511-515

68. The concordance rates for smokers were consistently higher in monozygotic (identical) then in dizygotic twins, even when the twins were brought up separately, supporting the idea of genetic component for the smoking habit.

The Tobacco Epidemic, p. 126

69. Adolescents with attention deficit disorder (formerly called hyperreactivity) have very high smoking rates, and adults with ADD have smoking rates of more than 40%. Paul Newhouse, M.D., Tenth National Conference on Nicotine Dependence, Minneapolis, October 17, 1997

70. In Japan, cigarette consumption among minors increased 16% after foreign transnational tobacco companies entered the market for the first time and began a massive advertising and promotional campaign. In Taiwan after the country opened to western brands, within two years the smoking rate among high school students had risen

from 19.5% to 32%, and cigarette consumption among women, almost nonexistent before, had skyrocketed. In South Korea, smoking rates among teenage boys rose from 18% to 30% in one year after import restrictions were removed, and among girls, smoking rates quadrupled. And in Thailand, the number of smokers aged 15 to 19 increased by 24% in the first three years after American brands first were sold.     INFACT Update, Summer 1994

71. In a study of 17,600 students from 140 four-year colleges, the smoking prevalence (smoking during the previous 30 days) was 22.3%. 25% were former smokers.     American Journal of Public Health, January 1998, pp. 104-107

72. By the mid-1980's, smoking was unusual in academically successful high school students. Only 5% of Harvard freshmen and 2% of Dartmouth freshmen are smokers.     Ellen Goodman column, December 10, 1995

73. In a 1994 poll, 88% of Americans favor banning free tobacco samples on public streets, 74% favor banning all cigarette vending machines, 59% favor banning all cigarette billboard advertising, 55% favor banning tobacco ads at sporting and entertainment events, and 51% favor banning tobacco ads in magazines and newspapers.
New York Times, February 1, 1995, p. A12

74. The weight control theme of cigarette ads plays into the preoccupation of many teenage girls with thin figures. Mistys are "slim and sassy", and a Virginia Slims ad says, "If I ran the world, calories wouldn't count."
Consumer Reports, March 1995, p. 143

75. Adolescents who begin to smoke share the risk factors of low socioeconomic status, poor school achievement, excessive rebelliousness and risk-taking, low self-esteem, dropping out of school, and not planning to go to college.                                                                                         Consumer Reports, March 1995, p. 145

76. An expert panel from the National Academy of Sciences recommends three major strategies to reduce the number of young people who begin to smoke: ban nearly all cigarette advertising and promotion, raise cigarette taxes to make smoking less affordable, and enforce laws against selling to minors.  Consumer Reports, March 1995, p. 146

77. An estimated 1.6 million children ages 12 to 17 are on tobacco company mailing lists for promotional items.
Tobacco Free Youth Reporter, Spring 1995

78. "Of all the things that will confuse historians of the next century, certainly the idea of a lethal product, a product of illness and despair, peddled to youngsters for the profit of the peddler, will be the most confusing."
William Forge, Proceedings of the 8th World Conference on Tobacco or Health, Buenos Aires, 1992

79. "Young smokers represent the majority opportunity group for the cigarette industry."
Marketing plan for Imperial Tobacco Ltd., 1971 (Washington Monthly, December 1995, p. 32)

80. "Realistically, if our Company is to survive and prosper, over the long term we must get our share of the youth market. In my opinion this will require new brands tailored to the youth market; I believe it unrealistic to expect that the existing brands identified with the an over-thirty 'establishment' market can ever become the 'in' products with the youth group." 1973 RJ Reynolds memo by Claude Teague (Washington Monthly, December 1995, p. 33)

81. The tobacco industry frames smoking as an "adult activity." This is an extremely effective strategy. First, adult activities are by definition attractive to many young people. Second, this strategy lumps smoking in with many other adult activities, such as making one's own choices, which are not inherently harmful. The tobacco industry has identified the "forbidden fruit" appeal as an important factor in adolescent experimentation with smoking. Youth access policies should not promote the status of smoking as the forbidden fruit, which is much more attractive to rebellious youth.                                              Quote from *Stop the Sale, Prevent the Addiction*

82. "Project Sixteen" was begun in 1976 by Imperial Tobacco of Canada, sister company to Brown and Williamson. The company in a 1977 summary discovered that serious efforts to learn to smoke occur at 12 or 13 years old. "Part of the thrill of adolescent smoking is the thrill of hiding it from parental wrath."
   • "In some cases, the beginning smoker is not just emulating the peer group in general, but copying a specific member of it that is respected and admired..."

•"More important reasons for this attraction are the 'forbidden fruits' aspect of cigarettes. The adolescent seeks to display his new urge for independence with a symbol, and cigarettes are such a symbol since they are associated with adulthood and at the same time the adults seek to deny them to the young."

•The company thus must ally itself with the children, against "adults" and aid the child in proclaiming "his break with childhood at least to his peers." *Smokescreen*, p. 83

83. "Evidence is now available to indicate that the 14-to18-year-old group is an increasing segment of the smoking population. RJR must soon establish a successful new brand in this market if our position in the industry is to be maintained over the long term." 1976 R.J. Reynolds internal memo (Tobacco Control, Autumn 1997, p. 234)

84. "Tobacco companies regularly and emphatically assert that 'we don't want kids to smoke', yet they spend billions on advertising campaigns featuring cowboys and cartoon characters. Not surprisingly, Marlboro and Camel are the brands most commonly smoked by kids; in California, 59% of 12 to 17 year old smokers smoke Marlboros and 23% smoke Camels." JAMA, February 10, 1993, p. 793

85. A 1974 RJR board of directors report states: "Winston and Salem show comparative weakness against Marlboro and Kool among these younger smokers. . . Thus, our strategy becomes clear. . . Direct advertising appeal to the younger smokers." American Medical News, February 2, 1998, p. 25

86. "If you are really and truly not going to sell to children, you are going to be out of business in 30 years." Bennett LeBow, Liggett Chairman Smoke Less States Tobacco News, Spring 1998

87. A 1950 item in the *United States Tobacco Journal* included the following: "A massive potential marker still exists among women and young adults, cigarette industry leaders agreed, acknowledging that recruitment of these millions of prospective smokers comprises the major objective for the immediate future and on a long term basis as well." *Smoke and Mirrors*, p. 177

88. One cigarette marketing plan noted, "The industry is dominated by the companies who respond most effectively to the needs of the younger smoker." British Medical Journal, August 23, 1997, p. 439

89. "However intriguing smoking was at 11, 12 or 13, by the age of 16 or 17 many regretted their use of cigarettes for health reasons and because they feel unable to stop smoking when they want to. By the age of 16, any peer pressure to initiate others to smoking is gone. In fact, smokers openly bemoan the sight of 11 or 12 year olds that they see smoking, and in effect, the 16 year olds now act towards their juniors as their own parents act towards them ..."

From "Project 16", a 1977 Canadian focus group report for Imperial Tobacco (*Smoke and Mirrors*, p. 167)

90. "...don't underestimate the industry's commitment to finding powerful nonverbal hooks, particularly for young beginning smokers. A lot of psychologists are reportedly on the payroll, and rumor has it that they include child psychologists, too." U.S. News and World Report, June 2, 1997, p. 18 (John Leo)

91. The message of Philip Morris to youth is "you shouldn't smoke unless you're a mature adult." That is nothing but a dare and an enticement or children to smoke. One of the main reasons children smoke is to appear mature and adult. New York Newsday, January 7, 1992

92. "While RJ Reynolds plasters 'Joe Camel' billboards and signs everywhere, they then go and hire actor Danny Glover to appear in ads that say the company *really* doesn't think that 'kids' should smoke. Do we really think that the fox truly cares about the safety of the chickens?"

Rev. Jesse W. Brown, Jr., (SCARC Action Alert, May 7, 1993)

93. Philip Morris sells more than $1 billion worth of Marlboro cigarettes to underage smokers each year just in the United States. JAMA, March 17, 1993, p. 1356

94. A study in the October 17, 1995 issue of the Journal of the National Cancer Institute refutes the tobacco industry's claim that peer pressure, not marketing, is the biggest factor in a teen's decision to smoke. Researchers at the Cancer Prevention and Control Program of the University of California, San Diego, found young adolescents are twice as likely to be influenced by cigarette advertising and promotion than by pressure from peers and family,

95. Another study by the San Diego researchers, published in the November 1995 issue of Health Psychology, found that each innovative tobacco marketing campaign since the 1890's has led to a major increase in the number of 14- to 17-year olds who became regular smokers. For example, in the late 19th century, when cigarette advertising was aimed exclusively at males, a major marketing war occurred between Allen and Ginter Co. and James Duke. Allen and Ginter incorporated suggestive pictures of a woman in each cigarette pack. This reportedly sent youths scrambling after them, and their smoking rates surged. In the mid-1920's, Chesterfield cigarettes introduced the first successful campaign directed at women with its "Blow Some My Way" slogan. The researchers documented a three-fold increase in the number of 14- to 17-year old girls who became smokers during the campaign.

American Medical News, November 6, 1995

96. There are more than half a million American children from age 8 to 11 who smoke.

*Tobacco and the Clinician*, p. 232

97. Children of smoking parents are four times more likely to smoke by age 13.

US News and World Report, September 25, 1995, p. BC29

98. Only 5% of smokers take up the habit after age 21.  Wall Street Journal, August 10, 1995, p. B2

99. Teenage smokers are more likely than nonsmokers to be socially precocious, rebellious, risk-takers, miss school, have low academic and career aspirations, and have low self-esteem and poor self-image.

*Interventions for Smokers*, p. 97

100. Half of all regular cigarette smokers who began as teenagers will die as a result of smoking, a quarter of them dying before age 70 and losing 20-25 years of life expectancy, and a quarter of them dying because of their habit in old age, losing about 8 years life expectancy.  *Tobacco and Health*, p. 83

101. Precancerous patches of tissue, or leukoplakia, are found in the mouth of about half of current teenage smokeless tobacco users. With continued use, about one in 20 such lesions will become cancerous within five years.

Consumer Reports, March 1995, p. 146

102. The likelihood of eventual smoking cessation is significantly higher in smokers who began smoking after age 13 than in those who had begun earlier.  American Journal of Public Health, February 1996, p. 214

103. This addiction, fundamental to the trade, does not develop among adults. Among those over the age of 21 who take up smoking for the first time, more than 90 percent soon drop it completely. It takes more than a year, and sometimes up to three years, to establish a nicotine addiction; adults simply don't stick with it. If it were true that the companies steer clear of children, as they say, the entire industry would collapse within a single generation. Put in market terms, the most important datum of the tobacco trade is that, among those who will be their customers for life, 89 percent have already become their customers by age 19. In fact three-quarters had already joined the ranks of users by age 17. Because of the companies' fears, over the years the tobacco folks have become less and less candid even in private about the fact that they cannot run their business without the children.  Quote from *Smokescreen*, p. 65

104. Religious conservatives are very intent about protecting children from dangerous drugs, but rarely say anything about smoking. In addition, smoking during pregnancy is responsible for an estimated 115,000 spontaneous abortions, or miscarriages, each year in the United States. The Rev. Patrick Mahoney, executive director of the pro-life Christian Defense Coalition, finds the oversight curious. "The pro-family, pro-life movement has been tragically silent on the whole issue of tobacco," says Mahoney. "You don't hear it from the Christian Coalition, you don't hear it from the 'Contract With the American Family,' you don't hear it from the National Right to Life Committee…. It's very disappointing that larger groups, people like Pat Robertson or Ralph Reed or others, have not been more forceful and articulate in addressing this issue."  Mother Jones, May-June 1996, p. 60

105. Among young adult current smokers, by age 18, 90% had smoked their first cigarette, and 70% already were smoking daily.                                              Nicotine Dependence Seminar, Mayo Clinic, May 1997

106. In the early 1960's, tobacco accounted for 40% of college newspaper ad revenues.
                                                                          JAMA, September 25, 1996, p. 998

107. Of high school seniors who smoke regularly, less than 2% began in their senior year of high school, and roughly two thirds began by the ninth grade.                                              *Nicotine*, p. 42

108. "More than 3000 adolescents in the United States begin to use tobacco every day. More than 8.5 million adolescents between the ages of 12 and 17 years, representing 42% of that age group, have tried smoking cigarettes, and 11% of high school seniors smoke at least 10 cigarettes daily. The mean age of initial tobacco use is 10.7 years for boys and 11.4 years for girls, and girls tend to have a more difficult time stopping than do their male counterparts. College-bound teens are less likely to smoke than non-college-bound teens (13.3% vs 29.0%).
                                                                          Pediatrics, October 1996, p. 659

109. 6000 young people try cigarettes for the first time each day; nearly 3000 will become regular smokers. Persons who smoke first try a cigarette at an average age of 13, and become daily smokers at an average age of 14 ½.
                                                              US News and World Report, November 25, 1996, p. 24

110. Each day, about 6000 young try a cigarette for the first time, and about 3000 become daily smokers. The estimated number of future smokers among persons ages birth to 17 in 1995 was 16.6 million in the United States. Of these, an estimated 5.3 million will die prematurely from smoking-related disease. This estimate includes 55% of the 16.6 million who will be lifelong smokers, and 45% who successfully quit in their adult lives. Although estimates of the number smoking-attributable deaths among former smokers range from 10% to 37%, a conservative estimate of
10% was used for this analysis. These projected patterns of smoking and smoking-related deaths could result in an estimated $200 billion (in 1993 dollars) in future health care costs (about $12,000 per smoker), and about 64 million years of potential life lost (12 to 21 years per smoking-related death).
                                                      Morbidity and Mortality Weekly Report, November 8, 1996, pp. 971-973

111. A study of high school students in Northern California concluded that knowledge of cigarette warning labels is not associated with reduced smoking, and that the current warning labels are ineffective among adolescents.
                                                      Archives of Pediatric and Adolescent Medicine, March 1997, p. 267

112. "The adolescent seeks to display his new urge for independence with a symbol, and cigarettes are such a symbol since they are associated with adulthood and at the same time adults seek to deny them to the young."
                                                                          Journal of Pediatrics, April 1997, p. 519

113. Under statutes passed in 1997 in Florida, Minnesota, and Texas, minors who violate tobacco laws could face suspension of driving privileges.                                              New York Times, December 7, 1997, p. 20

114. A South Dakota survey of students in grades 9 through 12 showed that 83% had tried smoking, 44% had smoked in the last month, and 18% had used chewing tobacco.                            USA Today, December 16, 1997, p. A6

115. The number of American youths smoking daily increased by 73% between 1988 and 1996. More than 1.2 million Americans under age 18 started daily smoking in 1996, up from 708,000 in 1988.
                                                                          USA Today, October 9, 1998, p. 10A

116. At present smoking rates, 5 million Americans under age 18 will die prematurely because they smoke.
                                                                          New York Times, August 25, 1999, p. A12
                                              (Michael Eriksen, director, Office on Smoking and Health, Centers for Disease Control)

117. In a survey from 116 colleges in 39 states by the Harvard School of Public Health, 28% of college students considered themselves smokers in 1997, up from 22% in 1993. However, fewer than 12% smoked a pack a day or

more. White students smoked more than other ethnic groups, and 90% of the college smokers said that they started smoking while in high school. New York Times, November 18, 1998, p. A18

118. Smoking among students in Canada in grades 7, 9, 11, and 13 rose from 22% in 1991 to 28% in 1999.
British Medical Journal, November 27, 1999, p. 1391

119. A 1999 survey in Oklahoma showed that 21% of middle school and 42% of high school students used tobacco products, including cigarettes, cigars, pipes and smokeless tobacco. USA Today, May 4, 1999, p. A9

120. One third of Louisiana high school seniors smoke cigarettes regularly. USA Today, May 28, 1999, p. A6

121. For adolescents beginning to smoke, smoking is strongly associated with adverse childhood experiences, including emotional, physical, and sexual abuse, parental divorce, and growing up with mentally ill or substance abusing family members. JAMA, November 3, 1999, p. 1652

122. Only 54% of eighth graders see "great risk" of harm in smoking a pack of cigarettes a day. This increases 71% by 12th grade. Washington Post National Weekly Edition, January 11, 1999, p. 34

123. In a 1999 survey of high school students conducted by the University of Michigan, 65% of current smokers chose Marlboro as their brand.

124. A 1998 survey showed the percentage of students who smoked in the previous month at 19.1% among eighth graders (down 1.9 percentage points from the previous year), 27.6% among 10th graders (down 2.8%), and 35.1% of 12th graders, down 1.4 percentage points from the 1997 survey.
Washington Post National Weekly Edition, January 11, 1999, p. 34

125. More than 4 million kids ages 12 to 17 in the U.S. are smokers. In 1997, 36.5% of high school seniors smoked, a 19 year high. During the decade of the 1990's, smoking among eighth and tenth graders increased by one third.
Data reported by Albert Hunt, Wall Street Journal, December 2, 1999, p. A23

126. 12.8% of middle school students (grades 6,7, and 8) in a 1999 survey were current tobacco product users, including 9.2% who smoke. 34.8% of high schoolers used some form of tobacco, including 28.4% who smoke.
Morbidity and Mortality Weekly Report, January 28, 2000, pp. 49-53

127. 22% of high school seniors reported smoking in the past 30 days in 1997, compared with 25% in 1996.
USA Today, July 9, 1999, p. A6

128. Smoking among students in sixth to eighth grades in Florida dropped 19% in one year, from 18.5% to 15%. These declines were larger than any seen nationally since 1980, after an aggressive state anti-smoking campaign that spent $70 million in 1998. Associated Press, April 1, 1999

129. Nearly 30% of college students, about 4 million in all, were current smokers in 1999 (defined by having smoked in the previous 30 days). This was an increase of 28% from six years earlier. USA Today, March 4, 1999, p. A1

130. Children ages 9 to 14 who want to lose weight are more likely than other children to experiment with cigarettes.
Associated Press, October 5, 1999 (from the journal Pediatrics)

131. In teenagers and preteens, there is an association between weight gain concern and smoking initiation. Girls and boys who reported a fear of weight gain or a desire to be as thin as possible were more than twice as likely to be smokers as their peers without these weight concerns. Pediatrics, October 1999, pp. 918-924

132. "Kids can't imagine themselves old. Health effects mean almost nothing to them." Stanton Glantz, PhD
(Washington Monthly, March 1999, p.8)

133. The 14th in the National Cancer Institute series, released in March 2002, dealt with "Changing Adolescent Smoking Prevalence." Its main conclusions:

•Smoking prevalence among adolescents increased during much of the 1990s, but has recently begun to decline. Female adolescents, Hispanic, and African-American adolescents have experienced a lower smoking prevalence than other subgroups.

•The increase experienced in the 1990s was accompanied by an increase in reports of friend's smoking, and this may indicate that teens are beginning to view smoking as normative behavior.

•Evidence on the relationship between tobacco advertising and promotion and youth smoking suggests that tobacco industry marketing practices are a causal factor in youth smoking initiation.

2002 AMA Annual Tobacco Report

134. Educational strategies, conducted in conjunction with community and media-based activities, can postpone or prevent smoking in 20 to 40 percent of adolescents.

Pharmacologic treatment of nicotine addiction, combined with behavioral support, will enable 20 to 25 percent of users to remain abstinent at one year posttreatment. Even less intense measures, such as physicians advising their patients to quit smoking, can produce cessation proportions of 5 to 10 percent.

Regulation of advertising and promotion, particularly that directed at young people, is very likely to reduce both prevalence and uptake of smoking.

An optimal level of excise taxation on tobacco products will reduce the prevalence of smoking, the consumption of tobacco, and the long-term health consequences of tobacco use.

Quote from Reducing Tobacco Use, 2000 Surgeon General report, p. 6

135. Referring to the tobacco industry's enunciated commitment to youth smoking prevention, health economist Kenneth Warner commented: "In 2000, industry behemoth Philip Morris, with domestic tobacco revenues of $23 billion, spent $115 million on such worthy endeavors – and then spent an additional $150 million on a national advertising campaign to inform the public about the company's largesse."

American Journal of Public Health, June 2002, p. 897

136. Dieting among middle school girls may exacerbate the risk of beginning to smoke. Frequent dieting in early adolescence increased by four times the risk for becoming a smoker, in a study from Boston. The same risk was not true for boys. American Journal of Public Health, March 2001, pp. 446-450

137. "It is important to know as much as possible about teenage smoking patterns and attitudes. Today's teenager is tomorrow's potential regular customer, and the overwhelming majority of smokers first begin to smoke while still in their teens. The smoking patterns of teenagers are particularly important to Philip Morris."

Philip Morris Companies Inc. 1981<br>The Tobacco Atlas, p. 28

138. "If younger adults turn away from smoking, the industry will decline, just as a population which does not give birth will eventually dwindle." RJ Reynolds researcher, 1984 The Tobacco Atlas, p. 28

139. "Evidence is now available to indicate that the 14-18 year-old group is an increasing segment of the smoking population. RJR must soon establish a successful new brand in this market if our position in the industry is to be maintained over the long term." RJ Reynolds document,

"Planning Assumptions and Forecasts for the Period 1976-1986," March 15, 1976

140. In adolescents, symptoms of nicotine dependence "typically develop rapidly with exposures of only a few cigarettes per week. Difficulty with cessation can occur within weeks of starting."

2002 National Conference on Tobacco or Health, Abstract CESS-41

141. In 1999, it was estimated that 3.76 million daily smokers ages 12 to 17 years consumed 924 million packs of cigarettes with a retail value of $1.86 billion. In an FDA compliance check study for curbing illegal sales to minors, clerk failure to request proof of age was most strongly associated with illegal sale, and the rate of illegal sale was 26.6% for all first compliance checks in stores selling cigarettes. JAMA, August 9, 2000, p. 729

142. Nearly 75% of black teens choose Newport as their brand, while more than half of young white and Hispanic smokers prefer Marlboro. Reuters, August 31, 2000

143. There is an increased risk for regular smoking among adolescents with a history of abuse, family violence, stressful life events, and depressive symptoms.

*Archives of Pediatrics and Adolescent Medicine* 2000;154:1025-1033

144. More than 90% of smokers who start smoking after the age of 21 "quickly drop the habit completely."

*Cigarettes* (Parker-Pope), p. viii

145. Guideline:  All schools should provide tobacco prevention education in kindergarten through 12th grade. The instruction should be especially intensive in middle and junior high and reinforced in high school.
Guideline:  Schools should provide instruction about the immediate and long-term consequences of tobacco use, about social norms regarding tobacco use and the reasons why adolescents say they smoke, and about social influences that promote tobacco use. Schools should provide behavioral skills for resisting social influences that promote tobacco use.

Quote from *Reducing Tobacco Use*, 2000 Surgeon General report, p. 81

146. Quote from the abstract/summary from the article "Tobacco Industry Youth Smoking Prevention Programs: Protecting the Industry and Hurting Tobacco Control"

(published in the American Journal of Public Health, May 2002, p. 917)
•Objectives. This report describes the history, true goals, and effects of tobacco industry-sponsored youth smoking prevention programs.
•Methods. We analyzed previously-secret tobacco industry documents.
•Results. The industry started these programs in the 1980s to forestall legislation that would restrict industry activities. •Industry programs portray smoking as an adult choice and fail to discuss how tobacco advertising promotes smoking or the health dangers of smoking. The industry has used these programs to fight taxes, clean-indoor-air laws, and marketing restrictions worldwide. There is no evidence that these programs decrease smoking among youths.
•Conclusions. Tobacco industry youth programs do more harm than good for tobacco control. The tobacco industry should not be allowed to run or directly fund youth smoking prevention programs.

147. "Smoking a cigarette for the beginner is a symbolic act. I am no longer my mother's child, I'm tough, I am an adventurer, I'm not square. Whatever the individual intent, the act of smoking remains a symbolic declaration of personal identity. As the force from the psychological symbolism subsides, the pharmacological effect takes over to sustain the habit."

Philip Morris (from 2001 publication "How do you sell death" from Campaign for Tobacco-Free Kids)

148. In a study from New Hampshire, it was found that adolescents are less likely to smoke if their parents (even if they smoke themselves) voice strong disapproval of smoking. These findings contrast with the widespread idea that there is little that parents can do to prevent their children from becoming smokers.Pediatrics, December 2001, p. 1256

149. The chance that a child will become an established smoker is significantly decreased if the child's parents make it clear that they strongly disapprove, even if the parents themselves are smokers. In a study from Vermont, smoking rates were 50% lower in students where both parents disapproved, as compared to "lenient" parents.

Pediatrics, December 2001, pp. 1256-1262

150. "…new research suggests teens are much less likely to smoke if they think their parents disapprove of the habit. Parental disapproval works even if the parents are smokers, and it can also blunt the effect of peer pressure…"

Associated Press, December 3, 2001

151. In a study from San Diego, adolescents who lived in smoke-free households were 74% as likely to be smokers as adolescents who lived in households with no smoking restrictions.        JAMA, August 9, 2000, p. 717

152. Children in fourth through sixth grades are almost three times a likely to have smoked cigarettes in the past 30 days if they lived with an adult smoker, and adolescents were about twice as likely to smoke daily if one or both parents smoked.        *Women and Smoking*, 2001 Surgeon General report, p. 468

153. In a study from San Diego, the promotion of smoking by the tobacco industry appeared to undermine the capability of authoritative parenting to prevent adolescents from starting to smoke. Adolescents in families with more-authoritative parents were half as likely to smoke as adolescents in families with more permissive parents (20% vs. 41%). In families with more-authoritative parents, adolescents who were highly receptive to tobacco industry advertising and promotion were at significantly higher risk of becoming smokers; an estimated 40% of adolescent smoking in this group was attributable to industry advertising and promotion, much higher than the attributable risk (8%) seen in families with less-authoritative parents.
American Journal of Preventive Medicine, August 2002, p. 73

154. In a study from California, "the promotion of smoking by the tobacco industry appears to undermine the capability of authoritative parenting to prevent adolescents from starting to smoke."
American Journal of Preventive Medicine 2002; 23:73-81

155. In a study from San Diego, youth ages 10 to 15 years old with greater exposure to television viewing had higher rates of smoking initiation. Those who watched more than 5 hours of TV each day were 5.99 times more likely to begin smoking than those who watched television less than two hours a day. Pediatrics, September 2002, p. 505

156. Teens and preteens whose parents restrict them from watching R-rated movies are only one third as likely to smoke or drink as are kids who do not have the restrictions. Time, February 25, 2002

157. States with strong anti-tobacco programs, including California, Florida, Arizona and Maine, have had the largest decreases in smoking rates among teenagers. San Francisco Chronicle, December 20, 2001, p. A2

158. Youth smoking declined from 1997 to 2001. In terms of high school smoking prevalence, current smokers (one day or more in the previous month) in 2001 were 28.5%, down from 36.4% in 1997, and frequent smokers (twenty days or more in the previous month) dropped from 16.7% to 13.8%. Factors contributing to the decline include a 70% rise in the price of cigarettes in this time period, more tobacco control programs, and increased state counter-advertising. Morbidity and Mortality Weekly Report, May 17, 2002

159. In a survey of 65,000 students on 150 college campuses in 1999, 35.5% of students had used tobacco in the previous 30 days. 2002 AMA Annual Tobacco Report

160. 28.5% of high school students reported that they had smoked a cigarette in the last month in 2001, a drop from the peak of 36.4% in a similar survey in 1996. This was the lowest rate since 27.5% in 1991. About 13.8% were frequent or daily smokers, down from 16.7% in 1997. The average price of cigarettes increased by 70% from 1997 to 2001, and this high price deterred many students from beginning the habit. Associated Press, May 17, 2002

161. In a 1999 survey of girls ages 12 through 17, the most popular brands chosen were Marlboro (55.6%), Newport (22.6%), and Camel (8.3%). Women and Smoking, 2001 Surgeon General report, p. 69

162. From 1997 to 2001, the percentage of teenage smokers dropped from 36% to 29% (CDC data).
San Francisco Chronicle, May 23, 2002, p. A24

163. Smoking rates for high school seniors (12th grade) declined from 25% in 1997 to 21% in 2000. For 10th graders, the decline was from 18% in 1997 to 14% in 2000, and eighth graders saw a decline from 10% in 1996 to 7% in 2000. 2002 AMA Annual Tobacco Report

164. Cigarette smoking among high school students continues to decline. In high school seniors (grade 12), 30-day smoking prevalence was about 29% from 1981 through the early 1990's, climbed to a peak of 38% in 1997, and dropped to 30% in 2001. Among 8th graders, 30-day use peaked at 21% in 1996 and fell to 11% in 2001, while daily smoking in this group declined from 10% in 1996 to 5% in 2001. JAMA, January 8, 2003, p. 163

165. Since 1994, the teenage smoking rate in California has declined by almost half, to 5.9%.
San Francisco Chronicle, July 3, 2002, p. A22

166. Teenagers exposed to the American Legacy Foundation's "truth campaign" television ads were much less likely to smoke than those who did not see the anti-smoking ads. Washington Post, September 22, 2002

# CHAPTER 16
# YOUTH ACCESS TO TOBACCO

1. Two programs introduced by tobacco companies in 1995, "Action Against Access," and "We Card," have not had any apparent impact on underage tobacco sales. Minnesota attorney general Hubert Humphrey says that if the tobacco companies were serious about keeping cigarettes away from minors, they would work with local officials instead of lobbying against them and trying to pass weak state preemption laws to take away local authority. "If they want something real, let's sit down and talk. Instead, we get full page ads...and excuses."

   USA Today, May 30, 1996, p. 221

2. "... if the tobacco industry is truly interested in keeping cigarettes out of the hands of minors, they would stop spending millions in states like Minnesota to defeat efforts to strengthen laws banning tobacco sales to kids."

   Hubert H. Humphrey III, Minnesota Attorney General (Wall Street Journal, June 28, 1995, p. A3)

3. The 1995 program Action Against Access was touted by Philip Morris to "prevent cigarette sales to minors." Nine of the ten promises were "useless and silly on their face," but one was potentially helpful: "Retail Payments. We will deny merchandising benefits to retailers who are fined for or convicted of selling cigarettes to minors."

   In 1995, an "anti-tobacco group in Minnesota, the Association for Nonsmokers of Minnesota, sent Philip Morris a list of recent convictions for underage sales in Minnesota. Philip Morris wrote back saying the company could not act because the citations from the anti-smoking group did not come from the proper authorities." The Minnesota Attorney General had an official list prepared.

   "Philip Morris replied that, though the notification was official, it was 'too early' to actually carry out its threat. 'We haven't finalized the actual proposal' to crack down on retailers, said company spokeswoman Ellen Merlo."

   "Asked whether the company would start enforcement actions after the proposal was finalized and sent out to retailers, she said not necessarily. 'First we hope to begin training and raise awareness,' she said."

   "Then, maybe in a store where training had been done, and a violation found, and a warning issued, and another two violations found, she said, possibly enforcement would take place if the program was still underway at that time."

   *Smokescreen*, pp. 99-101

4. Yet the tobacco industry continues, with great ferocity and dishonesty, to fight efforts to limit youth smoking. Philip Morris, for example, vowed more than a year ago to withdraw merchandising benefits from retailers convicted of selling cigarettes to minors illegally. The Philip Morris pledge was announced in big splashy national ads.

   Three states—Minnesota, Oregon and Massachusetts—decided to take Philip Morris up on its offer. They furnished the company with the names of stores that had been convicted of selling cigarettes to minors. The American Lung Association in Washington did the same.

   Then they waited for Philip Morris to act. And they waited. . . and waited. . . and waited. They're still waiting; in fact, Philip Morris has yet to punish a single dealer.

   "If anyone thinks that the tobacco industry can be trusted," Minnesota Attorney General Hubert Humphrey III was quoted as saying, "they should look at the pathetic grandstanding, foot-dragging and finger-pointing behind this public relations stunt." Quote from "...And the Kids Keep on Lighting Up," George Dessart

   (Washington Post National Weekly Edition, August 26-September 1, 1996, p. 28)

5. "It's the Law" programs are sponsored by Philip Morris, RJR, and the Tobacco Institute ostensibly for the purpose of encouraging merchant compliance with laws prohibiting tobacco sales to minors. However, a study from Massachusetts showed that these programs failed to produce a significant reduction in the illegal sale of tobacco to minors.

   American Journal of Public Health, February 1996, p. 221

6. "We conclude that the Tobacco Institute's 'Tobacco: Helping Youth Say No' program will *increase* the likelihood of tobacco use among children who are exposed to it."

   Journal of Family Practice 1992; 34:694 (Joe DiFranza)

7. In a study of 12-year-old seventh graders in Memphis, the students rated the components of the teenage smoking prevention programs of the American Lung Association and the Tobacco Institute. They perceived the Tobacco Institute program "Tobacco: Helping Youth Say No" to be much less effective than the Lung Association

pamphlet. The Tobacco Institute booklet suggests: "Smoking is not a choice for children because they do not have the maturity to make judgments that weigh all considerations." In marked contrast to the ALA approach, the Tobacco Institute program never mentions nicotine addiction, any health consequences of smoking, or the benefits of quitting, saying only that "Young people are aware of the claims that smoking presents risks to one's health."                                                                                        Tobacco Control, Spring 1996, pp. 19-25

8.   "By pretending to care about our nation's youth, their future customers, Philip Morris has once more demonstrated its ability to say one thing while doing another."     Rep. James Hansen (R-Utah), June 30, 1995

9.   The Philip Morris 1998 proxy statement regarding its "Action Against Access" program allegedly designed to keep underage smokers from purchasing cigarettes states: "We have initiated 60 programs against youth smoking in 36 countries and are increasing the momentum. We launched 18 new programs this year." Philip Morris ran an ad noting, "No one should be allowed to sell cigarettes to minors. Minors should not smoke. Period. That is why Philip Morris developed a comprehensive program to prevent sales of cigarettes to minors."
The protestations are too vehement, somehow.

   One newspaper series, in the Louisville Courier-Journal, looking into the gap between the companies' public statements and their day-to-day behavior, noted that in the places where strict licensing and strict enforcement have been used against store owners, they have been very effective. But the industry has fought fiercely against giving state health departments the power to carry out effective enforcement.

   The companies are on record as against most methods of enforcement, including inspections, sting operations, surveys, and holding merchants responsible for illegal sales. Instead they suggest punitive measures which would be certain not only to backfire, but to cast the enforcers in the worst possible light. They suggest targeting for arrest children who buy cigarettes rather than retailers who sell them. They also suggest arresting or fining the clerks in stores, not the managers or owners.

   What the industry is against is quite logical—anything that has been shown to be effective in any studies or in any actual town or state enforcement actions. The situation is similar to that of the CTR (Council for Tobacco Research)--maintain a public posture that appears honorable and in line with public opinion, and in practice prevent anything that would reduce sales in any way. It would be difficult to believe an industry could be so dishonest as to carry out such a two-faced program, but having seen the documents from 1954 to the present, and looking at one example after another when the companies' intentions have been tested, it is impossible to escape the conclusion that the industry is doing just that again.          Quote from *Smokescreen*, pp. 91, 94, and 95

10.   "The tobacco industry favors programs and policies penalizing youth for purchasing and possessing cigarettes. The reason for this is obvious—attention is diverted from the tobacco industry's own culpability, and blame is laid on children and parents. It also lessens the perceived responsibility of merchants. Effective youth access policies should avoid all appearance or effect of punishing youth."          *Stop the Sale, Prevent the Addiction*,
Centers for Disease Control and Prevention, 1995

11.   The tobacco industry's five major goals to ensure youth access are:
   •Use state level preemption to deny local governments the authority to regulate any aspect of tobacco use or distribution.
   •Put loopholes into youth access laws that prevent law enforcement officials from prosecuting merchants who sell tobaccoto children.
   •Hold children responsible for the fact that merchants violate the law (arrest the child, not the merchant).
   •Hamstring enforcement efforts as much as possible.
   •Outlaw public health research and investigative reporting about illegal sales to minors.
Tobacco Free Youth Reporter, Fall 1994, pp. 9-10

12.   "In many states, the tobacco industry has supported or engineered legislation that cripples enforcement of laws that could keep children from purchasing tobacco. The industry opposes licensing vendors; wants to bar local authorities from enforcement power; wants to fine only those who 'knowingly' sell tobacco to children; wants to outlaw public health research and investigative reporting about illegal sales; and wants to make the child-purchaser, not the merchant-seller, responsible for the illegal act."
North Carolina Medical Journal, January 1995, p. 21 (Tom Houston)

13. The tobacco industry "is strongly opposed to federal regulations requiring states to effectively enforce their laws prohibiting the sale of tobacco to minors. . . . the Tobacco Institute has circulated a model state bill concerning underage tobacco sales. These bills strip communities of enforcement authority while making effective enforcement by state officials virtually impossible."

    "The evidence strongly suggests an industry strategy to undermine efforts to enforce laws prohibiting the sale of tobacco to minors. As has been the case in the past, the tobacco industry is publicly endorsing a socially responsible goal while apparently taking action behind the scenes to ensure that the goal is not achieved."

    "Although the tobacco industry claims that it is working to halt the illegal sale of tobacco to minors, an examination…of the legislation it supports suggests that it is, in fact, doing a great deal to sabotage efforts to institute meaningful enforcement of laws prohibiting the sale of tobacco to minors. The enactment of so many weak, pre-emptive laws represents a severe blow to public health efforts to reduce the illegal sale of tobacco to children."
    Tobacco Control, Summer 1996, pp. 127-130 (Joe DiFranza)

14. Licensing system for tobacco retailers is a key component in implementing an effective policy for preventing youth access to tobacco. A licensing system has three major benefits: (1) it provides for license suspension or revocation as a penalty, which provides additional motivation for retailers to comply with the law (this process is similar to that used to control the sale of alcoholic beverages to minors); (2) it helps to identify most establishments that sell tobacco, thus facilitating compliance checks; and (3) licensing fees can generate a source of funds to pay for enforcement."

    "License suspension or revocation provides stronger economic deterrent than fines to retailers who violate youth access laws. With this greater economic stake in enforcement, retailers are more likely to monitor themselves and to provide or participate in merchant and employee education programs."
    *Stop the Sale, Prevent the Addiction*

15. In San Francisco, 35% of stores picked randomly in 1996 sold cigarettes without questions to 15- and 16-year-olds. The teenagers were recruited from high school anti-smoking programs and paid a small stipend. Statewide in California, 33% of the undercover kids who tried to buy cigarettes succeeded.
    San Francisco Chronicle, September 11, 1996, p. A13

16. In a study from Broward County, Florida, 33% of minors ages 12 to 17 years were successful in attempts to purchase cigarettes from vending machines. These success rates were lower than those conducted in Massachusetts (86%) and Minnesota (42%), and provide support for the FDA regulations that ban vending machines except in facilities where only adults are permitted.
    Morbidity and Mortality Weekly Report, November 29, 1996, pp. 1037-38

17. In a 1994 survey, only 28% of vendors consistently obeyed laws limiting sales of tobacco to children.
    American Journal of Public Health, February 1996, p. 156

18. In a 1997 survey of states and stores selling cigarettes to minors, Florida was the best in the nation, with teenagers able to buy tobacco only 7% of the time. Maine, New Hampshire, and Washington have also met the federal standard, under which less than 20% of underage smokers should be able to make tobacco purchases. California was at 29.7%. The five worst offenders were Louisiana, where minors were successful in purchasing cigarettes 72% of the time, Connecticut (70%), Kansas and Tennessee (63%), and Idaho (56%).
    San Francisco Chronicle, February 28, 1998, p. A3, and USA Today, February 27, 1998, p. A9

19. More than 40% of grade school students who smoke daily have at some time shoplifted cigarettes from self-service displays.
    NEJM, September 26, 1996, p. 991

20. A 1994 survey found that almost half of eighth and tenth grade tobacco users had shoplifted tobacco within the past year, and 12% of them "most often" obtained their tobacco this way.
    Fond du Lac (Wisconsin) school district survey,
    Addendum to the Michigan Alcohol and Drug Survey

21. Minors buy $1.6 billion worth of tobacco products each year, and 75% of teen smokers say that they have never been asked for an ID.
    San Francisco Examiner, February 28, 1997, p. A1

22. In the Chicago suburb of Woodridge, Illinois, more than 80% of its tobacco outlets sold tobacco products to minors. After using minors in sting operations to detect illegal sales, the sale rate dropped to 11%.

Associated Press, September 17, 1996

23. Generally, the only opponents to cigarette vending machine restrictions are the vending machine companies, often supported by the tobacco industry. Cigarettes comprised only 4.7% of total vending machine revenues in 1993, and cigarette vending machine sales average $10 per machine per day. For younger or less confident children, vending machines provide a less intimidating avenue for purchasing tobacco than over-the-counter sales; a study by the vending machine industry showed that 13-year olds use vending machines 11 times more frequently than do 17-year olds.

1997 STAT (Stop Teenage Addiction to Tobacco) Newsletter

24. In a study from Massachusetts, enforcement of laws prohibiting tobacco sales by merchants to adolescents under 18, as well as sting operations, resulted in only a small drop in the ability of adolescents to purchase tobacco, and no decline in tobacco use. The conclusion was that enforcing tobacco-sales laws improved merchants' compliance and reduced illegal sales to minors, but did not alter adolescents' perceived access to tobacco or their smoking. Reducing illegal sales to less than 20% of attempts, the goal of a new federal law, may therefore not be effective in decreasing young people's access to or use of tobacco.

NEJM, October 9, 1997, p. 1044

25. In a study from a low income area in East Baltimore just before implementation of a 1994 Maryland law prohibiting tobacco sales to minors, 14 to 16 year old adolescents were successful in purchasing cigarettes in 85.5% of corner stores. 58% of the stores displayed five or more cigarette advertisements outside their premises.

American Journal of Public Health, April 1997, p. 652

26. Surveys of illegal tobacco sales to children in California, monitored by 15 and 16 year olds attempting to purchase tobacco products over the counter, declined to 21.7% in 1997 from 29% of attempts in 1996, 37% in 1995, and 52% in 1994.

San Francisco Chronicle, September 3, 1997, p. A16

27. Illegal sales of tobacco products to minors in California dropped sharply to 13% in 1998.

California Department of Health Services press release, August 21, 1998

28. The 1992 Synar Amendment to the Public Health Service Act required states to adopt and enforce laws to reduce the sale of tobacco products to minors. States not complying may risk the loss of up to 40% of their block grant funds for substance abuse prevention and treatment; however, the law has gone unenforced so far.

Consumer Reports, March 1995, p. 146

29. Republican Representative Thomas Bliley of Richmond, VA, sometimes termed the "Congressman from Philip Morris," threatened "a challenge on constitutional grounds" if the Department of Health and Human Services required states to reduce the illegal sale of tobacco to children as mandated by the 1992 Synar amendment.

Letter to Gale Held, Center for Substance Abuse Prevention, October 25, 1993

30. About half of all teens and children who try cigarettes go on to become regular smokers. 60% of the 3 million teenagers who smoke buy their own cigarettes, even though underage sales are illegal now in all states and the District of Columbia.

Youth and Elders video program, March 24, 1994

31. Illegal tobacco sales to minors, about 947 million packs of cigarettes and 26 million containers of chewing tobacco in 1988, total $1.45 billion in sales and more than $221 million in profits each year. *Tobacco Use*, p.38

32. Minors illegally bought about one billion packs of cigarettes in 1989. The US Inspector General documented only 32 reported violations of the laws, however, a minimal level of enforcement by any criteria.

Smoking and Health Review, July 1990, p. 4

33. In a 1995 survey funded by the Robert Wood Johnson Foundation, U.S. adults strongly support specific actions to make tobacco less accessible to minors. 94% support identification and age verification by vendors, 78% support keeping tobacco products behind counters, and 74% support banning all cigarette vending machines.

34. Single cigarette pack self service displays in stores are easily accessible where customers can help themselves, and are often placed near candy and gum. Tobacco companies pay a premium, called slotting, often thousands of dollars to individual retailers to keep their displays in preferred placement areas up front. Only five states ban these self service displays. One third of all shoplifted items in supermarkets are cigarettes.

CBS evening news, April 12, 1999

35. A 1998 Maryland survey showed that underage students sent into stores to purchase tobacco were successful 35% of the time, down from 54% in 1996. USA Today, December 23, 1998, p. A5

36. An article reviewing impediments to the enforcement of youth access laws is in the summer 1999 issue of Tobacco Control, pages 152-155.

37. In a study from San Diego, 32% of adults agreed to buy cigarettes for underage smokers who requested them.

American Journal of Public Health, July 2001, pp. 1138-39

38. Regarding illegal sales to minors, the median retailer violation rate dropped from 40% in 1997 to 24% in 1999; violation rates in 1999 ranged from 4% in Maine to 47% in the District of Columbia.

Associated Press, December 7, 2001

39. Among youth smokers aged 12 to 17 in 2000, more than half (59.4%) reported that they personally bought cigarettes at least once in the past month. Approximately one-third of youth smokers (33.8%) reported buying cigarettes at a store where the clerk hands out the cigarettes. Among youth smokers aged 12 and 13 years old, 45.8% reported that they personally bought cigarettes in the past month. 2002 AMA Annual Tobacco Report

40. Nationwide, the number of retailers who are complying with state laws and refusing to sell tobacco products to minors increased from 59.4 percent in 1997 to 83.9 percent in 2001. The states with the highest compliance rates are Louisiana, Maine, South Dakota, and Washington. In Louisiana, compliance checks found that 94.3 percent of the 778 retailers in the state refused to sell tobacco products to minors last July and August. The compliance rate is an improvement over 1997, when fewer than 30 percent followed the law. In Maine, officials report a 95.9 percent compliance rate for 1999, while South Dakota had a 95.5 percent compliance rate in 2001. Washington had a 94.5 percent compliance rate in 1998. States are required to have a minimum compliance rate of 80 percent in order to maintain federal funds.

Quote from Associated Press, February 23, 2003,
Reported on tobaccofreekids.org website

JAMA is Journal of the American Medical Association
NEJM is New England Journal of Medicine

# CHAPTER 17
# SMOKELESS TOBACCO

## Historical

1.  In 1761, the British physician John Hill described five cases of nasal cancer that he attributed to nasal snuff use. He wrote "No man should venture upon snuff who is not sure that he is not liable to cancer, and no man can be sure of that."                                                                                              Pediatrics, December 1985, p. 1009

2.  In the 1800's an American national characteristic was a distended cheek, the identifying mark of the tobacco chewer. In a Lorillard ad, a happy farmer with a swollen jaw exclaims, "It ain't toothache--its Climax."
                                                                                              Health Education, June 1987, p. 8

3.  Charles Dickens wrote in *American Notes* (1842): "In the hospitals, the students of medicine are requested to eject their tobacco-juice into the boxes provided for that purpose, and not to discolour the stairs." He declared that he could not understand how Americans had won their reputation as riflemen, judging their poor aim when spitting tobacco. Another British writer sardonically commented that the national American symbol should not be the bald eagle, but rather the spittoon.                                                                     Health Education, June 1987, p. 8

4.  "At the turn of the century, it was discovered that tuberculosis was transmitted through expectoration, and the practice of chewing and spitting quickly became socially unacceptable and illegal in many public places. With the invention of the cigarette-rolling machine, it was possible to produce a cheap new tobacco product. By the early 1920's, cigarettes had replaced smokeless tobacco. Per capita consumption of cigarettes in the United States rose dramatically, from 50 cigarettes per year in 1900 to 4200 by 1965."                              NEJM, May 12, 1988, p. 1281

5.  In 1915, a Dr. Abbe described a series of oral cancer patients who were tobacco chewers, and postulated tobacco use as a risk factor.   *The Health Consequences of Using Smokeless Tobacco*, 1986 Surgeon General report, p. xix

6.  A 1921 article indicated that of 160 persons with cancer of the tongue, all but two were tobacco users.
                                                                                              JAMA, February 28, 1986, p. 1041

## General

1.  "It has not been scientifically established that smokeless tobacco causes adverse medical effects."
    Alan Hilburg, spokesman for the Smokeless Tobacco Council                    (New York Times, May 3, 1998, p. 17)

2.  The average age of initiation for "spit" or smokeless tobacco is age 9; 67% of a sample began at age 12 or younger, and 28% were 5 years old or younger when they first tried it. The highest spit tobacco use rates are in Native Americans, where female use rates sometimes equal males.
                                                      *Spit Tobacco and Youth*, US Dept. of Health and Human Services, 1992, p. 4

3.  Between 1972 and 1991, consumption of moist snuff and other smokeless tobacco products in the United States almost tripled, including an eight-fold increase in the 17 to 19-year-old group.
                                                                  Morbidity and Mortality Weekly Report, April 16, 1993, p. 263

4.  Smokeless tobacco users start early; use among preschool children has been reported, and in one study, 88% of users began by age 14. In the Native American Indian population, usage rates in adolescents (including females) are as high as 50%.                                                         American Journal of Public Health, March 1993, p. 468

5.  In the early 1990's, the prevalence of past year smokeless tobacco use among young males ages 18 to 24 in the military was 32.4%. This was much higher than the 18.5% for non-military males in this age group.
                                                                                              1992 Department Of Defense Survey

6. Former US Marine Corps Commandant (1986-1989) and four star General P.X. Kelley is a member of the Board of Directors of the US Tobacco Company, manufacturers of 80% of the nation's smokeless tobacco, including Copenhagen and Skoal. Almost half of male Marines under age 25 are daily users of smokeless tobacco, and the Marine Corps has the highest use rate of any of the military services.     Common Cause magazine, Summer 1993

7. "Once a kid is hooked, he doesn't leave." Smokeless tobacco company executive.
Journal of the American Dental Association 1980; 101:467

8. Each year in the United States, about 824,000 young people 11 to 19 years of age experiment with smokeless tobacco (2200 each day first trying it), and 304,000 (830 each day) become regular users.
American Journal of Public Health, January 1998, pp. 20-26

9. Cigar and pipe smoking has declined by 80% in the last 20 years. In the same period, use of smokeless tobacco by adolescent males has increased by 450% for chewing tobacco and by 1500%, or fifteen-fold, for snuff. From 1978 to 1984, there was a 15% compound annual growth rate in U.S. smokeless tobacco sales.
*Spit Tobacco and Youth*, p. B1

10. 30% of all male high school seniors in the southeastern United States were regular smokeless tobacco users in the early 1990's.                            Morbidity and Mortality Weekly Report, September 18, 1992, p. 699

11. 12 million Americans are "dippers" or "spitters"--regular users of smokeless tobacco (snuff and chewing tobacco). Three million of this group are under age 21. Use in children and adolescents doubled between 1970 and 1986.
NEJM, May 12, 1988, p. 1281

12. In 1990 in the states of Tennessee, Alabama, Montana, Colorado, and Wyoming, 31 to 34% of males in grades 9 through 12 were users of smokeless tobacco.
*Spit Tobacco and Youth*, Dept of Health and Human Services, 1992, p. 3

13. In the states of Alabama, Idaho, South Dakota, Colorado, Wyoming, and Montana, more adolescent males use smokeless tobacco than smoke cigarettes.
*Preventing Tobacco Use Among Young People*, 1994 Surgeon General report, p. 97

14. The spit tobacco use rate in NCAA college athletes rose from 20% in 1985 to 28% in 1989, a 40% increase.
*Spit Tobacco and Youth*, p. 3

15. In a 1990 statewide survey in Oklahoma, 13% of third grade and 22% of fifth grade boys reported regular use of smokeless tobacco. This increased to 33% of male high school freshmen and 39% of high school juniors.
*Smokeless Tobacco or Health*, p. 5

16. In a survey of adolescents in Arkansas, one quarter of smokeless tobacco users began the habit between ages 5 and 8.                                                                     Pediatrics, January 1993, p. 75

17. The 1990 Youth Risk Behavior Survey found that 24% of all white male high school students currently used smokeless tobacco. In Tennessee, Arkansas, Oklahoma, and Montana, a third of high school boys use it. Of the 10 million American users of smokeless or "spit" tobacco, 3 million are under age 21.
Tobacco Free Youth Reporter, Spring 1993, and Journal of Public Health Policy, Winter 1987, p. 501

18. Use of snuff and chewing tobacco by teenage males increased by 275% between 1970 and 1985.
Seminars in Oncology, August 1990, p. 407

19. 90% of smokeless tobacco users in high school report that they purchased their own supplies, and 94% said that although they were minors, it was either never or only rarely difficult for them to purchase smokeless tobacco.
*Preventing Tobacco Use Among Young People*, 1994 Surgeon General report, p. 141

20. As recently as 1975, only 3% of the US population used smokeless tobacco; use was primarily in older men at this time.                                                                    Preventive Medicine 1987; 16:402

21. 12 million American men used smokeless tobacco in the early 1990's. Of these, 90% were white, and 50% lived in the South. *Nicotine Addiction*, p. 263

22. Four classes of carcinogens in smokeless tobacco are N-nitrosamines, radioactive polonium-210, polycyclic aromatic hydrocarbons, and volatile aldehydes. Nitrosamines are found in smokeless tobacco in quantities between 10 and 1400 times greater than the allowable amounts for food and beverages. *Nicotine Addiction*, p. 265

23. The total concentration of carcinogenic nitrosamines in snuff is 10 to 100 times higher than the levels in the inhaled smoke of one cigarette and 20,000 times higher than the level allowed by the FDA and the Department of Agriculture in food. World Smoking and Health No. 1, 1994 and NEJM, April 17, 1986, p. 1023

24. The Food and Drug Administration (FDA) recommends limits on nitrosamine, a chemical strongly associated with cancer, at 10 parts per billion in bacon and half that in beer. The nitrosamine content of moist oral snuff is 1000 parts per billion and higher. Common Cause magazine, Summer 1993

25. 30,000 new mouth and throat cancers are detected in the United States each year. 50% of these are fatal within 5 years. Tobacco use causes about 75% of cases of oral cancer, and long term dipping increases the risk of oral cancer nearly fifty-fold. Tobacco Free Youth Reporter, Spring 1993

26. Within 30 minutes of smokeless tobacco use, heart rate increases 10-20 beats per minute, and blood pressure rises 5-10mm Hg. Postgraduate Medicine, January 1991

27. Men ages 35 to 54 who use smokeless tobacco are 2.1 times more likely to die of heart disease as those who do not use tobacco. Heavy smokers increase their risk by 3.2 times. American Medical News, April 18, 1994, p. 14

28. Leukoplakia (white wrinkled patches inside the mouth) and gum recession occur in about half of smokeless tobacco users. Oral leukoplakia is precancerous, and has a five-year malignant transformation potential of about 5%. 1994 Surgeon General report, p. 39

29. Regular use of smokeless tobacco causes foul-smelling breath and halitosis, periodontal disease and gum recession, tooth decay, and permanent staining and discoloration of teeth. Pediatrics, December 1985, p. 1009

30. Advertisements for smokeless tobacco have focused on changing the longtime image of dipping and chewing as an unattractive habit to a new image of an activity that is fun, and mark of virility, and as American as baseball and country music. NEJM, April 17, 1986, p. 1043

31. "Skillful television and magazine advertising featuring entertainers and sports personalities have transformed a habit previously considered dirty and unsociable into one viewed as attractive and healthful, with a strong youth appeal." Adweek, July 31, 1981

32. "Advertisements starring cowboys and sexy young women reinforce the he-man appeal of the smokeless tobacco user, ironically creating a sexually appealing image for a habit that women and girls rarely develop and usually find repugnant." C. Everett Koop M.D., NEJM, April 17, 1986, p. 1043

33. From the Washington Post of November 14, 1993: "Virginia's Dippin', Spittin' Governor. In electing George Allen governor, it has returned snuff dipping to the highest reaches of the Old Dominion. It has chosen a chief executive perpetually buzzed on nicotine and prone to randomly ooze brown juice." Newsweek (November 14, 1993, p. 7) reported: "Tobacco-chewing son of ex-Redskins coach soaks Dems. Virginia is for spitters."

34. Among Red Man chewing tobacco's sponsored activities are tractor pulls, country music concerts, and softball tournaments.

35. The health activist group DOC (Doctors Ought to Care) has sponsored a Dead Man Chew softball league in Omaha and an anti-smokeless tobacco monster truck in Seattle. American Journal of Public Health, March 1992, p. 353

36. Volvo has acquired a Swedish tobacco company that owns Pinkerton Tobacco, makers of Red Man chewing tobacco.
*Washington Post, January 11, 1994, p. 10*

37. The federal excise tax on smokeless tobacco is just under 3 cents per can, one-eighth the levy on a cigarette pack. 58 percent of the price of a can of snuff is pure profit.
*Common Cause magazine, Summer 1993*

38. A professor of dentistry at the University of Alabama at Birmingham has a controversial last resort solution for hard core smokers who cannot quit: switch to smokeless tobacco. Snuff or chewing tobacco can satisfy nicotine craving better than nicotine patches or gum, and has fewer health risks than cigarettes. Professor Brad Rodu concludes that if all US smokers switched to smokeless tobacco, the current 419,000 annual deaths would eventually drop to 12,000 from oral cancer.
*US News and World Report, July 11, 1994, p. 67*
(from American Journal of the Medical Sciences, July 1994)

39. Rodu was later quoted in March 2003: "Our research indicates that if all American smokers had instead used smokeless tobacco, the annual tobacco-related mortality in this country would be only 27% of the current figures."
from the Cleburne News, March 20, 2003

40. 81% of adolescents regard smokeless tobacco to be "much safer than cigarettes."
*Growing Up Tobacco Free, p. 155*

41. 43% of high school seniors who use smokeless tobacco also smoke cigarettes, and 32.5% of smokers in this group also use smokeless tobacco.
*Growing Up Tobacco Free, p. 166*

42. 25 to 30 percent of all regular smokeless tobacco users also smoke cigarettes.
*Smokeless Tobacco or Health, p. 283*

43. Between 1970 and 1985, the use of moist snuff increased by 30% among all Americans, but eightfold in the 17- to 19-year-old group.
World Smoking and Health No. 1, 1994, p. 13

44. Moist snuff sales grew 47% between 1986 and 1990 at a time when use of all other tobacco products was declining. The typical dose of snuff contains two to three times more nicotine than a cigarette.
Tobacco Control, Winter 1994, p. 299

45. "Users who are highly dependent on smokeless tobacco should be informed that what they may experience as heightened energy or strength are really elevations in heart rate and blood pressure, and that perceived relaxation is chiefly a relief from the craving associated with nicotine withdrawal."
NEJM, May 12, 1988, p. 1284

46. Users who consume two cans of snuff per week have cotinine levels equivalent to two pack a day smokers.
NEJM, May 12, 1988, p. 1281

47. A two can a week snuff dipper gets as much nicotine as a pack and a half a day smoker, but pays only 5 cents a week in federal taxes on the product, compared to $2.24 for the smokers.
Marines Semper Fit Health Promotion Office (1995)

48. In a Department of Health and Human Services survey of high school users of smokeless tobacco, 25% were unaware that it contained nicotine, 50% thought that it posed no health hazards, and 80% thought that it was safer than cigarettes.
Marines Semper Fit Health Promotion Office (1995)

49. Smokeless tobacco users are five times more likely to lose their teeth as a result of decay than a non-user.
Marines Semper Fit Health Promotion Office (1995)

50. There are no published mortality figures available for disease caused by smokeless tobacco use.
Editor

51. In 1985, Massachusetts became the first state to require a warning label for smokeless tobacco.
*Ashes to Ashes, p. 563*

52. While 4.0% of men older than age 18 use smokeless tobacco, 20.4% of boys in grades 9 through 12 were current users in 1993.                           *State Tobacco Control Highlights* 1996, Centers for Disease Control

53. "When You Can't Smoke, Introducing Skoal Flavor Packs. They're small, discreet pouches that are easy to use and control."                           Ad in Sports Illustrated, April 1, 1996, showing the pouches with a pack of cigarettes and pro basketball game tickets.

54. From 1980 to 1994, annual use of snuff in the U.S. increased from 25.2 to 59.5 million pounds. The amount of nicotine in a tin of snuff or a pouch of smokeless tobacco is equivalent to that in two and a half packs of cigarettes
.                                                         Reader's Digest, October 1996, p. 124

55. Sales of smokeless tobacco in the United States increased by 85% from $798 million in 1986 to $1.48 billion in 1993.                           American Journal of Public Health, September 1996, p. 1302

56. There are now 16 million smokeless tobacco users in the United States, and total consumption has increased to 61 million pounds in 1996 from 30 million in 1981. More than half of male high school seniors have tried chewing tobacco, and free samples are handed out at rodeos, rock concerts, and stock car races.
                                                         ABC evening news, October 7, 1997

57. In 1997, snuff for the first time exceeded the consumption of chewing tobacco for the first time in U.S. history. Moist snuff alone accounts for nearly 60 million of the 121 million total pounds of smokeless tobacco consumed.
                                                         Journal of the National Cancer Institute, November 5, 1997, p. 1573

58. An estimated 6.9 million Americans use smokeless tobacco.                           JAMA, January 20, 1999, p. 233

59. In 1998, 5.9% of men and 0.5% of women used smokeless tobacco. This rate has remained steady since 1991.
                                                         1998 National Household Survey on Drug Abuse

60. Among men, the prevalence of current smokeless tobacco use in 1997 was highest in West Virginia (18.4%) and Wyoming (14.7%); five states (Alabama, Alaska, Kansas, Kentucky, and Montana) reported prevalences of 9% to 12%.                           JAMA, January 6, 1999, p. 30

61. Smokeless tobacco manufacturers spent $150.4 million in advertising and promotional expenses in 1997, an increase of 21% from the previous year. Sales revenue was $1.82 billion in 1997.
                                                         Wall Street Journal, January 13, 1999, p. A13

62. About twelve million Americans are dependent upon chewing tobacco. Tobacco companies "worked the public health con of selling the product as a safe alternative to cigarettes. Young men, inspired by the example of pouch-lipped baseball demigods spitting long ropes of tobacco juice, were hardest hit by this escalation: from 1970 to 1985, chewing-tobacco usage increased nearly ten times among boys between the ages of sixteen and nineteen. Last year, the U.S. Smokeless Tobacco Company, Skoal's manufacturer, sold 650 million tins of chewing tobacco – one for every nine inhabitants of earth."                           Men's Journal, February 2002, p. 72

63. In a 2001 NCAA survey of student athletes, use of spit tobacco declined to 17.4%, from 22.5% in 1997 and 27.6% in 1989. Its use remains high in some specific sports, however: 41% of baseball players, 29% of football players and 18% of women skiers admit to using spit tobacco.                           2002 AMA Annual Tobacco Report

64. The prevalence of mouth leukoplakia, a white mucosal plaque, among smokeless tobacco users is very high, at least 50% by some reports.                           *Clearing the Smoke*, p. 563

65. Rates of smokeless tobacco use remained statistically unchanged between 2000 and 2001. In 2001, 4.0% of 8th graders, 6.9% of 10th graders, and 7.8% of 12th graders reported using smokeless tobacco in the past month.
                                                         2002 AMA Annual Tobacco Report

# Native Americans

1.  In 1988, there were an estimated 12 million smokeless tobacco users in the US, including 3 million teenage boys. The prevalence of current users in adults was 5% for men and less than 1% for women. The highest user group was young Native Americans; surveys reported regular use in 18% of children ages 5-11 and 55.9% in 9th and 10th graders in this ethnic group. In a Washington study, 40% of smokeless tobacco users also smoked cigarettes.
    Public Health Reports, March 1990, p. 196

2.  More than half of all Native Americans are smokeless tobacco users, including 45% of Native American adolescent girls. Native Americans are unusual in that female use rates sometimes equal males.
    *Spit Tobacco and Youth*, p.4, and JAMA, January 13, 1995, p. 195

3.  A survey of Native Americans living on reservations in Washington state showed that almost half of students ages 8 to 16 were smokeless tobacco users, including almost a third of the females.  *Nicotine Addiction*, p. 263

4.  Native Americans begin using smokeless tobacco products at much earlier ages than non-Native Americans. In a 1986 survey at the Rosebud Sioux Reservation in South Dakota, 21 percent of kindergarten children used smokeless tobacco products. A survey of Native Americans in the state of Washington indicated that 33 percent of former users and 57 percent of current users started using smokeless tobacco products before the age of 10.
    Federal Register, August 11, 1995, p. 41318

5.  According to the 1990-91 Youth Risk Behavior Survey, the smokeless tobacco product use rates among males in grades 9 through 12 were as high as 34 percent in Tennessee, 33 percent in Montana, 32 percent in Colorado, and 31 percent in Alabama and Wyoming. Native American youth are especially vulnerable to smokeless tobacco product use. The rates for both males and females are extremely high, ranging from 24 percent to 64 percent: rates in some areas are 10 times higher than those for non-Native Americans.
    Federal Register, August 11, 1995, p. 41317

# Baseball and Smokeless Tobacco

1.  " . . . when I see kids with these little cans in their back pockets and know what baseball has done to influence this, it makes me mad as hell."                                    Henry Aaron (National Spit Tobacco Education Flier)

2.  In a 1989 survey of major league baseball players, 45.6% were current smokeless tobacco users.
    *Smokeless Tobacco or Health*, p. 34

3.  35 to 40% of major league baseball players use chewing tobacco. 59% of a group of major league player tobacco users who volunteered for oral exams had tobacco-related mouth lesions, and 11% were serious enough to require a biopsy to rule out cancer and the need for surgery.                    USA Today, April 1, 1998, p. C3

4.  The American Dental Association has called for a ban on chewing tobacco at major league ball parks after a study showed that more than half of 91 National League baseball players who use smokeless tobacco had oral precancerous lesions.                                    Time, July 25, 1994, p. 18

5.  Babe Ruth smoked cigars and chewed tobacco, and died of throat cancer at age 53. He had been chewing tobacco since the age of seven.          NEJM, May 12, 1988, p. 1281, and Baseball, Ken Burns, 1994 (PBS film)

6.  Major League baseball teams once supplied free chewing tobacco to their players. During the 1980's, an industry marketing campaign delivered free samples to team clubhouses.    American Journal of Public Health 82:351, 1992

7.  Hall of Fame baseball player Rod Carew chewed tobacco from 1964 until he quit in 1992, when he had a growth in his mouth and spent more than $100,000 on remedial dental work.    San Francisco Chronicle, February 4, 1993

8. "Giants fans have reverently followed Barry Bonds' uncanny feats this season, and the same fans have also watched Bonds repeatedly return to the bench and pull out a big ol' wad of chewing tobacco. Baseball's best player, its most-watched role model, enjoys a good chew. He's not alone."

San Francisco Chronicle, August 18, 1993

9. Barry Bonds quit his smokeless tobacco habit in 1997. San Francisco Chronicle, May 13, 1997

10. During one game of the 1986 World Series, there were a total of 24 minutes on camera of televised images of players and coaches chewing and dipping smokeless tobacco. NEJM, April 9, 1987, p. 952

11. From 1986 to 1995, players and coaches in the World Series averaged 10.7 minutes of visible chewing tobacco use on TV. (The record was 23.9 minutes in a 1986 game.) US News and World Report, November 11, 1996, p. 16

12. In a poll of a professional baseball organization, 43% were smokeless tobacco users, and 37% of the year-round users had oral leukoplakia, a precancerous lesion. Journal of Family Practice, June 1992, p. 713

13. 37% of child and teenage spit tobacco users have a father who also uses. Use in NCAA college baseball players increased from 45% in 1985 to 57% in 1989. *Spit Tobacco and Youth*, p. 19

14. 39 year old Brett Butler, the Los Angeles Dodger's starting center fielder and a former tobacco chewer, was diagnosed with throat cancer in May 1996. He had 32 radiation treatments over six weeks, and 50 lymph nodes as well as the cancer surgically removed. He now has a scar from his right ear down his neck and across his throat. He returned four months later with great fanfare to the Dodger lineup. Sports Illustrated, September 16, 1996

# International Issues

1. In a study from Bombay, India, chewing tobacco use was responsible for 47% of all oral cancers, and the risk is increased six-fold compared to nonusers. In addition, the rate of stillbirths was tripled in tobacco users, and birth weights were decreased by an average of 4 to 8 ounces. JAMA, February 28, 1986, p. 1041

2. Australia, Hong Kong, Ireland, Israel, New Zealand, Saudi Arabia, Singapore, Thailand, as well as Great Britain and the 12 other European community nations have banned the manufacture, sale, and/or import of all smokeless tobacco products. Common Cause magazine, Summer 1993

3. The sale of smokeless tobacco has been banned in all European Union member countries since July 1992. Journal of the National Cancer Institute, September 4, 1996, p. 1189

4. A US Tobacco Company executive wrote Poland's minister of health asking permission to market oral snuff products there. "UST...is a community leader when it comes to accepting its social responsibilities". Common Cause magazine, Summer 1993

5. Hong Kong in 1987 became the first country in Asia and the second in the world to completely ban smokeless tobacco. "But there were more political pressures to come, in the shape of a letter from U.S. Senators Robert Dole, Christopher Dodd, Bob Kasten, and Lowell P. Weicker, Jr., to the Hong Kong government: 'We believe (a ban) would (be viewed in the United States as) an unfair and discriminatory restriction on foreign trade'. . . They continued that the ban could cause 'a potential barrier to our people's historic trade relationship'--words to make any trading partner tremble." *The Doctor-Activist*, Ellen Bassuk, Plenum Press, 1996, p. 46

6. Smokeless tobacco cannot be bought or sold in the U.K. British Medical Association

# U.S. Tobacco Company

1. A May 3, 1990 Wall Street Journal article "With the Help of Teens, Snuff Sales Revive" described US Tobacco, which controls 85% of the moist snuff market. "The company targets mostly white, blue-collar males who work in factories or on farms, or in such industries as lumber, steel and energy. To reach that audience, UST does little

print advertising. Instead, it and other smokeless tobacco makers have learned to fish where the fishing is good. They spend millions to sponsor such events as auto racing, rodeos, monster truck shows and tractor pulls, where their blue-collar customers are likely to gather."

2. Skoal and Copenhagen, the smokeless tobacco brands preferred by adolescents, are promoted on television by their sponsorship of "monster" truck shows, drag racing, stock car racing, and rodeos. "The harmful effects of tobacco are camouflaged against the backdrop and thrill of athletic victory".

.American Journal of Public Health, March 1992, p. 353

3. Celebrity athletes signed up by US Tobacco to promote the pleasures of dipping Skoal in advertisements and personal appearances have included football players Walt Garrison, Nick Buoniconti, Earl Campbell, Terry Bradshaw, and Lawrence Taylor, as well as baseball players Bobby Mercer and Carlton Fisk. A new "macho" image is now conveyed by these sports stars and other celebrity role models.

Common Cause magazine, Summer 1993, and *Smokeless Tobacco and Health*, p. xli

4. US Tobacco commands 87% of the US snuff market, and was the single most profitable company on the New York Stock Exchange in 1993, with profits of more than 50 cents for every dollar of revenue.

Tobacco Control, Winter 1994, p. 299

5. US Tobacco Company sales in 1991 rose 18% from the previous year to $773 million, and profits were $266 million. A Kidder Advisory on the stock market called UST "very well positioned in a high-growth, highly profitable industry."

*Spit Tobacco and Youth*, p. 9

6. US Tobacco Company sales reached $1 billion in 1992.

Common Cause magazine, Summer 1993

7. US Tobacco had a 153.5% return on equity in 1996, and an average of 73.9% a year return on capital in the previous five years.

Forbes, January 13, 1997, p. 161

8. The US Tobacco Company spent $1 million as an official sponsor of the 1980 Winter Olympics.

NEJM, May 12, 1988, p. 1281

9. US Tobacco, the major manufacturer of spitting tobacco, spends half its advertising budget on "young adults", although young adults make up only 2% of the company's market share. "The point is that unless you hook them young, you may not hook them at all."

JAMA, September 25, 1996, p. 998

10. US Tobacco "virtually invented a market for chewing tobacco beginning in 1970." Before this time, the habit did not exist among young people.

*Smokescreen*, p. 77

11. "Before the top smokeless tobacco company, US Tobacco (now called UST), launched a deliberate campaign to hook kids, the habit was confined to older men and was fast disappearing; fewer than 2 percent of young men ages 17 and 18 chewed or dipped tobacco. But then US Tobacco added sweet flavorings like cherry; created product lines with graduated nicotine strength; hired baseball players to flack that chewing tobacco was cool; sponsored rock concerts and rodeos; and through promotions for its starter product, Skoal Bandits, slyly implied that chew was a cool way for teens to rebel."

Mother Jones magazine, May-June 1996, p. 3

12. US Tobacco (UST) is the leading American seller of spit tobacco. A 1984 document, portions quoted below, shows that the company knowingly sought to create peer pressure to use its products, and then exploited that peer pressure to addict more young people and sell more product. UST sponsored a scholarship program for college rodeo athletes.
OBJECTIVES: To provide an introduction to our products through sampling (primarily SKOAL Bandits and SKOAL Long Cut) and peer pressure at a grassroots level in one of our primary markets, create brand awareness, reinforce brands to consumers (COPENHAGEN & SKOAL), introduction grounds for new products, and continue our association with the western lifestyle.
STRATEGIES: To sample college rodeo athletes and rodeo spectators at every possible sanctioned NIRA rodeo (within reason); to gain free publicity for our products, the company and the college program through all available media surrounding college rodeo; to create peer pressure through the use of U.S. Tobacco celebrity/spokesmen

where possible; to gain national recognition for the program, our products and associated lifestyle through the syndicated television show of the College National Finals Rodeo. To provide a base for direct advertising to potential consumers through the NIRA National program, newspaper ads, (local and on-campus), radio ads, banners, rodeo flags, Smokeless team jackets, etc. To tie-in our college sampling program through the use of on-campus activities. Our college program covers twenty-seven (27) states, mostly Midwestern and western. Our presence is national through syndicated television show, which covers approximately 80% of the United States…Major support via sixty minute, syndicated television show. Abundant local print and radio publicity around individual rodeos. Also, significant print support through national horse/rodeo/western publications

To have our college reps work hand in hand with the hosting rodeo club and supply the hosting school with logos and publicity information to encourage the hosting rodeo to include us in all print, radio and television advertising they purchase on site.

At the 1983-84 NIRA rodeos we reached 101,400 spectators, sampled 51,621 SKOAL Bandits envelopes and 3,960 cans of SKOAL Long Cut, which tabulates out that we reached 54% of the total attendance as potential new consumers. By attending 100 NIRA rodeos in 1984-85, we could hypothetically reach 510,700 potential new consumers, with 293,200 SKOAL Bandit envelopes and 36,000 cans of SKOAL Long Cut.

ON-CAMPUS REP JOB DESCRIPTION: GOALS:
1. Create new users of U.S. Tobacco's Smokeless Products.
2. Enhance the image of U.S. Tobacco and it's (sic) products on campuses.
3. Communications ideas, reservations and recommendations to the Area Manager.
4. Evaluate and report all college market and retail account conditions to the Area Manager.

OBJECTIVES:
1. The #1 priority of all college reps, is to sample as many SKOAL Bandits to cigarette smokers during each month.
2. Sampling should be conducted to all athletic events, frat parties, intramural games, and wherever students congregate.
3. College reps should vary their sampling locations to ensure all areas and peer groups on campus are thoroughly covered.
4. Promotional activities should be conducted to further create brand awareness and new consumers.

2003 AMA Annual Tobacco Report

13. In the six years between 1989 and 1994, UST and the Smokeless Tobacco Council paid a stunning $9.2 million in fees to "state legislative consultants."　　　　　　　　　　Washington Monthly, May 1996, p. 22

14. Sean Marsee, an Oklahoma high school track star, started using snuff at age 12 and died of mouth cancer at the age of 19. His family lost a subsequent lawsuit against US Tobacco Co., the manufacturers of Sean's brand Copenhagen.　　　　　　　　　　Beat the Smokeless Habit (National Cancer Institute), 1992, p. 6 and Wall Street Journal, May 3, 1990

15. "Don't discuss health issues with anyone." Quote from US Tobacco's college marketing manual. The company distributes free samples through the mail and at sponsored events, but only its low nicotine brands.　　　　　　　　　　Tobacco Control, Spring 1995, pp. 76-78

16. 400,000 free samples of Skoal Bandits were distributed in 1985.　　　American Medical News, May 15, 1995, p. 16

17. US Tobacco Company, the nation's largest producer of smokeless tobacco, set up a $100,000 fund to benefit firefighters as part of an aggressive new advertising campaign in Tennessee. The company plans to use publicity surrounding the fund to promote its products, including Copenhagen and Skoal.　　　　　　　　　　USA Today, September 15, 1994, p. 3B

18. US Tobacco and the Smokeless Tobacco Council contributed $975,000 to national parties between 1988 and 1992, most in soft money to the Republican National Committee.　　　Common Cause magazine, Summer 1993

19. Spokesperson Alan Hilburg of the Smokeless Tobacco Council says that there is no scientific proof "that smokeless tobacco causes any adverse health effects or human disease," or that nicotine is addictive.

Common Cause magazine, Summer 1993

20. In the early 1990's, Louis Bantle was the $2 million a year chairman of US Tobacco Company of Greenwich Conn., makers of Skoal and Copenhagen smokeless tobacco. His company contributed $100,000 to the 1992 Bush re-election campaign and hosted a $350,000 Bush fund-raiser. At the same time, UST got high-level Bush administration help in battling foreign governments that banned the import and sale of snuff.

Common Cause magazine, Summer 1993

21. Bantle and UST, ironically, give generously to the national Alcohol and Drug Abuse Council and are major backers of a drug treatment center in Baltimore. Louis Bantle cut the ribbon on Bantle Hall in Baltimore at a ceremony with guest speaker Betty Ford and former president Gerald Ford.Common Cause magazine, Summer 1993

22. Seconds after being told that users of oral moist snuff were fifty times more likely to develop oral cancer than abstainers, US Tobacco's president, Joseph Taddeo testified under oath to Congress: "Oral tobacco has not been established as a cause of mouth cancer".                                                              CSPAN, April 14, 1994

23. In testimony to Congress, Taddeo denied that low-nicotine Skoal Bandits are an introductory or "starter product" for new users before they move up to higher nicotine brands such as Copenhagen. ("Sooner or later, it's Copenhagen.")  This contradicted a memo from an executive vice president of US Tobacco that "Skoal Bandits is an introductory product."  Taddeo also revealed under questioning by Rep. Mike Synar that his total 1993 compensation was $5.5 million in salary, bonuses, and company stock.                     CSPAN, April 14, 1994

24. In 1993 and 1994, Senator Bob Dole took 26 flights aboard US Tobacco Company corporate jets. UST, the nation's biggest producer of smokeless tobacco has contributed $40,000 to Dole's political committee since 1987, and its senior vice president is a board member of the Dole Foundation charity. At the same time, Dole has worked to hold down taxes on smokeless tobacco. A Dole amendment in 1985 set the tax on smokeless tobacco at less than three cents a can.                                                          Newsweek, April 24, 1995, p. 32

# Low Nicotine Starter Products and "Graduated Nicotine Delivery"

1. UST distributes free samples of low nicotine-delivery brands of moist snuff and instructs its representatives not to distribute free samples of higher nicotine-delivery brands. The low nicotine-delivery brands account for 47 percent of UST's advertising dollars, but for only 2 percent of the market share. In contrast, Copenhagen, the highest nicotine-delivery brand, had only 1 percent of the advertising expenditures, but 50 percent of the market share. This advertising focus is indicative of UST's "graduation process" of starting new smokeless tobacco product users on low nicotine-delivery brands and having them graduate to higher nicotine-delivery brands as a method for recruiting new, younger users.                                         Federal Register, August 11, 1995, p. 41331

2. "The marketing strategy soon became clear. In 1983, UST concentrated nearly half of its advertising budget on its starter brand of smokeless tobacco, called Skoal, which provided the lowest dose of nicotine to the new, intolerant users. Despite the high level of advertising, Skoal accounted for only 2% of the market share by weight. In contrast, Copenhagen, the UST brand with the highest nicotine content, received only about 1% of the advertising budget but commanded half of the market. UST was seemingly successful in attracting users to Skoal and then, after nicotine tolerance and dependence on smokeless tobacco developed, moving users up to products with the highest nicotine content."                            Journal of Pediatrics, April 1997, pp. 521-22 (David Kessler)

3. "Cherry Skoal is for somebody who likes the taste of candy, if you know what I mean."
                      former US Tobacco sales representative (Tobacco Control, Autumn 1997, p. 249)

4. Control of pH is an important means by which manufacturers of smokeless tobacco control the speed of nicotine delivery of their products.                                           Tobacco Control, Autumn 1997, p. 224

5. ". . . manufacturers of moist snuff may have a strategy of marketing starter brands (Skoal Bandits and Hawken) that establish the initial nicotine dependence of young people. With time, the dependence increases and,

eventually, the young snuff user may switch to products with medium (Skoal, Fine Cut) and eventually high (Copenhagen, Kodiak) nicotine delivery, becoming thereby strongly dependent on nicotine.'

*Tobacco Control, Spring 1995, p. 62*

6. Tobacco companies control nicotine doses delivered in smokeless tobacco by manipulation of pH. Free nicotine per gram ranges from a low of 0.53 for the "starter product" Skoal Bandits Wintergreen to a high of 9.03 for Copenhagen Snuff.

*Tobacco Control, Spring 1995, p. 59*

7. The FDA learned that manufacturers of smokeless tobacco adjust the pH of their products to produce intentionally graduated nicotine deliveries. The industry's "starter" products for new users have a low pH and consequently deliver a low lever of "free" nicotine, limiting the absorption of the compound in the mouth. Smokeless-tobacco products intended for users who have already acquired a tolerance to nicotine have a high pH and consequently deliver a high level of free nicotine, increasing the amount of nicotine available for absorption. Indeed, internal documents from the United States Tobacco Company, the nation's largest smokeless tobacco manufacturer, refer to an explicit "graduation process" designed to encourage users to progress from low-nicotine brands to high-nicotine ones.

*Quote from NEJM, September 26, 1996, p. 990*

8. Low nicotine products such as Happy Days and Skoal Bandits are designed as "starter" products. It is expected that as a user becomes more addicted, he will move up to Skoal and finally to Copenhagen. *Nicotine Addiction, p. 269*

9. U.S. Tobacco's "starter" product Skoal Bandits delivers only 7% of its available nicotine; Copenhagen delivers 79%.

*San Francisco Chronicle, April 1, 1998, p. A16*

10. Oliver Twist smokeless tobacco comes in five strengths, from Freshman "perfect for beginners" to Senior.

*Tobacco Control, Spring 1995, p. 75*

11. Holding an average-size dip or chew in the mouth for half an hour delivers as much nicotine as smoking four cigarettes. A two-can-a-week snuff dipper gets as much nicotine as a pack and a half a day smoker. Each tin of snuff contains a lethal dose of nicotine. *Beat the Smokeless Habit, p. 7*

12. A pinch of snuff has 2 to 3 times the nicotine dose of a cigarette. UST's Copenhagen and Pinkerton's Red Man moist snuff have the highest levels of available nicotine. A user who consumes 8 to 10 dips or chews a day receives a nicotine dose equal to that taken by a smoker of 30 to 40 cigarettes daily. *Spit Tobacco and Youth, p. 5*

13. In 1978, the US Tobacco Company ran ads in Sports Illustrated for free samples of fruit-flavored, low-nicotine snuff products for beginners; the samples were accompanied by instructions on how to use the product.

*1994 Surgeon General report, p. 163*

14. The Skoal Bandit is a low-nicotine "tea bag" of snuff that is a teaching tool to allow novices to take up the habit and slowly develop a tolerance to tobacco. It is marketed with the slogan "Take a pouch instead of a puff."

*NEJM, May 12, 1988, p. 1281*

# CHAPTER 18
# PIPES AND CIGARS

## Historical

1.  In 1762, Israel Putnam returned to his Connecticut home from Cuba, where he had been a British army officer. Starting an American tradition, he brought back a cache of Havana cigars.
    *New York Times magazine*, June 29, 1997, p. 34

2.  Nineteen of the 41 presidents have smoked cigars. More enthusiastic smokers included Zachary Taylor (and his son-in-law Jefferson Davis), Ulysses S. Grant, Chester Arthur, Benjamin Harrison, William McKinley, William Howard Taft, and Calvin Coolidge (who smoked 12-inch super coronas). JFK was the last president to regularly light up.
    *San Francisco Examiner magazine*, December 15, 1996, p. 40

3.  In the mid-1800's, Pennsylvania became well known for a type of cigar named the "stogie" because the makers used the famous Conestoga wagon manufactured in the same region, as an advertising tie-in.
    *A Passion for Cigars*, p. 18

4.  Benjamin Harrison smoked half a dozen cigars a day, and William McKinley, 18 a day.
    *Tobacco Advertising*, p. 84

5.  General Grant's occasional cigar habit increased to 20 a day by 1862. He died of throat cancer in 1885, after losing 70 of his 200 pounds and becoming addicted to cocaine to ease the pain.
    *Newsweek*, December 2, 1996, p. 75

6.  In 1970, there were 235 cigar factories in the state of Connecticut.
    *A Passion for Cigars*, p. 18

7.  "I smoke in moderation. Only one cigar at a time."   Mark Twain (*The Cigar*, Barnaby Conrad, Chronicle, 1996)

8.  Rudyard Kipling wrote about Habana Puro cigars in his poem "The Betrothed." "And a woman is only a woman, but a good cigar is a smoke", he intoned, anticipating the man who, when asked what he would do if his wife objected his Cuban cigars, responded: "Get a new wife." Mark Twain said, or didn't say, "If I cannot smoke cigars in heaven, I shall not go."
    *San Francisco Examiner*, April 24, 1994, and *San Francisco Chronicle*, January 25, 1993, p. B4

9.  The newspaper editor Horace Greeley (1811-1872) called a cigar "a fire at one end and a fool at the other."
    *Thank You For Smoking*, Christopher Buckley p. 59

10. By 1900, an estimated four out of five men smoked cigars, and cigars accounted for nearly 60% of all tobacco sales. In 1903 in the US, there were twice as many cigars smoked as cigarettes, a total of 6.7 billion.
    *Tobacco Advertising*, p. 81

11. "Mark Twain. Albert Einstein. General Douglas MacArthur. Pipe smokers all. But pipes aren't just consigned to history. They're coming out of tweedy men's clubs and heading into the hottest nightspots."
    *USA Today*, December 10, 1996, p. 6D

12. American poet Amy Lowell, a cigar smoker, bought 10,000 Manillas in 1915 as a hedge against future wartime shortages.
    *San Francisco Chronicle*, August 10, 1997, p. 7

13. Cigars smoked in the US increased from 4 billion in 1907 to 8 billion in 1929.   *A Passion for Cigars*, p. 22

14. "What this country really needs is a good five-cent cigar."
    Thomas Riley Marshall, U.S. Vice-President, 1920, under Woodrow Wilson

15. "Sometimes a cigar is just a cigar."
    Sigmund Freud (Cigar Aficionado website)

16. Sigmund Freud smoked 20 cigars a day for the whole of his adult life and said to young nephew: "My boy, smoking is one of the greatest and cheapest enjoyments in life, and if you decide in advance not to smoke, I can only feel sorry for you." When he was 67, he developed cancer of the soft palate and jaw, but continued to smoke until his death in 1939 at age 83.

*Cigar Aficionado*, winter 1994, and *New York Times* magazine, June 29, 1997, p. 34

17. Winston Churchill smoked 8 to 10 cigars a day, primarily Cuban brands. "Not even the necessity of wearing an oxygen mask for a high altitude flight in a non-pressurized cabin could prevent Churchill from smoking."

*Cigar Aficionado*, December 1999

18. "As for cigars, they made some impact – particularly in America – after the British occupation of Cuba during the Seven Years' War (1756-63). Even so, it wasn't until Europe's soldiery got their hands on them while in Spain for the Peninsula War (1808-14) that cigars spread all over the continent – Britain imported 26 pounds of cigars in 1800, 250,000 pounds in 1830." *Faber Book of Smoking*, p. 58

19. Winston Churchill claimed to have smoked a quarter of a million cigars in his 91 years. "During the Nazi blitz of London in 1941, one of the Luftwaffe's raids destroyed the Dunhill tobacco shop on Drake Street, in which was stored a portion of the prime minister's treasured cache of Havanas... the store manager made a careful survey of the damage and rushed to the phone to report, 'your cigars are safe, sir." *A Passion for Cigars*, p. 24

20. In 1961, President John F. Kennedy ordered Pierre Salinger to purchase 1200 of Cuba's finest Petit Upmann cigars just before ordering a trade embargo on all imports from Castro's Cuba.

*San Francisco Chronicle*, January 25, 1993, p. B3

21. One day in 1961, shortly after the failed Bay of Pigs invasion, the president took legendary action that has become a classic anecdote of cigar lore. JFK called his cigar-smoking press secretary Pierre Salinger into the Oval Office and said, "I need a lot of cigars."
"How many, Mr. President?"
"About a thousand. Tomorrow morning, call all your friends who have cigars and just get as many as you can." Salinger rushed out and grabbed as many H. Upmann petits as he could find. The next morning there was an urgent message for him to enter the Oval Office immediately. "How did you do on the cigars last night?" asked Kennedy.
"Mr. President," replied Salinger, "I was very successful. I got eleven hundred." With that, Kennedy opened a drawer in his desk and pulled out a decree banning all Cuban products from entry into the United States. "Good," he replied. "Now that I have enough cigars to last awhile, I can sign this!"

Quote from *San Francisco Examiner* magazine, December 15, 1996, pp. 40-42 (Barnaby Conrad)

22. In April 1996, Cigar Aficionado editor and publisher Marvin Shanken bought JFK's walnut cigar humidor for $574,500 at a Sotheby's auction. *New York Times* magazine, June 29, 1997, p. 35

# General

1. In 1981, Al Goldstein, publisher of Screw magazine, started a new quarterly called Cigar. It folded after four issues, and Goldstein lost $200,000 on the venture. *New York Times* magazine, June 29, 1997, p. 34

2. Cuban cigar exports dropped from 120 million a year in the late 1980's to an estimated 50 million in 1994, mostly to Europe. 6 to 8 million make it into the United States despite being banned.

*San Francisco Examiner*, April 24, 1994

3. In 1985, Fidel Castro stopped smoking cigars after 44 years as part of Cuba's nationwide efforts to reduce tobacco use. For his role in this anti-tobacco campaign, he received an award from the World Health Organization.

*Cigar Aficionado*, Summer 1994, and *American Medical News*, June 13, 1994

4.   In 1983, the Ritz-Carlton hotel in Boston held a black tie cigar dinner, resurrecting an old custom. "By 1994, more than 2000 such evenings are being held in hotels, restaurants, bars and clubs across the country."
                                                                New York Times magazine, June 29, 1997, p. 34

5.   In 1970, 16% of men smoked cigars and 13% smoked pipes; in 1991, 4% smoked cigars and 2% smoked pipes.
6.                                                              Epidemiologic Reviews 1995; 17:55

7.   From 1964 to 1984, cigar smoking prevalence among American men declined from 29% to 6%, and pipe smoking form 19% to 4%.                    *Reducing the Health Consequences of Smoking*, p. 328

8.   Cigar sales declined from 5.5% of the tobacco product market in the early 1970's to 1.5% in 1991, but there were still 4 million cigar and pipe smokers in the US.
                                          Tobacco Control, Winter 1993, p. 57, and *Nicotine Addiction*, p. 17

9.   Cigars manufactured in the United States declined form a peak of 10 billion in 1972 to 3.2 billion in 1988, the lowest levels in more than a century.          Population and Development Review, June 1996, p. 223

10.  The cigar industry is now a billion-dollar business catering to an estimated 12 million American cigar smokers.
                                                                Contra Costa (Calif.) Times, February 6, 1998, p. D11

11.  Cigar consumption declined by 66% in the United States between 1964 and 1993. From 1993 to 1997, however, there was a dramatic increase of 50% overall in cigars consumed, including an estimated 250% increase in sales of premium cigars; 4 billion premium cigars were smoked in 1997.
                             Journal of the National Cancer Institute, April 15, 1998, pp. 562-563, and PBS television

12.  "In 1996, large inexpensive cigars (more than one dollar retail) and cigarillos accounted for the greatest share of cigar sales (60.3 percent) followed by small cigars (33.2 percent), and large premium cigars (6.5 percent). In recent years, cigar sales have increased in all three categories, but the fastest growing segment of the cigar market has been the premium cigar category where sales have increased by 154 percent since 1993."          *Cigars*, p. 52

13.  Total US cigar consumption was 9 billion in 1964. By 1994, it had dropped to 2.2 billion. However, the market for imported premium cigars costing $1.25 or more, mostly from Jamaica, Honduras, Mexico, and the Dominican Republic, increased from 88 million in 1989 to 122 million in 1994.    New York Times, January 30, 1995, p. C7

14.  About $1 billion worth of cigars were sold in the US in 1995; women account for 2% of the 10 million cigar smokers, up from 0.1% a decade ago. 170 million premium cigars were sold in 1995, up 32% from 1994.
                                                                USA Today, June 25, 1996, p. B1

15.  U.S. cigar consumption in the first five months of 1996 was up 51% from the same period the previous year. Total consumption increased from 3.4 billion in 1993 to 4 billion cigars in 1995.    USA Today, August 16, 1996

16.  In 1996, cigar consumption reached 4.4 billion, or $1.25 billion in retail sales. The market's peak was in 1973, when Americans smoked more than 11.2 billion cigars.          New York Times, February 16, 1997, p. F3

17.  1973 was the high-water mark of cigar consumption in American, with 11.2 billion smoked, an average of 54 cigars for every person in the country. In 1993, consumption bottomed out at 3.4 billion, the lowest annual total since records began being kept in 1920.          New York Times magazine, June 29, 1997, p. 34

18.  According to the editor of Cigar Aficionado, the number of cigar smokers in the United States increased from 3 million in 1992 to 10 million in 1996.          CBS evening news, January 26, 1997

19.  The average cigarette has approximately 0.68 grams of tobacco, 0.5 to 1.4 milligrams of nicotine, 0.5 to 18 mg of tar, and emits 0.5 to 18 mg of carbon monoxide. By contrast, a cigar has 8 grams of tobacco, 1.7 to 5.2 mg of nicotine, 16 to 110 mg of tar, and emits 90 to 120 mg of carbon monoxide.          Newsweek, July 21, 1997, p. 57

20. A large cigar is equivalent to four to five cigarettes in nicotine, 15 cigarettes in tobacco and 25 cigarettes in carbon monoxide.                    Texas Department in Health reported in Vitality magazine, December 1997

21. The smoke from one cigar equals the particle emissions of three cigarettes, and has thirty times the carbon monoxide of one cigarette.   Consumer Reports, March 1997, p. 8, and CNN Headline News, November 20, 1996

22. Cigars emit 22 times more carbon monoxide than cigarettes, and premium cigars have 15 to 20 times more tobacco than a cigarette.                                    USA Today, February 23, 1998, p. D10

23. Cigarettes generally contain less than one gram of tobacco and are smoked for about 7 to 8 minutes. Large cigars commonly contain 5-17 grams of tobacco and are smoked over intervals as long as 60 to 90 minutes. *Cigars*, p. 18

24. The tar in cigar smoke is more carcinogenic than the tar of cigarette smoke.                    *Cigars*, p. 3

25. Even an unlighted cigar held in the mouth can cause high levels of nicotine to be absorbed. Some cigars contain as much as 20 grams of nicotine, compared to about 15 grams in an entire pack of cigarettes.
USA Today, March 30, 1998, p. D1

26. Cigars and cigarettes, consumed in equal volumes, produce roughly equal risks of mouth and throat cancer. Heavy cigar smokers incur nearly three times the risk of lung cancer of nonsmokers, compared to nine times the risk for cigarette smokers.                    Newsweek, December 2, 1996, p. 75

27. Deaths from pipe and cigar smoking totaled 14,000 in 1991.
Internal Medicine World Report, September 15, 1991 p. 1

28. Celebrities with the cigar habit include David Letterman, Arnold Schwarzenegger, Danny De Vito, Tom Cruise, Bruce Willis, Tom Selleck, Rush Limbaugh, Jim Belushi, Gregory Hines, Linda Evangelista, Matt Dillon, Patrick Swayze, George Hamilton, Alec Baldwin, Demi Moore, James Woods, Whoopi Goldberg, Jack Nicholson, Bill Cosby, Paul Anka, Terry Bradshaw, Willie Mays, Claudia Schiffer, Pierce Brosnan, football coach Mike Ditka, Denzel Washington, Jesse Ventura, Milton Berle, Will Smith, John Grisham, and Robert DeNiro.
CBS News, October 24, 1995, and Cigar Aficionado

29. Bill Clinton occasionally enjoys wrapping his lips around an unlit cigar; he "smokes" Hoyo De Monterre Excalibur #1's, according to a local tobacconist.                    Time, July 4, 1994, p. 14

30. Supreme Court Justices Clarence Thomas and Antonin Scalia smoke cigars. Gangsters including Al Capone, Anthony "Fat Tony" Salerno, and Carmine "Lilo" Galante also were cigar smokers.
San Francisco Examiner magazine, December 15, 1996, pp. 42-44

31. Cigar Aficionado sponsored a $1000 a plate "Dinner of the Century" in Paris in 1994 one week after the World Conference on Tobacco and Health in the same city. Among those attending were cigar smoking film director Francis Ford Coppola and Rush Limbaugh.                    Tobacco Control, Spring 1995, p. 20

32. "Have you heard about the Tee-Gar? It's a plastic holder for one's cigar, affixed to a tee, so that before one hits a ball, stogies don't have to be tossed onto the turf, where they might pick up nasty things like pesticides and fertilizers."                    San Francisco Chronicle, July 13, 1996

33. A quarterly magazine, Cigar Aficionado, sold 100,000 of each of the first two issues in 1992. Advertisers for the magazine appreciate that the typical fine cigar smoker has a yearly income of $194,000 and a net worth of $1.5 million. 99% are males. A series of English Cigar smoker dinners at Ritz-Carlton hotels throughout the United States are priced at $300 per ticket.                    San Francisco Examiner, September 6, 1992, p. A8

34. The March 1997 issue of Cigar Aficionado features hockey star Wayne Gretzky and his wife, model Janet Jones, with stogies in hand. The magazine's circulation is now 413,000, up more than 71% from a year earlier. Celebrity

endorsements are way up, and actors James Belushi and Chuck Norris plan to develop a premium line of cigars and to build cigar lounges across the country
.
USA Today, February 11, 1997, p. 2B, and San Francisco Chronicle, March 9, 1997, p. 6

35. A sign was posted at LA's Hillcrest Country Club after member George Burns protested the club's new ban on stogies: "Cigar smoking prohibited for anyone under 95."
US News and World Report, November 22, 1993, p. 25

36. Christian Mortensen, who may have been the oldest man ever, died in 1998 in California at age 115. He had been a regular cigar smoker for more than 90 years.  San Francisco Chronicle, April 28, 1998, p. A15

37. Actor Jim Belushi owns four cigar stores.  USA Weekend, October 24, 1997, p. 18

38. "Dan Aykroyd and wife Donna Dixon stogied up during the John Belushi Memorial Cigar Night at L.A.'s House of Blues."  People magazine, October 14, 1996, p. 13

39. On the American black market, a box of 25 of Cuban top of the line cigars goes for $250 to $1000, or from $10 to $50 per cigar.  US News and World Report, April 14, 1997, p. 63

40. 800 cigar aficionados from around the world gathered at the Tropicana night club in Havana in early 1997 to celebrate the thirtieth anniversary of Cohiba, the world's most luxurious cigar. The fund raiser raised $2 million for Cuba's health care system, with $130,000 paid for a Cohiba-filled humidor signed by Fidel Castro.
Sunday Morning, Charles Osgood, March 23, 1997

41. In the last four years, charity cigar auctions in Cuba of humidors and boxes with Fidel Castro's signature have raised about $1 million for Cuban medical relief.  Cigar Aficionado, August 1997, p. 145

42. Cuba exported 100 million cigars in 1997, up from 70 million in 1996.  Reuters/CNN, December 23, 1997

43. In November 1997 at a Christie's auction in Geneva, an unidentified Asian buyer paid $16,400 for a box of 25 Trinidads, Cuba's "most exclusive cigar brand." This price, a record, comes out to U.S. $656 per cigar.
Cigar Aficionado website

44. A box of 25 coveted Cohiba cigars costs about $500 in Cuba, while the price ranges between $800 and $1000 in Europe.  Associated Press, February 24, 2001

45. As many as five million Cuban cigars were sold illegally on the black market in the United States in 1996.
Tobacco Control, Summer 1997, p. 86

46. A recent increase in the smuggling of Cuban cigars into San Diego has been linked to a weekly airline flight from Tijuana to Havana. "Nationwide, seizures of Cuban cigars have increased six-fold in the past three years, to more than $1.1 million worth in fiscal 1996." High-quality Monte Cristos can fetch $100 each.
San Francisco Chronicle, September 8, 1997, p. A22

47. The value of the 96,216 Cuban cigars seized by U.S. customs in fiscal year 1996 was $1.4 million, up from $142,000 in 1994. About half of the seizures were at Kennedy Airport in New York.
Cigar Aficionado, August 1997, p. 39

48. In the first half of 1997, there were 278 million cigars imported into the United States, an increase of 92% from the previous year.  NBC evening news, September 26, 1997

49. Premium cigars selling for $1 to $25 accounted for 40% of the $1.3 billion spent on cigars in the U.S. in 1996. The top selling brands are Macanudo and H. Upmann.
New York Times, August 24, 1997, p. 18, and July 22, 1997, p. D8

50. Premium cigar imports increased form 176 million in 1995 to 293.7 million in 1996; the market nearly tripled in four years.                                                  Cigar Aficionado, August 1997, p. 39

51. Consumption of premium cigars increased 65% in 1996, and 250% between 1993 and 1996.
                                                  Journal of the National Cancer Institute, July 16, 1997, p. 999

52. The number of premium cigars sold in the United States increased from less than 100,000 in 1992 to 274,000 in 1996. Americans consumed 4.6 billion cigars in 1996, an increase of 44% since 1993.
                                                  Newsweek, July 21, 1997, p. 57

53. An estimated 6 million (26.7%) of 14 to 19-year-olds reported having smoked a cigar in the previous year (37% of boys, and 16% of girls). 54% of cigarette smokers and 14% of nonsmokers of cigarettes reported having smoked a cigar.                                                  JAMA, July 2, 1997, pp. 17-18

54. Less than 15 percent of cigar smokers who have never smoked cigarettes report inhaling smoke into the lung. However, more than 20 percent of former cigarette smokers and about two thirds of concurrent cigar and cigarette smokers report inhaling.                                                  *Cigars*, p. 185

55. Most cigarette smokers report inhaling the smoke onto their lungs, while over three-quarters of the males who have only smoked cigars report that they never inhale. This difference in inhalation is likely due to the more acidic pH of cigarette smoke. The smoke of most cigars has an alkaline pH; and as a result, nicotine contained in the smoke can be readily absorbed across the oral mucosa without inhalation into the lung. The more acidic pH of cigarette smoke produces a protonated form of nicotine which is much less readily absorbed by the oral mucosa, and the larger absorptive surface of the lung is required for the smoker to receive the desired dose of nicotine. As a result, cigarette smokers must inhale to ingest substantial quantities of nicotine, the active agent in smoke, whereas cigar smokers can ingest substantial quantities of nicotine without inhaling. Individuals who have previously smoked cigarettes are more likely to inhale cigar smoke when they switch to smoking cigars, and this increased inhalation may reduce or eliminate any risk reduction with the change from cigarettes to cigars, particularly if cigars are smoked daily or as a means of satisfying an addiction to nicotine.
                                                  Quote from *Cigars*, pp. 4 and 10

56. As many as three quarters of cigar smokers smoke only occasionally, and there is no good data on adverse health effects in this group. A large, premium cigar is estimated to produce smoke equivalent to 15-20 cigarettes, and the lung cancer risk from inhaling moderately when smoking five cigars a day is comparable to that from smoking one pack of cigarettes a day.                                                  Journal of the National Cancer Institute, April 15, 1998, p. 563

57. The pattern of excess disease risk among cigar smokers is different from that observed in cigarette smokers. Mortality for cigarette smokers is much higher than cigar smokers for coronary heart disease, COPD and lung cancer. In contrast, mortality for oral and esophageal cancer are similar among cigarette and cigar smokers.
                                                  *Cigars*, p. 4

58. Cigar smokers have nearly twice the risk of dying from cancer and cardiovascular disease as do nonsmokers, and have a 25% higher mortality rate from all causes, in a study from Kaiser Permanente Hospital in Oakland.
                                                  Contra Costa (Calif.) Times, March 20, 1998, p. A12

59. Among adult males in California in 1996, 40% of current cigar smokers were never smokers. The highest rates of cigar use and the lowest rates of cigarette use occur in people with the highest educational attainment.
                                                  *Cigars*, p. 11

60. Men who smoke cigars have a death rate 34% higher than nonsmokers, and cigar smoking raises the risk of dying from cancers of the larynx, mouth, and esophagus by 4 to 10 times. These rates are similar to those associated with cigarette smoking.        Stop Teenage Addiction to Tobacco (STAT) fact sheet on cigars, February 1997

61. A case of "cigar smoke syncope" was reported in a man who smoked several cigars in a crowded cigar dinner, complained of feeling ill, and then lost consciousness for 12 minutes. On hospital admission, his oxygen saturation was 81% and carboxyhemoglobin level was 14.7%. The diagnosis was carbon monoxide poisoning

exacerbated by nicotine. JAMA, December 3, 1997, p. 1744

62. The Portuguese soccer team Benfica spent $26,000 on cigars in six months in 1997.
Sports Illustrated, December 1, 1997, p. 22

63. Former Prime Minister Binyamin Netanyahu of Israel listed an expenditure of $40,000 on cigars for one year on his expense account for himself and his guests. He apparently prefers Cuban cigars.
ABC radio news, April 13, 1998

64. "I reasoned with him, and we both smoked a couple of cigars," United Nations Secretary General Kofi Annan, describing his technique when negotiating with Iraqi dictator Saddam Hussein
San Francisco Chronicle, April 29, 1998

65. "The enjoyment of a cigar after a hard week gives me a feeling of well-being and relaxation that a Valium could not match. While there may be a more ideal form of stress reduction, I haven't yet discovered anything else as effective and easy."      Ear, Nose and Throat Surgeon M. Hal Pearlman, M.D., Cigar Aficionado, Spring 1993

66. An ad for cigarillo shows a couple each holding the product, with the copy reading, "For the women who say size doesn't matter, and the men who actually believe them." Another ad for the same brand shows a couple smoking, with the logo "when you only have time for a quickie." *Cigars*, p. 202

67. According to the Cigar Association of America, more than 10 million Americans smoked cigars in 1995, up from six to eight million in 1990. Wall Street Journal, February 16, 1996

68. In the first nine months of 1996, the cigar industry increased their ad expenditures by 438% over the previous year. Tobacco Control, Autumn 1997, p. 240|

69. Cigar sales in the US dropped from 9 billion in 1964 to 2 billion in 1992. However, the market for premium cigars costing $1.25 or more has recently increased. 38% of upscale cigar buyers are also millionaires; 60% wear a $500-plus watch, and 90% traveled abroad in the last year.
CBS News, November 30, 1993, and Time, May 11, 1992, p. 56

70. Men who smoke five or more cigars a day have a 220% greater risk of lung cancer and a 620% greater risk of throat and oral cancers than nonsmokers. Time, June 21, 1999, p. 83

71. Relative risk in cigar smokers compared with nonsmokers of heart disease is 1.27%, for COPD is 1.45, for oropharyngeal cancer 2.02, and for lung cancer 2.14. There was a synergistic relation between cigar smoking and alcohol consumption as risk factors for oropharyngeal and esophageal cancer. By comparison, relative risks associated with current cigarette smoking by men are much higher: 1.5 to 3.0 for coronary heart disease, 9 to 25 for COPD, 8 to 24 for lung cancer, and 4 to 12 for oropharyngeal cancer. NEJM, June 1, 1999, pp. 1773 and 1776

72. In a study from the Centers for Disease Control in Atlanta, current cigar smoking in men was associated with a five-fold increased risk of lung cancer mortality compared to never smoking men. The relative risk for cancer of the pharynx and oral cavity in the group was 4.0; it was 10.3 for cancer of the larynx and 1.8 for cancer of the esophagus. Journal of the National Cancer Institute, February 16, 2000, p. 333

73. In a study of lung cancer risk from three European countries, smoking cigars (odds ratio 9.0) or pipes (7.9) was only of moderately less risk for developing lung cancer than was smoking cigarettes only (odds ratio 14. 9)
Journal of the National Cancer Institute, April 21, 1999, p. 697

74. Total cigar consumption decreased from 8 billion in 1970 to 2 million in 1993, and then increased to 3.6 billion in 1997. Morbidity and Mortality Weekly Report, November 5, 1999, p. 989

75. Total U.S. cigar sales were 3.7 billion in 1998. US News and World Report, November 29, 1999, p. 55

76. Cigar Aficionado in December 1999 published an article "The top 100 cigar smokers of the Twentieth Century."

77. In 1998, 11.9% of men and 2.3% of women were cigar smokers, an increase from the previous year. 5.6% of youths ages 12 to 17, or 1.3 million, were current cigar users.     1998 National Household Survey on Drug Abuse

78. Cigar imports peaked at over 500 million in 1997, declining to 30 million estimated in 1999.

Newsweek, November 15, 1999, p. 8

79. The mainstream smoke from cigars, compared to mainstream cigarette smoke, contains greater concentrations of nicotine, benzene, aromatic hydrocarbons, hydrogen cyanide, lead nitrogen oxides, N-nitrosamines, ammonia, and carbon monoxide.     NEJM, June 10, 1999, p. 1779

80. Spending on cigars in the United States increased from $872 million in 1996 to $1.8 billion in 2000.

San Francisco Chronicle, July 1, 2000, p. E6

81. Cigar tobacco, compared to cigarette tobacco, is rich in the highly carcinogenic nitrosamines NNK and NNN. Between 1993 and 1997, US cigar consumption increased by 46.4%. A large cigar emits, when smoked, about 20 times the carbon monoxide, 5 times the respirable particles, and twice the amount of polycyclic aromatic hydrocarbon of a cigarette. In a study of a cigar banquet, the indoor carbon monoxide level averaged 10 parts per million for more than three hours; the EPA standard for carbon monoxide is a maximum permissible level of 9 ppm over an 8-hour period.     JAMA, August 9, 2000, pp. 735-738

82. "In terms of air pollution, even a medium-sized cigar can be the equivalent of five cigarettes; some large cigars contain an amount of tobacco equivalent to a pack of cigarettes."     *Nicotine and Public Health*, p. 193

83. Men who smoke three or more cigars daily and report moderate inhalation experience lung cancer death at about two thirds of the rate of men who smoke a pack of cigarettes a day. The death rate from oral (mouth and throat) cancers is nearly 8 times higher, and death from cancer of the larynx about 10 times higher, in male cigar smokers compared with lifelong nonsmokers; the death rate from esophageal cancer is 3 to 4 times higher.

JAMA, August 9, 2000, p. 738

84. Most significantly, the researchers found a five-fold overall increased risk of death from lung cancer among male cigar smokers – a much greater risk than had been previously reported in the US. That risk increased further among men who reported smoking three or more cigars a day (to 7.8 time the risk of men who have never smoked) and for men who inhale their cigar smoke (who have 11.3 times the risk of lung cancer death of nonsmokers). However, even men who said they did not inhale their cigar smoke had lung cancer death rates more than three times that of men who had never smoked. According to Eric Jacobs, PhD.: "We expected to find some increased risk of lung cancer, but we found that cigar smoking is much more lethal than we thought." Cigar smoking also increased risk of death from cancer of the larynx by more than 10 times and cancer of the oral cavity/pharynx by four times. Current cigar smokers who said they inhaled their cigar smoke were 2.7 times more likely to die of pancreatic cancer and 3.6 times more likely to die of bladder cancer than men who never smoked.

Quote from CA-A Cancer Journal for Clinicians, May/June 2000, p.138

85. Celebrities appearing on the cover of Cigar Aficionado have included Arnold Schwartzenegger (former chairman of the President's Council on Fitness and Sports), Tom Selleck, Pierce Brosnan, Wayne Gretzky, Michael Douglas, Lauren Hutton, Claudia Schiffer, Demi Moore, and Whoopi Goldberg.

86. A cigar can produce more than 25 times as much secondhand smoke as a cigarette.

ETR Associate brochure on cigars, 2001

# CHAPTER 19
# TOBACCO INGREDIENTS, ADDITIVES, AND RADIOACTIVITY

1.  There are 4000 different chemicals in cigarette smoke, including 43 that meet the stringent criteria for listing as known carcinogens. *Health Benefits of Smoking Cessation*, 1990 Surgeon General report

2.  Toxic components of cigarette smoke include carbon monoxide (used for suicides in garages with the car engine running), nicotine (active ingredient in bug sprays and pesticides), acetone (nail polish remover), naphthalene (active ingredient in mothballs), ammonia (toilet bowl cleaner), hydrazine (rocket fuel), methane (swamp gas), acetylene (blow torches), polonium-210 (radioactive particles), and hydrogen cyanide (active ingredient in San Quentin gas chamber). The leading source of lead exposure in buildings with smokers is environmental tobacco smoke. Stanton Glantz lecture, San Francisco, February 24, 1994

3.  Components of cigarette smoke include benzopyrene, hydrogen cyanide, dimethyl nitrosamines, and the radioactive element polonium-210. The polonium-210 in tobacco smoke may be the major source of exposure to radioactivity for the majority of Americans. American Journal of Public Health, February 1989, p. 209

4.  Tobacco plants are grown in soils with high phosphate fertilizers that are naturally contaminated with the alpha-particle emitting radionuclide polonium-210. In one year, the average smoker will irradiate the bronchial epithelium with 8 to 9 rem, the equivalent dose of radiation from 250 to 300 chest x-ray films per year. Pediatrics, September 1993, p. 464

5.  Radioactive constituents are present in both tobacco and tobacco smoke. The radioisotopes lead-210 and polonium-210 may contribute to the carcinogenicity of cigarette smoke. The radiation dose from polonium-210 in cigarettes has been variously estimated at one rad per year, 8 rem per year, and 80 to 100 rads over a lifetime. Clinics in Chest Medicine, December 1991, p. 633

6.  Alpha particles from polonium-210 are powerful mutagens, perhaps 100 times more than equal number of rads of gamma radiation. The lungs, blood, and liver of smokers contain a much higher concentration of polomium-210 than those of nonsmokers, and the radiation dose to the lower lobe bifurcations of the lung is estimated to be up to 200 REM each 25 years. NEJM 1965; 273:1344 and 1982; 307:311

7.  Tobacco leaves concentrate radioactive polonium-210 and lead-210 from the phosphate fertilizers that are commonly used in tobacco cultivation. C.R. Hill at the Institute for Cancer Research in England suggested that natural fallout from radon 222 might account for the radioactivity of tobacco smoke. R.T. Ravenholt of the Centers for Disease Control hypothesized that the radioactive elements in tobacco smoke might pass through the lungs and into the blood, causing cancers distant from the lung. He believes that smokers are exposed to "far more radiation from the smoking of tobacco than they are from any other source," and Dr. Joseph DiFranza states that the radiation from inhaled smoke could account for half of all lung cancers in smokers. *Cancer Wars*, p. 306

8.  Among the 700 chemical additives to cigarettes are ammonia, ethyl 2-furoate (which causes liver damage in animals and has been studied as a chemical warfare agent), sclareol (which can cause convulsions), and methoprene (a pesticide used on stored tobacco). Two others are megastigmatrienone and dehydromethofurolactone. Newsweek, April 18, 1994, p. 56 and San Francisco Examiner, April 15, 1994, p. A3 and April 9, 1994, p. D1

9.  Among the more than 2000 additives to cigarettes in Europe are methyl coumarin (rat poison), creosote (known carcinogen), naphthalene (active ingredient in mothballs), formaldehyde (embalming fluid), and arsenic. New South Wales Cancer Council, April 1994

10. Among chemicals on the top-secret list of about 700 additives to cigarettes reported to the US government are 13 not allowed in food (US FDA) and 5 designated as hazardous (US EPA). Most of the additives have not been scientifically investigated. National Public Radio report, April 1994

11. Two of the 700 additives in cigarettes are sclareol, which causes seizures in laboratory rats, and ethylfuroate, which was investigated in the 1930's as a possible chemical warfare agent.

American Medical News, May 2, 1994

12. Saccharin has received much attention as carcinogen, but the carcinogenic potency of benzopyrene in tobacco smoke is 50,000 times greater than that of saccharin.     North Carolina Medical Journal, January 1995, p. 5

13. Each tin of snuff delivers as much nicotine as 30 to 40 cigarettes. There is a lethal dose of nicotine in each can of spit tobacco, as well as lead (nerve poison), embalming fluid (formaldehyde), and radioactive particles.

*Quitting Spit*, National Cancer Institute, 1991, p. 5

14. Kretek, or clove cigarettes from Indonesia, are composed of cloves (up to 40%) and dark tobaccos. The local anesthetic in cloves, eugenol, permits the inhalation of the harsh smoke from the sun-cured dark tobaccos.

*Nicotine Addiction*, p. 15

15. Ammonia, an "impact booster" additive to cigarettes, changes the acidity of tobacco and produces free nicotine so that nearly twice the usual amount gets into a smoker's bloodstream.

New York Times, June 22, 1994, pp. A1 and C20

16. "Tar," the sticky brown substance condensing out of tobacco smoke, consists primarily of polycyclic aromatic hydrocarbons such as benzopyrene, an exceedingly potent carcinogen.

*Pharmacological Basics of Therapeutics*, Goodman and Gilman, 1990 edition, p. 545

17. Dr. John Slade, associate professor of medicine at the University of Medicine and Dentistry, New Jersey, advocates regulation of cigarettes to reduce the amount of soot, a term he prefers to "tar." One alternative would be to impose higher taxes on more toxic high-soot cigarettes, or to set limits on soot levels.

US News and World Report, December 30, 1996, pp. 66-67

18. The British Medical Journal (November 30, 1996, p. 1348) editorialized that the time has come for international standards for the "global cigarette" with a limit of 12 milligrams of tar, or soot, and 1 mg of nicotine. "This should be stated on all packets in every country along with health warnings." In 1997, the European Union mandated an upper limit of 12 mg tar to replace the current limit of 15 mg. Currently, the Lucky Strike brand delivers less than 15 mg soot in Europe but 27 mg in the United States.

19. In a study from Massachusetts, Marlboro was found to have 25.9 milligrams of tar per cigarette, compared to 16 milligrams in industry ratings. Merit Ultra Lights are rated by the Federal Trade Commission at 5 mg of tar, but the new study found that each Merit Ultra Lights delivers between 10.4 and 25.9 milligrams of tar for a smoker taking an "average" or "intense" puff, respectively.     Wall Street Journal, January 30, 1997, p. B1

20. Certain cigarettes advertised as having the lowest tar content actually contained the blends of tobacco richest in nicotine, suggesting that the manufacturers were compensating by using high-nicotine tobacco in the blends of their lowest tar products. One tobacco industry patent stated, "maintaining the nicotine content at a sufficiently high level to provide the desired physiological activity, taste, and odor…can thus be seen to be a significant problem in the tobacco art."     NEJM, September 26, 1996, p. 989

21. Tobacco smoke contains 13 billion particles per cubic centimeter, and is 10,000 times more concentrated than the aerosol resulting from automobile pollution at rush hour on a freeway.

*The Health Consequences of Smoking: Cancer and Chronic Lung Disease in the Workplace*, 1985 Surgeon General report

22. Smoking produces an estimated 2.25 million metric tons of gaseous and inhalable particulate matter each year. From 66 to 90% of cigarette smoke produced is sidestream smoke.

*Chronic Lung Disease in the Workplace*, 1985 Surgeon General report

23. Indoor tobacco burning produces an estimated 13,000 metric tons of respirable suspended particles each year.
*Chronic Lung Disease in the Workplace*, 1985 Surgeon General report

24. The government does not require the tobacco industry to list the chemicals it adds to cigarettes. In fact, it is a felony for any government official to mention any of the hundreds of chemicals on the list kept in great secrecy by the government.
ASH Review, March-April 1994, p. 7

25. Massachusetts was the first state to pass legislation requiring cigarette makers to disclose all the ingredients of their products including flavor enhancers, preservatives and nicotine levels. This information the manufacturers have heretofore zealously guarded as trade secrets.US News and World Report, August 5, 1996, p. 8

26. A federal judge has blocked a Massachusetts law that would have required tobacco companies to submit a list of ingredients used in their tobacco products. The case may go to trial for a final ruling in 1998, or be brought before a judge for a summary judgment.
Wall Street Journal, December 11, 1997, p. A6

27. Cigarette filters lauded for reducing inhaled tar may themselves be dangerous. The fibers in the filters may be inhaled and lodge in the lungs of smokers.
Associated Press, January 14, 1995

28. Lorillard produced 13 billion Kent micronite filter cigarettes from 1952 to 1957 with the ad touting "Just what the doctor ordered…maximum health protection." The filter was composed of 30% asbestos and 70% cotton and acetate. 20 out of the 36 workers of Specialties, Inc. which produced the filter subsequently died from lung cancer and asbestos poisoning; one of the worker's wives also died from inhaling asbestos fibers from her husband's clothing.
Rep. Mike Synar, CSPAN, April 14, 1994

29. SOME "REFRESHING" CHEMICALS IN TOBACCO SMOKE
**Nicotine:** the active ingredient in many bug sprays
**Cyanide:** the deadly ingredient in rat poison
**Formaldehyde:** the foul-smelling preservative found in dead laboratory frogs
**Ammonia:** a poisonous gas and a powerful cleaning agent used to clean toilets
**Arsenic:** a potent ant poison
**Methanol:** jet engine and rocket fuel
**Cadmium:** found in car batteries
**Butane:** a flammable chemical in lighter fluid
**Acetone:** a poisonous solvent and paint stripper
**Toluene:** a poisonous industrial solvent
**Polonium-210:** a highly radioactive element
**Carbon Monoxide:** an extremely poisonous gas found in auto exhaust
**Benzene:** the poisonous toxin that, in trace amounts, forced the global Perrier water recall.
reported in Tobacco Free Youth Reporter (STAT), Summer 1993

30. Cigarette additives include yeast, wine, caffeine, beeswax, coconut oil, chocolate, sclareolide, maltitol (a sweetener), ethyl furoate, dehydromethofurolactone, megastigmatrienone, and methoprene (an insecticide).
San Francisco Chronicle, April 14, 1994, p. A13

31. Other chemicals, which are used as additives in cigarettes, are safrole (mace), eugenol, D Limonene, benzyl acetate, cinnamaldehyde, and titanium dioxide (in the filter).
*The Cigarette Papers*, p. 227

32. The three classes of carcinogens in tobacco smoke are nitrosamines (including NNK), polynuclear aromatic hydrocarbons (PAH) including benzopyrene, and aromatic amines. Children of mothers who smoke have higher blood levels of PAH than children of nonsmoking mothers.
Journal of the National Cancer Institute, September 21, 1994, p. 1369

33. In 1990, Perrier halted its bottle water operation when traces of benzene were found. But there is more benzene in every pack of cigarettes than in hundreds of the contaminated Perrier water bottles.
Yale magazine, March 1991, p. 8 (Kenneth Warner)

34. In 1990, the FDA and EPA ordered Perrier water removed from the market when it was discovered to be contaminated with benzene. Ironically, benzene contained in a pack of cigarettes was up to 2000 times more than in each Perrier bottle.                                                                     *Ashes to Ashes*, p. 708

35. In 1988, the US government shut down all Chilean grape imports because of a small amount of cyanide found in two grapes. But there is ten times more cyanide in every puff from a cigarette than was found in the two Chilean grapes.          Yale magazine, March 1991, p. 8 (Kenneth Warner), and *Nicotine Addiction*, p. 129

36. Other chemicals identified in cigarette smoke are carbonyl sulfide, toluene, acrolein, hydrazine, methyl chloride, 1, 3-butadiene, acetic acid, and formic acid.          World Smoking and Health No. 1, 1993, p. 9

37. "Cigarettes contain ingredients so toxic that you could not dump them in a landfill under the federal environmental laws."          Rep. Ron Wyden (D-Oregon) (Reuters, April 9, 1994)

38. "Tobacco smoke is chemically complex and is usually analyzed in two parts, the particulate or solid and the gaseous phase. Some 4720 separate compounds have already been identified in the smoke. The gaseous phase contains many chemicals that are well known: carbon monoxide (5 percent), carbon dioxide, nitrogen oxide, ammonia, formaldehyde, benzene and hydrogen cyanide; the particulate phase includes nicotine,

39. phenol, naphthalene and cadmium among other compounds. The compounds in the particulate phase, excepting nicotine, are collectively called tar. The higher the nicotine yield, the higher the tar yield and vice versa. In the particulate phase, the free nicotine is suspended on minute droplets of tar. . . ."*Tobacco in History*, p. 5

40. The arsenic content of American tobacco was quite high until the early 1960's because of the use of arsenic-containing insecticides used on tobacco farms. Bowen's disease of the skin is associated with arsenic ingestion, and in a medical practice with 16 patients with the disorder, eleven had been smokers in the 1950's.
          Cutis, July 1996, p. 65

41. Of the EPA's list of class A carcinogens, vinyl chloride is reponsible for an estimated 30 deaths per year, asbestos about 15, and benzene seven or eight.          *Smokescreen*, p. 105

42. "Humectants, or moisturizing agents, are used in cigarette tobacco blends to assist with aerosol formation and thus make cigarette smoke 'milder.' The more that nicotine can be dissolved in the tar droplets, the less irritating the smoke is to the consumer's throat and the easier it is to inhale. Diethylene glycol, more familiar to most readers as automotive antifreeze, was introduced as a humectant in cigarettes in the 1930's by Philip Morris." It is unclear whether this additive is still used, since additives are trade secrets.
          *The Cigarette Papers*, pp. 223-225

43. Concentrations of 4–aminobiphenyl and dimethylnitrosamine in sidestream smoke exceed those of mainstream smoke by a factor of 30 to 100.          *The Tobacco Epidemic*, p. 114

44. 28 carcinogens have been identified in smokeless tobacco. The major carcinogens are the N-nitrosamines; others include volatile aldehydes, benzopyrene, lactones, urethan, hydrazine, coumarin, and radioactive polonium-210 and uranium-235 and 238.          *Smokeless Tobacco or Health*, p. 98

45. "Tobacco smoke is an aerosol of droplets (particulates) containing water, nicotine and other alkaloids, and tar. Tobacco smoke contains several thousand different chemicals, many of which may contribute to human disease. Major toxic chemicals in the particulate phase of tobacco include nicotine, benzopyrene and other polycyclic hydrocarbons, N-nitrosonornicotine, polonium-210, nickel, cadmium, arsenic, and lead. The gaseous phase contains carbon monoxide, acetaldehyde, acetone, methanol, nitrogen oxides, hydrogen cyanide, acrolein, ammonia, benzene, formaldehyde, nitrosoamines, and vinyl chloride. Tobacco smoke may produce illness via systemic absorption of toxins and/or by local pulmonary injury by oxidant gases."
          Cecil Textbook of Medicine, 1996 edition, p. 34

46. American smokers inhale 11 million pounds, or 5500 tons, of tar into their lungs each year (computed at 500 billion cigarettes with 10 milligrams of tar each, probably a low estimate for actual tar delivery per cigarette).

47. Polycyclic aromatic hydrocarbons that are implicated in smoking-induced cancers also appear to have atherogenic (plaque-forming) activity. *Cigarettes*, p. 28

48. About 76% of black smokers choose menthol brands compared to 23% of white smokers. Menthol brands are associated with higher cotinine levels and carbon monoxide concentrations, and appear to be associated with increased health risks compared to non-menthol brands. Chest, November 1996, p. 1194

49. Tobacco manufacturers add ammonia compounds to "liberate free nicotine from the blend, which is associated with increases in impact and 'satisfaction' reported by smokers." NEJM, September 26, 1996, p. 990

50. Ammonia, acetaldehyde, glycerin, and propylene glycol in cigarettes increase the rate and amount of nicotine getting to and enhancing its effects on the brain. British Medical Journal, January 13, 1996, p. 112

51. Liggett documents include a list of insecticides, fertilizers and additives that Liggett found in its products before 1969, including arsenic, DDT, and toxaphene (also known as toxokil). A 1958 entry also lists the insecticide Endrin, which the document calls "highly toxic." Federal guidelines cited in the log said that products for human consumption could not contain one part per million (ppm) of Endrin; cigarettes tested had 55ppm in the tobacco and 10ppm in the smoke. The EPA later banned Endrin.
Contra Costa (Ca.) Times, April 11, 1997, p. B2
(from the Washington Post, John Schwartz)

52. Tobacco additives and their definitions. Ammonium sulfide: "a corrosive chemical, contact with which can irritate nose, throat and lungs causing difficulty breathing." Camphene: "exposure can irritate eyes, nose and throat." Eucalyptol: "a human poison by ingestion." Wall Street Journal, April 14, 1997, p. A6

53. "A cigarette is like a little toxic waste dump on fire."
Stanton Glantz, Ph.D. The News Hour, PBS television, December 31, 1997

54. In late 1997, Liggett tobacco company for the first time listed the ingredients on cartons of its L&M cigarettes. Included along with tobacco was molasses, licorice flavor, chocolate flavor, vanilla extract, valerian root extract, oil of an East Indian mint called patchouli, cedarwood oil, menthol, sugar, high fructose corn syrup, phenylacetic acid, hexanoic acid, isovalenic acid, 3-methylpantanoic acid, glycerol, and propylene glycol.
San Francisco Examiner, December 4, 1997, p. A26

55. The amount of benzopyrenes in cigarettes have been reduced by half since the 1960's. However, in one unspecified American cigarette, the amount of NNK increased by 50% from 1978 to 1995.
10th World Conference on Tobacco or Health, Beijing, 1997 (Nigel Gray)

56. A poem relating to disclosure of tobacco ingredients was presented by Judy Knapp at the Tenth National Conference on Nicotine Dependence in Minneapolis on October 18, 1997:
"Say you wanna bum
   some cadmium?
Need a kick
   of arsenic?
Gotta get fried
   on formaldehyde?
Can we loan ya
   a bit of ammonia?
Can it go to your head
   a shot of lead?"

57. A federal judge struck down a 1996 Massachusetts tobacco ingredient disclosure law, the first of its kind in the nation. He ruled that the law forced tobacco companies to give away valuable trade secrets by ordering them to reveal the ingredients in cigarette and other tobacco products.
San Francisco Chronicle, September 9, 2000, p. A7

58. "Traces of cyanide, mercury, acetone, and ammonia have been discovered in a widely consumed product." After this black and white message appeared on French television, within hours one million viewers called the toll free number offered for more information. The were informed that "the product…is cigarettes."

Newsweek, July 22, 2002, p. 8

59. "Central estimates" are that radon exposure causes between 15,400 and 21,800 deaths from lung cancer in the United States each year, making it the second leading cause of lung cancer after cigarette smoking. Radon-222 is a colorless, odorless, radioactive gas that forms from the decay of naturally occurring uranium-238. Uranium-238 occurs in soil and rock, and radon exposure in the home is largely the result of radon-contaminated gas rising from the soil. Inhaled radon progeny reach the lungs and emit alpha particles, which can damage cells and thereby increase lung cancer risk. The EPA estimates that as many as eight million homes in the United States have elevated radon levels, mostly in the mid-Atlantic states from New York to Virginia, and in the upper midwest.CA--A Cancer Journal for Clinicians, November/December 2001, pp. 337-344

60. A pack a day smoker inhales 150cc (5 ounces) of thick brown gooey carcinogenic tar into the lungs each year.

Health Edco catalogue

# CHAPTER 20
# NICOTINE AND ADDICTION

## Historical

1.  Columbus noted when observing his sailors that "it was not within their power to refrain" from tobacco use.
    *Cigarettes* (Parker-Pope), p. 2

2.  A New Yorker cartoon from the 1940's showed Christopher Columbus smoking a peace pipe with the West Indian natives and the comment from one of his men: "Don't worry. If it turns out tobacco is harmful, we can always quit."

3.  "The use of tobacco...conquers men with a certain secret pleasure, so that those who have once become accustomed thereto can hardly be restrained therefrom."
    Francis Bacon, Historia Vital et Mortis, 1622 (Adolescent Medicine, June 1993, p. 305)

4.  "The fetid and nauseating smoke of tobacco was brought...by English infidels...pleasure-seekers and sensualists...became addicted, and soon even those who were not pleasure-seekers began to use it. Many even of the...mighty fell into this addiction."
    Turkish historian Ibrahim Pechevi, 1635 (Newsweek, July 29, 1996, p. 80)

5.  "It is better to take no snuff at all than a little; for it is certain that he who takes a little will soon take much, and that is why they call it 'the enchanted herb', for those who take it are so taken by it that they cannot go without it."
    Princess Elizabeth Charlotte of Orleans, about 1710 (*Licit and Illicit Drugs*, p. 211)

6.  "For thy sake, tobacco, I would do anything but die."
    Charles Lamb, 1820

7.  In 1828 the chemists Posselt and Reimann of the University of Heidelberg isolated nicotine as the major pharmacoactive ingredient in tobacco. In 1895, Pinner established the chemical structure of nicotine as that of 3-(1-methyl-2-pyrrolidinyl)pyridine.
    Quote from *Cigars*, p. 55

8.  "I have often wished that every individual afflicted with this artificial passion can force himself to try but for three months (to quit). I'm sure that it would turn every tobacco land into a wheat field and add five years to the average human life."
    John Quincy Adams, 1830 (*No Stranger to Tears*, p. 329)

9.  "Nicotine had been identified and accepted as the cause of tobacco's toxic properties as early as the 1860s. Laboratory experiments had graphically proven its poisonous qualities: A few drops of pure nicotine injected into a small animal was enough to kill it, and as an insecticide, nicotine had few equals."
    *Tobacco Advertising*, p. 238

10. "The habit once established gives rise to more or less craving for this form of indulgence."
    Ralph Waldo Emerson, about 1870 (*Ashes to Ashes*, p. 38)

11. "While all forms of smoking are injurious, it has been found that the use of the cigarette is more harmful than the cigar or pipe. It so seriously undermines the power of self-control that persons once addicted to its use very often find it impossible to break up and abandon the habit."
    *Primer of Physiology and Hygiene*, William Thayer Smith, about 1880

12. "A cigarette is the perfect type of a perfect pleasure. It is exquisite, and it leaves one unsatisfied."
    *The Picture of Dorian Gray*, Oscar Wilde, 1891

13. "The puffing of cigarettes...is a form of slight excitement; it feeds rather than satisfies the appetite; it is more like, in its effects and practice, the smoking of opium than of tobacco; the cigarette is a variety of the craving

from absinthe and morphia."     Late Nineteenth century description of smoking (*Cigarette Confidential*, p. 86)

14. It seems almost incredible that tobacco, the dried product of a common herb, possessing the properties of a narcotic stimulant, and in no way necessary for man's sustenance, should have from its first introduction progressively increased in consumption wherever used throughout the habitable globe; that, despite the opposition of the combined powers of the church, the state, and the moralist to its use, its consumers being the subject of ridicule, persecution, and even mutilation, and itself an object of universal taxation, it furnishes at the present time not only one of the largest staples of commerce, but provides as well one of the leading manufacturing industries of mankind.
     1895 quote from P. Lorillard, Jr., president of Lorillard Tobacco (*The Tobacco Epidemic*, p. 3)

15. A quote from 1896 on nicotine:
     Nicotine is a powerful poison, the physiological action of which seems dependent upon the dose. Small doses stimulate the pneumogastric; large doses paralyse it. Thus we find, in poisonous doses, an increased rapidity of the heart's action, followed by slowing of the pulse and a decrease in arterial pressure; whilst respiration, at first hurried, becomes slower than normal and finally ceases, the heart's action continuing for some time longer...Experience, as well as experimental research, shows us that a toleration to the toxic effects of the tobacco alkaloids may be acquired.     Practitioner 1896; 3:150-160

16. At the end of the nineteenth century, nicotine was isolated and its toxicity confirmed; it was in general use as an insecticide until the production of DDT until the early 1940's.     *Tobacco in History*, pp. 121-122

17. "Chewing tobacco, snuff, cigars, and pipes facilitate nicotine delivery through the oral or nasal mucosa because of the alkaline nature of the products. Cigarettes, a modern invention, use mostly flue-cured and sugared burley tobaccos, which provide a mildly acidic smoke that does not allow ready absorption of nicotine unless the smoke is inhaled into the lungs, where the absorption is quite efficient. Thus, cigarette users smoke cigarettes in a manner that is not only highly dependence producing but also highly toxic to the respiratory system.
     "Several technologies converged between the 1800's and 1913 to make the modern cigarette possible. New tobacco blends and curing processes were developed which produced a tobacco product that, when burned, produced a smoke that could be inhaled (that indeed had to be inhaled for nicotine absorption to occur). Machinery for cheaply manufacturing cigarettes was perfected; the safety match was invented; an efficient transportation system was developed, which allowed distribution of the product throughout the United States; and mass media advertising techniques were used to promote the purchase of Camel brand cigarettes."
     Epidemiologic Reviews 1995; 17:48-49

18. Sir Ernest Shackleton in his book *South* (p. 221) describes the rescue of his comrades from the Endurance Antarctic expedition on Elephant Island in 1916. "As I drew close to the rock I flung packets of cigarettes ashore; they fell on them like hungry tigers, for well I know that for months tobacco was dreamed of and talked of."
     Frank Wild, the leader of the shore party, gave this account (p. 242): "Before he could land, he threw ashore handfuls of cigarettes...and these the smokers, who for two months had been trying to find solace in such substitutes as seaweed...and sennegras, grasped greedily."

19. Dr. Sigmund Freud was an early prototype of tobacco addiction as he struggled for over 45 years to stop smoking. In his last 16 years of life, he endured 33 operations for cancer of the jaw and mouth, which finally killed him in 1939.     *Licit and Illicit Drugs*, p. 215

20. "How marvelous the ability to so camouflage its venom that millions of men are made to believe harmless a weed which almost every other living creature than man, great and small, recognizes and avoids as a baneful poison!"     *Tobaccoism*, John Harvey Kellogg, Modern Medicine Publishing Co., 1922

21. When the supply of cigarettes is limited, cigarette smokers behave much like heroin addicts. During extreme deprivation in Germany after World War II, "the majority of the habitual smokers preferred to do without food even under extreme conditions of nutrition rather than to forego tobacco. Thus, when food rations in prisoner-of-war camps were down to 900-1000 calories, smokers were still willing to barter their food rations for tobacco."     *Licit and Illicit Drugs*, p. 226

22. A British former World War II prisoner of war wrote: "The one thing that men were unable to give up was cigarette smoking. There was a very active market in bartering the handful of rice we received daily for the two cigarettes we were given. I have actually seen men die of starvation because they had sold their food for cigarettes."                                        *Smoking: the Artificial Passion*, David Krogh, W.H. Freeman, 1991

23. During the German siege of Leningrad in 1941, people refused to give up their ration of tobacco in exchange for chocolate or sugar in the city on the edge of famine.                        *Tobacco: A History*, V.G. Kiernan, 1991

24. In 1969, the Philip Morris vice president for research and development noted that smokers' craving for cigarettes is so strong that "the cigarette will even preempt food in times of scarcity."
                                                                                                        Lung Cancer, Vol. 18, 1997, p. 5

25. One internal Philip Morris report concluded that smokers crave nicotine more than food.
                                                                                                        Associated Press, July 25, 1995

# General

1. In a 1990 Gallup poll, 61% of smokers considered themselves addicted to nicotine.
                                                                                                        Clinics in Chest Medicine, December 1991, p. 820

2. Major recent studies have concluded that 77% to 92% of smokers are addicted to nicotine in cigarettes; about 75% of young regular users of smokeless tobacco are also addicted to nicotine.
                                                                                                        JAMA, February 5, 1997, p. 406

3. In one study of smokers, 90% of males and 75% of females were nicotine dependent.
                                                                                                        Tobacco Control, Spring 1996, p. 1

4. C. Everett Koop commented on the issue of cigarette warning labels during his tenure as surgeon general. "The interesting political thing is that there were five suggested warnings, the fifth of which was, tobacco contains nicotine, which is an addictive drug. That term addiction so bothers the tobacco people, that's the reason we got the other four with very little fight. They said 'if you drop the fifth one, we'll accept the other four'."
                                                                                                        St. Louis Times, July 1996, p. 14

5. "There is no conclusive proof that nicotine's addictive. . . and the same thing with cigarettes causing emphysema, lung cancer, heart disease."                        Rush Limbaugh on his radio program, April 29, 1994

6. Rush Limbaugh said in April 1994 that "It has not been proven that nicotine is addictive", despite the fact that in 1988, Surgeon General C. Everett Koop issued a 618-page report unequivocally saying that it is indeed addictive.                                                                        San Francisco Chronicle, July 5, 1994, p. E8

7. "Substantial evidence indicates that tobacco is not addictive. The effects of stopping are no different than those experienced upon discontinuance of any other pleasure."                        US Cigarette Export Association, 1988

8. William Farone, the former director of applied research at Philip Morris, informed the FDA "product developers and blend and leaf specialists at Philip Morris were responsible for manipulating and controlling the design and production of cigarettes in order to satisfy the consumer's need for nicotine."
                                                                                                        NEJM, September 26, 1996, p. 990

9. Smoking "is no more addictive than coffee, tea or Twinkies."
                                                                                                        1994 Congressional testimony from James Johnston, CEO of R.J. Reynolds

10. "It is simply not scientifically credible for anyone to conclude that nicotine is not addictive."
                                                                                                        David Kessler, MD (Wall Street Journal, July 5, 1996, p. A8)

11. In 1988, the Surgeon General's report *The Health Consequences of Smoking: Nicotine Addiction* declared that cigarette smoking is addictive by the same scientific standards that apply to heroin and cocaine.

New York Times, June 18, 1994, p. A12

12. Nicotine withdrawal peaks in 24 to 48 hours and is characterized by at some or most of the following signs: a craving for nicotine, irritability and frustration, anxiety, difficulty concentrating, restlessness, and increased appetite.

Chest, December 1991, p. 1485

13. Nicotine withdrawal is brief, with symptoms peaking 2 to 3 days after quitting, and disappearing after 10 to 14 days. After this time, cravings may occur, rarely lasting more than 30 seconds, and are related to situations and emotions, but not nicotine withdrawal.

Cleveland Clinic Journal, July 1990, p. 417

14. A person who smokes more than five cigarettes per day is likely to be addicted to nicotine; about 90% of all cigarette smokers are believed to be addicted.

NEJM, July 14, 1994, p. 124, and American Medical News, November 28, 1991, p. 11

15. Although the industry publicly says that nicotine is essential in cigarettes because of its taste, taste is irrelevant to nicotine as described in company internal documents.

*The Cigarette Papers*, p. 104

16. A 1965 Brown and Williamson memo discussed the push to "find ways of obtaining maximum nicotine for minimum tar." The methods being tried were adding nicotine powders to tobacco, soaking cigarette paper in nicotine, using chemical additives to boost nicotine release, and finally, altering leaf blends.

*Smokescreen*, p. 46

17. "…by the 1960s, BAT scientists had concluded that nicotine is addictive and company-sponsored laboratory tests showed that components of tobacco smoke cause cancer in animals. The company responded to these findings at first by attempting to create a 'safe' cigarette, although it publicly maintained that cigarettes had not been proven dangerous to health. When the scientists had concluded that they would not be able to create a 'safe' cigarette, the company retreated behind a stone wall of denial, where it remains to this day."

*The Cigarette Papers*, p. 32

18. The scientific basis for classifying nicotine as addictive was not highlighted until the 1988 Surgeon General report, *Nicotine Addiction*. However, by 1963 Brown and Williamson and British American Tobacco scientists and executives were internally acknowledging that nicotine is an addictive drug and that tobacco companies are essentially in the business of "selling nicotine."

*The Cigarette Papers*, p. 58

19. "Had we known then what the tobacco companies knew and had we been privy to their research on the addictive nature of nicotine, the 1979 Surgeon General's report would have found cigarettes addictive, and we would have moved to regulate them. Unfortunately, the president of the United States, the Secretary of HEW and the surgeon general were all victims of the concealment campaign of the tobacco companies."

Joe Califano, Secretary of Health, Education and Welfare in the Carter Administration

20. Researchers in Italy in a study published in the journal Nature noted virtually identical patterns of biochemical activity and increased dopamine levels in the brain following injections of cocaine, morphine, amphetamines, and nicotine. The brain thus appears to make no distinction between these addictive drugs.

Time, July 29, 1996, p. 65

21. Cigarette smokers who inhale absorb 92% of the nicotine available in the smoke. It takes about 7 seconds for nicotine absorbed through the lungs to reach the brain, compared to the 14 seconds it takes for blood to reach the brain from the arm after an intravenous injection.

*Tobacco in History*, pp. 5-6

22. Stress relief from smoking may actually be nicotine withdrawal relief; smoking may not produce positive moods, but only relieve negative moods produced by nicotine withdrawal. Psychopharmacology 1994; 115:389

23. "Chronic cigarette smokers maintain their habit not for any pleasure it adds to their lives, though they may rationalize that they do, but rather to avoid the unpleasantness that comes from not smoking."

Science 80, September 1980, p. 43

24. Chronic smokers are not made less irritable than other people by their habit; rather, they are protected from becoming more irritable.

Science 80, September 1980, p. 41

25. "Patients report that only a small minority of the cigarettes they smoke in a day are highly pleasurable. Experts believe that the remainder are smoked primarily to sustain nicotine blood levels and to avoid withdrawal symptoms."

FDA Commissioner David Kessler testimony to Congress, March 25, 1994

26. "Smokers regulate their nicotine dose to obtain desired effects; these include both intrinsic positive effects, such as pleasure and enhanced performance, and avoidance of the withdrawal syndrome. This syndrome is characterized by anger, anxiety, craving for tobacco products, difficulty concentrating, hunger, impatience, and restlessness. Most of these symptoms peak in 1 to 2 days and return to baseline within 3 to 4 weeks of quitting; however, craving for tobacco products and hunger may persist for extended periods."

Harrison's Principles of Internal Medicine, 1994 edition, p. 2433

27. "As the Philip Morris documents show, a certain amount of nicotine is expected and maintained, and is tested for hourly on the production line, and if not enough is there, they add some. It is simple, and it has nothing to do with the original levels of nicotine in plants. It has to do with their intent—the fact that they do control the level of nicotine precisely and purposefully."

*Smokescreen*, p. 115

28. "Many memos show an industry obsessed with nicotine and how to alter it." However, all the major tobacco producers have repeatedly denied that they manipulate or control nicotine levels in their cigarettes.

New York Times, March 1, 1998, p. 19

29. Internal documents from RJR suggest that the company manipulated nicotine levels in order to remain competitive with Marlboro (Philip Morris). In the 1970's, RJR researchers discovered that Marlboro contained higher levels of "free" nicotine than their Winston brand, and set out to provide the same levels in Winston. "Free" nicotine is more quickly absorbed than "bound" nicotine, and gives a quicker "kick" to the smoker.

New York Times, February 23, 1998, p. A1

30. "Any desired additional nicotine 'kick' could be easily obtained through pH regulation."

1973 R.J. Reynolds memo entitled "Cigarette concept to assure RJR a larger segment of the youth market."

31. Ammonia added to cigarette tobacco converts bound (unavailable) nicotine to pharmacologically active free nicotine. Acetaldehyde is another impact booster that augments the effect of nicotine. *Smokescreen*, p. 171

32. Ammonia is added to tobacco to increase the delivery of nicotine. Ammonia changes the acidity of tobacco and frees nicotine so that nearly twice the usual amount inhaled gets into a smoker's bloodstream.

New York Times, June 22, 1994, pp. A1 and C20

33. Several methods of enhancing nicotine delivery are commonly used in the manufacture of commercial cigarettes. Tobacco blending to raise the nicotine concentration in low-tar cigarettes is common. According to the vice chairman and chief operating officer of Lorillard Tobacco Co., for instance, "the lowest 'tar' segment is composed of cigarettes utilizing a tobacco blend which is significantly higher in nicotine." Another common technique for enhancing nicotine delivery in low-tar cigarettes is the use of filter and ventilation systems that by design remove a higher percentage of tar than nicotine. Yet a third type of nicotine manipulation is the addition of ammonia compounds that increase the delivery of "free" nicotine to smokers by raising the alkalinity or pH of tobacco smoke. These ammonia technologies are widely used within the industry.

Quote from JAMA, February 5, 1997, p. 407

34. "The secret of Marlboro is ammonia."  Scientist in 1989 B&W Tobacco Co. report (Smokeless States Tobacco News, Spring 1998)

35. "Ammonia technology is critical to the Marlboro character, taste, and delivery."
1993 Brown And Williamson memo (ASH Review, September-October 1995)

36. Adding ammonia to tobacco can dramatically increase the amount of "free" nicotine available to smokers, "similar to what occurs when cocaine is chemically converted to the more potent and smokeable drug known as crack."  New York Times, July 30, 1997, p. B7

37. Nicotine lowers the level of insulin in the blood and eases a smoker's craving for sweets. *Ashes to Ashes*, p. 418

38. Nicotine appears to suppress appetite for sweeter tasting food and to increase energy expenditure. Smokers weigh an average of 5 to 10 pounds less than non-smokers.  Goodman and Gilman, p. 546

39. Nicotine increases metabolism by 5% to 12%, depending on a person's level of activity. This metabolic effect may account for about 100 calories or more per day for the average smoker.
Journal of Respiratory Disease, May 1993, p. 636

40. "Chippers" are the 5 to 10% of all smokers who use fewer than five cigarettes a day.
*Tobacco*, Mark S. Gold, p. 47

41. While most consumers of alcohol are social drinkers, only 2% of smokers use cigarettes on an occasional basis.
JAMA 1985; 253:2999

42. Of those who ever experiment with cigarettes, about 75% eventually escalate to regular smoking. Fewer than 10% of smokers are able to smoke occasionally on a non-daily basis.
British Journal of Addiction 1990; 85:295

43. There are 15,000 cases a year reported to poison control centers of children eating cigarette butts or whole cigarettes. The number of cases of actual nicotine poisoning is unclear.
Dean Edell, MD, ABC News, San Francisco, March 1, 1996

44. "Cigarettes are as addictive as any substances we know."
Stanton Peele, author, *The Truth About Addiction and Recovery*, Washington Post National Weekly Edition, August 8, 1994, p. 38

45. A pack a day smoker receives 70,000 to 100,000 boluses or "hits" of nicotine per year, or two to three hundred a day. With inhalation, nicotine reaches the brain within 7 seconds, more than twice as rapidly as it takes for heroin to reach the brain from an injection site in the arm.
Pediatrics in Review, July 1993, p. 275, and Science 80, September 1980, p.41

46. 40% to 50% of smokers who have surgery for lung cancer, have a cancerous larynx removed, or suffer a heart attack resume smoking on discharge from the hospital.  Tobacco Control, Summer 1994, p. 149

47. Two thirds of smokers smoke within half an hour of awakening. Smoking the first cigarette of the day within 30 minutes of waking is a meaningful measure of addiction.  Tobacco Control, Summer 1994, p. 149

48. "Cigarette manufacturers....may be controlling smokers' choice by controlling the levels of nicotine in their products in a manner that creates and sustains an addiction in the vast majority of smokers."
FDA Commissioner David Kessler testimony to Congress, March 25, 1994

49. At a March 25, 1994 hearing, FDA Commissioner David Kessler testified that many modern cigarettes are "high technology nicotine delivery systems." At another hearing on April 14, 1994, seven tobacco CEO's testified under oath that nicotine is not addictive and that smoking has not been shown to cause cancer.
Tobacco Free Youth Reporter, Summer 1994, p. 4

50. "The tobacco industry may tell you that nicotine is important in cigarettes solely for 'flavor'. There is a great deal of information that suggests otherwise."                                             David Kessler testimony, March 25, 1994

51. "There is evidence that smokeless tobacco products with lower amounts of nicotine are marketed as 'starter' products for new users, and that advertising is used to encourage users to 'graduate' to products with higher levels of nicotine."                             FDA Commissioner David Kessler testimony to Congress, March 25, 1994

52. "Despite the buzzwords used by industry, what smokers are addicted to is not 'rich aroma' or 'pleasure' or 'satisfaction'. What they are addicted to is nicotine, pure and simple, because of its psychoactive effects and its drug dependence qualities."                                       David Kessler testimony to Congress, March 25, 1994

53. In a July 1962 research conference, Sir Charles Ellis, the chief researcher for British-American Tobacco, stated that nicotine is a "remarkable, beneficent drug that both helps the body to resist external stress and also can as a result show a pronounced tranquilizing effect. Nicotine is not only a very fine drug, but the technique of administration by smoking has considerable psychological advantages."
                                                                                    New York Times, June 16, 1994, p. D22

54. A 1972 Philip Morris internal memo read, "Think of the cigarette pack as a day's supply of nicotine. Think of the cigarette as a dispenser of a dose unit."                                             Newsweek, July 4, 1994, p. 45

55. In 1963 before the first Surgeon General's report was issued, a Brown and Williamson tobacco executive wrote: "We are, then, in the business of selling nicotine, an addictive drug." The industry also had research on the health hazards of cigarettes that it decided to withhold from the surgeon general. Instead, tobacco executives chose to launch a public relations campaign to dispute what they knew to be true.
                                                               Washington Post National Weekly Edition, June 6, 1994, p. 28

56. A 1972 internal memo by a Philip Morris scientist contended, "no one has ever become a cigarette smoker by smoking cigarettes without nicotine." That was proved when the company unsuccessfully introduced the nearly nicotine-free Next. The industry claimed that smokers turn away from such cigarettes because they lack "taste" or "flavor." But researchers say that these cigarettes taste no different; they merely lack the kick that nicotine provides.Time, April 18, 1994, p. 61, and Journal of the National Cancer Institute, January 17, 1990, p. 89

57. "A decade ago, Philip Morris spent more than $300 million on a factory designed to removed nicotine from cigarettes…The resulting product, DeNic, flopped in test marketing; without the nicotine kick, the cigarettes had all the appeal of smoking wheat."     Washington Post National Weekly Edition, June 30, 1997, p. 29

58. A scientist for Philip Morris, Victor DeNoble, discovered in the early 1980's an artificial version of nicotine that seemed to have few of the toxic effects on the heart that natural nicotine has. His research on rats also led him to believe that nicotine was addicting "on a level comparable to cocaine" and contrary to statements of Philip Morris executives. He was threatened with legal action if he published or talked about his nicotine research, and on April 15, 1984, he and his associates were abruptly told to halt their studies, close the lab, kill all the rats, and turn in their security badges by the next morning.           New York Times, April 27, 1994

59. A 1983 report by Philip Morris researcher Victor DeNoble accepted for publication in the journal Psychopharmacology concluded that nicotine is addicting. While it was awaiting publication, the scientist was forced to withdraw it, citing legal threats and a company injunction against its publication.
                                                                                       Washington Post, April 1, 1994

60. The Director of the Office on Smoking and Health, Michael Ericksen, abhors the strategy of tobacco companies to turn smoking from a health issue to a civil rights issue. "It just blows my mind to think that you could ever couch an addiction as a freedom, but they've been able to."                       Associated Press, November 7, 1994

61. "Cigarettes are no different then syringes. They are a drug delivery device for nicotine. They should be regulated just as we regulate morphine and heroin."
                                                      AMA trustee Randolph Smoak, M.D. (American Medical News, July 4, 1994, p. 16)

62. An investigative report suggests that cigarette companies, with annual U.S. revenues of $48 billion, cynically manipulate nicotine levels to keep their customers hooked.                    Day One, ABC News, March 7, 1994

63. "Smoking is habit forming...in the same way as watching T.V., eating your favorite foods and drinking coffee."
                    James Johnston, CEO, R.J. Reynolds, in testimony to Congress, April 14, 1994

64. "In a finding equivalent to a report that the Earth is not flat but round, an advisory panel to the FDA has concluded that the nicotine in cigarettes is addictive." One proposal is to gradually reduce cigarette nicotine levels. "But scientists testifying on behalf of the tobacco industry have balked at this proposal, saying that would produce cigarettes similar to a low-nicotine brand that proved to be unpopular. It may occur to them that it was probably unpopular because it lacked the level of nicotine required for addiction, though they are unlikely to acknowledge this seemingly obvious fact."     Editorial, Seattle Post-Intelligencer, August 20, 1994

65. 70% to 90% of smokers want to quit, but only one in three succeed by age 65. 40% to 50% of heart attack and lung removal for cancer patients resume smoking within days of hospital discharge. More than half of heroin and cocaine users and alcoholics rate smoking more difficult to give up.
                    Jack Henningfield, Ph.D., lecture in Atlanta, November 17, 1993

66. 74% of smokers believe that they are addicted to cigarettes. 86% of females and 77% of males would not start smoking if they had it all to do over again. 90% of smokers feel that smoking is harmful to their own health.
                    April 1993 Gallup Poll (reported by Gary Giovino at Nicotine
                    Dependence Conference, Atlanta, November 12, 1993)

67. 92% of the Americans believe that nicotine is addicting. Among those who smoke and have no plans to quit, the figure is 85%.                    New York Times, February 1, 1995, p. A12

68. 70% of current smokers in a 1991 Gallup poll consider themselves to be addicted to cigarettes. Each year, about 20 million US smokers try to quit, but only about 3% have long-term success.
                    1994 Surgeon General report, *Preventing Tobacco Use Among Young People*, p. 31

69. The 1990 edition of Goodman and Gilman's pharmacology textbook devotes only five of 1811 pages to nicotine and tobacco, but 42 pages to alcohol and illicit drugs. In other American pharmacology texts, alcohol and illicit drugs command an average of five and 40 times as much space, respectively, compared to nicotine and tobacco.
                    JAMA, February 23, 1994, p. 624

70. After 12 to 24 hours of tobacco deprivation, cigarette smokers' scores on tests of arithmetic and verbal skills are reduced by as much as 6%, with the time to complete the tests taking up to 1.5 times longer.
                    Drug Alcohol Dependence 1989; 23:259

71. Abstinence from smoking disturbs sleep and increases daytime sleepiness.                    Chest, April 1994, p. 1136

72. An average of one milligram of nicotine is inhaled and absorbed from each cigarette. As little as 20 mg taken at one time can cause death by respiratory arrest, and 60 mg is invariably fatal. There are about 631 tons of nicotine consumed in the US each year.                    Washington Post National Weekly Edition,
                    April 4-11, 1994, p. 37

73. The average nicotine dose from smoking a cigarette is 1 mg. The average dose per dip from oral snuff is 3.6 mg, and for chewing tobacco is 4.5 mg, or equivalent to more than 4 cigarettes.   *Growing Up Tobacco Free*, p. 39

74. Most cigarettes contain about 8 to 9 milligrams of nicotine, and the smoker inhales 1-2 milligrams per cigarette. A bolus of nicotine is delivered to the brain about 10 seconds after each inhalation.
                    *Preventing Tobacco Use Among Young People*, p. 31

75. Cigarettes contain 6 to 11 milligrams of nicotine. The smoker absorbs one to three milligrams, irrespective of the nicotine yield ratings provided by the tobacco companies. NEJM, November 2, 1995, p. 1196

76. Many cigarette brands have been purposefully engineered to test low in tar and nicotine content based on machine measurement, but generate much higher yields when smoked by people.

*Tobacco and the Clinician*, p. viii

77. Chewing tobacco, pipe, and cigar smoke is alkaline, and nicotine is absorbed through the oral mucosa or mouth without inhaling. However, cigarette flue-cured tobacco is slightly acid, and must be inhaled for nicotine to be absorbed because only in the lungs will the acid smoke be converted to alkaline. Cigarette tobacco is not only milder but more addictive then other tobaccos because of increased absorption of nicotine.

*Advertising, the Uneasy Persuasion*, p. 185

78. Pipe and cigar smoke is alkaline, and is absorbed through the mucous membranes of the mouth. The alkalinity makes the smoke irritating and deters inhalation. In contrast, cigarette smoke is slightly acid, is not absorbed from the mouth, and must be inhaled for the acidity to neutralized in the lungs and nicotine absorption to occur. The journey from lungs to brain takes seven seconds, where virtually all the delivered nicotine is taken up.

Science 80, September 1980, p. 40

79. Airline pilots are permitted to smoke, even though passengers cannot. The FAA maintains this policy not because smoking makes pilots more alert, but because nicotine withdrawal might cause mental impairment. Contrary to the myth that smoking enhances alertness and performance, nicotine withdrawal is responsible for dramatic mental dysfunction. Reader's Digest, March 1995, p. 129

80. The 1988 Surgeon General report *The Health Consequences of Smoking*: *Nicotine Addiction* concluded that:
    1. Cigarettes and other forms of tobacco are addictive.
    2. Nicotine is the drug in tobacco that causes addiction.
    3. The pharmacologic and behavioral processes that determine nicotine addiction are similar to those that determine addiction to drugs such as heroin and cocaine.

81. Brown and Williamson and the British American Tobacco Company "recognized more than 30 years ago that nicotine is addictive and that tobacco smoke is 'biologically active' (e.g. carcinogenic)."

JAMA, July 19, 1995, p. 219

82. Back in 1972, a high-ranking Philip Morris official, Dr. William Dunn, summarized a conference sponsored by the Council for Tobacco research:
    "The majority of the conferees would go even further and accept the proposition that nicotine is the active constituent of cigarette smoke. Without nicotine, the argument goes, there would be no smoking. Some strong evidence can be marshalled to support this argument:
    1) No one has ever become a cigarette smoker by smoking cigarettes without nicotine.
    2) Most of the physiological responses to inhaled smoke have been shown to be nicotine-related.
    3) Despite many low nicotine brand entries in the market place, none of them have captured a substantial segment of the market..." Federal Register, August 11, 1995, p. 41596

83. In 1994, a recently retired CEO of a major tobacco company openly stated that tobacco is addictive and that its addictive properties are why people smoke. In an interview for an article in the Wall Street Journal, the former executive of RJR Nabisco, F. Ross Johnson, was asked about nicotine in cigarettes, and he responded, "Of course it's addictive. That's why you smoke..." Federal Register, August 11, 1995, p. 41495

84. Tobacco manufacturers deliberately control the level of nicotine in cigarettes by monitoring and adjusting nicotine levels at each stage of the manufacturing process. The ultimate objective of these efforts is to ensure that the finished cigarette delivers the desired level of nicotine.

    Perhaps the best example of manufacturers' control of nicotine levels is the effort that the companies make to ensure that low-tar cigarettes deliver an adequate amount of nicotine. As described in the preceding subsection, tobacco industry research activities have focused on developing technologies for maintaining and increasing nicotine levels as tar is reduced. FDA's investigation has also shown that tobacco manufacturers actually use a number of techniques to ensure that nicotine levels in marketed products do not fall below a certain level, such as incorporating high nicotine tobaccos to ensure "adequate" levels of nicotine and using chemical additives to enhance nicotine delivery.          Quote from Federal Register, August 11, 1995, p. 41509

85. Further evidence of the ability of the tobacco industry to remove nicotine is seen in the marketing of a cigarette that was advertised as "de-nicotined." In 1989, Philip Morris test-marketed a cigarette, NEXT, that contained less than 0.1 milligrams of nicotine. The company's own advertisements for NEXT announced that a process called the "FreePLUS" system "naturally extract[s] nicotine from fine tobaccos...with rich tobacco flavor and less than 0.1 mg nicotine." This product was withdrawn from the market shortly after it was introduced for test marketing.

Despite this arsenal of nicotine-removing technologies, all brands of currently marketed cigarettes contain levels of nicotine that are sufficient to maintain a pharmacological response in smokers. Although cigarette manufacturers have the ability to market denicotinized tobacco products, to date there has not been any serious attempt, except for NEXT cigarettes, to market these types of products. All cigarettes on the market today have, and deliver, levels of nicotine that maintain an addiction to the product. These levels are deliberately maintained by the manufacturers.          Quote from Federal Register, August 11, 1995, p. 41783

86. Nicotine's psychoactive and addictive effects on tobacco users are plainly foreseeable to tobacco manufacturers, not only because they are widely known and published in scientific, governmental, and lay publications, but because for over 30 years the manufacturers themselves have engaged in intensive research on nicotine's psychoactive and addictive effects. In addition, tobacco industry documents reveal numerous statements by both industry researchers and executives in which they express their own views that nicotine in tobacco products acts as a psychoactive and addictive drug. Tobacco manufacturers' own research also demonstrates that consumers use cigarettes to obtain the pharmacological effects of nicotine. Finally, tobacco manufacturers have conducted numerous studies to identify the dose of nicotine that will elicit the psychoactive effects sought by tobacco users, and manipulate the amount of nicotine delivered by tobacco products.          Quote from Federal Register, August 11, 1995, p. 41491

87. Internal tobacco industry documents demonstrate the industry's long-standing knowledge of and extensive research on the significant addictive and pharmacological effects of nicotine. Moreover, manufacturers of tobacco products have conducted product development research regarding the levels of nicotine necessary to produce pharmacological effects in tobacco users and also on methods of manipulating the amount of nicotine delivered by cigarettes. FDA's investigation has revealed that tobacco manufacturers actively control the amount and rate at which nicotine from marketed cigarettes and smokeless tobacco is delivered to consumers. Smokeless tobacco manufacturers both manipulate the amount of nicotine delivered by their products and promote the graduation of smokeless tobacco consumers from the lowest to the highest nicotine products, demonstrating an intention to facilitate nicotine dependence.          Quote from Federal Register, August 11, 1995, p. 41465

88. Smokeless tobacco manufacturers control the delivery of nicotine from smokeless tobacco through a variety of additives and design features. Manufacturers use these additives and features to produce lines of smokeless products that deliver nicotine in increasing amounts. Evidence exists that smokeless tobacco manufacturers employ a "graduation process" to market these products. Low nicotine products are marketed to new users of smokeless tobacco. After these new users become tolerant to the low-nicotine products, manufacturer marketing encourages smokeless tobacco consumers to "graduate" to higher nicotine products. The goal of the graduation process is to establish and maintain a market for the smokeless tobacco products with the highest nicotine delivery. Smokeless tobacco manufacturers' deliberate manipulation of levels of nicotine delivery, and the marketing of low-nicotine products to new users and high-nicotine products to experienced users, demonstrates the manufacturers' intent to facilitate nicotine addiction. This evidence establishes that smokeless tobacco manufacturers intend to affect the structure and function of the body.          Quote from Federal Register, August 11, 1995, p. 41517

89. Dopamine is a mood-altering chemical causing a "feel good" sensation. Italian researchers have discovered that the dopamine surge in the brain produced by nicotine is almost identical to the surge seen with intravenous or smoked cocaine.          ABC News, July 17, 1996 (from Nature)

90. Smoking causes the brain to release noradrenaline and dopamine, which act as stimulants. Nicotine increases alertness, cognitive performance, and the ability to sustain performance while fatigued. *Cigarettes*, p. 113

91. Nicotine improves recall and memory by strengthening communications between neurons in the hippocampus, the brain area involved in learning and memory. Nicotine delivered by nicotine patch improves the performance of Alzheimer's patients on learning tests. Newsweek, November 3, 1996, p. 68

92. The severity of nicotine dependence in smokers can be illustrated by the fact that only 33% of self-quitters remain abstinent for two days, and fewer than 5% are ultimately successful on a given quit attempt. American Journal of Psychiatry, October 1996 Supplement, p. 3

93. In a survey reported in USA Today on May 28, 1997, 92% of current smokers believe that nicotine is addictive, and 88% believe that smoking causes cancer.

94. "The manufacturers employ a variety of methods to control nicotine delivery with great precision. They do so by: 1) adjusting tobacco blends, using high-nicotine tobaccos to raise the nicotine concentration in lower-tar cigarettes; 2) adding extraneous nicotine to tobacco stems, scrap and other waste materials, which are processed into 'reconstituted tobacco' and used in all major cigarette brands; 3) adding ammonia compounds to increase the delivery of 'free' nicotine to smokers by raising the alkalinity or pH of tobacco smoke; 4) using filter and ventilation systems that remove a higher percentage of tar than nicotine; 5) genetically engineering tobacco plants to increase nicotine content; 6) developing nicotine 'analogues' that retain nicotine's reinforcing characteristics; and 7) employing chemicals, such as acetaldehyde, that act synergistically to strengthen nicotine's pharmacological effects.

    The inevitable consequence of the tobacco industry's manipulation and control of nicotine is to keep consumers using cigarettes by causing and sustaining their addiction to nicotine." Lung Cancer, Vol. 18, 1997, p. 5 (Clifford Douglas)

95. In a 1963 letter, Brown and Williamson company counsel Addison Yeaman wrote: "We are, then, in the business of selling nicotine, an addictive drug effective in the release of stress mechanisms." In 1994, Brown and Williamson Tobacco corporation released a statement saying that cigarette smoking is not addictive. Washington Post, May 11, 1997, p. C2

96. "Then the industry created a public-relations disaster that its worst enemies could not have devised when a solemn assemblage of its top executives swore to Congress they did not believe tobacco was addictive. That ludicrous testimony earned the ridicule it deserved and convinced the public that these businesses respected neither facts nor fairness." New York Times editorial, April 17, 1997, p. A22

97. "The belated admissions by Liggett that it has lied in the past about the addictiveness of smoking can only bring added ridicule to all those industry executives who told Congress in solemn, straight-faced testimony that they did not believe tobacco is addictive." New York Times editorial, March 22, 1997, p. 22

98. "If they [cigarettes] are behaviorally addictive or habit forming, they are much more like caffeine, or, in my case, Gummi Bears." From an April 1997 legal deposition by James Morgan, CEO of Philip Morris

99. Andrew Schindler, president of R.J. Reynolds, told a plaintiff's lawyer that he didn't believe that tobacco was any more addictive than coffee or carrots. "Carrot addiction?" asked the lawyer. "Yes", replied Schindler. "There was British research on carrots." The Washington Monthly, October 1997, p. 4

100. In a House Commerce Committee hearing in January 1998, tobacco executives had very different testimony on the whether nicotine is addictive as compared to their predecessors in April 1994 testimony. Rep. Diana DeGette, D-Colo., asked: "Is tobacco addictive?" The answers followed.

    "That would be accurate." Vincent Grierer, CEO, U.S. Tobacco Co.

    "Yes, under the terms that people use today, I would say it is." Steven Goldstone, CEO, RJR Nabisco.

    "It would be." Laurence Tisch, CEO, Loews Corp., owner of Lorillard.

    San Francisco Chronicle, February 1, 1998

101. "...people who are nicotine-dependent are victims of addiction, and not social miscreants."

JAMA, October 1, 1997, p. 1090

102. "The main hazard of nicotine is that nicotine dependence maintains tobacco use. Nicotine per se does not substantially contribute to the medical complications of tobacco use, including cancer and heart and lung disease...nicotine is not a carcinogen." Conclusions from Round Table on Social and Economic Aspects of Reduction of Tobacco Smoking by Use of Alternative Nicotine Delivery Systems, Geneva, 24 September 1997

103. "At present, there is still no definitive evidence that nicotine directly contributes to human disease."

Neal Benowitz, M.D. Nicotine toxicity. Alternative Delivery Systems, Toronto, March 1997

104. Nicotine modulates the brain neurotransmitters dopamine (involved with pleasure), serotonin, and norepinephrine. With nicotine abstinence, there is a relative deficiency of these neurotransmitters, which produces some of the withdrawal symptoms. With smoking, arterial nicotine levels are 3 to 10 times higher than venous levels, and are reinforcing to the brain. Neal Benowitz, M.D., Tenth National Conference on Nicotine Dependence, Minneapolis, October 17, 1997

105. 10-15% of heavy smokers wake up in the middle of the night to smoke.

J. Taylor Hays, M.D., workshop, Tenth National Conference on Nicotine Dependence, Minneapolis, October 17, 1997 (and observations also by Linda Ferry, M.D.)

106. Nicotine may improve cognitive functioning in schizophrenia; 75 to 90% of schizophrenics are smokers.

Paul Newhouse, M.D., Tenth National Conference on Nicotine Dependence, Minneapolis, October 17, 1997

107. 40 milligrams of nicotine intravenously will cause death in about 20 seconds.

John Rosecrans, Ph.D., Tenth National Conference on Nicotine Dependence, Minneapolis, October 17, 1997

108. Dr. Cynthia Pomerleau from the University of Michigan Substance Research Center has evidence than many longtime smokers have an underlying psychiatric problem that nicotine may help to ameliorate. Nicotine can either sedate or stimulate, helping a person with anxiety to relax, but stimulate a depressed patient. The psychiatric disorder can be unmasked or worsened by nicotine withdrawal, which leads to higher relapse and lower successful quit rates. Different studies have shown (compared with people with no psychiatric disorder) rates of nicotine dependence twice as high among those with anxiety disorder as well as the diagnosis of attention deficit hyperactivity disorder, and smoking rates three times as high among those with major depression. New York Times, August 27, 1997, p. C8

109. "Cigarettes, it seems, give meaning to ordinary tasks and accentuate experiences. Unlike alcohol, which relaxes but can make a person groggy, or caffeine, which energizes but can give someone the jitters, tobacco has the chameleonlike ability to assuage bad feelings and intensify pleasurable ones. It calms and it invigorates."

Houston Chronicle, October 5, 1997

110. The new RJR nicotine delivery system Eclipse delivers similar amounts of nicotine and carbon monoxide as conventional cigarettes. As is the case for conventional cigarettes, standardized machine-determined nicotine yields for Eclipse are poor predictors of actual nicotine exposure.

American Journal of Public Health, November 1997, p. 1866

111. RJR began marketing Eclipse in Lincoln, Nebraska, in September 1997.     USA Today, October 1997, p. 1B

112. Eggplant and green and pureed tomatoes have high natural levels of nicotine.     JAMA, August 5, 1993, p. 437

113. Nicotine is contained in trace amounts in many plants, including tomatoes and eggplant. But vegetarians are unlikely to get addicted: they'd have to eat 100 pounds or more to get the nicotine in a single cigarette. Scientist speculate that tobacco evolved to contain more nicotine because it conveyed a measure of protection from herbivores and pests. In its natural form, nicotine causes a burning sensation in the mouth and throat,

which might deter animals from browsing. To insects, even a tiny dose is poisonous, so the pure chemical is still used as a pesticide in many countries. Even in this country, farmers sometimes make a folk insecticide by soaking cigarettes in water overnight. Quote from Baltimore Sun (Scott Shane)
reported in Contra Costa (CA) Times, November 15, 1997, p. A15

114. No vehicle carries it faster or more efficiently than tobacco smoke sucked from the 2,000-degree "micro blast furnace" of a glowing cigarette tip. The huge surface area of the lungs makes them an extraordinary absorption device, and the nicotine hits the brain within seconds. Initially, the body reacts to nicotine as a toxin. To prevent the big doses from doing harm, it boosts the number of nicotine "receptors," microscopic bits of protein on nerve cells coded to latch up with nicotine as a lock matches a key. Autopsies of some of the 425,000 Americans who die annually from smoking-related disease consistently show extra nicotine receptors. These additional receptors, many scientists believe, play a role in addiction. Once the body is accustomed to a steady dose of nicotine, the nicotine receptors apparently either get their drugs or start making physiological trouble. At a National Institute on Drug Abuse lab in Baltimore, scientists have observed the effect of nicotine addiction by injecting research subjects with radioactive water and using a PET scanner to watch brain activity. Smokers deprived of nicotine for 12 hours showed much greater brain activity during a memory test than nonsmokers. "They're still accomplishing the task, but the brain has to work much harder to do it," said Edythe D. London, director of the institute's brain imaging center. Quote from Baltimore Sun (Scott Shane)
reported in Contra Costa (CA) Times, November 15, 1997, p. A15

115. British physiologist Sir Henry Dale found in 1914 that nicotine mimics the effects of acetylcholine, a key neurotransmitter, one of the natural chemical messengers that carry nerve impulses.
Quote from Baltimore Sun (Scott Shane)
reported in Contra Costa (CA) Times, November 15, 1997, p. A15

116. But some anti-smoking activists say nicotine is relatively safe if ingested without the carcinogenic tar cocktail smokers inhale. They say government regulation of nicotine products has been exactly backward:
Cigarettes, incomparably the most dangerous way to take the drug, have been virtually unregulated, while nicotine chewing gum and nicotine patches were subjected to costly testing and made available without prescription only last year. Now the Food and Drug Administration is easing restrictions on safe nicotine products while seeking to regulate cigarettes. If courts uphold that power, the agency faces a paradox: forcing the level of nicotine in cigarettes down, to reduce addiction, would likely cause smokers to drag harder and smoke more to get their accustomed nicotine dose. "To keep their nicotine intake equal, they'll get more tar, carbon monoxide and other toxins," said Ronald Davis, a Michigan physician and editor of the journal Tobacco Control. "In the short term, that could actually make things worse." Quote from Baltimore Sun (Scott Shane)
reported in Contra Costa (CA) Times, November 15, 1997, p. A15

117. A report published in the journal Nature studied nicotinic receptors on neurons in the brain that respond to nicotine. Dr. John Dani said, "…as the nicotine first arrives, the neurons burst with activity. That burst causes dopamine release that contributes to the sensation of pleasure." After a night without nicotine, the receptors become more sensitive, and with the first cigarette of the day, the receptors are activated and "go wild", with the dopamine release providing the pleasure of the first morning cigarette. Dopamine is part of the reward and reinforcement cycle seen in addictive drugs such as cocaine.
United Press International, November 26, 1997, and Washington Post, December 1, 1997, p. A2

118. The FDA "found that cigarettes are a highly engineered product with components such as the tobacco blend, the filter, and the ventilation system that have been carefully designed to deliver controlled, pharmacologically active doses of nicotine to the smoker." JAMA, February 5, 1997, p. 407

119. "BAT should learn to look at itself as a drug company rather than as a tobacco company."
April 1980 memo by a team of BAT Co. scientists (Smokeless States Tobacco News, Spring 1998)

120. In California, 600 pounds of nicotine is used each year as a pesticide. Bruce Leistikow, M.D.

121. In a study from the Mayo clinic, transdermal nicotine was associated with improvement of 39% of nonsmoking patients with ulcerative colitis, compared to 9% of patients on placebo patches.

*Annals of Internal Medicine, March 1, 1997, p. 364*

122. 85% of cigarette smokers use the product daily, compared to only 10% of cocaine and 10% of alcohol users who do so every day.

John Slade, M.D.

123. 92% of American smokers think that their habit is addictive, and 70% want to quit.

C. Everett Koop lecture at Walter Reed Army hospital, 1998

124. A vaccine that works against nicotine is in the testing stage on animals. The product is designed to keep nicotine from reaching the brain.

Associated Press, December 18, 1999

125. Nicotine stimulates the release of the neurotransmitters dopamine and endorphin in the reward/pleasure centers of the brain.

Axel Stalcup, M.D., lecture, March 12, 1999

126. Twin studies estimate that the majority of the liability to become and remain a smoker is explained by genetic as opposed to environmental factors.

Journal of the National Cancer Institute, August 18, 1999, p. 1367

127. "Any action on our part, such as research on the psychopharmacology of nicotine, which implicitly or explicitly treats nicotine as a drug, could well be viewed as a tacit acknowledgement that nicotine is a drug. Such acknowledgement, contend our attorneys, would be untimely."

1980 Philip Morris memo by William Dunn, head of the company's "smoker psychology" group and known in-house as "the Nicotine Kid"(Washington Post National Weekly Edition, February 8, 1999, p. 7)

128. "Starters no longer disbelieve the dangers of smoking, but they almost universally assume these risks will not apply to themselves because they will not become addicted. Once addiction does take place, it becomes necessary for the smoker to make peace with the accepted hazards. This is done by a wide range of rationalization."

Quote from tobacco industry internal documents reported by David Simpson in Tobacco Control, Summer 1999, p. 132

129. Nicotine can improve some aspects of memory in patients with Alzheimer's disease.

*Nicotine Safety and Toxicity*, p. 141

130. Transdermal nicotine provokes gastroesophageal reflux and heartburn. Crohn's disease is primarily a disease of smokers, and smoking exacerbates symptoms. In contrast, nicotine promotes healing in ulcerative colitis, which is primarily a disease of nonsmokers.

*Nicotine Safety and Toxicity*, p. 165

131. Nicotine patch therapy shows promise in the treatment of children with Tourette's syndrome, a condition affecting 100,000 people in the United States and marked by facial tics and often uncontrollable movements and vocalizations.

San Francisco Chronicle, February 22, 2000, p. A2

132. The FDA has banned "Nico Water," a concoction of nicotine and water that had been marketed in early 2002.

2003 AMA Annual Tobacco Report

133. The inhalability of milder tobaccos used in cigarettes is the source of a second important distinction between cigarettes and other forms of tobacco. Because the smoke of pipes, cigars, and dark tobacco is relatively alkaline, its nicotine dose is absorbed through the linings of the mouth and nose. Flue-cured "blond" or light-colored tobacco, from which American cigarettes are normally blended, produces slightly acidic tobacco smoke; the nicotine dose thus must be inhaled to be absorbed. Drawn into the lungs through cigarette smoking, nicotine is absorbed into the systemic circulation more quickly than in other forms of smoking – hence the greater potential for nicotine addiction. quote from *Reducing Tobacco Use*, 2000 Surgeon General report, p. 35

134. Oral aphthous ulcers associated with Behcet's syndrome may in some cases be related to smoking cessation, and nicotine replacement therapy may be helpful in treatment.

New England Journal of Medicine, December 14, 2000

135. Chinese Americans metabolize nicotine 25% more slowly than do whites and Latinos, which might explain why they smoke fewer cigarettes and have a lower risk of lung cancer. Conversely, black smokers take in more nicotine per cigarette and metabolize it faster, which could explain a higher incidence of lung cancer in this ethnic group.
The Lancet, January 19, 2002, p. 234

136. In a study from San Francisco, Chinese smokers metabolized nicotine at only two thirds the rate of white and Latino smokers. Possibly because of this, Chinese Americans inhale less smoke per cigarette, and have much lower rates of lung cancer than white smokers.
San Francisco Chronicle, January 16, 2002

137. For some young smokers, it could take just a few cigarettes to become addicted. Dr. Joseph DiFranza from the University of Massachusetts conducted the study of 12 and 13 year olds, and said "…we have to warn kids that you can't just experiment with cigarettes for a few weeks and then give it up. If you fool around with cigarettes for a few weeks, you may be addicted for life."
Associated Press, September 12, 2000

138. In a study of middle school students in Massachusetts, teens became addicted to tobacco much faster than researchers had previously believed. In girls it took only an average of three weeks of smoking to get hooked. Boys are less easily addicted, half within six months of starting smoking. In contrast, adults take about two years and smoking half a pack a day to become addicted.
Los Angeles Times, August 29, 2002

139. Teens may become addicted to nicotine more quickly than adults, within a month, even without daily smoking. It had previously been thought that it took kids two years or so to progress from experimentation to becoming a confirmed smoker.
Tobacco Control, September 2000, pp. 313-319

140. The mechanism how the brain is "rewarded" by exposure to nicotine, and why cessation is so difficult, was reviewed in the March 2002 issue of Neuron. Nicotine hijacks the reward system by attaching to receptors on nerve cells and triggering the release of dopamine, a neurotransmitter that causes pleasant feelings. Nicotine also attaches to another receptor that triggers the release of a chemical called GABA, which stops dopamine. When GABA production is inhibited by nicotine binding these receptors, the body cannot stop the pleasure signal caused by dopamine.
2002 AMA Annual Tobacco Report

141. Management of Nicotine Addiction, pp. 97-155 in *Reducing Tobacco Use*, 2000 Surgeon General report, is a detailed review of nicotine addiction.

142. Genetically engineered very low nicotine biotech tobacco was introduced in 2002 in cigarettes made by Vector Tobacco of Durham, N.C.
Associated Press, February 17, 2002

143. An article in March 2002 in Newsday reports that Vector Tobacco planned to introduce a nicotine free cigarette called "Quest" in late 2002, complete with a $40 million ad campaign. 2002 AMA Annual Tobacco Report

144. "At this time, there is no definitive evidence that nicotine directly contributes to human disease, but there are several areas of concern."
*Nicotine and Public Health*, p. 65

145. Nonsmoked nicotine (such as in patches) has been found to stimulate the growth of blood vessels. This can be beneficial where the patient has circulatory problems, but nicotine can also encourage the growth of tumors.
Associated Press, June 30, 2001

146. In 1989, Philip Morris invested $300 million to develop a nearly nicotine-free cigarette called Next; it flopped and was withdrawn from the market.
*Cigarettes* (Parker-Pope), p. 130

147. Nicotine has not been shown to be carcinogenic, but it might promote tumor growth by several mechanisms, one by stimulating the development of blood vessels that supply the tumor. The Lancet, January 11, 2003, p. 146

148. Chinese Americans metabolize nicotine at lower rates than whites and Latinos, and take in less nicotine per cigarette. "The lower nicotine (and, therefore, tobacco smoke) intake per cigarette and fewer cigarettes smoked per day, which may result, in part, from slower clearance of nicotine, may explain lower lung cancer rates in Chinese-Americans."
Journal of the National Cancer Institute, January 16, 2002

149. Nicotine and its metabolite NNK may contribute to lung carcinogenesis by functioning as tumor promoters. There is no evidence, however, that nicotine replacement therapy is a risk for lung cancer.

Journal of Clinical Investigation, January 2003, pp. 81-90

# CHAPTER 21
## LOW TAR AND NICOTINE CIGARETTES:
## HEALTH AND SAFETY ISSUES

Editor note: many of the items in this section to some degree "say the same thing," but I have included a broad array because of the importance of the issue.

1.  "For more than 60 years, tobacco product manufacturers have made claims of reduced harm for some of their products; the first filter cigarette that claimed to reduce the acrolein content of smoke was marketed in 1930. When evidence linked cigarettes with lung cancer in the 1950's, harm-reduction claims became more blatant: filter cigarettes were advertised as reducing the risk of lung cancer. However, it is now known that the tobacco industry views filter and low-tar cigarettes as health-image (public relations tools, designed to calm smokers' anxieties) rather than health-oriented products (those that may reduce harm). Moreover, it is now common knowledge that low-tar cigarettes are smoked more vigorously, which undermines any potential benefit. Filter and low-tar cigarettes have thus been marketed with unregulated promises of reduced harm that have largely been unfulfilled; but for these innovations, there would be far fewer smokers today, given public awareness of smoking-related risks."  Reducing Tobacco-Related Diseases: Alternative Approaches, July 1996 Amsterdam workshop, p. 7 (John Slade)

2.  The tobacco industry has marketed low tar and nicotine cigarettes with the clear intention that by using them, a smoker can prevent or modify smoking-induced disease.  *Tobacco Use*, p. 54

3.  Increasing numbers of smokers have switched to lower tar and nicotine brands, rather than stopping smoking, in the misguided believe that they can smoke more safely.  NEJM, December 1, 1994, p. 1531

4.  75% of respondents in a Gallup poll believed that low tar cigarettes are less hazardous to health. However, when they switch to low-yield brands, smokers inhale more deeply, hold smoke longer in their lungs, smoke more cigarettes, or cover air holes in filters with their fingers. Low tar brands give smokers a false sense of security, and "the illusion that low tar brands are safer than regular cigarettes is all smoke and mirrors."  JAMA, September 2, 1993, p. 1399

5.  Many smokers intentionally block the ventilating holes in the cigarette and filter to get more smoke (and nicotine). As an example, Players Ultra Mild, normally a 0.8 mg tar cigarette, is transformed with the holes blocked into a cigarette that delivers 28.5 mg of tar. "This is nearly as much of the carcinogenic sludge you would have gotten smoking a straight Camel about 1955."  *Smokescreen*, p. 61

6.  Low tar and nicotine cigarette brands account for 60% of cigarettes sold in the U.S. However, they are no safer than "full-flavor" brands, since smokers make up for the "lighter" taste by drawing deeper and pulling in more smoke, or smoking more cigarettes to keep up the same blood level of nicotine. The result to the smoker is the same (or more) total amount of nicotine and tar absorbed.  San Francisco Chronicle, May 2, 1994, p. A3, and NEJM, June 15, 1989, p. 1569

7.  "Low-yield" cigarettes are not low in nicotine content and do not in general deliver less nicotine or tar to smokers than do higher-yield cigarettes. All cigarettes contain 6 to 11 milligrams of nicotine.  *Growing Up Tobacco Free*, p. 63 and JAMA, July 27, 1994, p. 312

8.  Low tar and nicotine brands of cigarettes increased in sales from 2% to 55% of the market in the last twenty years. But smokers of these brands have a false sense of security. There is no decrease in heart disease risk, and only a small decrease in lung cancer risk with these brands. Smokers compensate for lower yields by smoking more cigarettes, puffing more frequently, and inhaling more deeply. In summary, the health problems caused by smoking are not reduced by switching to low tar and nicotine brands.  JAMA, September 2, 1993, p. 1399, and American Journal of Public Health, January 1992, p. 17

9.  "You *can* switch down to lower tar and still get satisfying taste. Yes you can!"

    Philip Morris ad for Merit Cigarettes

10. The average cigarette delivers about one milligram of nicotine to the smoker. When the number of cigarettes available to heavy smokers was reduced from 38 to five per day, the intake of nicotine inhaled from each cigarette tripled.

    NEJM, July 14, 1994, p. 124

11. Switching from higher-yield to lower-yield cigarettes has been shown to result in smoking more cigarettes or smoking more intensively, both of which are associated with increased exposure to carbon monoxide and other toxins.

    NEJM, July 14, 1994, p. 125

12. Switching to low yield brands may even increase the health risk for smokers who compensate for reduced nicotine intake by increasing the number of cigarettes smoked per day, the frequency of puffing, and the depth and duration of inhalation.

    *Reducing Health Consequences*, p. 316

13. A 1993 Gallup survey found that 48.6 percent of adults think that smoking low tar brands is safer. But a wealth of scientific evidence contradicts this; low yield cigarettes can be a *greater* hazard. "Worried smokers are convinced that lower tar and nicotine means safer. The smoking public has bought the low tar bill of goods, and the cigarette makers are cashing in on the very health fear that they and their product have created. The tragedy is that their 'safer' alternative is not safe at all."

    Reader's Digest, April 1994

14. "Smoking low tar and nicotine cigarettes is the equivalent of jumping out of the 29th floor of a building rather than the 31st floor." American Journal of Public Health, January 1992, p.17 (Kenneth Warner and John Slade)

15. A major concern is that although machine-measured yields of tar and nicotine from cigarettes are lower in today's cigarettes than in those marketed in the 1950s, low yield cigarettes have little or no beneficial impact on health; indeed, smokers face a greater risk of dying from smoking-attributable disease than they did 40 years ago. Analysis of data collected from five of the world's largest epidemiological studies on smoking and health revealed that while the average tar level per cigarette has dropped by 70% since 1955, the relative risks for all smoking-related causes of deaths increased, the likely reason being that in order to obtain the same dose of nicotine smokers smoke more cigarettes and inhale more deeply. The risk of lung cancer doubled (from 11.9 to 23.2) in smokers overall, but was quadrupled for women (from 2.7 to 12.9). The increase in relative risk between the two generations of smokers is due to a greater lifetime dose of cigarette smoke; a result of starting smoking earlier in life (this was true especially for women) or because smokers are now smoking more cigarettes more intensively. These results are particularly worrying as most smokers believe that low tar and low nicotine cigarettes reduce the health risks associated with smoking.

    Moreover, the false sense of security generated by low tar and low nicotine cigarettes has increased the overall market of smokers; there would be far fewer smokers today, given public awareness of smoking related risks, if the unfiltered cigarettes of the 1950s were the only choice available.

    Quote from UICC/International Union Against Cancer paper "Clearing the Air Around Nicotine"

16. "Cigarette brands that deliver $\leq$ 15 mg of tar in official smoking-machine tests accounted for 72.7% of total cigarettes sales in 1995...Many of these brands use ventilated filters...air introduced through the vents dilutes the amounts of tar, nicotine, carbon monoxide, and other hazardous constituents of cigarette smoke...smokers who use reduced-tar cigarettes may be blocking some of the filter vents with their fingers or lips, therefore increasing their exposure to the carcinogens in cigarettes smoke...One study has estimated that 58% of persons who smoke cigarettes with $\leq$ 4 mg tar are blocking some filter vents. In tests conducted on cigarette smoking machines, blocking half of the ventilation holes on a cigarette with standard yields of 4 mg tar, 0.5 mg nicotine, and 5 mg CO increased FTC-rated tar yields by 60%, nicotine by 62%, and CO by 73%...An estimated two-thirds of U.S. smokers either are unaware of the presence of vents on cigarettes or do not know that tar yields increase when vents are blocked...These findings underscore the need for intensified efforts to educate smokers about the risks associated with smoking reduced-tar cigarettes."

    Morbidity and Mortality Weekly Report, November 7, 1997, pp. 1043-47

17. "...smokers of low-yield cigarettes often change the way they smoke to compensate for the nicotine they are missing. Compared with the standard machine-test method, smokers might take more puffs, take longer puffs,

smoke a cigarette closer to the butt, smoke more cigarettes, or even cover the ventilation holes in the filter. Thus, the reported quantities of tar and nicotine may be meaningless."

*Smoke and Mirrors*, p. 162 (Rob Cunningham)

18. If anything, ultra low nicotine delivery, with extremely mild and nontoxic smoke inhalation properties of little or no initial pharmacological toxicity, may, if anything, actually facilitate the initiation of a smoking practice that is otherwise generated primarily by psychological determinants or social factors... If smokers titrate smoking behavior to meet or accommodate their established nicotine dependency, however, they will ultimately have to smoke more of the lowered-nicotine delivery cigarettes and/or smoke them in a different manner, both of which may increase, rather than decrease, their health risks.

Quote from *The Tobacco Epidemic*, pp. 54-55 (Gary Huber)

19. Low tar and nicotine cigarettes may inhibit smokers from quitting, as 1978 internal documents from Imperial Tobacco Ltd. indicate: "We have evidence of virtually no quitting among smokers of those brands (of under 6 mg. of tar), and there are indications that the advent of ultra low tar cigarettes has actually retained some potential quitters in the cigarette market by offering them a viable alternative."

*Smoke and Mirrors*, pp. 163-164

20. Health concerns drove the 2 major previous paradigm shifts in cigarette architecture: filter-tipped cigarettes in the 1950's and low tar and nicotine (t&n) cigarettes at the end of the following decade, both presented to the public as radical design changes, much like the emerging generation of devices.

Filters were the industry's response to the then newly emerging public concern about smoking's relation to lung cancer. The cigarette companies marketed filters as trapping the dangerous components of cigarette smoke but letting the "flavor" through. Affording smokers an apparent alternative to quitting smoking, filters rapidly became the dominant product on the market. Their introduction and marketing were quickly followed by reversal of a 2-year decline in per capita cigarette consumption in 1953 and 1954 that had resulted from new evidence linking lung cancer to smoking, which then meant unfiltered cigarettes. Ironically, the most successful early filter, touted quite explicitly for its health protection properties, the Kent Micronite filter, used crocidolite asbestos as the filtering agent. That filter cigarettes were introduced primarily as a public relations gambit, rather than as truly less dangerous products, is suggested by the fact that some early filtered cigarettes used harsher tobaccos, so that the filtered smoke would taste like the unfiltered smoke of old.

The industry's next technological "fix" was the low t&n cigarette, marketed, often explicitly, with the theme that health-conscious smokers had the choice of either quitting smoking or switching to low t&n brands. By 1981, low t&n cigarettes had captured a majority of the market. Medical textbooks frequently recommended their use by patients unable or unwilling to stop smoking.

Since then, scientists have learned that smokers who switch from regular cigarettes to low t&n brands engage in "nicotine regulation," compensatory behavioral changes that greatly narrow the supposed gap between high- and low-yielding cigarettes. Low t&n smokers may consume more cigarettes, take larger and more frequent puffs, inhale more deeply, smoke to a shorter butt length, and subvert the technologies that lower machine-measured t&n yields (by blocking ventilation holes in filters that, unoccluded, dilute smoke by mixing it with air).

Low t&n cigarettes could reduce health risks if smokers did not engage in nicotine regulation to a significant degree and if they would have continued to smoke even if low t&n cigarettes were not on the market. However, most smokers who "switch down" to low t&n cigarettes do engage in nicotine regulation. Further, the availability of low t&n cigarettes has probably substantially impeded smoking cessation. On balance, therefore, low t&n cigarettes may well have increased the aggregate societal burden of smoking, primarily by reducing the number of people who would have quit in the absence of their availability, and secondarily by switchers smoking more cigarettes.

Quote from JAMA, October 1, 1997, p. 1088
(Kenneth Warner, John Slade, and David Sweanor)

21. In the late 1970's, medical textbooks advised physicians to recommend low tar cigarettes if a patient was not able to stop smoking.

*The Cigarette Papers*, p. 360

22. An estimated two thirds of U.S. smokers either are unaware of the presence of vents on cigarettes, or do not know that tar yields increase when vents are blocked. Cigarette brands delivering less than 15 mg of tar accounted for almost 73% of total cigarette sales in 1995.

JAMA, February 11, 1998, pp. 424-425

23. Sales of filter cigarettes increased from 1% of the total market in 1950 to 51% in 1960 and 95% of the market by 1988. The proportion of "low tar" brands increased from 2% in 1967 to 54% in 1988 and 69% in 1992
*Reducing the Health Consequences of Smoking*, p. 328
and New York Times, April 12, 1996, p. D17

24. Filter cigarettes increased from 0.3% in 1949 to 51% in 1960 and 97% by 1992. Cigarettes yielding less than 15 milligrams of tar rose from 2% in 1967 to 69% in 1992 and 73% in 1995.
Epidemiologic Reviews 1995; 17:49

25. Filter cigarette sales in China increased from 40% of cigarettes sold in 1989 to 77% in 1995.
New York Times, August 27, 1997, p. A7

26. "Yishou healthy cigarette was especially recommended at the 10th World Conference on Tobacco or Health," states a brochure. "A finest selection of Chinese herbs and natural spices serves as a substitute of tobacco and helps to give up smoking addiction in an easy manner."          10th World Conference, Beijing, China, 1997

27. Cigarettes made from lettuce are being marketed as an adjunct for patients who are trying to stop smoking.
Neal Benowitz, M.D., Tenth National Conference on Nicotine Dependence, Minneapolis, October 17, 1997

28. A cigarette called Bravo made from enzyme-treated lettuce was successfully re-introduced in 1997 after a failed marketing attempt in 1969. It is advertised as a nicotine and tobacco-free safer alternative to standard cigarettes.          U.S. News and World Report, October 27, 1997, p. 66

29. "Low tar cigarettes are a fraud."          John Slade, M.D.

30. The Federal Trade Commission protocol for machine – smoking analysis of smoke "underestimates nicotine and carcinogen doses to smokers and overestimates the proportional benefits of low-yield cigarettes."
Journal of the National Cancer Institute, January 19, 2000, p. 106

31. First, the tobacco market is dominated by cigarettes that readily deliver high levels of tar and nicotine, regardless of their claimed yields and regardless of whether their brand names and advertising indicate that they are "light" or "reduced" in tar and nicotine delivery. Second, the epidemiologic data show that, despite their labeling and advertising, so-called "light" cigarettes are not associated with any important health benefits compared with currently available "regular" or "full-flavor" cigarettes.

Smokers adjust a variety of their smoking behaviors, such as puff frequency, depth of inhalation, and ventilation hole blocking, thereby ingesting high levels of nicotine and tar irrespective of the advertised yields of the cigarettes. Moreover, the results show that cigarettes branded as "lights" can provide deliveries of tar and nicotine that are similar to those of the regular versions. It is highly unlikely that the small differences in tar and nicotine deliveries found across brands have any toxicologic significance.
Quote from the Journal of the National Cancer Institute, January 19, 2000, pp. 90-91

32. Low tar cigarette U.S. market share increased from 3.6% in 1970 to 44.8% in 1980 and 72.7% in 1995. (It was 87% in 2001 – editor).          Journal of the National Cancer Institute, April 21, 1999, p.. 687

33. "...proposed legislation must not include provisions that allow the industry to continue to label and promote their 'light' and 'low-tar' products, thus continuing the low-tar, low-nicotine scam."
JAMA, October 7, 1998, p. 1180 (Richard Hurt)

34. A detailed article about safer cigarettes, their manufacture, and the politics of the issue written by John Schwartz was published in the Washington Post National Weekly Edition, February 8, 1999, pp. 6-10.

35. In November 2001, the National Cancer Institute (NCI) released the 13th in its "Smoking and Tobacco Control Monograph" series. Titled "Risks Associated with Smoking Cigarettes with Low Machine-Measured Yields of Tar and Nicotine," the monograph concludes that:

There has not been a public health benefit from changes in cigarette design and manufacturing over the last 50 years.

There appears to be complete compensation for nicotine delivery among brand switchers, reflecting more intensive smoking of low-yield cigarettes.

Low-yield cigarettes have not prevented the sustained increase in lung cancer in older smokers.

Many smokers use low-yield products as an alternative to smoking cessation, and believe that the products are less risky. Tobacco company advertising and marketing of low-yield products seems to promote initiation and impede cessation.

The Federal Trade Commission (FTC) measurements of tar and nicotine do not provide meaningful information for smokers on the amount of these substances actually delivered while smoking, or from smoking different brands.
2002 AMA Annual Tobacco Report

36. A 2001 National Cancer Institute monograph reports that reduced tar cigarettes carry no health benefits, and that the adoption of lower-yield cigarettes have not prevented the continued increase in lung cancer in the United States. Cigarettes labeled "low-tar" do not generally deliver lower tar to smokers, and smokers of low tar brands cannot expect to have fewer smoking-related health problems.
American Medical News, May 6, 2002, p. 39

37. The European Parliament has approved a measure requiring tobacco makers to reduce tar and nicotine levels in cigarettes, and to print larger health warnings covering almost half of the pack.
San Francisco Chronicle, June 15, 2000

38. 87% of the 47 million U.S. smokers choose low tar brands.
NBC Evening News (Tom Brokaw), November 28, 2001

39. "Considering all I'd heard, I decided to either quit or smoke True. I smoke True."
1976 ad (New York Times, April 20, 1997, p. E3)

40. A study from London compared nicotine yields from machine-smoked cigarettes with actual nicotine intake in smokers of brands with varying nicotine content. The authors' conclusion was that the actual nicotine intake did not correspond to the machine-smoked yields, and concluded that "smokers' tendency to regulate nicotine intake vitiates potential health gains from lower tar and nicotine cigarettes. Current approaches to characterizing tar and nicotine yields of cigarettes provide a simplistic guide to smokers' exposure that is misleading to consumers and regulators alike and should be abandoned."
Journal of the National Cancer Institute, January 17, 2001, p. 134

41. Vector Tobacco in 2001 introduced Omni, "the first reduced carcinogen cigarette that tastes, smokes and burns just like any other premium cigarette."     Ad from San Francisco Chronicle, November 13, 2001

42. Both Vector Tobacco and Brown & Williamson rolled out "reduced carcinogen" cigarettes in November 2001. Vector's nationally-marketed offering is called "Omni," a product that claims to have less polycyclic aromatic hydrocarbons (PAHs), nitrosamines and catechols, three major carcinogens in tobacco smoke. Vector uses a "catalytic" approach to removing the chemicals, with palladium and other elements. Omni is promoted as having "great taste" with less risk, at least by inference. The ads have a second warning in addition to the standard Surgeon General wording, which says, "Smoking is addictive and dangerous to your health. Reductions in carcinogens (PAHs, nitrosamines, and catechols) have NOT been proven to result in a safer cigarette. This product produces tar, carbon monoxide, and other harmful by-products."

Brown and Williamson began test-marketing in Indianapolis with "Advance." This product claims that differences in curing reduce the tobacco specific nitrosamines, and the use of a 3-stage filter with an "ion exchange" mechanism further reduces "toxins across several categories."     2002 AMA Annual Tobacco Report

43. "When filter ventilation holes are blocked on 'low tar' cigarettes, the tar yield can increase dramatically, up to 12 times in some cases."     British Medical Association (www.tobaccofactfile.org)

# CHAPTER 22
# SMOKING AND TOBACCO CESSATION

"Stopping smoking is easy to do; I have done it thousands of times!" Statement attributed to Mark Twain.
*Clinics in Geriatric Medicine*, May 1986, p. 337

1. "No-Ta-Bac" was introduced in the 1890's as a "guaranteed tobacco habit cure." It was advertised to permanently stop the craving for all forms of tobacco and was guaranteed to cure 99 out of 100 cases.
*Tobacco Advertising*, p. 253

2. In 1990 and 1991, 42% of all smokers abstained for at least a day, but 86% of this group subsequently resumed smoking. About 1.2 million persons (2.5% of smokers) quit permanently and become former smokers each year.
Morbidity and Mortality Weekly Report, September 4, 1992, p. 505

3. In the United States, only 7.6% are successful of the 17 million smokers who attempt to stop smoking each year.
Mayo Clinic Proceedings, October 1997, p. 917

4. In the United States, 70% of smokers want to quit, 33% try to quit each year, but only 3% succeed, and only one third ever quit before age 65.     10th World Conference on Tobacco or Health, Beijing, 1997 (Saul Shiffman)

5. If only half of office-based physicians in the US delivered a brief intervention to each of their smoking patients, and achieved only a 10% sustained quit rate, the national cessation rate would more than double, increasing from 2 million to 4.5 million new ex-smokers each year.     *Nicotine Addiction*, p. 214

6. 70% of smokers see a physician at least once a year. Two to four minutes of firm physician advice to quit leads to long term cessation rates of about 10%. This simple step would yield about two million new ex-smokers each year, and 20 million over a decade.     How to Help Your Patients Stop Smoking,
National Cancer Institute, 1991, and *Advances in Cancer Control*, pp. 11-25, 1990

7. One of the national health objectives for the year 2000 (DHHS No. 3.16, 1991) was to increase to at least 75% the proportion of primary care health workers who routinely advise cessation and provide assistance and follow-up for patients who use tobacco.

8. Having a heart attack produces 50 to 60% one year quit rates, the most effective known smoking cessation "treatment." The fear of imminent death is a strong motivator to stop smoking.     *Nicotine Addiction*, p. 148

9. 38% of smokers who had been off cigarettes for over a year report relapsing at some point.
*Nicotine Addiction*, p. 150

10. About a third of smokers who have been abstinent for one year will relapse at some time in the future.
Clinics in Chest Medicine, December 1991, p. 640

11. In a survey from San Diego, the likelihood of remaining continuously abstinent for two years was about 90% for former smokers who had quit for three months or longer, and 95% of those who had quit for one year or longer.     Journal of the National Cancer Institute, April 16, 1997, p. 572

12. 17 million Americans each year make a serious attempt to quit smoking, but 15 million fail. 38% of smokers who have a heart attack begin smoking again as soon as they leave the hospital, as do 40% of patients who have had cancerous larynxes removed.     Washington Post National Weekly Edition, April 4, 1994, p. 27

13. 48% of all California smokers quit for at least a day during the previous year, but more than 80% of these attempts did not last a full year.     *Tobacco Use in California*, p. 58

14. The 1.3 million successful quitters each year in the US are almost compensated for by a million new smokers each year.                                                                JAMA, January 6, 1989, p. 61

15. More than two thirds of all college graduates who ever smoked have now quit.

16. In 1990, the King Country Blue Cross/Blue Shield, the largest medical insurer in Washington state, became the first Blue Cross/Blue Shield company to formally reimburse physicians for outpatient treatment of nicotine dependence.                                                Family Practice News, December 1990, p. 25

17. Most smokers persist in their habit to satisfy a craving for nicotine, not because there is any inherent pleasure in it. If smokers are given cigarettes made from de-nicotinized tobacco, almost none choose to continue.
                                                Journal of the National Cancer Institute, January 17, 1990, p. 89

18. In 1964, golfer Arnold Palmer quit smoking and gave up the $10,000 a year he was being paid to throw an L&M on the green and then pick it up and take a puff after putting. Within 6 months, he had gained 20 pounds and resumed smoking, not to quit for good until 1975.                          Reader's Digest, April 1992

19. Senator Jesse Helms of North Carolina, a leading champion of the tobacco industry, quit smoking when he underwent coronary bypass surgery.                          Tobacco Free Youth Reporter, Fall 1992, p. 21

20. 10.8 million of the nation's 46 million smokers participated in the American Cancer Society's Great American Smokeout in 1992. Of these, 3.3 million stopped for 24 hours, and 1.5 million were still not smoking 5 days later.                                                                SCARC, November 5, 1993

21. During the 1993 Great American Smokeout, an estimated 2.4 million smokers (6%) reported quitting for at least a day, and 6.0 million (15%) reduced the number of cigarettes smoked on that day.
                                                Morbidity and Mortality Weekly Report, November 4, 1994, p. 785

22. At the 1996 Great American Smokeout, 6% of smokers quit at least for the day, and 20% reduced smoking.
                                                Morbidity and Mortality Weekly Report, September 19, 1997, p. 869

23. The 1996 Great American Smokeout was associated with helping an estimated 7400 persons quit smoking.
                                                Morbidity and Mortality Weekly Report, November 7, 1997, p. 1037

24. In a 1992 Gallup poll, two thirds of adolescent smokers reported that they wanted to quit, and 70% indicated that they would not have started smoking if they could choose again.          JAMA, December 7, 1994, p. 1649

25. Among smokers who stop the habit, almost half who stayed off cigarettes for two weeks were able to successfully quit for at least six months. On the other hand, for those who smoked even a single puff during the critical first two weeks, 90% were back to smoking full time after six months.
                                                American Medical News, March 14, 1994

26. "...any cigarettes at all smoked following a target quit day have extremely poor prognostic implication for the long-term success of that attempt. Even an isolated cigarette smoked more than 2 or 3 days into a quit attempt seems to lead almost invariably to long-term relapse."                          The Tobacco Epidemic, p. 162

27. In a "success curve" for a single attempt to quit smoking, by the end of one week, only 46 percent of smokers were still off cigarettes; in other words, 54 percent had relapsed within seven days of stopping. By the end of four weeks, only 25 percent remained abstinent; by the end of six months, ten percent; and at one year, only eight percent were still successful.                          *Deadly Choices*, p. 167

28. 32% of current smokers quit for at least a day in the previous year, and 81% have tried to quit at some time in the past. There are 15 million unsuccessful quitters in the US each year.          *Deadly Choices*, p. 250

29. 70% of the nation's 46 million current smokers want to stop smoking and 34% attempt to quit each year, but only 2.5%, or about a million people, are actually successful.                    JAMA, February 1, 1995, p. 370

30. Guidelines for the physicians to help patients stop smoking stress the "Four A's": ASK about smoking at every opportunity, ADVISE all smokers to stop, ASSIST the patient in stopping, and ARRANGE follow up visits.How
To Help Your Patients Stop Smoking,
Thomas Glynn and Marc Manley, National Institutes of Health, 1991

31. The level of stress is predictive of the likelihood of smoking relapse, and one study attributed about 80% of relapses to interpersonal conflict.                    Clinics in Chest Medicine, December 1991, p. 716

32. Intensive smoking cessation programs cost about $2000 per year of life saved, and for this reason are considered to be very cost-effective by public health authorities. In contrast, mammographic screening for breast cancer costs about $50,000 per year of life saved.                    JAMA, October 23/30, 1996, p. 1291

33. Estimated cost effectiveness of smoking cessation programs: for men ages 35 to 69, $4113 to $6465 when the method is nicotine chewing gum with physician counseling; $705 to $988 when the physician provides only brief advice and a self-help booklet.                    American Medical News, January 9, 1995, p. 14

34. In a study of smoking cessation, a combination of carbon monoxide breath measurement and spirometry yielded a quit rate twice as high as that attained using a simple educational message without reinforcers.
Federal Practitioner, April 1996, p. 20

35. Adults who start smoking in their early teens are less likely to have quit by age 30 than those who start later. Only 4.4% of smokers who began before age 14 quit by age thirty; the percentage is 9.6% for those who began between ages 14 and 16, and 13.6% for those who began after age 16.        USA Today, March 11, 1996, p. 1

36.        Quit smoking. At a pack a day, there's $700 a year right there, plus a big savings on your life insurance. Tell your teenager you don't care about her health or her soon-to-yellow teeth, you care about her money. The decision to develop a saving rather than a smoking habit makes a huge difference. One way, she puts $700 a year into Marlboros and, at age 65, has cancer. The other way, she puts into a mutual fund that compounds at 12% a year and, at 65 has $896,000.
Quote from *The Only Investment Guide You'll Ever Need*, Andrew Tobias, Harcourt Brace, 1996, p. 31

37. Taking high doses of Prozac for ten weeks raises the odds for successful smoking cessation. The drug seems to ease cravings and reduce the irritability that often accompanies quitting.        Time, May 5, 1997, p. 28

38. It has been suggested that after stopping smoking, withdrawal symptoms peak in one to two weeks and then decline. However, in a study from the Center for Tobacco Research in Madison, Wisconsin, 30 to 60% of subjects showed withdrawal that persisted over 7 weeks, or withdrawal that peaked at 4 to 8 weeks post-cessation.        Abstract 1A, Tenth National Conference on Nicotine Dependence, Minneapolis, October, 1997

39. In a study of exhaled carbon monoxide breath samples from University of North Carolina, the average level for smokers was 16.5 parts per million, and for nonsmokers, 3 parts per million. The usual cut-off of 8ppm to differentiate smokers from nonsmokers is probably too high, and 4 to 5 ppm was proposed as a more appropriate cut-off level. The authors reported that a level of 8ppm failed to identify almost one in four pregnant smokers who misrepresented their smoking status as having quit.
Abstract 5A, Tenth National Conference on Nicotine Dependence, Minneapolis, October 1997

40. The national health promotion and disease prevention objectives for the year 2000 as set forth in Healthy People 2000 propose to increase to 100 percent the proportion of health plans that offer treatment of nicotine addiction.
Clinical Practice Guideline on Smoking Cessation,
US Department of Health and Human Services, 1997

41. The risk of death is 70% higher in cigarette smokers who switch to pipes and cigars compared to smokers who give up smoking altogether. However, the risk of death in the "switchers" was 50% better than in men who continued to smoke cigarettes and did not opt for a safer substitute.                  Times of London, July 3, 1997 (from The British Medical Journal, June 28, 1997)

42. 1.3 million Americans successfully quit smoking each year, only 10% of those who attempt to stop. While 70% quit after one or two tries, 22% make three to five attempts before they are successful, and 9% try six or more times before succeeding.          American Lung Association data reported by the Detroit News, April 16, 1997

43. Among patients seeking smoking cessation treatment, as many as 25 to 40% have a past history of major depression. This is triple the rate for nonsmoking adults.
                                      American Journal of Psychiatry, October 1996 supplement, p. 21

44. In a study from Purdue of smokers in their 30's who were casual drinkers, those who drank alcohol (compared to a "placebo" nonalcoholic drink) had a 35% higher level of cigarette cravings than those who did not drink alcohol. The researchers concluded that alcohol alone can prompt smokers to crave a cigarette.
                                                                  CNNfn (from Internet), June 14, 1997

45. Dr. Richard Hurt, director of the Nicotine Dependence Center at the Mayo Clinic, estimates that "at best" only 30% to 40% of managed care plans cover smoking cessation services.   American Medical News, May 20, 1996

46. Although virtually every medical insurance plan pays for the adverse outcomes of tobacco use, fewer than half of such plans pay for smoking cessation services.               Tobacco Control, Autumn 1997, p. S7

47. In 1997, only 22 states and the District of Columbia reported coverage for nicotine addiction treatment services under Medicaid.                                                Tobacco Control, Spring 1998, p. 92

48. In a survey of 105 large health-maintenance organizations in 1995, two thirds reported offering some level of smoking cessation program. However, only 23% of the plans offered nicotine replacement therapy as a standard drug benefit. Few corporations include coverage for smoking cessation services as a benefit. The Medicare program does not pay for either special smoking cessation programs or for nicotine replacement therapy; as of 1997, only five state Medicaid programs provided reimbursement of smoking cessation counseling or group programs.                          Morbidity and Mortality Weekly Report, December 26, 1997, p. 1219

49. In a study from the Mayo Clinic, 63% of smokers who had a percutaneous coronary revascularization procedure for coronary artery disease continued to smoke after the procedure.
                                                                  Mayo Clinic Proceedings, March 1998, p. 205

50. Increased anxiety has been reported to follow smoking cessation in most studies. However, in a group of 70 patients who stopped smoking, "results weaken the view that increased anxiety is a ...central element of the nicotine withdrawal syndrome and suggest that giving up smoking is quite rapidly followed by reduction in anxiety that may reflect removal of an anxiogenic agent, nicotine."            JAMA, January 21, 1998, p. 178
                                      (Abstract from American Journal of Psychiatry 154:1589-92, 1997)

51. In encouraging smoking cessation, most authorities recommend emphasizing the good things that will happen if a smoker quits, rather than the bad things that will happen if the smoker does not quit. Nagging and "scare tactics" are not recommended.               Michael Wall, M.D. lecture in Oakland, Calif., April 21. 1998

52. Obtaining lung function values in smokers and converting the volumes into "spirometric lung age" is helpful for motivating smoking cessation.                                    Preventive Medicine 1985; 14:655-662

53. In a study from the Journal of Family Practice, only 25% of smokers were counseled by their doctors about how to quit. The authors offered reasons why doctors often fail to talk to patients about smoking. They worry that it may take too much time, that their advice will be perceived as nagging, and that good smoking cessation programs are not available.                                          Washington Post, September 15, 1998

54. Investment in research and development in tobacco control in 1990 amounted to $50 per death. In contrast, HIV research and development received about $3000 per 1990 death. *Curbing the Epidemic*, p. 82

55. In the mid 1990's the average medical school education curriculum devoted a total of one hour to smoking cessation. Kevin Ferentez, M.D., University of Maryland Medical School, 1998 lecture

56. In a survey of 122 medical schools in the United States, 69.2% did not require clinical training in smoking cessation techniques. 31.4% of the schools spent 3 hours or less on smoking cessation over the entire four years of medical school. Only 5.8% of the medical schools provided more than 5 hours of instruction on tobacco intervention in the clinical (third and fourth) years. The study authors concluded that the majority of U.S. medical school graduates are not adequately trained to treat nicotine dependence. JAMA, September 1, 1999, pp. 825-829

57. After surgery for lung cancer, about 50% of patients resume smoking; after laryngectomy (vocal cord removal), about 40%, and in smokers with heart attacks, 70% take up the habit again within a year. *Faber Book of Smoking*, p. 179

58. 38% of people with diagnosed emphysema continue to smoke, as do almost 25% of those with asthma. Associated Press, December 25, 2002

59. A study from the Mayo Clinic suggests that just cutting down on cigarettes instead of quitting will not help a smoker's health. Associated Press, January 2, 2001

60. In a study from Minnesota, smoking cessation interventions during physician visits were associated with increased patient satisfaction with their care among those who smoked. This information should reduce concerns of physicians about providing tobacco cessation assistance to patients during office visits. Mayo Clinic Proceedings, February 2001, p. 138

61. A Historical Review of Efforts to Reduce Smoking in the United States. see *Reducing Tobacco Use*, 2000 Surgeon General report, Chapter 2, pp. 29-57

62. In a 2000 survey, only 29% of health and welfare funds associated with large labor unions provided insurance coverage for smoking cessation treatment to their union members. American Journal of Public Health, September 2001, p. 1412

63. In 2000, 11.5 million low income smokers were enrolled in the federal and state Medicaid health insurance program. About 73% of this population in 33 states had some degree of coverage for tobacco dependence treatments. However, Oregon was the only state to offer all the pharmacotherapy and counseling services recommended in the 2000 Public Health Service clinical practice guideline on treating tobacco use and dependence. The following states did not offer any coverage for tobacco dependence treatments in 2000 for their Medicaid patients: Alabama, Alaska, Connecticut, Georgia, Idaho, Iowa, Kentucky, Mississippi, Missouri, Nebraska, Pennsylvania, South Carolina, South Dakota, Tennessee, Utah, Washington, and Wyoming. 2002 AMA Annual Tobacco Report

64. In 1997, only 31% of American medical schools required training in smoking cessation techniques. JAMA, April 26, 2000, p. 2174

65. A majority of medical school graduates are still not adequately trained to treat nicotine dependence, and US medical schools inadequately teach tobacco intervention skills. JAMA, September 4, 2002, p. 1102

66. An estimate is that smoking cessation is 17 times more cost effective than the use of statins to lower cholesterol in terms of cost per life-year gained. The Lancet, March 24, 2001, p. 897

67. In a study of British smokers, 83% said that they would not take up smoking if they had it to do over again. Those 45 to 64 were most regretful, with 90% saying that they were sorry they took up the habit, but even in the groups ages 16 to 24, 78% would not smoke if they could make the decision again. Smokers in this survey had

inappropriate expectations related to cessation; 53% expected to stop within two years, while in reality only 6% manage to do so.
British Medical Journal, March 8, 2002

68. Teachers seemed to be the most successful at stopping smoking, perhaps partially due to schools' no-smoking policies. Twice as many teachers were former smokers than were current smokers.
2002 AMA Annual Tobacco Report

69. A summary of the US Public Health Service report Treating Tobacco Use and Dependence: A Clinical Practice Guideline was published in the Journal of the American Medical Association, June 28, 2000, pp. 3244-3254. It details recommendations for brief clinical interventions and intensive interventions in the treatment of tobacco dependence.

70. Smokers with a history of major depression who attempt to stop smoking have a higher risk of failure or relapse than do smokers without depression. In addition, smokers with a history of depression who successfully abstain are at significantly increased risk of developing a new episode of major depression; this risk remains high for at least 6 months after quitting.
The Lancet, June 16, 2001, p. 1929

71. Substantial reductions in hospital admissions can be achieved by interventions to prevent smoking and helping smokers quit. Eliminating smoking would reduce annual rates of all-cause hospitalization among older adults by 8.9% twenty years after baseline.
American Journal of Preventive Medicine 2001; 20: 26-34

72. In a Mayo Clinic comparison of smoking abstinence outcomes between smokers treated in a residential (inpatient) program and an outpatient program, the inpatient group had a 12-month abstinence rate of 45%, almost double the success rate of 23% for the outpatient group.
Mayo Clinic Proceedings, February 2001, p. 124

73. In an era when there is less time available to see each patient, almost 40% of pediatricians and family physicians in a survey felt that talking about smoking cessation with parents was too time consuming.
Archives of Pediatrics and Adolescent Medicine, January 2001, p. 15

# Nicotine Replacement and Pharmacologic Treatment

1. Nicotine patches were used by 5 million Americans and had $1 billion in sales in 1992, the year that they were first marketed.
JAMA, May 26, 1993, p. 2615

2. The 1997 market for smoking cessation products, after the nicotine patch was approved for over the counter sale, is expected to be $500 million to $1 billion, compared with about $250 million in 1996.
Wall Street Journal, June 25, 1997, p. B1

3. The 21- or 22-milligram nicotine patches release about the amount of nicotine that a smoker would get form 10 to 20 cigarettes a day, depending on the brand. 14-milligram patches are roughly equivalent to smoking 5 to 10 cigarettes a day.
San Francisco Chronicle, April 1, 1992, p. D3

4. Three-month nicotine patch therapy, even when used with virtually no behavioral treatment component, can produce one-year sustained abstinence rates of 11%. Though modest, this figure was a solid five-fold increase over placebo patches.
Journal of Smoking-Related Disease 5:183, 1994 (supplement)

5. "Transdermal nicotine is safe and easy to use, has very good compliance, and increases quit rates by a factor of 2.5 even when smokers do not attend concurrent behavior therapy... At 3 months after their quit day, 29% of subject who ever used the patch reported not smoking currently... For these reasons, we believe state health departments, Medicaid, and Medicare programs, and health maintenance organizations should fully reimburse transdermal nicotine for poor smokers. It is ironic that in many states the poor can receive free treatment for non-life-threatening disorders such as otitis media, but can not receive free treatment for a dependence that has a 40% chance of causing their death."
JAMA, July 19, 1995, p. 214 (John Hughes)

6. Even with the aid of nicotine replacement therapy (patch or gum) which can triple the rate of successful smoking cessation, only two to three percent of smokers successfully quit each year.

NEJM, November 25, 1995, p. 1215

7. Smoking abstinence rates were 27% for the active nicotine patch compared to 13% for the placebo patch at the end of 4 to 8 weeks of treatment, and 22% compared to 9% at six months.        JAMA, June 7, 1995, p. 1657

8. A meta-analysis of nicotine replacement therapy found the following one-year effectiveness in achieving abstinence from smoking. For the nicotine patch, 16% (vs. 9% placebo controls); nicotine gum, 19% (11% placebo); and nasal spray, 24% (vs. 11% in the placebo or control population). All these results, while showing only modest effectiveness, were highly clinically significant (p<0.001).  ACP (American College of Physicians) Journal Club, November/December 1996, p. 70

9. In a study from 10 Veterans Affairs Medical Centers, use of transdermal nicotine patches was shown not to cause a significant increase in cardiovascular events in high risk patients with cardiac disease.

NEJM, December 12, 1996, p. 1792

10. Nonprescription over the counter nicotine replacement products are estimated to yield from 114,000 to 304,000 new former smokers annually in the United States. Their use has increased by 152% compared to prior prescription use, and the cost for a three month supply of nicotine patches is $300 to $350.

Tobacco Control, Winter 1997, pp. 306 and 563

11. Actor James Garner, 68, was successful in 1996 in stopping after 55 years of smoking, and now serves as a spokesperson for the Nicotrol brand of nicotine patches.        USA Today, February 14, 1997, p. 2D

12. Nicotine patches help in reducing symptoms in patients with ulcerative colitis, a chronic condition that eventually results in nearly 30% of colitis sufferers having their colons surgically removed. The condition affects 320,000 Americans and results in rectal bleeding, severe diarrhea and cramping. It is much less common in smokers.        Associated Press, March 1, 1997

13. Nicotine NS, a nasal spray delivering one milligram per squirt (about as much as an average cigarette) was approved by the FDA in March 1996.        American Medical News, April 15, 1996

14. A Federal advisory committee has recommended approval of a metered dose oral nicotine inhaler as a fourth alternative source of nicotine for people trying to give up smoking.        Associated Press, December 14, 1996

15. In a study from Iceland, by adding nicotine nasal spray to the nicotine patch, abstinence rates were doubled at 6 months, tripled at 12 months, and remained double at the end of a five year follow up period compared to use of the transdermal nicotine patch alone.

10th World Conference on Tobacco or Health, Beijing, 1997 (Thorsteinn Blondal)

16. In a study from Iceland, use of nicotine nasal spray combined with the nicotine patch was a more effective method of stopping smoking than use of a patch only.        British Medical Journal 1999; 318:285

17. Heavy smokers have plasma cotinine levels averaging 300, although there is wide variability. Nicotine patch replacement therapy requires on average about 44 milligrams a day to attain this cotinine level, or "100% replacement level."

Richard Hurt, M.D., Tenth National Conference on Nicotine Dependence, Minneapolis, October 17, 1997

18. Nicotine patch therapy can increase cognitive function in patients with Alzheimer's disease, and there is some evidence of a protective effect of smoking for the development of Alzheimer's, particularly for people with a strongly positive family history of the disease.        Paul Newhouse, M.D., Tenth National Conference on Nicotine Dependence, Minneapolis, October 17, 1997

19. Nicotine patches can help in children with Tourette's syndrome, which consists of involuntary movements and tics.Paul Newhouse, M.D., Tenth National Conference on Nicotine Dependence, Minneapolis, October 17, 1997

20. "In any event, the absurd irony of the contemporary nicotine regulatory environment must be reversed: new pharmaceutical products currently face a long and expensive marketing approval process, while the most dangerous nicotine-delivery devices ever invented, tobacco products, are introduced and sold without regulatory impediments. In essence, the deck of competition has been stacked heavily in favor of conventional tobacco products. A manufacturer who wishes to introduce a new cherry-flavored smokeless tobacco product does so with no regulatory obstacles. If a pharmaceutical company wants to add mint flavoring to nicotine gum to make it more palatable as a nicotine-replacement product, the company must endure years of expensive regulatory hurdles. At a minimum, rationality recommends comparable treatment of the 2 situations."
   JAMA, October 1, 1997, p. 1091 Kenneth Warner, John Slade, and David Sweanor)

21. The FDA in 1997 approved the antidepressant bupropion (marketed by Glaxo as Zyban) as the first nicotine-free antismoking drug. It appears to reduce the desire for tobacco.             Associated Press, May 16, 1997

22. In a study from the Mayo Clinic on smoking cessation, the antidepressant bupropion at 150 milligrams twice a day for seven weeks, beginning one week before the quit date, was found to be similar in clinical efficacy to nicotine replacement therapy. At the above dose, the rate of smoking cessation was 44% at six weeks and 23% at one year on bupropion (Zyban), compared to 23% and 12.4%, respectively, in the placebo group. The drug was well tolerated, with the most common side effects being headache, dry mouth, and difficulty sleeping. The average weight gain was only 1.5 kilograms, compared with the typical weight gain associated with successful smoking cessation of 3 to 4 kg.             NEJM, October 23, 1997, pp. 1195-1202

23. Zyban sales were $151 million in the United States in 1998, and were expected to increase to $250 million in 1999.             New York Times, March 19, 1999, p. C1

24. In a new approach with 4000 smokers, 40% to 60% remained smoke-free a year after completing a program combining nicotine replacement delivered through patches, gum, nasal spray or inhalers, the antidepressant buproprion (Zyban), and individual counseling. The 40 to 60% success rates compare with 10 to 20% success at one year among smokers who try to quit by using nicotine replacement alone.
   New York Times, March 2, 1999, p. D1

25. In a study from the Mayo Clinic, nicotine patch therapy plus minimal behavioral intervention was ineffective for smoking cessation in adolescent smokers; the 6-month successful abstinence rate was only 5%.
   Archives of Pediatric and Adolescent Medicine, January 2000, p. 35

26. Nicotine replacement via patch, nasal spray, and inhaler are equally effective, but compliance is much higher with the patch.             Archives of Internal Medicine, September 27, 1999, p. 2033

27. Combining nicotine patch therapy with nicotine gum or nasal spray or inhalers, or combining patch with bupropion, may increase smoking cessation rates compared with any single treatment.
   JAMA, January 6, 1999, pp. 72-76

28. Over the counter nicotine patch therapy is effective for smoking cessation; active patch users have double the cessation rates over placebo control subjects in most clinical trials. In a study from the Mayo Clinic of nicotine patch therapy without behavior modification treatment, smoking cessation rates were 18.4% and 11.0% at 12 weeks (end of patch therapy) and 26 weeks, respectively. This compared to 7.0% and 4.2% cessation rates at 12 and 26 weeks in the placebo groups.             American Journal of Public Health, November 1999, pp. 1701-1706

29. Nicotine inhalers delivering 4 milligrams of nicotine per cartridge were introduced in late 1998 to join nicotine patches, sprays, and gum in the $725 million a year nicotine replacement industry.
   San Francisco Chronicle, September 9, 1998

30. A smoking vaccine is in development; it is a nicotine derivative attached to a large protein that works by preventing nicotine from reaching the brain.                    *Respiratory Reviews*, March 2001, p. 17

31. Clinical trials began in 2001 on a nicotine addiction vaccine which would stop nicotine from crossing the blood-brain barrier. The nicotine molecule is too small by itself to generate an immune response, so it is bound to cholera vaccine. The combined molecule generates circulating anti-nicotine antibodies that render nicotine too large to effectively pass the blood-brain barrier, and preventing or blunting the nicotine "hit" that smokers get.
                    2002 AMA Annual Tobacco Report

32. In 1999, smokers spent $730 million on smoking cessation products such as nicotine patches and gum.
                    *Cigarettes* (Parker-Pope), p. 139

33. With or without nicotine replacement therapy, most withdrawal symptoms disappear within three to four weeks.
                    *Reducing Tobacco Use*, p. 117

34. "A review of tobacco industry documents written in the 1980's and 1990's alleged that ties between the industry and pharmaceutical companies may have led to a scaling back of the marketing of such smoking cessation products as nicotine gum and patches…One case study demonstrated how tobacco companies pressured drug companies to scale back the smoking cessation educational materials and resources that had accompanied the nicotine gum, Nicorette."                    *American Medical News*, September 9, 2002, p. 26

35. Methoxsalen, a medication used to treat psoriasis, may help a smoker light up less by partially blocking the body's ability to metabolize nicotine.                    *JAMA*, August 16, 2000, p. 822

36. In a study from California, there was no significant benefit from nicotine replacement therapy (NRT) in either the short or long term for smoking cessation for the nearly 60% of California smokers classified as light smokers (less than 15 cigarettes per day). The study concluded that "since becoming available over the counter, NRT appears no longer effective in increasing long-term successful cessation in California smokers."
                    *JAMA* September 11, 2002, p. 1260

37. Oral nicotine inhalers are effective in long term reduction in smoking.
                    *British Medical Journal* 2000; 321: 329-333

38. A low-dose nicotine patch may be useful in treating Tourette's syndrome.
                    *American Medical News*, March 20, 2000, p. 33

39. The FDA has prevented the sale of NicoWater, water laced with nicotine that was billed as a "refreshing break to the smoking habit." The FDA also in 2002 ordered nicotine-laced lip balm and lollipops off the market, calling them unapproved drugs that had enough nicotine to endanger children lured by their resemblance to candy.                    *San Francisco Chronicle*, July 3, 2002

40. In a study reported in the August 2002 issue of *Chest* (p. 403) the anti-depressant drug Nortriptyline significantly increased the smoking cessation rate in chronic smokers.

41. In a study from New York, of seven smokers who went through a single session of breathing nitrous oxide, or laughing gas, four were successful in quitting a month later.                    *Associated Press*, May 18, 2000

42. Acupuncture can be of benefit in smoking cessation.
                    *American Journal of Public Health*, October 2002, p. 1642

43. Bupropion is associated with a relatively high risk, 3% to 4%, of allergic skin rashes. There are also case reports of erythema multiforme and serum sickness associated with the use of the antidepressant.
                    *Mayo Clinic Proceedings*, June 2001, p. 664

44. "Big Tobacco Pressured Drug Companies To Soften Quit-Smoking Message" According to tobacco industry documents, from 1982 through 1992, tobacco companies used coercion and economic intimidation to muffle aggressive anti-smoking messages by the makers of cessation products, such as the nicotine patch or gum. In 1984, Phillip Morris canceled chemical purchases from Dow Chemical after one of Dow's subsidiaries, Merrell Dow, introduced Nicorette and prepared literature for doctors' offices urging smokers to quit. Dow Chemical eventually got the Philip Morris account back, but only after Dow assured Philip Morris it was "committed to avoiding contributions to the anti-cigarette effort," and Merrell Dow president David Sharrock informed tobacco executives that he would personally begin to "screen advertising and promotional materials to eliminate any inflammatory anti-industry statements."                    quote from news summary regarding the article
"Big Tobacco Threatened Drug Manufacturers With Reprisal"
by Myron Levin in Los Angeles Times, February 14, 1999

45. Nicotine replacement products are promoting a manner certain to minimize conflict with cigarette manufactures... for at least a decade (from 1982 to 1992), Philip Morris sought to intimidate drug firms marketing the stop-smoking products, using the threat of economic reprisals to make them tone down their ads and refrain from supporting the anti-smoking cause, according to once-secret documents..." Internal memos showed that the cigarette industry threatened to cancel supply contracts with the corporate parents of the drug firms. The February 14, 1999 article by Myron Levin in the Los Angeles Times gives details of the tobacco industry's successful efforts to water down the anti-smoking message by Merrell Dow and Ciba-Geigy in their marketing campaigns for nicotine replacement products. The National Association of State Fire Marshals received $50,000 a year from Philip Morris for "administrative expenses." The tobacco industry for decades has courted firefighters to weaken their support for the manufacture and regulation of fire-safe cigarettes.
Baltimore Sun, February 16, 1999, p. 287

# Weight Gain

1. The average smoker is 2.4 to 4.0 kg (5.8 to 9.6 pounds) lighter than the average nonsmoker. Past smokers have a 33% higher prevalence of obesity by comparison with their currently smoking siblings.
Archives of Internal Medicine, November 8, 1993, p. 2457

2. 79% of smokers who quit do gain some weight. Smoking generally suppresses body weight below "normal", and smoking cessation allows weight to return to this normal level.                    *Nicotine Addiction*, p. 344

3. The average weight gain associated with the cessation of smoking is 4.4 kg (9.7 lbs) for men and 5.0 kg (11 lbs) for women.                    NEJM, November 2, 1995, p. 1215

4. The average woman who successfully quits smoking gains 8 pounds, and the average man, about 6 pounds, a weight gain associated with minimal health risk. The ex-smoker would have to gain 60 to 80 pounds to counteract the health benefits of quitting.
Time, March 25, 1991, p. 55 and Journal of Respiratory Disease, May 1993, p. 636

5. The health risks of a modest weight gain after cessation are insignificant compared to the health risks of continued smoking.                    New York Times, September 14, 1995, p. A11

6. The health risk of smoking one pack per day is equal to being 100 pounds overweight. A smoker would have to gain more than 100 pounds after quitting to equal the health risk of heavy smoking.
Journal of Family Practice, Vol. 34, No. 6, 1992, p. 691

7. Smoking cessation is associated with a net excess weight gain of about 2.4 kilograms (6 pounds) in middle-aged women. However, this weight gain is minimized if smoking cessation is accompanied by a moderate increase in the level of physical activity.                    American Journal of Public Health, July 1995, p. 999

8. Smoking cessation interventions that promote dieting to control weight have not been successful in preventing cessation-related weight gain.                    Annals of Behavioral Medicine 1995; 17:234

9. Increased metabolic rate explains at least some of smokers' leaner body weights. Smoking increases metabolic rate by approximately 2 to 10 percent. However, an increased metabolic rate doesn't account for the total difference in body weight between the average smoker and the average non-smoker. Overall, smoking-induced metabolic rate increases are thought to account for about half of the difference. Another likely mechanism is that smoking alters the body-weight set point – the weight toward which a person tends to return despite vigorous attempts to gain or lose weight. This means that the changes in caloric intake that occur with changes in smoking status are actually secondary to a change in the regulation of body weight around a different set point. Experts believe that smoking cessation returns the set point to normal.     Quote from *Cigarettes*, p. 137

10. "Smoking tobacco…can make people thinner by raising metabolism and deadening the senses of taste and smell and, hence, the urge to eat."                                               San Francisco Chronicle, April 16, 1997

11. Smoking appears to augment satiety from food, but does not change the metabolic rate. After quitting, intake increases by 400 calories per day on average. Dieting and rigid weight control efforts increase the risk for relapse, and are not recommended during the initial cessation phase. Nicotine replacement therapy may delay, but does not eliminate, this weight gain                                               J. Taylor Hays, M.D., workshop, Tenth National Conference on Nicotine Dependence, Minneapolis, October 17, 1997

12. A June 15, 1997 article "Hooked on Smoking, Hooked on Thinness" in the Washington Post reported on a poll which indicated that four out of ten smokers who want to stop, say that they would not quit smoking if it meant that they would gain more than five pounds. One in four (more women than men) said that they would not stop if it meant gaining any weight at all. In fact, two thirds of all quitters do gain more than five pounds, and 20 to 30% gain more than 15 pounds.

13. In a study in the Archives of Internal Medicine, women who exercised vigorously while trying to quit smoking gained only about half the weight of those who did not exercise.               Associated Press, June 18, 1999

14. "On average, cigarette smokers weigh 4kg less than nonsmokers, and when smokers quit, their body weight increases, on average, that amount."                               *Nicotine Safety and Toxicity*, p. 11 (Neal Benowitz)

15. Vigorous exercise facilitates smoking cessation in women as well as reducing weight gain, when the exercise is combined with a behavioral smoking cessation program.     Archives of Internal Medicine 1999; 159: 1229-1234

16. A study of young adults by researchers at the University of Memphis Prevention Center found minimal evidence of a weight control benefit from smoking, disputing widespread perceptions, particularly among young people, that smoking controls weight. American Psychological Association press release, November 22, 1998

17. Dieting while trying to stop smoking significantly worsens outcomes, and it is recommended not to attempt caloric restriction until several months after successfully stopping smoking.
CA-A Cancer Journal for Clinicians, May/June 2000, p. 147

# Health Benefits of Quitting

1. Smoking cessation even after many years of the habit has immediate positive health benefits. The risk of coronary heart disease is reduced 10 to 15 years following cessation to that of lifelong nonsmokers. A lifelong smoker who quits at age 50 reduces by 50% his or her chances of dying before age 65. One year after quitting, half of the excess heart disease risk is gone.
*The Health Benefits of Smoking Cessation*, 1990 Surgeon General report

2. Male smokers who quit between ages 35 to 39 add an average of 5 years to their lives; female quitters in this age group add 3 years. Even lifelong smokers (male and female) who quit at age 65 to 70 increase their life expectancy by one year.                                               1990 Surgeon General report

3. Ten years after quitting, the death rate of former smokers declines to about the same as those who never smoked. 1990 Surgeon General report

4. Smoking cessation would increase overall life expectancy by 2.4 to 4.4 years among men, and from 2.6 to 3.7 years among women. Archives of Internal Medicine, August 8, 1994, p. 1697

5. "On stopping smoking, former smokers removed one-third of the excess risk of total coronary heart disease incidence within 2 years of cessation. The risk among former smokers declines to the level of never-smokers during the interval of 10 to 14 years following cessation. The risk of total stroke incidence among former smokers approaches the level of never-smoker during the interval of 2 to 4 years following cessation." *Changes in Cigarette-Related Disease Risks*, p. 562

6. One third of the excess coronary artery disease risk in smokers is eliminated within two years after smoking cessation. Within 3 to 5 years after stopping smoking, the risk of myocardial infarction in former smokers declines to almost the level of those who have never smoked. Mayo Clinic Proceedings, March 1998, p. 292

7. The years of life gained for a two pack a day smoker who quits are 7.84 years for a 30 year old, 4.88 years for a 50 year old, and 1.13 years for a 70 year old. Wall Street Journal, February 27, 1998, p. B1

8. A study from Canada concluded that stopping smoking, even after lung cancer has developed, can lengthen survival. Two years after treatment of lung cancer, 28% of nonsmokers were still alive, compared to 16% of patients who continued to smoke. After five years, 9% of nonsmokers survived, compared to only 4% of smokers. The reason why stopping smoking during lung cancer treatment can be beneficial is not known. San Francisco Chronicle, May 19, 2002 (from the New York Times)

9. Stopping smoking, even after lung cancer has developed, can lengthen survival, a study from London, Ontario has found. Similar benefits were shown in an earlier study involving head and neck cancers. New York Times, May 19, 2002, p. 19

10. For patients with congestive heart failure, smoking cessation is at least as effective, and perhaps more so, in reducing mortality as is treatment with beta-blocker drugs or angiotensin-converting enzyme inhibitors. Journal of the American College Of Cardiology 2001; 37: 1677-1682

11. As soon as you snuff out that last cigarette, your body will begin a series of physiological changes:
   - Within 20 minutes: Blood pressure, body temperature and pulse rate will drop to normal.
   - Within eight hours: Smoker's breath disappears. The carbon monoxide level in blood drops, and the oxygen level rises to normal.
   - Within 24 hours: Chance of heart attack decreases.
   - Within 48 hours: Nerve endings start to regroup. Ability to taste and smell improves.
   - Within three days: Breathing is easier.
   - Within two to three months: Circulation improves. Walking becomes easier. Lung capacity increases up to 30 percent.
   - Within one to nine months: Sinus congestion and shortness of breath decrease. Cilia that sweep debris from your lungs grow back. Energy increases.
   - Within one year: Excess risk of coronary heart disease is half that of a person who smokes.
   - Within two years: Heart attack risk drops to near normal.
   - Within five years: Lung cancer death rate for average former pack-a-day smoker decreases by almost half. Stroke risk is reduced. Risk of mouth, throat and esophageal cancer is half that of a smoker.
   - Within 10 years: Lung cancer death rate is similar to that of a person who does not smoke. The precancerous cells are replaced.
   - Within 15 years: Risk of coronary heart disease is the same as a person who has never smoked.
     data from American Cancer Society reported in Ann Landers column, August 6, 2001

12. In the first year after quitting, weight gain averages 4.9kg for men and 5.2kg for women. British Medical Association (www.tobaccofactfile.org)

13. Smokers tend to be overly optimistic about their chances of quitting, particularly women and younger smokers. "Slightly more than half expected to stop smoking within two years, but the odds are that only 6% will do so... More than 80% of smokers wished that they had never started."

Wellness Letter (University of California Berkeley), October 2002

14. The FDA is investigating the legality of over the counter (non-prescription) sales of nicotine-laced lollipops with names such as likatine and nicostop.

Time, April 15, 2002, p. 62

15. In 2003, only four states have designated funding for tobacco prevention programs at a level that meets the CDC's minimum recommendation. They are Maine, Maryland, Minnesota, and Mississippi.

CA-A Cancer Journal for Clinicians, March-April 2003, p. 68

16. The "5 A's" for doctors seeing patients who smoke:

| | |
|---|---|
| ASK: | Identify tobacco users at every medical visit. |
| ADVISE: | Urge all users to quit. |
| ASSESS: | Determine willingness to make "quit attempt." |
| ASSIST: | Aid the patient with a plan. |
| ARRANGE: | Schedule follow up contact. |

17. Since the launch of an anti-smoking campaign in California in 1989, the number of smokers has dropped by 21%, and lung cancer cases by 14%. This contrasts with a nationwide drop in lung cancer of only 2.7% in the same time period.

Time, December 11, 2000, p. 41

JAMA is Journal of the American Medical Association
NEJM is New England Journal of Medicine

# CHAPPTER 23
# TOBACCO, ALCOHOL AND ILLICIT DRUGS

1.  Tobacco kills more Americans every week than cocaine, crack, heroin, and illicit "hard drugs" do in an entire year.

2.  "Although tobacco kills nearly 500,000 Americans every year, the federal government spends only about $100 million a year on tobacco control. Yet it spends $12 billion to fight illicit drug use, which is responsible for only 10,000 to 20,000 deaths a year." There is $2.5 billion allocated for AIDS (34,000 deaths) and $300 million for alcohol abuse (105,000 deaths).                    JAMA, May 11, 1994, p. 1390 (Stanton Glantz)

3.  About 9000 deaths a year in the US are attributed to illicit use of drugs. If indirectly related factors such as homicides, accidents, infections with HIV, and hepatitis are added, the total rises to about 20,000 per year.
                                                JAMA, November 10, 1993, p. 2207

4.  The Premier "smokeless cigarette" developed by RJ Reynolds can be used as a delivery device for crack cocaine. Partly because of this adverse publicity, it was never put on the market.
                                                JAMA, January 6, 1989, p. 41

5.  98% of people who have used both cocaine and cigarettes smoked cigarettes first. Cigarette smoking is likely to precede the use of alcohol or illegal drugs, and illegal drug use is rare among those who have never smoked. Virtually all illegal drug users had previously used cigarettes, alcohol, or both.
                                *Preventing Tobacco Use Among Young People*, 1994 Surgeon General report, p. 35

6.  Of adolescents in inpatient substance abuse treatment facilities, 85% were also smokers. About 90% of adult alcoholics also smoke cigarettes.                                Pediatrics, April 1994, p. 561

7.  In a study of cocaine-dependent patients enrolled in drug abuse treatment, the prevalence of smoking was 75%
                                                JAMA, December 14, 1994, p. 1724

8.  Of teens who smoke, 88% also are drinkers, 45% have used marijuana, 33% used smokeless tobacco, and 11% used cocaine.        *Preventing Tobacco Use Among Young People*, 1994 Surgeon General report, p. 87

9.  Among adolescents who have never smoked, only 3% had binged (had 5 or more drinks in a row) in the last month, whereas nearly 40% of daily smokers in the 12- to 17-year-old age group had binged in the previous month.                                        1994 Surgeon General report, p. 35

10. According to the 1994 Surgeon General's report 12-17 year olds who smoke were three times more likely to use alcohol, eight times more likely to smoke marijuana, and 22 times more likely to use cocaine, compared to nonsmokers of the same age.
                        American Lung Association Fact Sheet--Teenage Cigarette Smoking (August 1997 Update)

11. 92% of adolescent marijuana smokers also smoke cigarettes.                National Institute on Drug Abuse

12. The National Institute of Drug Abuse, National Household Survey on Drug Abuse reports that smokers between the ages of 12 and 17 are 23 times more likely to use marijuana, 12 times more likely to use heroin, 51 times more likely to use cocaine and 57 times more likely to use crack. Tobacco use thus serves as a gateway drug for later illegal narcotic use.                        Baltimore Sun, March 11, 1994, p. 12A

13. Children ages 12 to 17 who smoke have a risk 14 times greater of having an alcohol abuse problem than their nonsmoking peers.                        Audio Digest Internal Medicine, May 17, 1995 (J. Kirchner)

14. A child who smokes more than 15 cigarettes a day is more than twice as likely to use an illicit drug and 16 times more likely to use cocaine that one who smokes but on less than a daily basis. They are 10 times more likely to use an illicit drug and 104 times more likely to use cocaine than someone who never smokes. Adults

who started smoking as children are three times more likely to use marijuana and four times more likely to use cocaine, compared to adults who did not smoke during childhood.

*Cigarettes, Alcohol, Marijuana: Gateways to Illicit Drug Use, Center on Addiction and Substance Abuse at Columbia University, October 1994*

15. The relative risk of alcoholism among smokers is estimated to be 10 times that of nonsmokers. Cirrhosis of the liver is three times more common among alcoholics who also smoke. And pancreatitis is increased ten-fold among alcoholics who smoke compared to those who do not. It is hypothesized that cyanide from cigarette smoke is toxic to the pancreas and that alcohol interferes with its detoxification.

*Nicotine Addiction*, pp. 311 and 313

16. 90% of adolescent smokeless tobacco users also drink alcohol. 31% of smokeless tobacco users also smoke marijuana, and 7% use cocaine. For this reason, smokeless tobacco as well as cigarettes is often considered a "gateway" drug.                                 1994 Surgeon General report, p. 102

17. Over 85% of alcoholics also smoke. The combined cost to society of alcohol abuse and tobacco exceed $140 billion annually in the United States.                    Tobacco Control, Winter 1993, p. 520

18. The relative risk of alcoholism is increased ten-fold among smokers, and the percentage of heavier smokers who develop problems with alcohol might be greater than 30%.             1994 Surgeon General report, p. 36

19. The "war on drugs" budget proposed for 1996 was $14.6 billion, including $9.3 billion for the effort to cut off the flow of drugs into the country. Money for tobacco control is less than one percent of this amount.

Contra Costa Times, February 15, 1995, p. 13A

20. Federal government expenditures for drug control increased from $1.8 billion in 1981 to $6.6 billion in 1990, $12 billion in 1993, and $18 billion in 1998.

21. Both cofounders of Alcoholics Anonymous, Bill Wilson and Dr. Bob Smith, died from their tobacco use; Wilson from emphysema, and Smith, a cigar smoker, from throat cancer.

Professional Counselor, December 1996

22. In 1965, 90% of male alcoholics in the Untied States were smokers compared to 60% of men in the general population. In 1990, 82% of male alcoholics smoked, compared to 33% of adult men overall. Heavy smokers (more than 20 cigarettes, or one pack per day) comprise 9% of the general population, but 72% of alcoholics are heavy smokers. 35% of heavy smokers have a lifetime history of alcoholism, including 13% with current alcoholism. There is evidence that smoking cessation does not increase relapse to alcoholism; successful alcohol quitters are more likely to be successful in smoking cessation.             John Hughes, M.D., Tenth National Conference on Nicotine Dependence, Minneapolis, October 17, 1997

23. A bumper sticker on a pickup truck in Virginia says "Tobacco money paid for this vehicle" pasted next to another bumper sticker "Say No To Drugs."             Washington Post magazine, October 25, 1992, p. 24

24. Smoking teens were 17 times more likely to use marijuana, 26.5% compared to 1.5% of nonsmokers. Cocaine use was reported in 3.5% of smokers and less than 0.5% of nonsmokers.             Associated Press, May 15, 1995

25. Teenage smokers were more than twice as likely to have carried a gun, knife, or club in the last month, 26% vs. 10%. For girls, the difference was 11% for smokers vs. 2.6% for nonsmokers. 80% of the teen smokers had had sexual intercourse, compared with 41% of nonsmokers.             Associated Press, May 15, 1995

26. More Colombians are killed every year from American cigarettes than there are Americans killed by Colombian cocaine.             Scientific American, May 1995, p. 51

27. More than 40% of patients who leave chemical dependency treatments sober later die of a tobacco-related disease.             *Tobacco and Health*, p. 777

28. For every one person who dies from a heroin overdose, 90 die from tobacco-related disease.

Tobacco Free Youth monograph, Rick Kropp, p. 50

29. A study from the Mayo Clinic of alcoholics showed that tobacco-related causes of death accounted for 50.9% of the deaths, and alcohol-related conditions accounted for 34%. Many of the patients conquered their alcoholism, only to die of nicotine dependence. 75% of the alcoholics were smokers, and at 20 years, their observed overall mortality was 48% versus an expected 18.5%.

JAMA, April 10, 1996, p. 1097

30. Alcohol consumption has an enormous synergetic effect on the risk for developing esophageal cancer among cigarette smokers.

*Cigarettes*, p. xiii

31. Cocaine addicts in treatment tend to find cigarettes harder to give up than cocaine.

JAMA, February 10, 1989, p. 898

32. A lower fraction of smokers even than of heroin addicts have successfully quit.

JAMA, September 25, 1996, p. 998

33. In the United States, each year illicit drugs lead to about 11,000 deaths, direct government expenditures of $27 billion (1991 data), and over half a million drug-related hospital emergency visits. In addition, nearly 900,000 people receive drug-related rehabilitation treatment each year, and law enforcement results in more than one million arrests.

JAMA, March 18, 1996, p. 827

34. Marijuana smokers get about four times as much tar in their lungs per puff as tobacco smokers. About one quarter of people who smoke three to four marijuana cigarettes a day have chronic bronchitis, slightly less bronchitis than is seen in a pack-a-day cigarette smokers.

Washington Post National Weekly Edition, December 9-15, 1996, p. 35

35. "Not a single death has ever been credibly attributed directly to smoking or consuming marijuana in the 5000 years of the plant's recorded use."

Atlantic Monthly, August 1994, p. 48 (E. Schlosser)

36. "…the quarter century since large numbers of Americans began to use marijuana has produced remarkably little laboratory or epidemiological evidence of serious health damage done by the drug."

American Journal of Public Health, April 1997, p. 585 (Mark Kleiman)

37. "Marijuana is unique among illegal drugs in its political symbolism, its safety, and its wide use. More than 65 million Americans have tried marijuana, the use of which is not associated with increased mortality."

NEJM, August 7, 1997, p. 435 (George Annas)

38. In a survey from Austria, more than 90% of former heroin addicts were smokers already prior to opiate dependence.

Abstract PO56, 10th World Conference on Tobacco or Health, Beijing, 1997

39. 40 times as many Americans die from tobacco as from the use of all illegal drugs combined.

World Watch, July-August 1997, p. 23

43. In his ABC radio program on January 15, 1998, Dr. Dean Edell stated that if he had to choose between being addicted to alcohol, cigarettes, marijuana, cocaine, or heroin, he would choose heroin as the least harmful to his health of this group. (This assumed that the supply was pure and was available legally without having to resort to crime to obtain.)

44. Smoking marijuana increases the heart rate by 40 beats per minute, and causes an increase in blood pressure when recumbent. A middle-aged person's risk of a heart attack increases nearly five-fold in the first hour after smoking marijuana.

New York Times, March 3, 2000 (from American Heart Association conference in San Diego)

45. Between 80 and 95% of alcoholics also smoke cigarettes, a rate three times higher than the general population. And about 70% of alcoholics are heavy smokers, more than a pack a day, compared with only 10% of the general population.                                    Alcohol Alert newsletter, January 1998

46. Recovering alcoholics often receive less than optimal tobacco cessation counseling out of fear that attempts to stop smoking might jeopardize their sobriety. However, recent research does not support this idea, and instead suggests that smoking cessation may actually enhance abstinence from alcohol.
American Family Physician, April 15, 1998, p. 1869

47. Teenagers who smoke were 11.4 times more likely to use illicit drugs and 16 times more likely to drink heavily than nonsmokers in the 12 to 17 year old age group.          1998 National Household Survey on Drug Abuse

48. 1999 "drug war" expenditures were $18 billion, and drug czar Barry McCaffrey estimated 14,000 deaths from illicit drugs.

49. About 9% of marijuana users become dependent, compared to 15% of drinkers who become dependent on alcohol.                                               Time, November 4, 2002, p. 64

50. 9% of the U.S. population regularly smokes marijuana. 16% of eighth graders, 32% of tenth graders, and 37% of high school seniors have tried pot, and it is no longer a pathway to more serious addiction or "hard drugs." In the 1960's, marijuana users moved on to hard drugs 20% of the time; in the 1970's and 1980's, the progression to hard drugs decreased to only 6%.                    NBC evening news (Tom Brokaw), May 14, 2001

51. Former Surgeon General C. Everett Koop, 86 years old in 2003, urged the nation's drug czar to focus on "the burden of abuse of legal drugs like tobacco and alcohol instead of concentrating solely on illicit drugs." He said in an address to addiction specialists: "What is the difference between a drug lord in Columbia, his lieutenant in Miami, or an executive of a cigarette company? None...they are the real terrorists."
Reuters Health, February 12, 2003

52. In a study released in Australia, tobacco, alcohol and illicit drugs were responsible for about 8.9% of the total global burden of disease in 2000. Tobacco was responsible for 71% of the total drug-related deaths in 2000, 4.9 million total, and accounted for 61.2% of the costs to society of drugs. Alcohol accounted for 26% of drug-related deaths, 1.8 million worldwide total, and 22% of total costs; illicit drugs caused 223,000 deaths, 3% of the total, and accounted for 17% of total drug-related costs to society.
New York Time and Reuters, February 25, 2003 and British Medical Journal, February 1, 2002, p. 242

53. From Doonesbury, Garry Trudeau, February 2, 2003, where Mr. Butts is talking to Mr. Jay, the marijuana cigarette: "So how about you? How many did you kill? Uh.none. None? Zippo. The only thing that I caused was 735,000 arrests."

54. Yearly U.S. arrests for marijuana possession are 641,000, and another 82,000 arrests for marijuana sale.
Dean Edell, M.D., ABC radio, February 12, 2003

# CHAPTER 24
# WOMEN AND SMOKING

## Historical

1. American women began to smoke in great numbers shortly after the country became independent. A 1799 pamphlet in Massachusetts blamed the rise in fires on "the smoking of cigars by women in bed."
San Francisco Chronicle, January 19, 1997, p. 7

2. English women of high social class began to smoke cigarettes in public in the 1880's, and in 1906, English railroad officials adopted special smoking cars for women. At about this time, the "new spirit of liberation" spread to upper class women in the United States, including Alice Roosevelt Longworth, daughter of T.R.
Tobacco Advertising, p. 212

3. In the early 1900's, smoking by female school teachers was considered grounds for dismissal. In 1910, Alice Roosevelt Longworth, President Roosevelt's daughter, was scolded for smoking in the White House and retorted she would smoke on the roof. She would later appear in an advertisement for Lucky Strikes. The first images of women in cigarette ads appeared in 1919. First Lady Eleanor Roosevelt smoked in public in the 1930's.
NY State Journal of Medicine, July 1985, p. 335

4. In 1910 a picture of Alice Roosevelt Longworth, TR's daughter, appeared on the front page of the Woman's Daily, as she was accused of the dastardly act of smoking in public. In 1927, society had changed, and she posed for an ad for Luckies.
Tobacco Advertising, p. 218

5. The first ad showing women smoking was in 1919 for Helmar's cigarettes.
Tobacco in History, p. 107

6. Lucy Page Gaston in 1899 founded the Anti-Cigarette League with the goal of "Abolition of the Cigarette in America." She campaigned tirelessly until her death in 1924. Cigarette consumption in the Untied States had increased fifty-fold between 1899 and 1924.
Tobacco Advertising, p. 205

7. The first cigarettes marked specifically to women appeared between 1910 and the early 1920's. They included Milo violets, Blue Peter, Ulissa, Gold Tip, and Marlboro.
Tobacco Advertising, p. 221-223

8. Advertising genius Albert Lasker in 1922 was hired to boost sales for the American Tobacco Co. After the suggestion "Get women to smoke, and you'll double your market," he hired actresses and opera sopranos to endorse Lucky Strikes. For women worried about their weight, he coined the slogan "Reach for Lucky Instead of a Sweet." Lucky Strikes sales increased by 312% in the following year.
US News and World Report, March 7, 1994, p. 21 and NEJM, November 19, 1987, p. 1343

9. In 1924 women accounted for only 5% of national cigarette consumption. This rose to 12% by 1929.
Tobacco in History, p. 106

10. "Women - when they smoke at all - quickly develop discriminating taste…That is why Marlboros now ride in so many limousines, attend so many bridge parties, repose in so many hand bags."
1927 ad for Marlboro, a new women's cigarette

11. In 1929 a US senator declared: "Not since the days when the vendor of harmful nostrums was swept from our streets, has this country witnessed such an orgy of buncombe, quackery and downright falsehood and fraud as now marks the current campaign promoted by certain cigarette manufacturers to create a vast woman and child market."
Preventing Tobacco Use Among Young People, 1994 Surgeon General report, p. 166

12. In the 1920's tobacco companies viewed the prospective female market as "opening a new gold mine right in our front yard." The American Tobacco Company promoted cigarettes as "symbols of freedom," and organized women in the 1929 New York Easter parade to carry placards identifying their cigarettes as "torches

of liberty."

13. In 1929 a band of glamorous Manhattan debutantes marched down Fifth Avenue in the New York Easter Day parade. They brandished "torches of freedom" – Lucky Strike cigarettes. This was a public relations coup for the American Tobacco Company.                        Harvard Magazine, July-August 1996, p. 19

14. "At a time when women rarely smoked in public, (public relations guru Edward) Bernays arranged for 19 pretty debutantes to march up Fifth Avenue in New York's 1929 Easter Parade while smoking cigarettes. The women waved their cigarettes, proclaiming them 'torches of liberty,' an image that was captured by photographers and displayed in newspapers around the world. The strategy worked. By 1931, women accounted for 14 percent of U.S. tobacco consumption, up from just 5 percent in 1924."

*Cigarettes* (Parker-Pope), p. 86

15. In 1930, actress Constance Talmadge in an American Tobacco ad said, "Light a Lucky, and you'll never miss sweets that make you fat." Another ad showed a fat woman with the slogan "When Tempted To Overindulge, Reach for a Lucky Instead."                        *They Satisfy*, p. 101

16. "Women, because their throats are more delicate than men's, particularly appreciate...relief from the hot smoke of parched dry-as-dust tobacco, and are switching to Camels everywhere."

Text from a color ad on the back cover of the January 8, 1932 issue
of the Harvard Alumni Bulletin, depicting a young woman clutching skates and a pack of Camels.

17. The US Tobacco Journal reported in 1950: "A massive potential market still exists among women and young adults, cigarette industry leaders agreed, acknowledging that recruitment of these millions of prospective smokers comprises the major objective for the immediate future and on a long basis as well."

1994 Surgeon General report, p. 166

18. In 1968 with its introduction of Virginia Slims, Philip Morris had an ad depicting a Victorian-era scene with a girl in an old-fashioned bathing suit saying, "Just you wait. Someday we'll be able to wear any bathing suit we what. Someday we'll be able to vote. Someday we'll be able to smoke just like any man. Someday we'll even have our own cigarette."                        *Ashes to Ashes*, p. 316

19. In the late 1960's, cigarette advertisements in women's magazines increased rapidly, particularly the "You've come a long way, baby" campaign for the new Virginia Slims brand. By 1973, smoking rates in girls younger than age 17 had increased by 110% from 1967 levels, white initiation rates in women 18 or older remained unchanged. "Tobacco advertising plays an important role in encouraging young people to begin this lifelong addiction before they are old enough to fully appreciate its long-term health risks."

JAMA, February 23, 1994, p. 611

20. In 1968, Philip Morris introduced the Virginia Slims brand with a major promotional campaign targeting young females. Between 1968 and 1974, the proportion of teenage girls smoking cigarettes nearly doubled from 8.4% to 15.3%.                        Journal of Public Health Policy, Winter 1987, p. 500

21. From 1967 to 1975, billions of dollars of sales accumulated for Virginia Slims, Silva, and Eve. These were all new brands, which went from nothing in 1967 to $16 billion in 1976 sales.

"...from 1967, coinciding with the new ad campaigns targeting young girls, the girls 11 to 17 years old showed a sudden, large rise. The jump was 110 percent in 12-year-olds; 75 percent among 15-year-olds; 55 percent among 16-year-olds; and 35 percent among 17-year-olds. Those over age 17 showed no increase, but instead the steady decline continued. So the ad blitz targeting girls either was fantastically successful, if the companies were aiming at girls 17 and under, or the campaign was a complete disaster, missing altogether the company's stated target of young adults over 21."                        *Smokescreen*, p. 69

22. One of the early Virginia Slims models was Cheryl Tiegs, who went on to become a well-known fashion model. In 1989, an American advertising account executive for a leading brand said, "We try to tap the emerging independence and self-fulfillment of women, to make smoking a badge to express that. The irony

today, however, is that the women who are the most emancipated in terms of education and career are those least likely to smoke."

Quote from Smoke and Mirrors, p. 177

# General

1.  "Cigarette ads promise emancipation, whereas in reality smoking is yet another form of bondage for women."
    Judith Mackay, M.D. (The Doctor-Activist, Ellen Bassak, 1996, p. 42)

2.  Tobacco advertising links smoking with women's emancipation and achievement of equality with men. Themes like "You've come a long way, baby" and the introduction of a new cigarette "For women who know the meaning of free" testify to the continuing marketing appeal of stressing independence and equal right to enjoyment.
    NEJM, November 19, 1987, p. 1343

3.  Currently, about 12% of women smoke worldwide, compared to 42% of men. But the World Health Organization estimates that the prevalence of female smoking will rise to 20% by the year 2025 based on current trends. The number of women smokers will increase from the current 187 million to about 532 million in 2025, 80% of whom will live in developing countries. And lung cancer, now the fifth leading cause of cancer deaths among women in the world, will become the number one cause, as it already is for men (and American women).
    American Medical News, August 10, 1998, p. 20

4.  The tobacco companies say that their advertising is not aimed at attracting new smokers, but only to get established smokers to switch to their brand. In 1984 Virginia Slims was introduced to Hong Kong, where only 1% of women smoked. It was clearly targeted at young women, with the usual images of beauty, slimness, and desirability, combined with clear messages of emancipation. But because so few women in Hong Kong smoked, the number who could brand switch was negligible, and the expensive advertising blitz seemed to be a clear attempt to create a new market. The same type of promotion aimed at women is seen in many developing countries, where currently only an average of 5% of women are smokers.
    Thorax 1991; 46:153

5.  A columnist noted in Vogue magazine a mini-catalogue of upbeat fashion items from "Virginia Slims Promotional Services." She remarked: "Maybe they ought to drop the stuff about fetal death and lung cancer and go with something like 'WARNING: Smoking cigarettes dramatically reduces the glamour value of your clothes and forces you to take them to the cleaners more often, which can damage the fabric.' Millions would quit tomorrow."
    Ann Conway, LA Times, March 4, 1994, p. E1

6.  In February 1994, Josephine Camel made her debut in multi-page spreads in major magazines. "It's a reckless and dangerous campaign to lure more young female smokers into the fatal confines of Joe's place."
    Sidney Wolfe, Public Citizen

7.  For a given number of cigarettes smoked in a lifetime, women may run twice the risk that men smokers do for developing lung cancer.
    Associated Press, September 22, 1993

8.  The executive director of a major women's organization commented: "Philip Morris is probably (our) first corporate contributor… Politics is about taking care of the people who have been with you since the beginning, and they have.
    Tobacco Use, p. 29

9.  By interfering with the body's production of estrogen, smoking increases a woman's risk for fractures and for osteoporosis by making her bones less dense. If a woman smokes a pack a day, by the time she reaches menopause, her bones will be 5% to 10% less dense than they otherwise would have been.
    American Medical News, March 7, 1994

10. Women who smoke a pack a day have a 5-10% deficit in bone mass by the time they reach menopause. Teenage girls who smoke have a lower bone mineral density than similar-aged girls who don't smoke.
    Cigarettes, p. 63

11. Smoking lowers estrogen levels in a woman's body. As a result, women who smoke have an earlier menopause, which translates into an increased risk of osteoporosis and an increased risk of heart disease.

*Cigarettes*, p. 136

12. In women, smoking is associated with an earlier menopause. The onset of menopause raises heart-disease risk because postmenopausal women produce much less estrogen, a hormone known to protect against heart disease. Even female smokers who have not yet reached menopause have estrogen levels that are lower than normal, a factor that increases their heart-disease risk. Postmenopausal smokers who undergo estrogen replacement therapy do not achieve as high a level of blood estrogen as do nonsmokers. Smoking "induces" enzymes from the liver to break down estrogen at a faster rate than occurs in nonsmokers.

Quote from *Cigarettes*, p. 29

13. In a group of 117,000 female registered nurses ages 30 to 55 years, the risk of coronary heart disease was increased more than nine-fold in smokers who started smoking before the age of 15.

Archives of Internal Medicine, January 24, 1994, p. 169

14. In a study of coronary heart disease in 120,000 female nurses ages 30 to 55, the risk of fatal or nonfatal coronary events in heavy smokers (more than 25 cigarettes a day) was more than five times the risk of nonsmokers. More than 80 percent of heart attacks in this group were attributable to smoking.

NEJM, November 19, 1987, p. 1344

15. The annual number of female deaths in the US attributable to smoking was only 30,000 in 1965, but rose to 147,000 by 1988. 1995 estimates were 240,000, or half of the total number of female deaths from smoking in the entire developed world.

Washington Post, March 1992

16. Adolescent girls who diet or who are concerned about their weight initiate smoking at higher rates than those with fewer weight concerns.

American Journal of Public Health, November 1994, p. 1820

17. 58% of female smokers expressed concern about gaining a lot of weight if they quit smoking, compared with 26% of male smokers.

American Journal of Public Health, September 1993, p. 1203

18. Women's groups were outraged by an aborted plan to market a new brand of cigarettes called Dakota to young, poorly educated, white women described as "virile females" who "do what their boyfriends tell them to do." Native Americans were also incensed at the misuse of the word Dakota, which means friend. The RJ Reynolds brand was never introduced.

Washington Post National Weekly Edition, February 16, 1990, p. 22, JAMA, September 26, 1990, p. 1505, and Lancet, March 3, 1990, p. 537

19. "Dakota: A Case Study in Marketing Failure," is detailed in *Women and Smoking*, 2001 Surgeon General report, pp. 512-513.

20. Smoking is a risk factor for the development of pelvic inflammatory disease in women.

American Journal of Public Health, October 1992, p. 1352

21. In women who quit smoking, relapse rates are much higher for the group with the lowest income and the least education, as well as for unmarried women.

Internal Medicine News, January 15, 1992, p. 40

22. "Something is out of whack when women who smoke are more terrified of breast cancer, about which they can do very little, than of lung cancer, which they can effectively prevent - and when one of the main reasons they continue to puff away is that they fear modest weight gain often attendant on quitting."

Kathy Pollit from *Dr. Nancy Snyderman's Guide to Good Health*, William Morrow, 1996, p. 107

23. "For more than twenty years, advertisements for Virginia Slims in magazines such as Cosmopolitan and Vogue included sepia-toned vignettes that contrasted subjugated, male-dominated housewives of the 19th century with the liberated superwomen of today - who smoke Virginia Slims. Recollection of the fact that black women were enslaved in the 19th century doubtless led the cigarette advertiser to make a different

approach to their descendants; advertisements for Virginia Slims in Ebony and Essence magazines stuck strictly to models holding cigarettes." Journal of Medical Activism (DOC), December 1995

24. Tobacco now causes almost one third of all US female deaths in middle age. The US has only 5% of the world's females, but it has 50% of the world's female deaths from smoking.
9th World Conference on Tobacco or Health, Paris, 1994 (Imperial Cancer Research Fund Press Release)

25. "During the 1990's, smoking is going to kill about a quarter million women in the United States each year. That's out of a worldwide total of half a million women a year killed by tobacco. The United States may have only 4% of the female population of the world, but it's going to have 50% of the deaths from tobacco in the world among women. If the women smoke like men, then they're going to die like men."
JAMA, June 24, 1992, p. 3255 (Richard Peto)

26. Tobacco is responsible for the deaths of 300,000 women each year in the developed countries. The World Health Organization estimates that this figure will rise to a million women each year by 2020.
*Tobacco and Health*, p. 7

27. More than 140,000 American women die each year as a result of cigarette smoking, compared to "only" 30,000 in 1965. Journal of the American Medical Woman's Association, January 1996, p. 69

28. The Virginia Slims theme "You've come a long way, baby" in use since the brand's introduction in 1968, is being changed to "It's a woman thing." New York Times, April 10, 1996, p. D6

29. The number one cigarette brand among women is Marlboro Lights.
Eric Solberg, July 9, 1996, seminar in St. Louis, Missouri

30. Supermodel Kate Moss, the "new Twiggy", was featured in a "Feed the Waifs" spoof in Esquire magazine. Prominent in the photograph are her cigarette and pack of Marlboro Lights. JAMA, January 23, 1994, p. 629

31. "Cigarettes are like girls; the best ones are thin and rich."
Pitch for now-defunct Silva Thins (New Yorker May 13, 1996, p. 42)

32. Many women's cigarette brands use code words for weight control such as thin, slim, superslim, and long. These "diet terms" are effective in luring women to smoke because of the strong societal pressure to be thin.
*Tobacco Use: An American Crisis*, p. 29

33. Ads for Super Slims from Virginia Slims have photographs of ultra thin young women whose images have been elongated and bodies made to appear even more slender through trick photography. And ads for Capri Super Slims have the slogan "The Slimmest Slim." *Tobacco Use*, p. 65

34. "Marketing experts have shrewdly promoted smoking as a way of remaining slim in a culture that this obsessed with thinness. Incorporation of 'slims' in the name of many current brands, prominent advertisements in Weight Watchers magazine, and pictures of very trim models in advertisements… suggest that cigarettes may help a woman lose weight or avoid gaining weight." NEJM, November 19, 1987, p. 1343

35. Between 1960 and 1986, the rate of lung cancer increased fourfold among women smokers.
*The Harvard Guide to Women's Health*, p. 582

36. The number of female smokers ages 12 to 18 doubled between the mid-1970's and mid-1980's.
*The Harvard Guide to Women's Health*, p. 582

37. Smoking accounts each year for 25% of all deaths among American women, or about 106,000 deaths each year. *The Harvard Guide to Women's Health*, p. 582

38. A middle aged woman who smokes is three times more likely to die of coronary artery disease and five times more likely to die of a stroke than a nonsmoking woman of the same age.

*The Harvard Guide to Women's Health*, p. 582

39. Girls who smoke attain a lower maximal level of pulmonary function than nonsmokers.

NEJM, September 26, 1996, p. 936

40. 1999 estimated deaths from lung cancer in the U.S. women were 68,000, compared to 43,400 deaths from breast cancer.                                               NBC evening news, April 12, 1999

41. The number of female deaths from smoking in the European Union countries increased from 10,000 in 1955 to more than 110,000 in 1995.                   Journal of the National Cancer Institute, February 3, 1999, p. 213

42. The countries with the highest female smoking prevalence (age 15 and over) are Denmark (37%), Norway (35%), the Czech Republic (31%), Fiji (30.6%), and Israel and Russia (30%). Countries with a female smoking prevalence of 4% or less include China, India, Sri Lanka, Pakistan, Indonesia, Thailand, Malaysia, Singapore, Egypt, Saudi Arabia, Lesotho, Uzbekistan and Turkmenistan.

*Tobacco or Health: a Global Status Report*, World Health Organization, 1997

43. Smoking prevalence is 32.9% in women with only 9 to 11 years of education, compared to 11.2% for women with a college education.                    *Women and Smoking*, 2001 Surgeon General report, p. 7

44. In a study from Sweden, postmenopausal women who smoked had a 66% increased risk for hip fracture.

Archives of Internal Medicine, August 2001, p. 983

45. Postmenopausal women who smoke have double the risk for rheumatoid arthritis compared to nonsmokers and women who had quit smoking for more than 10 years.         American Journal of Medicine 2002; 112:465-471

46. Many women do not know about the health dangers of smoking, according to a British study released in 2001. The Smoking Cessation Action in Primary Care (Scape) surveyed 1,757 men and women who were smokers or ex-smokers. Figures show that 14-year-old girls are twice as likely to smoke as their male peers. And last year, lung cancer overtook breast cancer as the biggest killer of women in Britain (it has had that distinction in the U.S. since 1986). But the Scape study showed 8% of women did not believe smoking was linked to increased risk of lung cancer. Two thirds did not think smoking increased the risk of SIDS. A quarter did not know smoking increases the risk of heart disease, and 2/3 did not believe smoking increases the risk of miscarriage. Other survey findings:

> 89% were unaware smoking is associated with cervical cancer.
> 42% did not believe it increased the risk of stroke.
> 88% did not believe it increased the risk of osteoporosis.
> 30% did not think smokers had an increased risk of developing throat and mouth cancer.

2002 AMA Annual Tobacco Report

47. The number of female smoking related deaths in the European Union countries increased from 10,000 in 1955 to 113,000 in 1995.                        British Medical Association (www.tobaccofactfile.org)

48. Women account for 39% of smoking-related deaths in the United States, a proportion that has more than doubled since 1965.                                            Chicago Tribune, March 28, 2001

49. In women in 2003, breast cancer will account for 32% of all new cancer cases in the United States (211,300), and 15% of all cancer deaths (39,800). Lung cancer, with its much higher mortality, had 12% of new cancer cases in women (80,100), but accounted for 25% of the estimated deaths (68,800).

CA A Cancer Journal for Clinicians, January/February 2003, pp. 7-9

50. Deaths from lung cancer among white women in the United States increased by 600% between 1950 and 2000. In 1950, lung cancer accounted for only 3% of all female cancer deaths, whereas in 2000 it accounted for an estimated 25%.                                            British Medical Journal, March 31, 2001, p. 752

(from 2000 Surgeon General report, *The Health Consequences of Smoking for Women*)

# CHAPTER 25
# AFRICAN AMERICANS AND SMOKING

1.  Black Americans have higher rates of morbidity and mortality from smoking-related diseases than do other races. It is possible that the anesthetic effects of the menthol cigarettes used by 76% of this group facilitate deeper and longer inhalation of smoke, thus increasing exposure and toxicity.
    *Nicotine Addiction*, pp. 341 and 356, and American Journal of Public Health, October 1989, p. 1416

2.  Blacks absorb as much as 30% more nicotine than whites or Hispanics with every cigarette that they smoke; this may explain why they have more difficulty stopping smoking and have a higher rate of lung cancer.
    New York Times, July 8, 1998, p. A16

3.  About 76% of black smokers choose menthol brands compared to 23% of white smokers. Menthol brands are associated with higher cotinine levels and carbon monoxide concentrations, and appear to be associated with increased health risks compared to non-menthol brands.                          Chest, November 1996, p. 1194

4.  Lung cancer is the leading cancer killer in African Americans, accounting in 2003 for an estimated 29% of cancer deaths in men and 20.7% in women. In terms of new cancer cases, lung cancer accounted for 15.5% in men (second behind 39% for prostate cancer) and 13.1% in African American women (second behind 31.3% for breast cancer).          CA-A Cancer Journal for Clinicians, November-December 2002, p. 329

5.  Black smokers have a 50% higher incidence of lung cancer as well as death from lung cancer compared to whites. One reason might be that blacks have a poorer capacity than whites to detoxify NNK, one of the most important tobacco-related carcinogens linked to lung cancer. Another reason is that black smokers are more likely to choose brands with higher tar and nicotine levels.
    American Medical News, November 15, 1993, and May 2, 1994

6.  Cigarette smoking is a major contributor to the short life expectancy of inner city black men. Black men in Harlem are less likely to reach the age of 65 than are men in Bangladesh.          NEJM, January 18, 1990, p.173

7.  The American Cancer Society in 1981 published a brochure entitled Smoking and Genocide. The word genocide was removed from subsequent editions of the ACS brochure because of fear of offending potential contributors.                          *Minorities and Cancer*, Lovell Jones, Springer-Verlag, 1989, p. 152

8.  The years of potential life lost before age 65 attributed to smoking for African Americans is twice that for whites. The lung cancer death rate is 2.3 times higher in blacks than for whites. And from 1980 through 1990, lung cancer increased 99% for African American females compared to 86% for white females, and 32% for African-American males compared to 21% for white males.          *Tobacco Use: An American Crisis*, p. 44

9.  A billboard produced by the National Medical Association in white tombstone letters on a black background says: "Last year 45,000 African Americans died for a cigarette. To die for smoking is to die for nothing."
    JAMA, September 8, 1993

10. Cigarette smoking accounts for 40% of all deaths among adult black men, as well as 30% of all deaths of persons over age 20, in the District of Columbia, and is a major contributing cause for the black-white disparity in health status. A brown cigarette called "More" is targeted to black women, so that "more" black women smoke "More" cigarettes, and "more" black women get cancer, and of course, the tobacco industry makes "more" money.
    Journal of the National Medical Association, November 1989, pp. 1119-1121 (Reed Tuckson, M.D.)

11. "By deciding to conceal and deny the deadly consequences and addictive nature of smoking (in the 1960's), tobacco companies bought time to scrounge for new markets. They chose two targets, women and minorities."
    Joe Califano, Washington Post National Weekly Edition, June 6, 1994, p. 28

12. During the 1970's, about 70% of black smokers were smoking Kool menthol cigarettes. By the 1990's Newport, also a menthol brand, had become the most popular.                    Tobacco Control, Winter 1993, p. 512

13. The African American publications Jet, Essence, and Ebony are read by 47% of black women and 38% of black men. Despite frequent discussions of health topics in lead articles, Essence has never published an article on smoking, and in 40 years, Ebony has never published a major article on tobacco, which is the leading cause of death among African Americans. The leading advertiser in these three magazines is the tobacco industry.
*Tobacco Use*, p. 65

14. In 1993 the California Department of Health tried to place an ad in Essence magazine showing three famous African American musicians who died from tobacco use. Essence declined the ad because it was "too controversial." The director of Woman and Girls Against Tobacco, which was to have co-sponsored the ad, said: "There is an understanding in the ad industry that magazines that accept tobacco ads do not run derogatory articles about tobacco."                    *Tobacco Industry Strategies*, p. 10

15. In the 1980's, football players Earl Campbell and Lawrence Taylor promoted the use of Skoal Bandits spit tobacco.                    *Minorities and Cancer*, p. 157

16. Brown and Williamson presents annual "Kool Achiever" award (named for Kool cigarettes) to people who want to improve the "quality of life in inner-city communities."                    *Minorities and Cancer*, p. 159

17. A 1993 winner of a $5000 "Kool Achiever" award was Ronald Johnson, a former gang member now working in a gang prevention program. At an awards ceremony, he declined the prize in front of a stunned audience, citing nicotine addiction as having turned into "a war on black men." He called nicotine the "number one most addictive drug on the planet," and the audience of 150 gave him a standing ovation.
Tobacco Control, Spring 1994, p. 11

18. "With massive, deceptive advertising and promotions in African American communities, the tobacco industry spreads its pervasive and deadly addiction."                    Rev. Jesse Brown, National Association of African Americans for Positive Imagery (SCARC, April 29, 1994)

19. "While RJ Reynolds plasters 'Joe Camel' billboards and signs everywhere, they then go hire actor Danny Glover to appear in ads that say that the company really doesn't think that 'kids' should smoke... Do we really think that the fox truly cares about the safety of the chickens?"
Rev. Jesse Brown, The Uptown Coalition for Tobacco Control

20. In St. Louis, 62% of billboards in the black community advertised cigarettes and alcohol, compared with 36% of billboards in the white community. In a poor black area of Philadelphia, 66 out of 73 billboards in one 19-block area advertised alcohol or tobacco.
Journal of the National Medical Association, November 1989, p. 1121

21. In Baltimore, 20% of billboard ads in white communities are for tobacco or alcohol. In black neighborhoods, 76% of billboards promoted these products. [Billboards advertising tobacco are no longer permitted in the United States – editor]                    Time, January 29, 1990

22. Billboards advertising tobacco products are placed in African-American communities four to five times more often than in white communities. The tobacco industry spends 70% of its billboard advertising dollars in black and Hispanic communities. In many ethnic neighborhoods, as much as 80% to 90% of all billboard advertising is for tobacco and alcohol products.
JAMA, September 8, 1993, p. 1168, and Journal of Medical Activism (DOC), September 1995

23. Men and women in lower socioeconomic groups are more responsive than are those in higher socioeconomic groups to changes in the price of cigarettes, and less responsive to health publicity.
British Medical Journal, October 8, 1994, p. 923

24. Philip Morris donates heavily to black groups and politicians. "The tobacco companies target African-Americans with the intensity of fanatical hunters on the trail of very special game... The tobacco companies are buying the silence of black leaders... The leaders of these organizations should have been fanatical in their opposition to smoking, which slaughters their memberships. Instead they lined up before the tobacco companies with their lips zipped and their hands out for their share of the industry's hush money."

New York Times, November 28, 1993 (Bob Herbert column)

25. Philip Morris has been a bonanza for black groups and politicians. In 1988, Philip Morris gave to the NAACP, the Urban League, Associated Black Charities, Black Women in Publishing, the United Negro College Fund, the New York Coalition of 100 Black Women, the Central Harlem Meals on Wheels Coalition, the Harlem YMCA, and the National Association of Black Social Workers, to name a few.

San Francisco Chronicle, November 30, 1993, p. A19

26. In 1987, Philip Morris gave $2.4 million and RJ Reynolds $1.9 million to African-American groups including the United Negro College Fund, the NAACP, and the congressional Black Caucus Foundation. In 1988, Philip Morris paid for a conference of presidents of black colleges on Martin Luther King's birthday; a PM spokesman said, "Good citizenship is as important as is investment in research and development."

Journal of the National Medical Association, November 1989, p. 1122
and *Growing Up Tobacco Free*, p. 46

27. In 1991, Philip Morris handed out $17.3 million in "philanthropic" contributions, including $86,000 to the Congressional Black Caucus and another $837,000 to the NAACP, National Urban League, and other black organizations. They also gave $569,000 to Hispanic organizations.     *Tobacco Use: An American Crisis*, p. 46

28. In 1993, the tobacco industry increased their contributions to the Congressional Black Caucus Foundation to $155,000.                                                                Common Cause magazine, Spring 1995, p. 22

29. RJR Nabisco in 1989 gave $250,000 to the United Negro College Fund. The NAACP receives about $250,000 each year from the tobacco industry.        American Medical News, November 15, 1993, p. 15

30. In November 1985, Philip Morris hosted three publishers of African American newspapers at its corporate headquarters in New York for a forum on preserving freedoms in American life. Several months later, these publishers voted to condemn the AMA's call for a ban on tobacco advertising. The National Association for Hispanic Publications made a similar statement in 1990.      *Tobacco Use: An American Crisis*, p. 65

31. Congressman Charles Rangel, a Harlem Democrat, has been a major recipient of tobacco money, as has Rep. Edolphus Towns, a Brooklyn Democrat who is so close to the tobacco industry he's known as the "Marlboro Man."                                    New York Times, November 28, 1993 (Bob Herbert column)

32. The tobacco industry heavily markets menthol cigarettes (primarily Newport, Kool, and Salem) to African Americans. The percentage of menthol cigarettes advertised in Ebony, Jet, and Essence was 66%, compared to 15% in general market magazines. In 1985, cigarette companies spent $3.3 million in ads in Ebony alone, including most of the back covers.                                                      *Tobacco Use*, p. 45

33. Dr. Louis Sullivan, former Secretary of Health and Human Services and now dean of the Morehouse School of Medicine in Atlanta, has been unsuccessful in his efforts to persuade the Congressional Black Caucus Foundation not to accept money from tobacco companies.

San Francisco Chronicle, February 21, 1998, p. A18 (Cynthia Tucker)

34. Led by Health and Human Services Secretary Louis Sullivan, health advocates in 1990 aborted a plan to market a new brand of RJ Reynolds cigarettes called Uptown to urban blacks. It was to have been a high-tar, high-nicotine menthol brand tailored to the tastes of black smokers.     JAMA, September 26, 1990, p. 1505,
and American Medical News, November 15, 1993, p. 16

35. Further information on the "Uptown Story" may be found in *Reducing Tobacco Use*, 2000 Surgeon General report, p. 399

36. Another new cigarette brand "Menthol X" was sold for a year in the East before being withdrawn from the market. African Americans protested that its packaging used images associated with Malcolm X and racial pride to lure buyers from the black community. The cigarettes were sold in black, red and green boxes labeled with a large white "X" and resembled a poster used to promote Spike Lee's movie about the slain Black Muslim leader. Black, red and green also symbolizes racial pride to many African Americans.

San Francisco Chronicle, March 17, 1995

37. Black leaders have mobilized their communities against cigarettes marketed at black teens. Several years ago, Harold Freeman, the director of surgery at Harlem Hospital, installed posters in New York subways showing a skeleton resembling the Marlboro man lighting up a cigarette for a black child. The poster legend read: "They used to make us pick it. Now they want us to smoke it."

Newsweek, May 1, 1995, p. 76 and Journal of the National Cancer Institute, September 2, 1991, p. 1315

38. The Rev. Calvin Butts in Harlem has led "billboard beautification projects" to whitewash tobacco and alcohol billboards.

American Medical News, November 15, 1993, p. 18

39. A predominately black neighborhood on the south side of Chicago was found to have 118 billboards advertising cigarettes and liquor, compared with just three in a nearby white neighborhood of similar size. When a local parish priest organized a "billboard beautification project" which painted some of them over, he had his car doused with paint and tires slashed.

Audubon, August 1991, p. 18

40. Among African American males in urban areas, the smoking prevalence rates are about 40-50%, and up to 50% in unemployed men. In women it is about 35%.

Tobacco Control, Autumn 1995, p. 515

41. From 1960 to 1990 in African Americans, lung cancer increased by 170% in males and 464% in females. The increase for cancer of the larynx was 77% for males and 210% for females.

CA-A Cancer Journal for Clinicians, March/April 1996, p. 115

42. An estimated 48,000 African Americans die from smoking-related diseases yearly.

American Lung Association Fact Sheet, Targeted Populations and Smoking (August 1997 Update)

43. African American smokers have more than a threefold higher rate of cancers of the upper respiratory and digestive tracts than whites. The incidence of oral and pharyngeal cancer in black men increased by 47% between 1977 and 1988, compared to a decline in oral cancer of 9% for white men in the same time period.

Western Journal of Medicine, March 1997, p. 189

44. 75% to 90% of African Americans prefer menthol cigarettes, compared to 23% to 25% of whites. Among African American teenagers, 70% choose Newport and 12% choose Kool, both menthol brands. "Menthol cigarettes were introduced in the 1930's, but did not exceed 3% of the total market until 1949. By 1963 the market share was 16%, and by 1976 it was 28%. Sales to African Americans accounted for the vast majority of this increase."

Western Journal of Medicine, March 1997, p. 191

45. Among smokers younger than age 18, blacks are much more likely than whites to smoke menthol brand cigarettes – 70% of blacks compared to 9% of whites choose Newport, and 12% of blacks and less than 1% of white adolescents prefer Kools.

1993 TAPS data reported by Campaign for Tobacco-Free Kids

46. "The majority of blacks... do not respond well to sophisticated or subtle humor in advertising. They related much more overt, clear-cut story lines."

From a 1981 Reynolds marketing plan (San Francisco Chronicle, February 6, 1998, p. A5)

47. African-Americans absorb significantly more nicotine per cigarette smoked than do whites.

Journal of the National Cancer Institute, August 18, 1999, p. 1367

# CHAPTER 26
# TOBACCO AND THE MILITARY

## Historical

1. The superintendent of the Naval Academy at Annapolis, Commodore Parker, in 1879 lifted a regulation that had barred the use of tobacco by midshipmen. *Tobacco Advertising*, p. 16

2. In 1898, Surgeon General Rixey of the U.S. Navy expressed alarm at the increased cigarette smoking by sailors during the Spanish-American War. He threatened to ban cigarettes aboard ships, but backed down in the face of a possible mutiny. *Tobacco Advertising*, p. 115

3. In 1900, cigarettes were banned in the U.S. Navy at the same time that the cigar was widely accepted. The cigarette was regarded as "a debasement of manhood." *Advertising, the Uneasy Persuasion*, p. 184

4. During the first and second World Wars, tobacco companies gave away billions of free cigarettes to the troops. This practice coincided with the most rapid increases in overall smoking prevalence and in cigarette sales at any time in the United States.

5. General John J. Pershing, Commander of American forces in France in 1918, cabled Washington D.C.: "Tobacco is as indispensable as the daily ration: we must have thousands of tons of it without delay. It is essential for the defense of democracy." On another occasion he was quoted: "You ask me what we need to win this war. I answer tobacco as much as bullets." *Cigarettes*, p. 40 and *Advertising*, p 186

6. American soldiers first received tobacco rations (0.4 ounces with 10 cigarette papers) in World War I. When the War Department approved the rations, "a wave of joy swept through the American Army." Until 1975, cigarettes were included in all k-rations and c-rations provided to soldiers and sailors. *Advertising, the Uneasy Persuasion*, p. 186 and *Reducing Health Consequences of Smoking*, p. 278

7. In World War I, wounded soldiers were allowed to smoke while being operated on. An army surgeon described the calming effect of cigarettes. "Wonderful. As soon as the lads take their first whiff, they seem eased and relieved of their agony." *Tobacco Advertising*, p. 184

8. In World War II, cigarettes were sold at military stores tax-free for usually a nickel a pack, and were distributed free in overseas areas. *Reducing the Health Consequences of Smoking*, p. 425

## General

1. The Pentagon, the world's largest office building, became smoke free in March 1994.
American Medical News, April 4, 1994

2. On April 8, 1994 when the Department of Defense banned indoor smoking, the Pentagon's central courtyard became the primary designated smoking area. This area had been nicknamed "Ground Zero" during the cold war. JAMA, April 6, 1994

3. "Achievement of a non-smoking environment is the greatest, single and most immediate health care service we can provide our sailors." Message from VADM Anthony Less, Commander, Naval Air Force, to Atlantic-based carriers, February, 1993 (Navy Times, March 8, 1993)

4. Since 1989, tobacco use has been prohibited in all Navy and Marine Corps health care facilities.
Bureau of Medicine and Surgery, US Navy

5. In January 1987 the Naval Hospital at Camp Pendleton, California, became the first military hospital to become totally smoke free and to ban all tobacco sales. (The Naval Hospital San Diego followed a year later).
San Diego Union, February 19, 1987, p. B3

6. In 1991, the nation's 172 veteran's hospitals banned all tobacco sales and became smoke-free in all indoor areas.
JAMA 267:87, 1992

7. The Coast Guard has banned smoking in all buildings, ships, aircraft, and vehicles under their control, as well as in housing units occupied by more than one family. Coast Guardsmen who complained received a letter stating: "Your right to smoke indoors was weighed against the right of your shipmates to breathe air relatively free of carbon monoxide, carcinogens and other harmful products of tobacco smoke. The right to breathe unpolluted air took precedence."
Navy Times, April 13, 1992

8. Philip Morris sponsored 15 country music concerts in 1992 under the banner "Marlboro Music." 10 of these were on military bases.
JAMA, May 27, 1992, p. 2720

9. During Operation Desert Storm in 1990-1991, Philip Morris made Christmas cards for relatives and friends to send recorded messages to the troops. It featured a Marlboro man on the front and a picture of a pack of Marlboros on the back.
Navy Times, 1991

10. A shipment of 200,000 donated magazines in late 1990 bound for US military personnel in the Persian Gulf was held up because the promoter had the magazines wrapped in special cover advertising Camel Filters.
American Medical News, October 19, 1990

11. Before the Pentagon prohibited the practice, Philip Morris donated 2 million free cigarettes to the Desert Shield armed forces.
American Medical News, October 19, 1990

12. At a 1991 Blue Angels show at Miramar Naval Air Station in San Diego, a popular attraction was a 15-foot high inflatable pack of Camels and its "spokesman," a giant cartoon Joe Camel with a three foot long cigarette. Free cigarette lighters, hats, and tote bags bearing the Camel logo were handed out.
David Moyer, M.D.

13. In 1988, Philip Morris published for a time a monthly newsletter called "The Military Smoker." It featured articles opposing restrictions on smoking and on cigarette sales in military facilities; readers were urged to call a toll-free "Military Smoker" hot line telephone number.
*Reducing the Health Consequences of Smoking*, p. 278

14. The tobacco industry attempts to link patriotism, toughness, and military service with smoking. But the "macho" image of the hard charging cigarette-smoking military man or woman is slowly changing to a hard charging, physically fit, non-smoking image.
Navy Times editorial, 1991

15. Philip Morris tested a new cigarette brand called Player's Navy Cut, featuring a stalwart sailor wearing a cap labeled "Hero."
New York Times, April 10, 1996, p. D6

16. The Defense Department estimates that its 448,000 smokers (32 percent of the 1.4 million active duty force) incur about $530 million a year extra in health expenses and $345 million in expenses for lost productivity attributable to smoking.
New York Times, October 25, 1996

17. The estimated extra annual cost in lost productivity and extra medical costs of one active duty Army smoker is $3050.
1992 ODCSPER calculations and 1991 Draft AR 600-63

18. After 62 hours submerged in a submarine which allowed smoking, the carbon monoxide levels in the exhaled breath of nonsmokers had increased to a level about the same as the initial level in crew members who smoked 21 cigarettes a day. There are now six smokefree US Navy submarines.
Navy Medical Corps Update, Fall 1995 (LCDR Kevin Seufert)

19. "Military imagery in smoking is an old story. The famous Marlboro chevron is a military insignia. Both Marlboro and Pall Mall carry military mottoes of conquering Roman emperors on every pack."
US News and World Report, June 2, 1997, p. 18 (John Leo)

20. A 1993 general counsel decision, reaffirmed in 1997, states that any veteran with a smoking-related illness may be entitled to benefits if the veteran first became addicted to smoking during military service. If all tobacco claims could be processed immediately, it would cost the government $4.4 billion in fiscal year 1998, and $23.8 billion over the next five years. "Veterans' health and benefit claims for tobacco-related illness soon could overwhelm the Department of Veterans Affairs with as many as 2.5 million claims over the next 10 years."
US Medicine, December 1997, p. 3

21. The Department of Veterans Affairs spends up to $4 billion a year treating veterans for smoking-related health problems.
Navy Times, July 10, 2000, p. 6

22. In a study of army recruits, smokers were 1.5 times more likely to suffer fractures, sprains, and other physical injuries during an eight-week basic training program than were non-smokers. Smokers also had lower levels of physical fitness.
American Journal of Preventive Medicine 2000; 18:96-102

23. A 1998 Pentagon survey showed a smoking prevalence of 30% among active duty military members. The Defense Department spends nearly a billion dollars a year for health care costs and lost productivity from tobacco use among military beneficiaries.
Navy Times, November 26, 2001, p. 28

24. In a study of 29,000 Air Force recruits at Lackland AFB, Texas, smoking appeared to be the best predictor of whether the recruits would be prematurely discharged from the military. A year after service entry, 19.8% of the smokers had been discharged early, compared to 11.8% of non-smokers. The reasons for this surprising finding is unclear, but smoking can make it more difficult to keep up with the rigorous physical training. Applying these findings to all branches of the military, the authors concluded that smoking costs the country $130 million a year, or about 1% of the armed forces' $14 billion a year training budget.
Tobacco Control 2001; 10:43-47

25. In December 2002, recreation facilities joined other buildings on military bases by either becoming smoke free or providing specially ventilated designated smoking areas. Most bases have chosen to go smoke free.
Navy Times, December 23,2002, p. 21

26. U.S. Marines in Iraq are growing irritable as their supply of cigarettes and chewing tobacco has run dry. "Some are so desperate for a cigarette that they are begging them from local farmers." Associated Press, April 1, 2003

# Prevalence Data

1. Smoking prevalence in US military forces decreased from 51 percent in 1980 and 1982 to 46 percent in 1985, 41 percent in 1988, 35 percent in 1992, 32 percent in 1995, and 30 percent in 1998..
*1992, 1995, and 1998 Worldwide Surveys of Substance Abuse Among Military Personnel*

2. In a 1985 DOD survey, 44% of military men and 40% of military women were smokers. The civilian rates at that time were 32 and 27%, respectively.

3. In a 1987 survey of Navy men assigned to shipboard duty, 60% of those older than age 35 were smokers, and more than 69% of the group without a high school diploma were smokers.
Military Medicine, April 1988, p. 175

4. 28% of Navy recruits smoked on entry to basic training, and 50% of shipboard men were smokers in a 1987 survey, many not beginning to smoke until after entering the Navy.    Military Medicine, April 1988, p. 175

5.   In 1990, 41% of service people smoked, including 47% of enlisted personnel and 18% of officers. By 1992, smoking rates in the military dropped to 35% overall. In the Army (overall rate 37%), 13% of officers but 49% of E1 to E3 (junior enlisted) personnel were smokers. Rates for the Marine Corps were 39%, Navy 37% and Air Force 29%.                                                                            *1992 Worldwide Survey*

6.   In 1992, 17.4% of military personnel used smokeless tobacco, including 36% of Marines, figures unchanged from 1988. Use in Marine Corps males under age 25 was nearly half, or 47.4%.
                                                                                             *1992 Worldwide Survey*, p 6-11

7.   One of the Healthy People 2000 objectives was to reduce the prevalence of current cigarette smoking to no more than 20% of military personnel. The 1995 DOD survey released in February 1996 showed a decline in overall smoking prevalence in the military to 31.9% from 35.0% in the previous 1992 survey. This included 34.9% for the Navy, 35.0% for the Marine Corps, 34.0% for the Army, and 25.1% in the Air Force. The lower Air Force prevalence was attributable to the fact that Air Force personnel were more likely to be older, better educated, and married. The data were extremely discouraging for younger military personnel; of those age 20 or younger, 40.8% smoked, despite universal prohibition during recruit training, and the same percentage, 40.8%, of those in pay grades E1 to E3 were smokers. This group was almost six times more likely to smoke than officers O4 and above (7.1%).

8.   In the 1995 DOD survey, males were significantly more likely than females to be current smokers (32.7% vs. 26.3%). Young women in the Marines, however, had a 35.4% smoking prevalence. Whites (34.4%) were more likely than blacks (23.4%) to be smokers, and those with a high school education only were much more likely to smoke (41.0%) than personnel with a college degree or higher (11.5%).

9.   In the 1995 DOD survey of the US military, overall the prevalence of cigar or pipe use was 18.7%, ranging from 12.8% in the Air Force to 28.4% in the Marine Corps.

10.  In the 1995 DOD survey of the US military, overall prevalence of smokeless tobacco use was 13.2%, ranging from 7.9% in the Air Force to 24.0% in the Marine Corps. 30.6% of Marine Corps males under age 25 were regular smokeless tobacco users, down from 47% in this group in the 1992 survey.

11.  The Coast Guard Academy had only three smokers out of their 206 graduates of the Class of 1991. The Class of 1994 did not have a single smoker.                                                             Navy Times, April 13, 1992

12.  In a 1990 survey by David Moyer, M.D., of 800 students at the Naval School of Health Sciences in San Diego, 41% were current tobacco users. Despite their work as navy hospital corpsmen, only 10% who used tobacco before service entry elected not to resume the habit after their two months of forced abstinence during recruit training.

13.  In a survey by John Kelso, M.D. of a Marine battalion in Saudi Arabia in 1991 during Operation Desert Shield, 60% of enlisted personnel and 34% of officers were tobacco users.

14.  In a 1991 survey by David Moyer, M.D. of 9000 Marine Corps recruits, 52% were tobacco users before service entry. All tobacco use is prohibited for three months during recruit training, but 91% intended to restart the habit as soon as they graduated from "boot camp."

15.  Former US Marine Corps Commandant (1985-1989) General P.X. Kelley is a member of the board of directors of the US Tobacco Company, manufacturers of 80% of the nation's smokeless tobacco. A third of male Marines under age 25 are daily smokeless tobacco users, and the Marine Corps has the highest use of any of the military services. Both General Kelley and his successor, General Al Gray, were public smokeless tobacco users.                                                                                Common Cause magazine, Summer 1993

16.  In a 1995 survey by Jon Bayer, M.D. of 15,000 Navy recruits at Great Lakes, Illinois, 36% identified themselves as smokers prior to Navy enlistment (36.5% of males, and 30.5% of females). The average age of smoking initiation was 15.2 years, although 34% of male smokers began before age 10. The rate for

Caucasians was 43.5%, and was 27.6% for non-Caucasians.

17. In 1992 survey aboard the aircraft carrier USS Lincoln, 45% of the crew used tobacco. In a 1995 survey of the carrier USS Carl Vinson, 44% of the crew were current tobacco users.
                          Oakland Naval Hospital Red Rover, August 1993 and Lamont Berg, M.D.

18. The aircraft carrier Theodore Roosevelt became the Navy's first smoke-free carrier in July 1993 after a series of incremental steps. Tobacco products were not sold aboard, and the crew of 5482 was prohibited from any tobacco use. The Roosevelt was on deployment in the Adriatic Sea off Yugoslavia at the time of the ban, and returned to home port in Norfolk in September 1993. In late 1993, Congressional pressure lead to reversal of the ban.                          JAMA, June 16, 1993, p. 2960 and Navy Times, March 8, 1993

19. 56% of Vietnam veterans with high combat experience are smokers. Smoking-related diseases were present in 42% of veterans in a study from Denver, and another study documented smoking-related diseases in 35% of outpatients in veteran's hospitals.                          Federal Practitioner, February 1995, p. 11

20. The 1996 Air Force smoking rate was 23%, down from 43% in 1985. The 1996 Navy smoking rate was 35%, and 35% for males and 27% for females in the Army.                          US Medicine, February 1997

21. 36% of female Navy recruits ages 17-18 are current smokers, compared to only 13.8% of their non-military age group peers. Among entering female recruits age 19-23, 41% are smokers, compared to 24.8% of their civilian counterparts. The reason why the U.S. Navy attracts young women who smoke is not known.
                          Tobacco Control, Summer 1999, pp. 222-223

22. Smoking in the military dropped to 30% overall in 1998.                          US Medicine, June 1999, p. 21

# Military Store Pricing Issues

1. In 1986, Defense Secretary Caspar Weinberger overruled a decision by his assistant secretary for health affairs to eliminate discounts on cigarette purchase in military stores. Military groups had protested that this would have provided a "dangerous precedent" for cuts in other benefits. Then-Surgeon General C. Everett Koop commented: "How could this be viewed as a reduction in benefits, when the only benefits would be a lifetime of illness and early death?"                          Associated Press, February 27, 1986 and Koop, p. 178

2. "It's time for the Pentagon to ...raise the price of tobacco products in military stores to match those of civilian retailers, and divert the extra income to military-sponsored fitness programs. The signal sent to military people would be strong and clear."                          Navy Times editorial, June 17, 1991

3. Selling discount cigarettes to members of the armed services encourages smoking and costs the Pentagon nearly a billion dollars a year in tobacco-related health and work expenses. Associated Press, November 12, 1996

4. The military "commissary benefit" provides savings averaging 23% over outside retail stores on hundreds of items. However, the discount approaches 60 percent on tobacco products. The Pentagon says that is up to Congress to raise military tobacco prices, but Senator Jeff Bingaman (D-New Mexico) says that the Defense Department "has the authority to change this tomorrow morning."                          Common Cause magazine, Fall 1995

5. Tobacco sales in military commissaries, or grocery stores, totaled $529 million in 1992, or 10% of sales. The average discount was 52% over "outside" prices. In addition to commissaries, Navy exchanges or stores sold $133 million worth of tobacco products, and Marine Corps exchanges $37 million in 1992.
                          Navy Times, July 15, 1993

6. In 1995, tobacco sales accounted for about 11% of total retail sales at military commissaries that sell tobacco products, ranging up to 49% of retail sales at Fort McCoy, Wisconsin. In civilian supermarkets and grocery stores, tobacco accounts for about 3% of sales.                          Navy Times, December 2, 1996, p. 8

7. In 1996, the cheapest cigarettes for sale at Travis Air Force Base, California, were only 57 cents a pack.

8. Vice Admiral Donald Hagen, Surgeon General of the Navy at the time, in a letter commented on August 31, 1993 on the controversy about raising prices of tobacco products in military stores to "civilian levels" and the perceived "erosion of benefits" for service personnel: "It is an oxymoron to say that reduced tobacco sales (and therefore possibly reduced smoking) would produce a negative impact on the overall quality of life."

Bureau of Medicine and Surgery, US Navy

9. Rep. Norman Sisisky D-VA complained at an April 1995 House National Security committee meeting that cigarettes in Navy exchanges are priced higher than in Army and Air Force stores. He also questioned policies that limit where sailors may smoke aboard ships.  Navy Times, April 24, 1995, p. 14

10. Prices of tobacco products in military commissaries (grocery stores) were raised on November 1, 1996 to equal prices in exchanges (retail stores). In some cases, this meant a one-third increase, while the average increase was 18%. Military commissaries have $458 million in yearly sales of tobacco products.

Air Force Times, September 2, 1996, p. 12 and US Medicine, February 1997

11. The tobacco industry is campaigning on Capitol Hill to block a Pentagon plan to raise the price of discounted cigarettes sold in scores of military grocery stores around the world. The military sells $458 million of cigarettes and chewing tobacco a year in government-subsidized commissaries, at 30 percent to 60 percent less than prices in commercial grocery stores. Commissaries sell 58 million cartons of cigarettes a year. Government budget analysts estimate the plan could cut tobacco sales at commissaries in half and cost tobacco companies as much as $200 million a year in sales. Under the Pentagon's plan, which is scheduled to take effect on Nov. 1, the government would end its subsidy of commissary tobacco products in an effort to discourage tobacco consumption... A Defense Department report estimated that tobacco use by military personnel costs the agency more than $900 million a year in medical expenses and lost productivity. But at the urging of the tobacco industry's powerful lobby, a panel of the House National Security committee in a letter signed by all 12 members, has demanded that the Pentagon cancel the price increase... 70 percent of the tobacco products are being bought by retirees. Diseases attributed to tobacco use accounted for about 16 percent of the deaths in the military last year, according to the inspector general's report.

Quote from San Francisco Examiner, October 20, 1996 (Eric Schmitt, New York Times)

# CHAPTER 27
# INTERNATIONAL

## General

1. A comprehensive reference for global trends and data on individual countries is *Tobacco or Health, a Global Status Report*, World Health Organization, 1997

2. *Tobacco Control Country Profiles* (American Cancer Society, 2000) has detailed information on smoking prevalence, tobacco economy, and infrastructure for tobacco control for all the countries of the world. However, prevalence data for this chapter is adopted from the more recent
*The Tobacco Atlas*, published in October 2002.

3. World production of cigarettes increased from 3.18 trillion in 1970 to 4.58 trillion in 1983 and 6 trillion in 1997.

4. The world's top five tobacco producers are China (2.9 million tons per year), the US (698,000 tons), India (445,000), Brazil (440,000), and the Soviet Union (242,000 tons). The top consumers are China, the United States, and the former Soviet Union.
Los Angeles Times, June 5, 1990, p. H1 and International Journal of Health Services 1986; 16:281

5. From 1975 to 1995, total tobacco consumption dropped 5% in developed countries, but more than doubled in developing countries. 9th World Conference on Tobacco or Health, Paris, 1994 (Greg Connolly)

6. "Whereas in most industrialized countries the smoking habit is decreasing and becoming socially less acceptable, in developing countries it is on the increase, fueled mainly by intensive and ruthless promotional campaigns on the part of the transnational tobacco companies."
World Health Organization press release, January 1986

7. Consumption in the third world is growing by more than 2% per year. With current smoking rates, the number of smokers dying from their habit each year in poor countries will increase from 1 million per year in 1992 to 7 million deaths a year thirty years from now. In the rich countries, deaths will increase from the current 2 million to 3 million per year. 9th World Conference on Tobacco or Health, 1994 (Richard Peto)

8. The World Health Organization has said, "Deaths caused by smoking in the developing world will soon wipe out gains made in preventing deaths from malnutrition and communicable diseases." This future epidemic "will result in the loss of more lives than those lost from all previous world epidemics."
The New Yorker, September 13, 1993, p. 81

9. "Failing immediate action, smoking diseases will appear in developing countries before communicable diseases and malnutrition have been controlled, and the gap between rich and poor countries will thus be further expanded." World Health Organization, 1978

10. "It is reprehensible for industrial nations to export disease, death and disability in the way of cigarette smoking to developing countries, putting on their backs a health burden that they will never be able to pay for 20 or 30 years from now." C. Everett Koop, M.D., NEJM, September 12, 1991, p. 816

11. Between 1970 and 1985, per capita tobacco consumption fell by 9% in the United States and 25% in Great Britain. In the same period, it increased by 22% in Asia, 24% in Latin America, and 42% in Africa.
British Journal of Addiction 1989; 84:1398

12. From 1970 to 1980, cigarette consumption doubled in Pakistan, Egypt, Libya, and Kenya, and quadrupled in India. International Journal of Health Services 1986; 16:281

13. From 1970 to 1980, cigarette consumption increased by 28% in Latin America, 30% in Asia, and 77% in Africa. The Lancet, October 6, 1990, p. 865

14. Smoking rates are falling 1.1 percent a year in the developed world, but are rising 2.1 percent a year in the developing world.                                                                                    Washington Post, October 21, 1995

15. In 1994, the World Health Organization announced that in developed countries per capita cigarette consumption had fallen by 10% since 1970. But in the developing countries, it increased by 67% over the same period. A spokesman for BAT industries, one of the major cigarette exporters, said: "The notion that we play any role in increasing tobacco usage is fanciful."                       British Medical Journal, November 18, 1995, p. 1321

16. On average, about 50% of men and 8% of women in developing countries are smokers. About 800 million of the world's 1.1 billion smokers (73% of the total) are in developing countries.Tobacco Control, Winter 1995, p. 327

17. During the 1980's, while per capita cigarette consumption was declining an average of 1.4% per year in developed countries, it rose an average of 1.7% annually in less-developed countries. In 1970, per capita consumption was 3.25 times higher in developed countries as in less-developed countries. By 1992, the ratio had fallen to 1.75, and it is expected to be equal by 2005 or 2010.                       *Smoke and Mirrors*, pp. 209-210

18. While low tar and nicotine cigarettes are popular in developed countries, most cigarettes available in underdeveloped countries are very high in tar and nicotine.                       NEJM, March 28, 1991, p. 918

19. 1990 smoking prevalence in the Philippines was 64% of men and 19% of women; in India, 53% of men and 3% of women; in China, 61% of men and 7% of women; in Russia, 50% of men and 12% of women; and in Saudi Arabia, 53% of men and only 2% of women.                       American Medical News, October 3, 1994, p. 14

20. "A white supremacist racism is explicit in much Third World tobacco advertising. . . with products in Western settings with Caucasian models...Such advertising...offering vicarious participation in wildly fantastic jet-setting lifestyles to populations often living in the world's worst squalor and shanty-town degradation."
                       *Tobacco Control in the Third World*, p. 78

21. "Stevie Wonder...Luciano Pavarotti, Tom Berenger, Roger Moore, James Coburn, Jimmy Connors, and John McEnroe have all endorsed cigarettes overseas, either directly or indirectly. And they don't get any grief about it here, because nobody sees it."       *Thank You for Smoking*, Christopher Buckley, Random House, 1994, p. 205

22. In the Third World, tobacco is often used by the very poor as an appetite suppressant.
                       *Tobacco Control in the Third World*, p. 16

23. North America comprises only about 5% of the world's tobacco market.
                       American Medical News, October 20, 1997, p. 30

24. Multinational companies control 75% of the cigarette market in Latin America, 85% in Eastern Europe, but only 1% in China. (The companies first entered the China market in 1995.)
                       10th World on Tobacco or Health, Beijing, 1997 (Greg Connolly)

25. Tobacco marketing is exemplified by the types of brand names that have been available: Long Life (Taiwan), Life (Malawi, Chile), Hollywood (Brazil), Sport (Mexico), Ambassade (Zaire), Diplomat (Ghana), Casino (Latin America), Parisiennes (Argentina), Charms (India), High Society (Nigeria), Full Speed (Ecuador), Sportsman (Kenya), Olympic (Cote d'Ivoire), and Double Happiness (China)...In Abidjan, Cote d'Ivorie, a Marlboro advertisement occupies the highest point in the city's skyline. In Malaysia, Taiwan, South Korea, and Hong Kong, the Marlboro Adventure Team program is a competition offering lucky entrants a 9-day adventure in the American "Wild West". In the Philippines, where the population is predominantly Roman Catholic, promotional calendars feature cigarette brands under a picture of the Virgin Mary.
                       Quote from *Smoke and Mirrors*, p. 226 (Rob Cunningham)

26. In 1990-1992, the countries with the highest annual per capita cigarette consumption per adult 15 years of age and older were Poland (3620), Greece (3590), Hungary (3260), Japan (3240), Korea (3010), Switzerland (2910), Iceland (2860), the Netherlands (2820), Yugoslavia (2800), Australia (2710), and Spain and the United

States (2670). Countries with the lowest reported consumption included the Sudan, Niger, Burma (Myanamar), Afghanistan, and Ethiopia, all with 170 cigarettes per capita per year or less.

*Tobacco or Health: a Global Status Report*, 1997, pp. 25-27

27. The countries with the highest smoking prevalence for men are Korea (68%), Latvia and Russia (67%), the Dominican Republic (66%), Tonga (65%), Turkey (63%), China (61%), Bangladesh (60%), and Fiji and Japan (59%). (Individual country surveys were between 1988 and 1994.)

*Tobacco or Health: a Global Status Report*, 1997, p. 14

28. The countries with the highest female smoking prevalence (age 15 and over) are Denmark (37%), Norway (35%), the Czech Republic (31%), Fiji (30.6%), and Israel and Russia (30%). Countries with a female smoking prevalence of 4% or less include China, India, Sri Lanka, Pakistan, Indonesia, Thailand, Malaysia, Singapore, Egypt, Saudi Arabia, Lesotho, Uzbekistan, and Turkmenistan.

*Tobacco or Health: a Global Status Report*, World Health Organization, 1997

29. Worldwide, tobacco provides an estimated 47 million jobs, including 30 million in growing the crop. (15 million of the agricultural jobs are in China.)

10th World Conference on Tobacco or Health, Beijing, 1997 (Kenneth Warner)

30. Average 1999 prices in U.S. dollars for a pack of cigarettes are $3.88 in Hong Kong and $5.50 in the United Kingdom.

CBS evening news, July 8, 1999

31. Of the half billion deaths from tobacco expected among people alive today, about 100 million are expected to be in Chinese men.

*Curbing the Epidemic*, p. 23

# Canada

1. Adult smoking rates for Canada are 25% of adults (27% of men and 23% of women). In the United States, the rates are 23.6% (25% of men and 21.5% of women).

data from *The Tobacco Atlas*

2. "The tobacco industry, those who sell tobacco to our children, are kissing cousins to those who push marijuana, or hashish, or crack, or heroin. It is time we treated them as such."

Marcian Fournier, M.D., President, Canadian Medical Society,
Canadian Medical Association Journal, January 1, 1990, p. 58

3. "We recommend the prohibition of all forms of tobacco advertising and promotion in Canada, including advertising in conjunction with athletic events. We also support the taxation of tobacco products at a level to discourage their purchase, with tax revenues earmarked for health budgets." Canadian Medical Association policy statement, 1985. By 1990, all these objectives had been enacted.

Canadian Medical Association Journal, June 15, 1985, p. 1440A

4. The government of British Columbia received $505 million from tobacco taxes and $579 million from alcohol taxes in 1995. While it allocated more than $50 million to address alcohol problems, only $350,000 went to fund tobacco control efforts.

Canadian Medical Association Journal, January 15, 1996, p. 163

5. Cigarettes cost an average of five to six dollars a pack in Canada by 1991; taxes averaged $3.72 per pack, or 18.6 cents per cigarette.

Canadian Medical Association Journal, July 1, 1991, p. 45

6. If the United States taxed cigarettes at the same level as Canada, $40 billion per year in tax revenue would be collected, and 120,000 lives per year would eventually be saved because of reduced consumption.

Canadian Medical Association Journal, 1993

7. In Canada, the 1980 annual average of 3800 cigarettes smoked per capita in adults fell to 2600 in 1990, down by about a third. During that time, teenage smoking fell by two-thirds.

American Medical News, September 2, 1991, p. 8

8.  There are at least 45,000 tobacco-related deaths in Canada each year among the country's 5.4 million smokers, and smoking-related health care costs total nearly $3 billion annually.
    Canadian Medical Association Journal, August 1, 1994, p. 338 and *Smoke and Mirrors*, p. ix

9.  36% of French Canadian adults smoke, compared with 26% of English Canadian adults. Quebec has the highest smoking rate, 32% of the teenage and adult population, of any of the Canadian provinces. "For decades, Quebec has held out as a guilt-free, laissez-faire smokers' paradise in North America's increasingly prohibitionist sea."
    New York Times, January 25, 2000, p. D8

10. Philip Morris threatened Canada with divestment and future economic reprisals if Canada were to pass a tombstone packaging law, which would allow only for plain black and white packaging. In addition, PM said that it would file a suit under the North American Free Trade Agreement claiming that the packaging law would be an unfair trade barrier, threatening Canada with millions of dollars in trade penalties.
    *Tobacco Industry Strategies*, p. 9

11. In Canada, smoking is part of the "Navy culture." 53% of junior enlisted Navy personnel are smokers, more than twice the national rate of 26%; cigarettes on board Navy ships cost $1.50 a pack compared to over $6 a pack on the "outside."         Canadian Medical Association Journal, December 15, 1992, p. 1827

12. In response to smoking rates of 45% in the Canadian Navy, largely because cigarettes are sold for $1.50 per pack compared to $6 in civilian stores, the Navy discontinued sales of all tobacco products from shore facilities as well as ships in port.         Tobacco Control, Fall 1993, p. 191 and JAMA, October 27, 1993, p. 1932

13. In Canada, smoking prevalence in 15- to 19- year olds dropped from 46% in 1979 to 16% in 1991, a decrease of almost two thirds, largely as a result of a 2.6-fold increase in the inflation-adjusted cigarette price.
    Adolescent Medicine, June 1993, p. 310

14. The large increases in cigarette taxes in Canada led to a 35% reduction in adult consumption and a 62% decrease in consumption by teens between 1985 and 1991.
    *Preventing Tobacco Use Among Young People*, 1994 Surgeon General report, p. 273

15. In Canada, cigarette sales declined from 71.3 billion units in 1981 to 40.1 billion in 1992, a 44% drop in sales. Taxes per pack rose in this time from 96 cents to an average of $3.58. Despite the drop in sales, tax revenue rose from $3.4 to $7.2 billion during this time.         Washington Post, September 15, 1993

16. About 30% of cigarettes smoked in Canada in the early 1990's were smuggled in, including contraband cigarettes accounting for up to 75% of the market in Quebec. Because of this, Prime Minister Jean Chretien slashed federal tobacco taxes by $11 per carton in February 1994.         JAMA, March 2, 1994, p. 647

17. By early 1994, two-thirds of the cigarettes sold in Quebec and one-third of those sold in Ontario were contraband. In February, the federal government in Ottawa cut the tax, and the price of a "legal" carton of 200 cigarettes sold in Quebec fell from $47 to $22.73 overnight. Public health authorities warned that despite cutting smuggling from the United States, the price decreases will induce additional 245,000 Canadian teenagers to begin smoking.         Canadian Medical Association Journal, April 15, 1994, p. 1295

18. In 1994, five eastern provinces in Canada lowered cigarette taxes, dropping the price from (Canadian) $47 a carton to $26 or less. The provinces in western Canada, British Columbia, Alberta, Saskatchewan, and Manitoba, kept their taxes high, and a carton still costs from $45 to $48. This resulted in smuggling and contraband sales; an estimated 20% of cigarettes sold in British Columbia are contraband, resulting in a tax revenue loss of up to $125 million each year.     Canadian Medical Association Journal, January 13, 1998, p. 97

19. The average price of cigarettes in Alberta is now (Canada) $64 a carton.     Edmonton Journal, March 20, 2002

20. For the indigenous (Inuit) peoples of Canada, the average adult cigarette smoking prevalence rate is 62%. The prevalence is 72% in the age 20-24 group. 11th Conference on Tobacco or Health, Chicago, 2000, Abstract SR02

21. Between 1982 and 1992, total per capita cigarette consumption in Canada fell by 38%. And between 1979 and 1991, smoking prevalence among Canadians over age 14 decreased from 38% to 26%, as teenage smoking declined from 42% to 16%. *Growing Up Tobacco Free*, p. 186

22. "Can a vigorous national policy that includes high taxation and strong legislation toward smoking bring about significant declines in tobacco consumption? In Canada, the answer is yes... For policymakers, the conclusions are simple. Although education and smoking cessation programs can result in moderate declines in tobacco consumption, major declines can be achieved through increased taxation and advertising bans." American Journal of Public Health, July 1991, p. 902

23. In Canada, smoking prevalence in men peaked at 62% in 1960. Among women, prevalence peaked at 40% in 1974. *Smoke and Mirrors*, p. 14

24. The first completely smoke free Olympics were the 1988 Calgary Winter Games. *Smoke and Mirrors*, p. 190

25. George Knudson, Canada's most famous golfer who won eight PGA events in the 1960's and 1970's, died of lung cancer at age 51. JAMA, May 28, 1997, p. 1652

26. Of every 1000 Canadians age 20 who smoke, about half (500) will eventually die from smoking if they continue, 250 of them before the age of 70. In contrast, 9 of the 1000 will die in traffic accidents, and one will be murdered. National Clearinghouse on Tobacco and Health (Canada) Fact Sheet

# Latin America

1. Latin America and Caribbean adult smoking rates (percentages) from *The Tobacco Atlas*, 2002

| Country | Total | Male | Female |
|---|---|---|---|
| Argentina | 40.4 | 46.8 | 34.0 |
| Bahamas | 11.5 | 19.0 | 4.0 |
| Bolivia | 30.4 | 42.7 | 18.1 |
| Brazil | 33.8 | 38.2 | 29.3 |
| Chile | 22.2 | 26.0 | 18.3 |
| Columbia | 22.3 | 23.5 | 21.0 |
| Costa Rica | 17.6 | 28.6 | 6.6 |
| Cuba | 37.2 | 48.0 | 26.3 |
| Dominican Republic | 20.7 | 24.3 | 17.1 |
| Ecuador | 31.5 | 45.5 | 17.4 |
| El Salvador | 25.0 | 38.0 | 12.0 |
| Guatemala | 27.8 | 37.8 | 17.7 |
| Haiti | 9.7 | 10.7 | 8.6 |
| Honduras | 23.5 | 36.0 | 11.0 |
| Jamaica | 14.6 | -- | -- |
| Mexico | 34.8 | 51.2 | 18.4 |
| Panama | 38.0 | 56.0 | 20.0 |
| Paraguay | 14.8 | 4.1 | 5.5 |
| Peru | 28.6 | 41.5 | 15.7 |
| Trinidad | 25.1 | 42.1 | 8.0 |
| Uruguay | 23.0 | 31.7 | 14.3 |
| Venezuela | 40.5 | 41.8 | 39.2 |

2. 37% of men and 20% of women in Latin America are smokers. San Francisco Chronicle, December 26, 1994, p. A17

3. Fidel Castro, a long-time cigar smoker, has stopped smoking, and has also made well-publicized public statements supporting smoking control. Social Science and Medicine 1993; 38:109

4.  The smoking prevalence in Cuba (age 15 and older) declined from 42% in 1984 to 37% in 1995.
                                    Abstract PO 114, 10th World Conference on Tobacco or Health, Beijing, 1997

5.  Total cigarette consumption in the Dominican Republic rose by 44% between 1976 and 1990, with aggressively
    promoted Marlboros accounting for most of the increase.          World Watch, July-August 1997, p. 21

6.  Puerto Rico has much higher smoking prevalence rates than the rest of the United States, and Winston has 80% of
    the market share. In Hispanic areas all over the United States, Skoal Bandits are a heavy promoter of Cinco de
    Mayo events.                          10th World Conference on Tobacco or Health, Beijing, 1997 (Alan Blum, M.D.)

7.  "Mexicans have enjoyed smoking for a long time. Ceramic figurines found recently in a tomb in central Mexico
    dating from A.D. 135 depict two people puffing on cigarettes and grinning."
                                    New York Times, June 30, 1996, p. 14 (Travel Section)

8.  Cigarette ads were banned on television and radio in Mexico as of January 2003.
                                    Contra Costa Times, June 1, 2002, p. A16

9.  "During Nicaragua's civil war, when most vehicles wandering into battle zones were considered fair game, the
    contra rebels refused to fire on distribution trucks from tobacco companies. In a nation of heavy smokers,
    sabotaging the cigarette supply was no way to win hearts and minds."
                                    San Francisco Chronicle, December 26, 1994, p. A1

10. "Brown and Williamson has virtually redecorated Managua with the red-white-and-black logo of its Lucky Strike
    brand. Hundreds of restaurants, pool halls and grocery stores are garnished with Lucky Strike neon signs, wall
    clocks and ash trays."                      San Francisco Chronicle, December 26, 1994, p. A17

11. In Columbia, Marlboro is the most popular brand, and Marlboro Man billboards are all over in its cities. Although
    Marlboros in most cases can be bought legally only in duty-free shops, only an estimated 4% of the brand smoked in
    the country got there legally; the remaining Marlboros are smuggled in.          Newsweek, July 31, 2000, pp. 38-39

12. In a survey of medical students in Columbia, 26% were current smokers.
                                    11th World Conference on Tobacco or Health, Chicago, 2000, Abstract, PO 200

13. In a survey from Argentina, 38% of physicians and 33% of registered nurses were current smokers.
                                    11th World Conference on Tobacco or Health, Chicago, 2000, Abstract PO 115

14. In a survey from Buenos Aires, 20% of 8th graders were current smokers, as were 43% of 11th graders.
                                    American Journal of Public Health, February 2001, p. 219

15. Brazil is the fourth largest tobacco producer in the world, and in 1999 exported 341,000 tons of tobacco generating
    U.S. $884 million in income.          11th World Conference on Tobacco or Health, Chicago, 2000, Abstract NT 18

16. The smoking prevalence in Brazil in 1996 was 30.6 million smokers in the country of 150 million people. Total
    yearly deaths are 80,000 caused by tobacco. 36% of pregnant women are smokers.
                                    Abstracts PO 323 and 324, 10th World Conference on Tobacco or Health, Beijing, 1997

17. There are about 209,000 tobacco farmers in Brazil cultivating 750,000 acres of land; in 1997, 300,000 tons of
    tobacco worth almost a billion dollars was exported, representing one third of Brazil's agricultural income, after
    soybeans and coffee. Tobacco companies make high profits on fertilizers and pesticides (many of the latter highly
    toxic and banned in Europe and the U.S.) that they sell to tobacco farmers. 9540 cases of pesticide poisoning and
    919 deaths were reported from 1986 to 1997; in Southern Brazil, tobacco workers were the main victims.
                                    Earth Island Journal, Fall 1998, p. 28

18. Total employment from tobacco cultivation, manufacturing, and distribution in Brazil is about 2.5 million. The price
    of a pack averages $1.07.     Abstracts OS 155 and 156, 10th World Conference on Tobacco or Health, Beijing, 1997

19. "Brazil is the main exporter of tobacco leaves and the 4<sup>th</sup> major world producer, behind only China, USA and India. In 1994/1995 there were 1,040,000 farmers employed in the tobacco crops."
Abstract PO 322, 10th World Conference on Tobacco or Health, Beijing, 1997

20. In the Brazilian state of Rio Grande do Sul, high-nicotine tobacco is grown on 20,000 acres. Farmers call it fumo louco, or crazy tobacco, because it has been genetically altered to have twice the nicotine of standard tobacco leaf. The plants are 12 feet tall, 7 feet higher than regular varieties.
Associated Press, December 21, 1997

21. B.A.T. industries has opened an $80 million tobacco processing plant in Santa Cruz do Sul, Brazil, about 800 miles southwest of Rio de Janeiro. Its annual capacity is 120,000 tons, greater than any other facility of its kind in the world, and "just down the road, Philip Morris is working on its own $220 million expansion." Unlike most of Brazil, the area economy is booming.
Wall Street Journal, July 21, 1997, p. B1

22. In 1985, the World Health Organization named smoking as the leading cause of death in Brazil, the first developing country to gain this distinction.
*Tobacco Control in the Third World*, p. 15

23. In Brazil, $68.2 million was spent on tobacco advertising in 1988, the highest per capita amount of any developing country in the world. "On the South Atlantic coast, deforestation is virtually total, with the tobacco industry being the main culprit."
Tobacco Control

24. Brazil's 100,000 tobacco farmers alone need annually the wood of about 60 million trees, or the equivalent of 1.5 million acres of forest, to cure their tobacco, according to one estimate. In 1991 alone, 20,000 new curing barns were built.
*No Smoking*, RE Goodin, University of Chicago Press, 1989, p.118,
*Smoke Ring: the Politics of Tobacco*, P. Taylor, Bodley Head, 1984, and Panos Briefing, September 1994

25. "In one of the widest attacks on smoking in the Third World, Brazil's Health Ministry has announced a ban on cigarette advertising in sporting and cultural events and on television until 11 p.m. Prime-time shows...will also be forbidden from showing people smoking...For those who cannot read, a graphic warning will cover one quarter of the front of each cigarette pack. One of the eight designs shows a black cloud hanging over a fetus carried by a smoking woman."
New York Times, January 15, 1995

26. In Brazil, nine new picture-based warnings must be placed on cigarette packs beginning January 1, 2002. The warnings will cover 100% of the back of the pack, and will have text warnings that include several topics, including cancer, heart disease, impotence, addiction, and the effects of smoking on pregnancy. Words like "light" or "suave" will no longer be permitted on packs. A toll-free number for those wishing to quit will also be provided. The tobacco industry publication, *Tobacco Journal International*, calls the new law "a serious blow to the country's tobacco industry."
2002 AMA Annual Tobacco Report

27. Cigarette consumption in Brazil dropped rapidly in the early 1990's, from 164 billion in 1990 to 103 billion in 1994, a per capita drop of 40 percent taking into account population growth.
New York Times, January 15, 1995

28. In 1993, Brazil overtook the US as the world's largest exporter of raw tobacco. In 1994, Brazil exported $1 billion worth of tobacco, double the level of five years earlier.
New York Times, January 15, 1995

29. From 1973 to 1993 in Chile, prevalence of smoking for women increased from 25% to 35%. About 45% of women smokers continue the habit throughout their pregnancies.
Panoscope, October 1994, p. 20

30. In Chile, smoking rates are 35%, but the prevalence is 55% in the 15 to 16 year old group. Popular brands are "Life" and "Advance". Cigarettes can be bought individually, and sales to children are legal. The total yearly budget for tobacco control is $20,000, donated by the World Health Organization. In a Lucky Strike campaign, a poster of a man on a motorcycle in Monument Valley, Arizona with the slogan "An American Original" greets visitors on every available space at the Santiago airport.
Tobacco Control, Summer 1994, p. 161

31. The Chile Ministry of Public Health estimates that 40% of the 13 year olds in Santiago are smokers
Reader's Digest, April 1993, p. 55

# Australia, New Zealand, and the Pacific

1.  Australia and the Pacific adult smoking rates (percent) from *The Tobacco Atlas*, 2002

    | Country | Total | Male | Female |
    |---|---|---|---|
    | Australia | 19.5 | 21.1 | 18.0 |
    | Fiji | 20.5 | 24.0 | 17.0 |
    | New Zeeland | 25.0 | 25.0 | 25.0 |
    | Papua New Guinea | 37.0 | 46.0 | 28.0 |
    | Samoa | 23.3 | 33.9 | 12.7 |
    | Tonga | 38.3 | 62.4 | 14.2 |

2.  Smoking prevalence in Australia (age 14 and older daily smokers) had dropped to 19.5% in 2001, compared to 58% of men and 28% of women in the 1960's.        Simon Chapman, Ph.D., lecture, San Francisco, November 20, 2002

3.  Cigarettes sold in Australia have warning labels covering a third of the back and one quarter of the front of each pack.                              9th World Conference on Tobacco or Health, Paris, 1994 (M. Swanson)

4.  A controversy eruption in May 1994 in Australia over the appointment of Bronwyn Bishop as shadow minister of health. Her first public statement was: "If a product is legal then it should be able to be advertised. It can be cigarettes today, alcohol tomorrow, Mars bars the day after...I say to those people who believe [tobacco] is a dreadful product to make your case. They have not done so." The president of the Australian Medical Association called for her resignation, and a press commentator termed her comments "one of the most absurd statements any spokesperson for health has ever issued."                              British Medical Journal, June 18, 1994, p. 1590

5.  In 1992, tobacco consumption was estimated to have cost more than 19,000 lives in Australia and $9.2 billion for health care and loss of productivity.                              The Lancet, February 10, 1996, p 390

6.  "Philip Morris in Australia argued persistently that its small, inexpensive packs of 15 cigarettes were not marketed with children in mind, despite an overtly teenage oriented advertising campaign. A quick survey comparing schoolchildren and adults from the same area showed otherwise: 57% of smoking children had bought a pack of 15s in the past month compared with only 8% of adult smokers. As a result, Philip Morris's argument was quickly diffused and the small packs banned in South Australia, causing a domino effect around all the other Australian states in the following few years."
    *The Fight for Public Health,* Simon Chapman, BMJ Publishing Group, 1994, p. 245

7.  In a 1990 survey of the cigarette brand preferences of Australian children ages 12 to 17 in four different states, the preferences corresponded perfectly and dramatically with the brands of cigarette that sponsored the major football team in each of the four states. This information refuted the tobacco industry's claim that tobacco sponsorship of football was not a form of advertising, and that even if it were, it did not influence children in any way. In 1992, the federal government supported a legislative ban on tobacco sponsorship.
    *The Fight for Public Health*, Simon Chapman, BMJ Publishing Group, 1994, p. 162

8.  In 1980, the Australian Advertising Standards council prohibited actor Paul Hogan from participating in a major advertising campaign for Winfield Cigarettes because of his enormous popularity with children.
    British Medical Journal, November 1, 1980, p. 1197

9.  "I'm going to try to be the healthiest health minister in Australia – by eating well, exercising and drinking in moderation." New Year's resolution of the New South Wales health minister, a heavy smoker.
    Tobacco Control, Summer 1997, p. 143

10. In Australia, the Northern Territory has the country's highest smoking rate, 28%, down from 37% a decade ago. The national prevalence is 23%. [The prevalence dropped to 19.5% in 2001 –editor]
    The Australian, December 24, 1997

11. In New Zealand, tobacco is responsible for 4500 deaths each year, and in Australia, an estimated 18,000. In Australia in 1993, 29% of men and 21% of women smoked, compared to 60% of men and 28% of women in 1964.

World Health Organization Regional Office for the Western Pacific

12. In New Zealand between 1984 and 1992, consumption per adult fell 42 percent and smoking prevalence from 32 to 27 percent. In 1990 the Smoke-free Environments Act was passed, banning tobacco advertising and restricting smoking at work, in shops, transport and other enclosed public places. *Tobacco and Health*, p. 169

13. "Just over half of all Maori over the age of 15 smoke (54%); Maori men at a rate of 45%, Maori women 57%. As many as 68% of our pregnant Maori women smoke. Smoking rates for our young Maori women in their 20s is as high as 77%, and 12% of Maori children aged 10-14 are regular smokers."

*Tobacco and Health*, p. 908 (Marewa Glover)

14. Among New Zealand Maori, smoking causes one in three deaths, including 42% of all deaths from cancer. Two thirds of Maori women smoke during pregnancy. *Tobacco: the Growing Epidemic*, pp.73 and 468

15. In New Zealand, about one in three deaths in the Maori native population are due to smoking.

Abstract OS 2, 10th World Conference on Tobacco or Health, Beijing, 1997

16. Pacific Island smoking rates for French Polynesia are 41% of men and 27% of women (1986 data), 40% prevalence in Guam (1989), 46% of men and 28% of women in Papua New Guinea (1990), and 65% of men and 14% of women in Tonga (1991). World Health Organization Regional Office for the Western Pacific

17. In Samoa in 1994, the smoking prevalence was 53% of men and 19% of women, as well as 50% of male doctors. In Fiji, 59% of Melanesian men and 51% of Fijian Indian men smoke, as do 31% of Melanesian women and 14% of Fijian Indian women (1988 data). World Health Organization Regional Office for the Western Pacific

# Western Europe

1. Western Europe adult smoking rates (percent) from *The Tobacco Atlas*, 2002:

| Country | Total | Male | Female |
|---|---|---|---|
| Austria | 24.5 | 30.0 | 19.0 |
| Belgium | 28.0 | 30.0 | 26.0 |
| Denmark | 30.5 | 32.0 | 29.0 |
| Finland | 23.5 | 27.0 | 20.0 |
| France | 34.5 | 38.6 | 30.3 |
| Germany | 35.0 | 39.0 | 31.0 |
| Iceland | 24.0 | 25.0 | 23.0 |
| Ireland | 31.5 | 32.0 | 31.0 |
| Italy | 24.9 | 32.4 | 17.3 |
| Malta | 23.9 | 33.1 | 14.6 |
| Netherlands | 33.0 | 37.0 | 29.0 |
| Norway | 31.5 | 31.0 | 32.0 |
| Portugal | 18.7 | 30.2 | 7.1 |
| Spain | 33.4 | 42.1 | 24.7 |
| Sweden | 19.0 | 19.0 | 19.0 |
| Switzerland | 33.5 | 39.0 | 28.0 |
| United Kingdom | 26.5 | 27.0 | 26.0 |

2. In Europe, the smoking prevalence for men has stabilized to 38% (34% in western Europe and 47% in eastern Europe) and 24% for women (25% western European and 20% for eastern European women.)

The Lancet, February 16, 2002, p. 585

3. The 15 European Union nations with 375 million people agreed to adopt in October 2002 one of the world's toughest anti-smoking laws. Cigarette companies will be required to disclose all ingredients and limit tar to 10 milligrams and nicotine to no more than one milligram per cigarette. The law also bans manufacturers from using terms such as "mild" and "low tar" on the grounds that they falsely suggest lower toxicity. As well, health warnings will become much larger and more explicit, and (as in Canada) graphic pictures of scarred lungs, rotting teeth, and other smoking-induced afflictions will begin.                    Washington Post National Weekly Edition, May 21-27, 2001, p. 16

4. Smoking kills 114,000 women in the European Union each year.
                    11th World Conference on Tobacco or Health, Chicago, 2000, Abstract EM 01

5. The World Health Organization estimates that the deaths of 571,000 persons in 1994 in the European Community will be attributable to smoking.                    JAMA, March 2,1994, p. 643

6. At present smoking rates, 20 million out of Europe's 250 million children will be killed by tobacco.
                    The Lancet, September 21, 1991, p. 748

7. In Europe in the early 1990's, overall smoking prevalence was 45% for males and 25% for females. Highest rates for men was over 60% in Greece, Hungary, and Turkey, and 57% in Spain and 56% in Poland. The highest rate for women was in Denmark (47%).                    Tobacco Alert (WHO), July 1993, p. 5

8. The number of deaths from smoking in Europe just in the age group 35 to 69 years doubled from 700,000 in 1965 to almost 1,400,000 in 1995. Central and Eastern Europe have the highest rates of smoking-related mortality in the world.                    *Interventions for Smokers*, pp. 323 and 344

9. In the European Union each year, over 130,000 individuals die from lung cancer, and approximately 450,000 premature deaths are caused by tobacco-related diseases. Of every three premature deaths (in the 35 to 65 year age group), one is caused by tobacco. In spite of these health effects, in the European Union, tobacco consumption has decreased only slightly in men and has markedly increased in women over the past ten years.
                    *Tobacco and Health*, p. 213

10. There are 2,000 "Marlboro Classics" clothing stores in Europe.
                    Eric Solberg, tobacco seminar lecture of July 10, 1996, St. Louis

11. In 1993, the European Union gave $1.44 billion in price supports to tobacco producers.
                    *Tobacco and Health*, p. 208

12. The European Commission (European Common Market) spends $14 million each year to promote information on the health hazards of smoking. But it spends $1600 million, or more than 100 times as much, for price supports and subsidies to Europe's tobacco growers each year.
                    The Lancet, November 2, 1991, p. 1138 and British Medical Journal, April 9, 1994, p. 938

13. European price subsidies to encourage tobacco production are 684.5 million pounds a year, more than sixty times the amount (10.3 million pounds) spent for programs designed to reduce smoking. There is no domestic demand for the poor quality highly subsidized European Union tobacco, so most of it is sold in Eastern Europe or in North Africa at prices which are less than a fifth of the original subsidy.                    British Medical Journal, November 16, 1996, p. 1228

14. The European Union countries in 1994 produced 328,000 tons of tobacco, much of it of poor quality, and imported 490,000 tons to meet demand. The Union spends $1.24 billion a year on tobacco subsidies, but only $1.85 million on smoking prevention.                    British Medical Journal, March 30, 1996, p. 832

15. The European Commission in 1992 proposed a total ban on the advertising of tobacco products, but a blocking minority of the United Kingdom, Germany, Denmark, and the Netherlands until late 1997 prevented implementation. Countries with advertising bans and restriction of smoking in public places are France, Italy, Portugal, Finland, and

Sweden. (Norway also does, but is not a member of the European Union.)  The United Kingdom, Denmark, Germany, and Spain, on the other hand, have no general regulation covering smoking in public places.

Journal of the National Cancer Institute, September 4, 1996, p. 1189

16. The United Kingdom, Germany, and the Netherlands until late 1997 repeatedly defeated the European Union draft directive for a tobacco advertising ban. A billion dollars is spent each year subsidizing tobacco growing, including much that is of worthless quality that is dumped in Eastern Europe. This compares to less than $2 million for anti-tobacco work, and the grant to fund BASP (Bureau for Action on Smoking Prevention) has not been renewed.

Tobacco Control, Spring 1996, p. 9

17. The 15 European Union member nations in December 1997 voted to eliminate most tobacco advertising within three years, all advertising in six years, and sponsorship of sporting events and the arts within eight years.

Los Angeles Times, December 5, 1997

18. Philip Morris is the largest seller of cigarettes in Europe, controlling a third of the market.

New York Times, December 5, 1997, p. A1

19. Since Great Britain's first cigarette pack warnings in 1962, tobacco has been responsible for four million deaths in the country.

NBC evening news (Tom Brokaw), February 1994

20. There are 13 million adult smokers in the United Kingdom.

Journal of the National Cancer Institute, January 20, 1999

21. Smoking causes 120,000 deaths each year in the United Kingdom, and smoking prevalence is 28% in adults.

British Medical Journal, January 16, 1999, p. 182

22. In 1991 in Great Britain, there were smokers in three quarters of the families receiving income support from the government, and one seventh of their disposable income was spent on cigarettes.

British Medical Journal, November 7, 1998, p. 1266

23. In the United Kingdom, 10% of women and 12% of men in the highest socioeconomic group are smokers. The figures for the lowest socioeconomic groups are 35% for women and 40% for men.     *Curbing the Epidemic*, p. 16

24. In the United Kingdom, 350 deaths a year are due to illicit drugs, 25,000 deaths from alcohol, and 100,000 deaths a year from smoking. (By 1994, deaths had increased to 138,000--Richard Peto.)

British Journal of Addiction 1990; 85:313

25. In England in 1992, 25% of girls and 21% of boys at the age of 15 years were regular smokers.

Tobacco Control, Spring 1995, p. 103

26. Smoking among British 15-year-olds dropped from 30% in 1996 to 23% in 1999; a pack of cigarettes in the UK costs about $6.

Associated Press, November 3, 2000

27. One in four 15 year olds in the UK are regular smokers, as are 35% of the population ages 20 to 34.

British Medical Association (www.tobaccofactfile.org)

28. Benson and Hedges cigarettes in the UK have "by appointment to her Majesty the Queen" printed on each package.

29. Prince Charles' friend Camilla Parker Bowles is a Marlboro smoker.     Time, September 7, 1998, p. 48

30. In the United Kingdom, over half of persons over 60 years old previously smoked regularly.

NEJM, February 12, 1998, p. 471

31. In the UK, smokers pay an extra 25% to 70% supplement for life insurance. In Norway, drivers are prohibited from smoking behind the wheel in urban areas, and in Spain, drivers are prohibited from lighting a cigarette while the engine is running.

Nonsmokers Pay Less, Europe Against Cancer, 1992, pp. 18 and 20

32. Only 4% of general practice physicians in Great Britain are smokers, but this figure is 32% for GPs in France. More than 50% of the male doctors in several European countries still smoke     Tobacco Control, Fall 1993, p. 187

33. Victims of tobacco include Queen Elizabeth's father, King George VI, her grandfather, King George V, and her uncle, King Edward VIII, the Duke of Windsor. The Queen Mother, a nonsmoker, when she died at age 101 in 2000 had outlived her husband King George VI by more than 50 years.

34. Every king of England in the 20th century died from tobacco-related disease.
     Canadian Medical Association Journal, January 15, 1993, p. 243

35. Cambridge University has accepted a $2.25 million donation from British American Tobacco (BAT) to fund the Sir Patrick Sheehy chair in international relations, named after BAT's retiring chairman.
     British Medical Journal, July 27, 1996, p. 186

36. "Are the finances of Cambridge University really so desperate that it will succumb to one of the more audacious tobacco advertising ploys attempted in recent years?" The university proposes to accept 1.5 million pounds from British American Tobacco to fund a new chair in international relations. The company's profits went up to 56% to a record 1.56 billion pounds in 1995, most of the growth coming from selling 100 billion more cigarettes in developing countries than it had in 1994.     British Medical Journal, March 26, 1996, p. 72

37. When she was Prime Minister, Margaret Thatcher was a vigorous antismoking activist. After her retirement, she was hired as a consultant to Philip Morris for a reported fee of $2 million. One of her specific agreements was to try to open up markets in the Third World, particularly Asia, for Philip Morris cigarettes.
     60 Minutes, August 18, 1996

38. In 1985, "a U.S. company" opened a smokeless tobacco factory in Scotland and began a marketing strategy in the U.K., where oral tobacco use was almost unknown. In 1988, the U.K. government announced its intention to ban the product. The tobacco company challenged the decision in court, but the ban went into effect in 1990, and the European Commission instituted a community-wide ban (with the exception of Sweden) in 1992 on spit tobacco.
     Tobacco Control Fact Sheet 8, International Union Against Cancer

39. The annual cost of smoking to the National Health Service in England is estimated to be 1.5 billion pounds.
     British Medical Association (www.tobaccofactfile.org)

40. All tobacco advertising is now banned in Great Britain.     San Francisco Chronicle, February 15, 2003, p. A13

41. In Norway, the peak prevalence of smoking in men born between 1915 and 1930 was close to 80%. In the mid-1950's, smoking prevalence in Norwegian men was almost 70%.
     9th World Conference on Tobacco or Health, Paris, 1994 (K. Lund)

42. In Norway in 1996, 34% of adult males and 32% females were smokers. The price of cigarettes in Norway is $7 a pack, compared to an average of $1.91 in the United States, and smoking is banned in schools, hospitals, and government offices.     Wall Street Journal, June 12, 1997, pp. B1 and B13

43. Norway bans smoking in all public buildings.     San Francisco Chronicle, September 2, 2001, p. T3

44. More than half the cigarettes smoked in Norway, and almost half in the Netherlands, are hand-rolled or the "RYO" variety.     *Tobacco or Health: a Global Status Report*, 1997, p. 20

45. In Sweden the smoking prevalence is only 19%, one of the lowest rates of any developed country. However, there is also a 9% rate of smokeless tobacco use, and Sweden is the only country in Europe where smokeless tobacco is used to any degree. There is a long tradition of snuff use in Sweden, which has been exempted from the European Union ban on smokeless tobacco.     Abstract S6/3, 10th World Conference on Tobacco or Health, Beijing, 1997

46. In a 1997 survey in Sweden, smoking prevalence rates had dropped to 17% in men and 21% in women. In addition, about 20% of adult men, but very few women, use "snus" daily (oral moist smokeless tobacco).     Internet Sources

47. Only 19.7% of Swedes over age 15 were daily smokers in 1998, down from one in three in 1980. Sweden is the first and only country in the world to meet the World Health Organization's goal for smoking prevalence of 20%.

Associated Press, September 17, 1999

48. In Sweden between 1969 and 1996, smoking prevalence among doctors decreased from 46% to 6%.

Abstract PO 152, 10th World Conference on Tobacco or Health, Beijing, 1997

49. Sweden now has giant-size health warnings that occupy the entire back of the cigarette package.

American Medical News, April 1991

50. Miss Sweden 1996, Annika Duckmark, is a well-known smoke-free ambassador for Sweden, and attended the 1997 World Conference on Tobacco or Health in Beijing. Beginning in 1996, all candidates for Miss Sweden had to be nonsmokers. Abstract OS 35, 10th World Conference on Tobacco or Health, Beijing 1997

51. In contrast to Sweden, Denmark had a 33% smoking prevalence rate in 1995.

Abstract OS 35, 10th World Conference on Tobacco or Health, Beijing 1997

52. Finland was an early pioneer in the international antismoking campaign, in 1976 banning all tobacco advertising and sales to children. JAMA, June 22, 1994, p. 1957

53. In 1994, Philip Morris Europe ran a massive ad blitz about secondhand smoke, claiming that ETS is less dangerous than eating cookies or drinking milk. USA Today, June 28, 1994, p. 13A

54. Legal action by French biscuit manufacturers has succeeded in halting publication of an advertisement that claims that eating a biscuit a day is a greater cardiovascular risk than breathing secondhand tobacco. The biscuit manufacturers took their case to the highest civil court, the Paris tribunal de grande instance, where Jean-Pierre Marcus, vice president of the tribunal, promptly ruled against Philip Morris Europe. Philip Morris [had] launched a European advertising campaign in which it compared the risk of passive smoking to that of eating biscuits, drinking milk or chlorinated water, using too much pepper, or frying food with rapeseed oil.

Quote from British Medical Journal, July 6, 1996, p. 7

55. Tobacco kills about 60,000 people in France each year.

11th World Conference on Tobacco or Health, Chicago, 2000, Abstract PS03

56. In a 1999 survey from France, 32% of physicians were current smokers (34% of men and 25% of women).

11th World Conference on Tobacco or Health, Chicago, 2000, Abstract PO 120

57. In France in 1953, 77% of men and 12% of women smoked. By 1990, young women smoked as much as young men, and per capita consumption had doubled; deaths in 1990 in France were 55,000 males and 5000 females.

9th World Conference on Tobacco or Health, Paris, 1994 (C.Hill)

58. In France, 76% of the retail cost of a pack of cigarettes is tax. The money spent to educate people about the dangers of smoking is less than $400,000 a year. Nonsmokers worried about passive smoking are frequently dismissed as antisocial fanatics, despite a largely unenforced law making smoking illegal in cafes, public workplaces, restaurants, and train stations, except for designated areas. Los Angeles Times, January 26, 1997, p. A8

59. In France in 1998, Marlboro had a 29.6% market share as the leading brand, and Camel had a 5.6% market share.

Revue des Tabacs, May 1998, pp. 25-26

60. In France, there are no restrictions on cigarette sale to children, and 37% of people between the ages of 12 and 25 are smokers. A law which would ban sales to children under 16 is being considered.

New York Times, February 12, 2003, p. A6

61. French President Jacques Chirac, a former chain-smoker, has announced a "war on smoking" as part of an aggressive campaign to prevent cancer. He said France would continue to raise cigarette prices, and pledged to spend half a billion euros over five years in the fight against cancer. Reuters, March 24, 2003

62. At least 40% of physicians in France, Italy, Spain, Greece and Japan smoked in the early 1990s.
American Medical News, October 3, 1994, p. 14
and Morbidity and Mortality Weekly Report, May 12, 1993, p. 365

63. In France, sales of American cigarettes have surged. Marlboro had an 18% market share in 1995, just behind Gauloises Brunes with 19%. The proportion of French smokers who favor the dark tobacco of Gauloises and Gitanes has dropped from 46% to 27% in the last decade. New York Times, January 11, 1997, p. 4

64. The French government collected $5.48 billion in 1990 in tax revenues from tobacco sales. The annual cost to the country for health care related to smoking is estimated at $8.8 billion, plus $2.6 billion in lost productivity, for a total social cost per year of $11.4 billion.
9th World Conference on Tobacco or Health, Paris, 1994 and Atlantic Monthly, November 1991, p. 50

65. A tobacco counterad televised in France had a macho cowboy riding a horse on the range with inspirational western music playing. He dismounted and, instead of pushing Marlboros, advised listeners not to smoke. In a lawsuit against the ad, Philip Morris asked $3 million in damages, but was awarded the sum of one French franc. However, they were successful having the message taken off the air. American Medical News, April 20, 1992, p. 22

66. In France between 1953 and 1991, smoking prevalence in adult men decreased from 72% to 38%; in women during the same period, it increased from 17% to 26%. The highest current smoking rates are for young adults age 20 to 34; 69% of men and 62% of women in this age group were current smokers in the early 1990's.
*Tobacco and Health*, p. 122

67. In the Netherlands in 1990, 20% of medical students, 28% of interns and residents, and 34% of practicing physicians were smokers. European Respiratory Journal, April 1992

68. "Germany: tobacco industry paradise" from Tobacco Control, December 2001, pp. 300-303, describes the continued social acceptability of smoking in Germany, where 37% of men and 28% of women smoked in 1998. There are 800,000 cigarette vending machines with free access to all, and voluntary restrictions on tobacco advertising are largely ignored. Formula One motor racing champion Michael Schumacher, the world's highest paid sports figure "is the definitive Marlboro Man."

69. The German government collects almost $20 billion each year in tobacco taxes, or about 5% of the federal budget. It has balked at raising tobacco taxes, and has rebuffed efforts by the European Union to restrict tobacco advertising.
American Medical News, November 4, 1996, p. 6

70. Germany is Europe's largest producer of cigarettes, manufacturing one third of the 625 million cigarettes consumed in Western Europe each year. New York Times, December 5, 1997, p. C8

71. The German Parliament rejected a bill that would have restricted smoking in public buildings and workplaces.
Washington Post, February 6, 1998, p. A36

72. Frankfurt's international airport in 1998 became smoke-free in most of its passenger areas. This ban was seen as a bold and controversial move in a country where there are almost no limits on smokers. CNN, December 22, 1997

73. In Germany, the average age of starting smoking is 13.6 years. There are 800,000 cigarette vending machines in the country. Tobacco Control, December 2002, p. 292

74. In Switzerland in 1990, there were 10,550 deaths linked to tobacco, compared to 959 in auto accidents and 300 from illicit drugs. *Tobacco and Health*, p. 181

75. The Austrian government tobacco monopoly Austria Tabak has bought the Head ski company. Tabak recently introduced Head Lights cigarettes, featuring the classic ski-top logo and the "revolutionary Head filter system".
Ski Magazine, October 1995

76. In Italy in the early 1990's, 30% of female college graduates and 40% of university graduates smoked. The prevalence among physicians was 25.4%.                *Tobacco or Health, a Global Status Report*, 1997, p. 334

77. Italy has 18 million smokers, or 36% of the adult population. The Italian government produces a third of the cigarettes smoked, and is the sole legal distributor of tobacco products, earning $8 billion each year from tobacco sales. San Francisco Chronicle, August 16, 2000

78. "Italians are thinking what was once unthinkable: that it may be time to clamp down on tobacco users." The Italian Senate has approved a measure to forbid smoking in public places and confine restaurant smoking to special sections.                New York Times, November 12, 2002, p. A10

79. Smoking was banned in all indoor spaces in the Vatican in July 2002.                Reuters, June 27, 2002

80. In a survey in Italy of career military physicians and medical corpsmen at a military health school, 40% were smokers. Rates for military personnel at the La Spezia naval base were 46%, and 54% in a survey from three military commands.                *Tobacco and Health*, p. 914

81. In Italy, tobacco advertising was banned in the 1960's, and taxes are high, leading to "the flourishing contraband of American cigarettes from which a substantial part of Naples earns its living."
The Lancet, November 5, 1994, p. 1290

82. In November 1992, 14,000 striking tobacco workers in Italy blocked the supply of cigarettes to stores for several weeks, causing traffic into Switzerland to increase seven-fold as some of Italy's 13.5 million smokers (one-third of adults) headed north to buy cigarettes. The resulting black market resulted in prices of up to $125 a carton. Prostitutes were reportedly accepting 200-cigarette cartons as payment.                New York Times, November 28, 1992, p. A1

83. Italian tax fraud experts are investigating claims that Philip Morris, which holds 46% of the Italian cigarette market, took part in a $6.4 billion tax evasion scheme dating back to 1987.                Associated Press, July 6, 1996

84. Chocolate candy cigarettes packaged to look like real cigarettes are sold in Italy.
British Medical Journal, February 8, 2003, p. 302

85. In Spain, smoking prevalence declined from 40% in 1978 to 36% in 1993. However, in the same period, the percentage of male smokers declined from 65% to 48%, but the prevalence of smoking among women increased from 17% to 25%. In 1995, an estimated 46,000 men died from tobacco, up from 7,200 in 1955.
*Tobacco or Health: a Global Status Report*, p. 381

86. In Spain in the 1980's, 65% of male physicians smoked, and in the Netherlands, 56% did. In contrast, fewer than 10% of physicians smoke in the United States, the United Kingdom, Canada, Australia, and Norway.
British Journal of Addiction 1989; 84:1397

87. In a survey of medical students in Santiago, Spain, the prevalence of "habitual smokers" dropped from 58% in 1985 to 20% in 1996. Prevalence was also 20% in medical students from Zaragoza.
Abstracts PO 61 and 71, 10th World Conference on Tobacco or Health, Beijing, 1997

88. In a 1999 survey of medical students in Spain, 22% were smokers.
11th World Conference on Tobacco or Health, Abstract PO 200

89. In Greece, 44.9% of adults smoke daily, the highest percentage in Europe. In 2003, outdoor tobacco advertising will be banned, and for the first time, no-smoking sections will be available in restaurants. The Greek health minister is himself a smoker.                Contra Costa (CA.) Times, May 31, 2002, p. BC

90. Greece has the highest per capita yearly cigarette consumption in Europe (3800 cigarettes), and 51% of men are smokers.    *Taxes on Tobacco Products*, European Bureau for Action on Smoking Prevention, December 1992, p. 4

# Eastern Europe

1.  Eastern Europe adult smoking rates (percent) from *The Tobacco Atlas*, 2002

    | Country | Total | Male | Female |
    |---|---|---|---|
    | Albania | 39.0 | 60.0 | 18.0 |
    | Bosnia | 48.0 | -- | -- |
    | Bulgaria | 36.5 | 49.2 | 23.8 |
    | Croatia | 33.0 | 34.0 | 32.0 |
    | Czech Republic | 29.0 | 36.0 | 22.0 |
    | Greece | 38.0 | 47.0 | 29.0 |
    | Hungary | 35.5 | 44.0 | 27.0 |
    | Moldova | 32.0 | 46.0 | 18.0 |
    | Poland | 34.5 | 44.0 | 25.0 |
    | Romania | 43.5 | 62.0 | 25.0 |
    | Slovakia | 42.6 | 55.0 | 30.0 |
    | Slovenia | 25.2 | 30.0 | 20.3 |
    | Yugoslavia | 47.0 | 52.0 | 42.0 |

2.  In central and eastern Europe, smoking rates are high in men and rapidly increasing in women, while in northwestern Europe, smoking rates are similar in men and women.
    British Medical Association (www.tobaccofactfile.org)

3.  Five Eastern European nations are among the top ten consumers of cigarettes per capita (1993 data, cigarettes smoked per person per year). The top countries are, in order: Greece (2800 per capita), Hungary, Japan, Poland (2600), South Korea, Switzerland, Bulgaria, Yugoslavia, Spain, and the Czech Republic and Slovakia (approximately 1950 cigarettes per capita per year).
    Washington Post National Weekly Edition, December 9-15, 1996, p. 9

4.  42% to 45% of premature deaths in men ages 35 to 69 are attributable to smoking in the countries of Hungary, the Czech Republic, Poland, and Russia.    International Union Against Cancer (Geneva) newsletter, January 1995

5.  In Eastern Europe, the chance of a 15 year old boy living to age 60 is lower than a child growing up in China, Latin America, or even India.    Multinational Monitor, July-August 1997, p. 25

6.  "The tobacco epidemic in Eastern Europe is worse than anywhere else in the world. Consumption in some countries is about twice the world average and still increasing. High smoking rates have been around for decades. WHO estimates that in Eastern Europe there are now 763,000 tobacco-related deaths a year, about one quarter of the world's total. In Eastern Europe, as many as 80% of these tobacco-related deaths occur before the age of 70; the comparable rate in Western countries is estimated at 50% or less. In some parts of Eastern Europe, lung cancer rates in men are the highest ever recorded anywhere in the world."    *Smoke and Mirrors*, p. 237 (Rob Cunningham)

7.  In Eastern Europe, Philip Morris is involved in nine joint ventures in seven countries and is investing $80 to $100 million in a new plant in St. Petersburg, Russia. RJ Reynolds has invested a total of $300 million in the area since 1992, and together, the two companies' Eastern European operations manufactured nearly 157 billion cigarettes in 1994.    American Medical News, October 3, 1994, p. 14

8.  155 million of the 425 million people in Eastern Europe are smokers of 700 billion cigarettes a year. In 1989, only 3% of the market in Eastern Europe was controlled by the multinational companies, but they have now purchased a total of nine plants for $640 million with a manufacturing capacity of 200 billion cigarettes a year.
    9th World Conference on Tobacco or Health, Paris, 1994 (Greg Connolly)

9. In Turkey in the early 1990's, 30% of senior medical students were smokers, as were 63% of men and 25 to 50% of women depending upon the area of the country. 30% of teens ages 15 to 18 also smoked. Philip Morris and RJ Reynolds have invested half a billion dollars in new factories in Turkey.

*Tobacco Control*, Fall 1994, pp. 202 and 208

10. Half of men and one third of women in Turkey are smokers. 56% of male physicians ages 30 to 44 are smokers.

*Tobacco: the Growing Epidemic*, p. 898

11. Poland had one of the world's highest smoking rates, 62% of men and 30% of women in 1982, but has since seen rates fall to about 40% of men and 20% of women.

Associated Press, June 1, 2001

12. In Poland in the early 1980's, 70% of male physicians smoked, as did more than 50% in the Netherlands, Greece, France, Spain, and Hungary.

European Journal of Respiratory Disease 1986; 69:209

13. In Poland in 1994, up to 50% of all billboard and press advertisements were for tobacco, and the tobacco industry was the source of 50% of the entire profit of advertising companies.

International Union Against Cancer (Geneva) newsletter, January 1995

14. Poland has since 1991 organized a health promotion campaign that has led to significant decreases in smoking. Prevalence rates for men dropped from 62% in 1982 to 52% in 1992 and 42% in 1996; in women the corresponding rates for these years were 30%, 25% and 21%, respectively.

Abstract OS 171, 10th World Conference on Tobacco or Health, Beijing, 1997

15. An ad for L&M cigarettes in Poland features red Mustangs and the logo "Discover a taste of freedom."

San Francisco Examiner, April 18, 1998, p. A1

16. Lady Di brand cigarettes are available in Poland, manufactured by the Polish Tobacco Co.

Tobacco Control, Spring 1999, p. 17

17. In the Czech Republic in the mid-1990's, 40% of doctors, 70% of the members of parliament, and the health minister were smokers.

10th World Conference on Tobacco or Health, Beijing, 1997 (Hana Sovinova)

18. In the Czech Republic, cigarette consumption is increasing by 4% per year. 43% of men and 31% of women smoke, including a third of the doctors, half the nurses, and the country's minister of health. Philip Morris has bought the state tobacco company and has locked up 80% of the Czech market; Philip Morris officials refused to speak to CBS news for the report.

CBS evening news, May 8, 1997

19. In the Czech Republic, 41% of nurses and 29% of doctors, but only 15% of senior medical students are smokers.

*Tobacco the Growing Epidemic*, pp. 893-894

20. In Prague, Czechoslovakia, an electric streetcar decorated as a pack of Camels runs its route with another tram resembling a Marlboro pack.

9th World Conference on Tobacco or Health, Paris, 1994 (Greg Connolly)

21. A survey in Romania found that 43.2% of doctors were current smokers, compared to 28% of adults in the general population. 54% of Romania's doctors are women, and the cheapest cigarettes cost only U.S. 25 cents a pack.

The Lancet, October 21, 2000, p. 1420

22. In a survey of pulmonary specialists in Romania, the prevalence of smoking was 60.5 % in men and 40% in women.

Abstract PO 66, 10th World Conference on Tobacco or Health, Beijing, 1997

23. "I am sure that Camel and the other splendid products of RJ Reynolds will prosper in Romania."

US Ambassador Alfred H. Moses, opening an RJ Reynolds factory in Bucharest.

Associated Press, "Smoking Spreads Across Europe," 27 April 1999

24. In Bucharest Romania, the yellow or amber filters of many of the city's traffic lights advertise Camels in silhouette when the light is on. *Tobacco Control, Spring 1994, p. 14*

25. Hungary has instituted a total ban on direct and indirect advertising for tobacco products, to include print media and outdoor posters and billboards. *Tobacco Control, March 2002, p. 79*

26. Hungary now has one of the most progressive tobacco control policies in the world, and in 2002 banned almost all forms of tobacco advertising. *2002 AMA Annual Tobacco Report*

27. 35% of secondary school students in Budapest, Hungary, including 48% of 18-year-olds, reported current smoking in a 1995 survey. Marlboro was the brand choice for 41% of this group. *JAMA, April 9, 1997, p. 1110*

# Russia and the Former Soviet Union

1. Russia and former Soviet Union adult smoking rates (percentages) from *The Tobacco Atlas*, 2002

| Country | Total | Male | Female |
|---|---|---|---|
| Armenia | 32.5 | 64.0 | 1.0 |
| Azerbaijan | 15.7 | 30.2 | 1.1 |
| Belarus | 29.8 | 54.9 | 4.6 |
| Estonia | 32.0 | 44.0 | 20.0 |
| Georgia | 37.5 | 60.0 | 15.0 |
| Kazakhstan | 33.5 | 60.0 | 7.0 |
| Kyrgyzstan | 37.8 | 60.0 | 15.6 |
| Latvia | 31.0 | 49.0 | 13.0 |
| Lithuania | 33.5 | 51.0 | 16.0 |
| Russian federation | 36.5 | 63.2 | 9.7 |
| Turkmenistan | 14.0 | 27.0 | 1.0 |
| Ukraine | 35.3 | 51.1 | 19.4 |
| Uzbekistan | 29.0 | 49.0 | 9.0 |

2. In Russia, 59.8% of men older than 15 years old are smokers, including 72% of men ages 30 to 34. Among women, only 9.1% of those over age 15 are smokers. In 1999, 63,000 Russians died from lung or throat cancer, 90% smoking related, and 2.35 million from cardiac disease, 25% blamed on smoking.
*Los Angeles Times, August 13, 2000*

3. Russians smoke 265 billion cigarettes each year; 59.8% of men older than 15 years smoke, as do 9.1% of women.
*San Francisco Chronicle, August 18, 2000, p. D3*

4. In Moscow, 59% of men and 18% of women are current smokers. *Tobacco: the Growing Epidemic, p. 53*

5. A pack of Pall Malls or Winston cigarettes costs just 50 cents in Russia, and domestic brands are even less. Almost two thirds of Russian men are smokers. *Washington Post National Weekly Edition, September 3-9, 2001, p. 16*

6. There are about 70 million smokers in the former Soviet Union, or 26% of the population. 90% of the cigarettes produced are of the high tar variety, and 700 billion are consumed each year. (Another source estimates consumption at 450 billion). *Tobacco: A Major International Health Hazard, p. 75,*
*NBC News, March 10, 1994, and American Medical News, September 28, 1992*

7. There are 280,000 yearly deaths from smoking in Russia. *CNN news, August 26, 1997*

8. A 1993 survey found that 48% of male and 14% of female medical students in Russia were smokers.
*Tobacco or Health: a Global Status Report, p. 372*

9. The Marlboro Man, long banned from US television, is riding freely over the Russian airways. Also on Russian television many nights, a sexy young couple in the wide-open American desert share a sensual moment with a

Lucky Strike--"the real America", Russians are told. Western cigarettes are advertised as the key to a free and romantic lifestyle. Tanya Rydlevich, a Moscow City Council member, says: "If they want to introduce an American way of life, fine, but it should be a healthy way, not something Americans have already rejected. What do they have, a wish to destroy our people?"    Quote from Washington Post National Weekly Edition, August 23, 1993, p. 18

10. Russian television viewers and readers of magazines and newspapers have been deluged with Western-style advertisements for cigarettes and alcohol, mostly foreign brands, since the late 1980's. On February 18, 1995, President Boris Yeltsin issued a decree banning all tobacco and alcohol advertising as a threat to public health.

Reuters, February 19, 1995

11. "Downtown Kiev has become the Ukrainian version of Marlboro country, with the gray socialist cityscape punctuated with colorful billboards of cowboy sunsets and chiseled faces."

Washington Post National Weekly Edition, November 25-December 1, 1996, p. 6

12. A new cigarette brand called Lolita has been introduced in Russia. It is packed in a gold box and features on the cover a reclining bare-breasted young woman apparently dressed only in black stockings and stiletto heeled shoes.

Tobacco Control, Winter 1995, p. 328

13. A new cigarette in Russia, "Peter the First", is named after the 17th century tsar who introduced tobacco and other western customs to Russia. It comes in a black and gold package featuring the double-headed eagle, the symbol of Russian imperialism. The cigarettes are manufactured by the R. J. Reynolds tobacco company at a plant near St. Petersburg. RJR acquired its first Russian factory in 1992, and now has 20% of the country's cigarette market.

Oakland Tribune, September 14, 1997, p. A14 (Cox News Service)

14. In a survey from Yerevan, Armenia, 57% of physicians were smokers (81% of males and 42% of females), and 39% smoked near their patients. 39.6% of pregnant patients and 37% of teenagers also smoked.

Abstract OS 253, 10th World Conference on Tobacco or Health, Beijing, 1997

15. Cigarette brands in Russia include standard American brands plus new ones that glamorize the Western way of life. These include Hollywood, West, and Apollo Soyuz (depicting the joint ventures in space programs).

Mayo Clinic Proceedings, October 1995, p. 1007

16. Almost 50% of the male physicians in the former Soviet Union smoke, and 40% of Polish medical students are smokers.    American Medical News, October 3, 1994, p. 14

17. From 1965 to 1989, the number of cigarettes imported into Russia has doubled to more than 73 billion per year, and Russia is now the largest importer of tobacco products in the world. In 1990 during the Russian economic crisis, RJ Reynolds, Philip Morris, and the British American Tobacco Company made "emergency" shipments of an estimated 38 billion cigarettes to Russia.    Mayo Clinic Proceedings, October 1995, p. 1007

18. In 1995, an estimated 45% of the deaths of middle aged Russian men were tobacco related. On the basis of current rates, about 5 million tobacco-related deaths will occur in Russia in the decade of the 1990's.

Mayo Clinic Proceedings, October 1995, p. 1009

19. In the summer 1990 Soviet Union cigarette shortage, President Mikhail Gorbachev pleaded with the West for help, and the American tobacco industry agreed to deliver 34 billion cigarettes. R. J. Reynolds now sells 50 billion cigarettes a year in the former Soviet republics, an increase from zero at the beginning of the decade. "When Philip Morris hired former British Prime Minister Margaret Thatcher as a part-time consultant on a three-year contract reportedly worth $2 million, one of her first tasks was to travel to Kazakhstan to sell a major stake in its state tobacco company to Philip Morris."    Washington National Weekly Edition, December 9-15, 1996, p. 8

20. In the former Soviet Union a severe shortage of cigarettes in 1990 resulted from a breakdown in the distribution system and closure of 24 plants for repair, resulting in the Russian Republic purchasing 20 billion cigarettes from PM and 15 billion from RJR for $1.8 billion. PM renewed the contract for 1992 to ship 11 billion cigarettes. The availability of these brands increases consumer demand for them and pressures governments to allow overseas tobacco companies to manufacture locally.    *Tobacco and Health*, p. 52

# Middle East and Egypt

1. Middle East adult smoking rates (percent) from *The Tobacco Atlas*, 2002

| Country | Total | Male | Female |
|---|---|---|---|
| Bahrain | 14.6 | 23.5 | 5.7 |
| Cyprus | 23.1 | 38.5 | 7.6 |
| Egypt | 18.3 | 35.0 | 1.6 |
| Iran | 15.3 | 27.2 | 3.4 |
| Iraq | 22.5 | 0.0 | 5.0 |
| Israel | 23.5 | 33.0 | 24.0 |
| Jordan | 29.0 | 48.0 | 10.0 |
| Kuwait | 15.6 | 29.6 | 1.5 |
| Lebanon | 40.5 | 46.0 | 35.0 |
| Oman | 8.5 | 15.5 | 1.5 |
| Qatar | 18.8 | 37.0 | 0.5 |
| Saudi Arabia | 11.5 | 22.0 | 1.0 |
| Syria | 30.3 | 50.6 | 9.9 |
| Turkey | 44.0 | 62.0 | 22.0 |
| United Arab Emirates | 9.0 | 18.0 | 1.0 |
| Yemen | 44.5 | 60.0 | 29.0 |

2. Cigarette consumption in Egypt is increasing by about 8% per year, and an individual smoker spends an average of almost 22% of total income on tobacco. The average income in Egypt is about $1200 per year.

    2002 AMA Annual Tobacco Report

3. Water pipe smoking is common among men in Egypt, but the fad is now increasingly popular among young women. [It is also becoming a fad in some bars in the United States--editor].

    San Francisco Chronicle, October 27, 2002, p. F7

4. Egypt is the "leading" Third World country in importing tobacco, losing $178 million a year in balance of trade from tobacco imports.                    *Tobacco Control in the Third World*, p. 43

5. The gross domestic product of Egypt in 1992 was $33.6 billion. Worldwide Philip Morris sales that year were $50.2 billion.                    World Watch, July-August 1996, p. 39

6. Muslims who were found smoking in Arab countries during February could be thrown in jail. The faithful observed a month-long fast from dawn to dusk following the law of Ramadan that banned smoking.

    Tobacco Free Youth Reporter, Spring 1995

7. In a survey from Riyadh, Saudi Arabia, 31% of male secondary students ages 18 and 19 were smokers.

    Tobacco Control, Spring 1996, p. 26

8. In Kuwait, 65% of high school teachers smoke, as do 50% of their students (including 37% of girls). 58% of Kuwaiti dentists are smokers.                    *Tobacco and Health*, p. 462

9. In the late 1980's, 51% of doctors in Jordan were smokers, including the director of the government's antismoking program as well as the Jordan Health Ministry's chest disease specialist. 27% of Jordan's 10th graders and 45% of

    university students were smokers, and King Hussein smokes an American brand in public.

    Los Angeles Times, August, 3, 1988

10. Jordan's King Hussein and Israel's Yitzhak Rabin beamed while lighting up each other's cigarettes, Marlboro Lights, after signing a peace treaty on October 26, 1994.                    New York Times, February 8, 1999, p. A11

11. 16.6% of 13 to 15 year olds in Jordan are current smokers, and 24.8% of teens in this age group have been offered free cigarettes by tobacco companies.

Time, September 3, 2001, p. 26

12. In a study of school children ages 11 to 17 years in Jerusalem, 14% were current smokers, including 36% of 15 and 16 year olds (tenth graders).

Chest, October 1996, p. 921

13. 28% of Israel's 5.6 million people smoke, and 5,000 die each year from smoking-related disease. In the country's first smoking-related lawsuit, lawyers representing 15 people are suing for $4 million in damages from Dubek, the country's only cigarette manufacturer. As well, the Israel Health Ministry plans to file an $8 billion damage suit against the tobacco industry (both Israeli and foreign companies), with the proceeds to be used to treat sick smokers.

American Medical News, October 6, 1997

14. The government of Iran has banned tobacco advertising and smoking in public buildings, including restaurants and hotels.

The Advocacy Institute, October 31, 1997

# Africa

1. Africa adult smoking rates (percentages) from *The Tobacco Atlas*, 2002

| Country | Total | Male | Female |
|---|---|---|---|
| Algeria | 25.2 | 43.8 | 6.6 |
| Botswana | 21.0 | -- | -- |
| Cameroon | 35.7 | -- | -- |
| Cote d' Ivoire | 22.1 | 42.3 | 1.8 |
| Djibouti | 31.1 | 57.5 | 4.7 |
| Ethiopia | 15.8 | -- | -- |
| Gambia | 17.8 | 34.0 | 1.5 |
| Ghana | 16.0 | 28.4 | 3.5 |
| Guinea | 51.7 | 59.5 | 43.8 |
| Kenya | 49.4 | 66.8 | 31.9 |
| Libya | 4.0 | -- | -- |
| Malawi | 14.5 | 20.0 | 9.0 |
| Mauritius | 23.9 | 44.8 | 2.9 |
| Morocco | 18.1 | 34.5 | 1.6 |
| Namibia | 50.0 | 65.0 | 35.0 |
| Nigeria | 8.6 | 15.4 | 1.7 |
| Rwanda | 5.5 | 7.0 | 4.0 |
| Senegal | 4.6 | -- | -- |
| South Africa | 26.5 | 42.0 | 11.0 |
| Sudan | 12.9 | 24.4 | 1.4 |
| Tanzania | 31.0 | 49.5 | 12.4 |
| Tunisia | 34.8 | 61.9 | 7.7 |
| Uganda | 34.5 | 52.0 | 17.0 |
| Zambia | 22.5 | 35.0 | 10.0 |
| Zimbabwe | 17.8 | 34.4 | 1.2 |

2. In the Sahara desert of Africa, the Tuareg people often give their camels a snort of tobacco as a "pick me up" before long desert journeys.

"Desert Odyssey," National Geographic film shown on PBS television, September 16, 2001

3. In Senegal, West Africa, the amount of money that consumers spent on cigarettes doubled between 1985 and 1990. "On the streets of Senegal, billboards for L&M cigarettes show well-dressed, smiling white young people with the caption, 'Go For It!' An American flag and a red, white and blue color scheme support the ad's most explicit claim, 'real American taste'."

New York Times, April 23, 1997, p. A23

4. In Senegal, a very poor country in West Africa, "most store counters sport the Marlboro man's image along with the phrase 'The cigarette sold most around the world!' Camel advertises itself on automobiles as 'the taste of action' and plays up the fact it is 'made in the U.S.A.!' ...At least 90% of all cigarette billboards in Senegal show Caucasians only, a striking phenomenon in a country whose only light-skinned people are essentially albino or tourists." When people were asked to estimate the percentage of smokers in the United States, the average estimate was 60%.                                                                 Tobacco Control, Autumn 1997, pp. 243-245

5. In Kenya, cigarettes with brand names such as "Life" and "Sportsman" are promoted as the passport to success, health, and a Western lifestyle.                                                                 NEJM, March 28, 1991, p. 917

6. In Kenya, the tobacco industry is using loan incentives to switch peasant farmers from food production to tobacco growing. Each year, about 10,000 new farmers from the most productive parts of the country sign contracts to cultivate tobacco.                                         9th World Conference on Tobacco or Health, Paris, 1994 (J. Nkuchia)

7. In Kenya, adult per capita cigarette consumption increased by 28% between 1970 and 1985.
                                                                                                                                            *Tobacco and Health*, p. 295

8. British American Tobacco ads being screened in Kenya on TV and cinema "ranged from scenes of footballing prowess and leaping Masai tribesmen, and promises of just reward for hard toil, to a depiction of a highly upwardly mobile young couple, replete with sportscar, high fashion clothing, romantic poses, and under the table gropings."
                                                                                                                    British Medical Journal, January 15, 1994, p. 191

9. The environmental damage is considerable in developing countries from the cultivation of tobacco, where it is flue cured by wood. In Tanzania, 12% of all trees felled annually are used for tobacco curing, and neighboring Malawi has already cut down one third of its forested land for this purpose.                     NEJM, March 28, 1991, p. 918

10. About half the tobacco grown in the world is flue cured over wood fires, significantly contributing to deforestation.
                                                                                                                                            *The Real Cost*, Richard North, p. 99

11. Since 5 to 7 acres of forest are needed to flue cure one ton of tobacco, tobacco cultivation has substantially contributed to deforestation in many Third World countries. Other estimates are one to two acres of forest to cure one ton of tobacco.                     International Journal of Health Sciences 1986; 16:288 and NEJM, March 28, 1991, p. 918

12. Zimbabwe has 100,000 people employed in the tobacco industry and is the major tobacco distributor in Africa. Tobacco comprises more than 50% of total agricultural exports, and earns 25% of the country's foreign exchange. The export income is a total of $400 million from 200,000 tons of tobacco.
                                                                                                                    International Journal of Health Sciences 1986; 16:281

13. In Zimbabwe, tobacco provides 30% of all export revenue ($580 million in 1992), and finances a considerable portion of the government's budget.                                         San Francisco Examiner, August 28, 1994, p. C16

14. Tobacco is the principal export earner and largest employer of labor in the African countries of Zimbabwe, Malawi, and Tanzania. It is also the major non-food crop in Nigeria and Kenya.
                                                                                                                    International Journal of Health Sciences 1986; 16:281

15. 94% of all export earnings from tobacco in Africa went to Zimbabwe and Malawi. These countries produce 74% of the continent's total crop (Zimbabwe 44%, Malawi 30%), although Africa grows just 6% of the world total of 8.148 million tons of tobacco each year.
                                                                                        British Medical Journal, January 15, 1994, p. 190, and Simon Chapman, Ph.D.

16. The African country of Malawi increased its tobacco production from 20 million pounds in 1981 to 200 million pounds in 1991.                     *Tobacco Control in the Third World*, p. 43, and American Medical News, June 29, 1992

17. The economy of Malawi, in central Africa, depends heavily on tobacco, which accounts for 75% of the country's total export earnings. 93% of all fuel used in Malawi is wood, with 23% of the total (420,000 cubic meters a year) consumed by the tobacco industry, mostly to dry and cure burley tobacco leaves.         Panoscope, October 1994, p. 16

18.  South Africa has about 89,000 yearly deaths from tobacco. Smoking prevalence there declined from 34% in 1992 to 28% in 1997.                                                                 *Tobacco Control*, Summer 1999, p. 132

19.  In South Africa, the highest percentage of tobacco ads were in a man's "soft porn" magazine, with 26 of 30 issues having these ads on the back cover.          9th World Conference on Tobacco or Health, Paris, 1994 (D. Yach)

20.  British American Tobacco organized a seminar to try to "restore the balance" of public perception of the health risks of smoking. The company paid for senior journalists from southern African countries to attend the conference at the luxurious Mount Sheva resort in the Eastern Transvaal. The move worked; coverage was widespread under headlines such as "smoking risk exaggerated--health message simplistic" in the Cape Times of Capetown, South Africa.                                                                 *Tobacco Control*, Spring 1994, p. 76

21.  In 1994, there was only one person in all of Africa working full time on tobacco control. *Smoke and Mirrors*, p. 229

# Asia

1.  Asia adult smoking rates (percent) from *The Tobacco Atlas*, 2002

| Country | Total | Male | Female |
|---|---|---|---|
| Bangladesh | 38.7 | 53.6 | 23.8 |
| Cambodia | 37.0 | 66.0 | 8.0 |
| China | 35.6 | 66.9 | 4.2 |
| India | 16.0 | 29.4 | 2.5 |
| Indonesia | 31.4 | 59.0 | 3.7 |
| Japan | 33.1 | 52.8 | 13.4 |
| Korea | 35.0 | 65.1 | 4.8 |
| Laos | 38.0 | 41.0 | 15.0 |
| Malaysia | 26.4 | 49.2 | 3.5 |
| Mongolia | 46.7 | 67.8 | 25.5 |
| Myanmar (Burma) | 32.9 | 43.5 | 22.3 |
| Nepal | 38.5 | 48.0 | 29.0 |
| Pakistan | 22.5 | 36.0 | 9.0 |
| Philippines | 32.4 | 53.8 | 11.0 |
| Singapore | 15.0 | 6.9 | 3.1 |
| Sri Lanka | 13.7 | 25.7 | 1.7 |
| Thailand | 23.4 | 44.1 | 2.6 |
| Vietnam | 27.1 | 50.7 | 3.5 |

# India and Bangladesh

1.  Tobacco was introduced to India by Portuguese traders about 1600. Of the 400 million people age 15 or over in India, 47 percent use tobacco in some form, including 16 percent who use smokeless tobacco. Including Pakistan, there are an estimated 100 million smokeless tobacco users on the subcontinent.
                                                                 *Smokeless Tobacco or Health*, pp. 51 and 315

2.  In India and Southeast Asia, cancer of the oral cavity represents about 35 percent of all malignant tumors.
                                                 CA-A Cancer Journal for Clinicians, November-December 1995, p. 352

3.  In India, the adult smoking rate is 16% (29.4% of men and 2.5% of women).          *The Tobacco Atlas*, 2002

4.  Tobacco is responsible for about 800,000 deaths in India each year. About 194 million men and 45 million women in India use tobacco.                                                 *Tobacco: The Growing Epidemic*, p. 459-460

5.  China produces 30%, the United States 9% and India 7.9% of the world's tobacco. 450 to 500 million kilograms of tobacco are grown in India, out of a total of 6 billion kg globally. India produces 120 million cigarettes and 900

million bidis each day. 30% of the tobacco grown is for bidis, 15% for cigarettes, 20% for chewing, and 6% for export.                                                                                                   *Tobacco: the Growing Epidemic*, p. 41

6.  About 65 percent of men in India are tobacco users.                                                   *Tobacco* (Gately), p. 360

7.  About 70% of the tobacco smoked in India is in the form of bidis; the tobacco they contain has as much as three times the nicotine concentration of American tobacco, and more tar and carbon monoxide. The tendu leaf wrapping is nonporous, and prevents outside air from mixing with the inhaled smoke and diluting it. Flavors include grape, strawberry, lemon, mint and vanilla.
                            Time, December 16, 2002, p. 87, and NBC evening news (Tom Brokaw), December 16, 2002

8.  In India, 200 million men and 50 million women use tobacco in various forms. Most of this is in the form of bidis, and traditional cigarettes make up just 20% of tobacco consumed. India is the third largest world producer of tobacco, and it provides livelihood for 6 million farmers and 20 million industry workers. Tobacco also contributes U.S. $1.5 billion to government earnings.                               British Medical Journal, February 17, 2001, p. 386

9.  In a survey of adults over age 34 in Bombay, the prevalence of smokeless tobacco use among men was 56% and women 59%.                                    11th World Conference on Tobacco or Health, 2000, Abstract NT 02

10. "Prompted by a slick and many-tentacled advertising campaign, gutka, an indigenous form of smokeless tobacco, has become a fixture in the mouths of millions of Indians over the last two decades." Up to 20% of teenage boys use the product, sales increased fivefold in the 1990's, and oral cancers in young people have increased dramatically. About 30% of all cancers in India are in the head and neck, compared with 4.5% in the West
                                                                          New York Times, August 13, 2002, pp. A1 and A9

11. In India, 6 million children 4 to 14 work full time in the bidi industry.                     *The Tobacco Atlas*, p. 49

12. India's Supreme Court directed all states and centrally ruled territories, on Nov. 2, 2001, to immediately issue orders banning smoking in public places and on public transport. Public places where smoking has been banned include hospitals, health institutes, public offices, and libraries. Hotels and amusement parks were excluded from the ban.
                                                                                              2002 AMA Annual Tobacco Report

13. The Supreme Court of India in 2002 directed the states to ban smoking on all public transportation and in all public places including educational institutions, libraries and auditoriums.            2003 AMA Annual Tobacco Report

14. "Delhi's air is the most polluted of any city in the world. Breathing it is as dangerous as smoking twenty cigarettes a day."                                            *The Ends of the Earth*, Robert Kaplan, Random House, 1996, p. 350

15. India is the world's third largest producer of tobacco, with an annual crop of 500,000 tons. 142 million men and 72 million women in India regularly use tobacco (often chewing tobacco), including 4 million children under age 15
                                                                                     British Medical Journal, June 11, 1994, p. 1523

16. Only 3% of women smoke cigarettes, but 50% to 60% of women chew tobacco in many areas of India.
                                              Journal of the American Medical Women's Association, January 1996, p. 48

17. Tobacco causes 600,000 to 1 million deaths each year in India; oropharyngeal cancer is diagnosed in 100,000 patients each year.                             The Lancet, March 10, 1990, p. 594 and Tobacco Control, Fall 1994, p. 201

18. Oral cancer accounts for about a third of all cancers in Bangladesh, India, Pakistan and Sri Lanka; tobacco is the greatest single risk factor. Betel quid ("pan") chewing is very common in these countries.
                                                                                              Tobacco Alert (WHO), July 1996

19. Oral cancers comprise 50 to 70% of all cancers diagnosed in India, where use of chewing tobacco is very high. A third of the 650,000 cancer deaths each year are tobacco-related.            JAMA, February 28, 1986, p. 1042
                                                                   and Journal of the National Cancer Institute, December 7, 1994, p. 1752

20. In India, 635,000 deaths each year are attributed to tobacco. Tobacco is responsible for half of all cancers in men and about 20% of cancers in women. Cigarettes account for only 18% of tobacco use, bidis for 50% and chewing tobacco the rest. The "tobacco sector" employs 7 million people, and nearly 10% of the government's excise tax revenue comes from tobacco.                                                            The Lancet, October 10, 1998, p. 1204

21. Annual bidi sales in India are around $1.4 billion; eight are consumed for each conventional cigarette. A bundle of 25 costs about 8 cents, and they are considered the poor man's cigarette. Bidi-making employs about 5 million Indian women who wrap the tobacco in tendu leaf and who typically earn only about 80 cents for a full day's work making about 1000 bidis, or $18 a month, below average for the country where the average monthly household income is $40. Even though exports to the United States have doubled in the last year, exports account for less than 1% of sales.                                                            Wall Street Journal, August 17, 1999, pp. B1 and B4

22. The cheap smoking brands for tens of millions of poor people in India and Bangladesh are bidis, or thin, tapered sticks of tobacco wrapped in a leaf or paper treated with molasses or artificial fragrance. "Millions of bidis are churned out every day by a vast army, mainly children, squatting in suffocating sheds across the subcontinent." Each rolls about 4000 bidis in an eight hour day and is paid just over a dollar a day for the work.
                                                            Panoscope, October 1994, p. 23

23. Bidis consist of a small amount of tobacco (0.2-0.3 grams) wrapped in a temburni leaf and tied with a small string. Their tar and carbon monoxide are similar to manufactured cigarettes. About 675 billion bidis are smoked each year in India, 50 billion in Bangladesh, and 25 billion in other countries in the region. Smokers in India consume eight times more bidis than manufactured cigarettes, and in Bangladesh, nearly four times more.
                                    *Tobacco or Health: a Global Status Report*, World Health Organization, 1997, pp. 7 and 20

24. "In India, tobacco is available in more than a dozen forms: cigarette, cigar, pipe, cheroor, bidi, chutta, dhumti, chilum, and hookah (all consumed by smoking); chewing tobacco, sometimes in the form of betel quid (tobacco mixed with lime and areca nut, rolled in a betel leaf); snuff; mishri; and tobacco toothpaste." Among smokers, the majority smokes hand rolled bidis, not cigarettes. About 40% of consumption is in the form of smokeless tobacco.
                                                            *Smoke and Mirrors*, p. 230, and Abstract OS 186,
                                                            10th World Conference on Tobacco or Health, Beijing, 1997

25. Betel quid, or pan, chewing is common in India and Southeast Asia. The ingredients are tobacco, areca nuts, and slaked lime wrapped in a betel leaf.                                    *Tobacco or Health: a Global Status Report*, 1997, p. 8

26. In 1985-6, 45% of men and 7% of women aged 25-64 years smoked in Delhi, urban India. Lack of education was the strongest risk factor for smoking: men with no education were 1.8 times more likely to be smokers than those with college education, and women with no education were 3.7 times more likely. There are two subpopulations of smokers in India: the affluent, white collar cigarette smoker and the less affluent laborer who smokes bidi and chutta.                                                            British Medical Journal, June 22, 1996, p. 1579

27. In a study from Bombay, prevalence of tobacco use was 57.5% among women, almost solely in the form of smokeless tobacco. Among men, 69% used tobacco, including 24% who smoked. About half of the smokers smoked cigarettes, and half bidis.                                    Tobacco Control, Summer 1996, p. 114

28. Harvard brand cigarettes are available in India.                                    Yale alumni magazine, March 1999

29. In Pakistan, 36% of men and 9% of women are smokers.                                    *The Tobacco Atlas*, 2002

30. Said, a television and film actor, is promoting British American Tobacco's Gold Street cigarettes in Pakistan, where he is "known to millions through his starring role in one of the country's most popular television drama series."


Also in Pakistan, Philip Morris ads for its Red and White brand feature BMW's and are in journals such as the Cricketer, which covers the country's most popular sport. Cricket's most ardent fans are teenage boys.
                                                            Tobacco Control, September 2002, pp. 172-173

31. There are 22 million tobacco users in Pakistan. The FBI has been distributing matchbooks there since early 2000 with a picture of Osama bin Laden and the notice in Arabic "Up to $500,000 Reward." (This is a printing error: the amount is actually $5 million). *Parade Magazine, September 9, 2001, p. 9*

32. In Sri Lanka, smoking rates are high for males but very low in females. The national tobacco monopoly, Ceylon Tobacco Company (CTC), is a subsidiary of British American Tobacco (BAT), and markets Bristol, the "popular" brand, and John Player Gold Leaf, the "premium" brand. The company has been aggressively marketing their Benson and Hedges brand in discos with free samples, and publishes "Golden Tone News", a weekly pop music supplement. CTC sponsors many popular sporting events, and by report has hired young women to drive around in "Gold Leaf" cars to give out free cigarette samples and promotional items in places such as school campuses and shopping malls. As in India, chewed betel and tobacco is widely used by both men and women. *Reported by Garrett Mehl, Johns Hopkins School of Public Health, December 1997*

33. In 1993, BAT's subsidiary, the Ceylon Tobacco Company, organized a news conference to dispute the alleged health effects of smoking. A report of the session in *The Island* newspaper was headlined "Anti-smoking campaign comes under heavy fire" and "Consultants rule out lung cancer, heart disease." Here are excerpts from the article:
    "An international team of consultants hosted by Ceylon Tobacco Company last week insisted that smoking could not be linked to lung cancer and heart disease. They accused the mass media of being biased against smoking. Dr. Sharon Boyse, head of the Smoking Issues Department of the British American Tobacco Corporation in the United Kingdom, said there is 'absolutely' no laboratory proof that smoking is directly related to lung cancer or heart disease. Lung cancer, she pointed out, could be caused by various other factors also – keeping pet birds and ethnic factors for instance....The issue of passive smoking was dealt with by Philip Witorsch of the George Washington University Medical Center. According to him, passive smoking or inhaling what he calls 'Environmental Tobacco Smoke' is not hazardous to one's health." *Quote from Smoke and Mirrors, p. 215*

34. 43% of all cancers in Sri Lanka are tobacco related. An advertising ban was imposed in 1999. *The Lancet, October 10, 1998, p. 1204*

35. In Bangladesh, 54% of men and 24% of women are smokers. *The Tobacco Atlas, 2002*

36. In Bangladesh, cigarette consumption more than doubled in the last 10 to 15 years. The popular film hero is seldom to be seen in a moment of crisis without a cigarette. The most important tobacco health risk may be the reduction in nutritional status of young children that results from expenditure on tobacco in households whose income for food purchase is already marginal. *The Lancet, May 16, 1991, p. 1090*

37. Low-income people in Bangladesh who smoke have to cut food purchases to pay for tobacco, leading to a reduction of daily caloric intake to 1700 from an already low 2000. *Panos Briefing, September 1994, p. 9*

38. In Bangladesh, the perinatal mortality is 27% for children of smoking mothers, more than twice the rate for babies of nonsmokers. *NEJM, March 28, 1991, p. 918*

39. In Bangladesh, as many as 20-30% of women in rural areas use smokeless tobacco. *Tobacco and Health, p. 178*

40. "Nepal has already one of the highest prevalence rate of tobacco smoking and unlike many other Asian countries, the rate of tobacco smoking in women is also very high." *Abstract P 4/3, 10th World Conference on Tobacco or Health, Beijing, 1997*

41. The Jumla district of western Nepal has adult smoking rates of 86.6% for men and 76.7% for women *11th World Conference on Tobacco or Health, Chicago, 2000, Abstract PR 07*

# Japan

1. "In a world turning against smoking, Japan is still the land that time forgot." *CBS evening news, May 8, 1997*

2. The most recent reported smoking prevalence in Japan was 33.1% (52.8% of men and 13.4% of women).

*The Tobacco Atlas*, 2002

3. 60% of Japanese men smoked regularly in the early 1990's, the highest prevalence of any developed country, as did 13% of Japanese women. The prevalence of smoking in Japanese doctors is 44%, exceeded only by Spain's 45% (WHO data).

The Japan Times, July 27, 1993, p. 16

4. Japan Tobacco, the world's third largest cigarette manufacturer after Philip Morris and British American Tobacco, has argued in and out of court that health risks from tobacco are not scientifically proven. There are 630,000 cigarette vending machines in Japan, eight inside the Health Ministry, and as many as 76% of high school smokers buy their cigarettes from machines. The Health Ministry does not have a single fulltime official working on smoking issues, a practice that kills 95,000 Japanese a year, and the budget for anti-smoking awareness is $180,000 a year, compared to $94 million for AIDS prevention, which kills 45 Japanese a year. Tobacco contributes $19 billion a year in tax dividends to the government, and 49% of men and 14% of women are smokers.

San Francisco Chronicle, December 12, 2002, p. A11

5. In Japan in 1998, 53% of men and 3.4% of women were smokers; per capita consumption per year in 1999 was 2600 cigarettes, the same as in 1980. (Per capita consumption per year in the United States dropped from 2800 in 1980 to 1600 in 1999, by comparison.) In Japan, tax revenues from cigarette sales are $18 billion each year.

New York Times, June 13, 2001, p. A10

6. In Japan, twenty-two percent of death from all causes, 25% of all cancer, and 17% of all circulatory system disease deaths, could be attributed to cigarette smoking in males, and 5%, 4%, and 11% of all deaths, cancer deaths, and circulatory system deaths in females, respectively.

2002 AMA Annual Tobacco Report

7. In Japan, the legal age to buy cigarettes is 20, but the law is almost meaningless considering that there are half a million vending machines on the streets.

Washington Post National Weekly Edition, October 2, 2000, p. 17

8. In Japan, 27.1% of male physicians and 6.8% of women doctors are smokers, about half of the prevalences of the general Japanese population. This compares to smoking prevalence among doctors in the United Kingdom of 4%-5%, and 3%-10% in the United States.

JAMA, May 23/30, 2001, p. 2643

9. In a 1999 survey, 36.7% of male and 10.4% of female medical students in Japan were smokers.

JAMA, August 22/29, 2001, p. 917

10. There were 810,000 more women smokers in Japan in 1990 than in the previous year, and the total number of smokers in the country increased by 890,000 to 33,190,000. Sales that year totaled $26.89 billion for 322 billion cigarettes.

Wall Street Journal, September 23, 1991, p. B1

11. In Japan, the number of men who smoke has declined to 60 percent from 80 percent in the 1960's, but the percentage of women who smoke is now at 14 percent and rising steadily.

San Francisco Chronicle, July 30, 1994, p. D1

12. Smoking prevalence among Japanese men peaked at 84 percent in 1967.

New York Times, June 30, 1996, p. 12 (Travel Section)

13. In 1993, Japan's total cigarette sales rose to a record 332.6 billion "units", with foreign (mostly American) brands increasing by 6 percent in a year to 18 percent of total sales.

San Francisco Chronicle, July 30, 1994, p. D1

14. Japan Tobacco has revenues of more than $32 billion a year. A company spokesman has said: "Cause and effect between smoking and lung cancer has not been proved pathologically, but we do not deny the risk that smoking may affect physical health."

The Lancet, January 00, 1999, p. 1456

15. From 1990 to 1996, smoking rates for 17 year olds in Japan increased from 5 to 15% in girls and from 26 to 40% in boys.

*Global Aggression*, p. 24

16. "Philip Morris aimed at Japanese women with Virginia Slims: Japan Tobacco fought back with Misty, a thin, mild-blended cigarette. When RJR wooed young smokers with Joe Camel, JT countered with Dean, named after fabled actor James Dean. Cigarettes became the second most-advertised product on television in Tokyo--up from 40th just a year earlier. Today, imported brands control 21 percent of the Japanese market and earn more than $7 billion in annual sales. Female smoking is at an all-time high, according to Japan Tobacco's surveys, and one study showed female college freshmen four times more likely to smoke than their mothers."

The Washington Post National Weekly Edition, November 25-December 1, 1996, p. 8

17. Two years after the American tobacco companies entered the Japanese market in 1986, cigarette television ads had increased ten-fold. Five years after the market was opened, female smoking prevalence increased from 8.6% to 18.2%. Prevalence is now 27% among Japanese women in their twenties. *Tobacco Use: An American Crisis*, p. 73

18. In Japan, cigarette ads rose from fortieth to second place in total commercial television airtime from 1986 to 1988 following the entry of US companies into the Japanese market. Two thirds of the ads were for American brands. On an average day, 60 ads for US brands appear on Japanese TV. By 1988, 26% of Japanese female high school seniors smoked, compared to 13% of adult women.

Reader's Digest, April 1993, and Tobacco Control, Autumn 1995, p. 239

19. 25% of the physician members of the Japan Society of Chest Diseases admit to being smokers.

Chest, February 2, 1991, p. 526

20. Warnings on cigarette packages in Japan read: "Let's be aware of smoking too much, as there is a danger it could harm your health."   NEJM, January 12, 1991, p. 815

21. In Japan there are 5.5 million vending machines, of which 500,000 dispense cigarettes. Life insurers in Japan offer no discounts for nonsmokers, and no-smoking sections in workplaces and restaurants remain curiosities.

New York Times, October 17, 1993, p. F1

22. Japanese law forbids smoking by children and teenagers, but this age group smoked 40 billion cigarettes in 1990, a six-fold increase from 1978.   Wall Street Journal, September 23, 1991, p. B2

23. Designed to attract young smokers, candy-flavored cigarettes called Nova went on the market in Japan in 1983. Flavors available included mint, orange, lime, and cinnamon.   *Nicotine*, p. 39

24. There is "little tangible evidence of efforts on Japan's part to open your doors to more U.S. tobacco products. This inaction is causing a growing sentiment among my colleagues in the U.S. Congress to take strong action against Japan in matters of trade."   Letter from Sen. Jesse Helms of North Carolina to Prime Minister Nakasone, 1985.

JAMA, January 6, 1989, p. 29

25. Since the end of the tobacco import ban in Japan in 1986, there has been a ten-fold increase in the number of television ads for cigarettes, and concomitant sharp increase in smoking among Japanese women and adolescents.

NEJM, March 28, 1991, p. 918

26. "Why are Americans trying to encourage Japanese to smoke? The advertisements we have every night are an assault, like the old B-29 bombings. The term 'Ugly American' is coming back." Takeshi Hirayama, Director, Institute of Preventative Oncology, Tokyo.   New York Times magazine, July 10, 1988, p. 20

27. From 1955 to 1991 in Japan, rates of lung cancer increased tenfold from seventh to second place among cancer deaths, just behind stomach cancer. 60% of Japanese men and 44% of physicians are smokers; overall, 36% of adults smoke, compared to 25% in the US. Lung cancer deaths in Japan doubled between 1950 and 1991, and by 1994, lung cancer overtook stomach cancer as the most common cancer killer for men.

New York Times, October 17, 1993, p. F1
and 9th World Conference on Tobacco or Health, Paris, 1994 (H. Thai)

28. "There could be no mistake about the intended target audience for Philip Morris's latest TV ad in Japan featuring the American actor Charlie Sheen, who is wildly popular among young people here."

San Francisco Chronicle, July 30, 1994, p. D2

29. Tobacco and cigarettes are the number one American agricultural export, and Japan is the number one importer of American cigarettes.

In Health, May 1991, p. 14

30. The total government antismoking activity in Japan in 1993 consisted of one doctor and two staff employees of the Health and Welfare Ministry operating on a total yearly budget of less than $200,000.

New York Times, October 17, 1993, p. F1

31. The Japanese Ministry of Health and Welfare has only two employees in the "Health Promotion and Nutrition Section", and the 1994 budget to implement smoking regulation policies is only $180,000, 600 times less than the budget for AIDS problems. The Tobacco Business Law has the purpose "to promote the sound development of the Japanese tobacco industry, thereby securing stable national revenues." All tobacco policies are determined by the Ministry of Finance, not the Ministry of Health, and no Japanese law regulates smoking in the workplace.    Topic

Tobacco Problems Information Center, B. Watanabe
(9th World Conference on Tobacco or Health, Paris, 1994)

32. Japan's state-owned tobacco monopoly was disbanded in 1985, but the government still owns two-thirds of its successor, Japan Tobacco. The company is regulated by the Ministry of Finance, which collects $16 billion a year in revenue from cigarette sales. 40% of all sales are from vending machines.

San Francisco Examiner, May 18 1997, p. A1

33. "Taxes on cigarettes are big revenue sources for the central and local governments. I will smoke as much as possible, while watching my health, and avoid imposing a burden on the medical insurance system budget."

Japanese Prime Minister Ryutaro Hashimoto, a chain smoker
(U.S. News and World Report, April 7, 1997, p. 15)

34. Smoking rates among 17-year-old boys in Japan increased from 26% in 1990 to 40% in 1996. Among girls the same age, rates increased from 5% to 15% in the same time period. Dr Judith Mackay notes, "Every other government has top-down policies to try to reduce smoking. But there's complete inertia in Japan."

The Charlotte Observer, October 18, 1997

35. Smoking prevalence in Japanese men dropped from 82% in 1965 to 59% in 1995, while the female prevalence remained at 15%. Female smoking prevalence is declining for women over age 40, but is increasing steadily for young women. Total cigarette consumption was 322 billion in 1995, or 3200 per capita; 21% of sales were imported cigarettes, up from 2% in 1985.

Abstract S 1/3, 10th World Conference on Tobacco or Health, Beijing, 1997

36. In Japan there were 115,000 deaths from smoking in 1990, with a social cost of $56 billion. The deaths are expected to rise to 200,000 per year by 2010.

Abstract OS 158, 10th World Conference on Tobacco or Health, Beijing, 1997

37. The world's second most popular brand after Marlboro is Japan Tobacco's Mild Seven; Japan Tobacco's cigarette exports have increased from 1.5 billion in 1987 to 16.4 billion in 1993.       *Smoke and Mirrors*, p. 213

38. "Since smoking might injure your health, let's be careful not to smoke too much."

Warning label on cigarette packs in Japan (Time, June 25, 2001, p. 19)

39. Japanese tobacco companies have agreed to stop tobacco advertising on TV, radio, movie screens, and the Internet.

The Advocacy Institute, November 11, 1997

# China

1.  1.5 trillion (1,500,000,000,000) cigarettes were smoked in China in 1988, 29% of the total world consumption.
    *Nicotine Addiction*, p. 97

2.  66.9% of men and 4.2% of women in China are smokers (adult prevalence 35.6%).     *The Tobacco Atlas*, 2002

3.  China has 340 million smokers in a population of 1.1 billion, and yearly per capita cigarette consumption doubled in the decade of the 1980's. In 30 years, two million Chinese will die annually from tobacco-induced disease, including 900,000 per year from lung cancer alone.
    JAMA, January 6, 1989, p. 28 and Los Angeles Times, January 27, 1988

4.  Smoking is expected to eventually kill one third of all the young men in China. Smoking causes many more deaths from chronic lung disease than lung cancer, the reverse of what happens in the West.
    Associated Press, August 16, 2001

5.  "No discussion of the tobacco industry in the year 2000 would be complete without addressing what may be the most important feature on the landscape, the China market. In every respect, China confounds the imagination."
    Rene Soull, Vice President, Philip Morris Asia  (Tobacco Control, Summer 1997, p. 77)

6.  China consumes one-third of the world's cigarettes, and total consumption has tripled in the last 10 years. Estimates are that 50 million children alive in China today, none of whom yet smoke, will eventually die from tobacco-induced disease.
    Thorax, March 1991, p. 153, and Journal of the National Cancer Institute, November 18, 1992, p. 1689

7.  The world now has an estimated 1.1 billion smokers, about one third of the global population aged 15 years and over. Most of these smokers (800 million) live in developing countries. China alone has 300 million smokers (90% men), about the same number as in all the developed countries combined. About one third of regular smokers in developed countries are women, compared with only about one in eight in the developing world. Total world consumption is 6.05 trillion cigarettes annually.                     British Medical Journal, July 13, 1996, p. 97

8.  British American Tobacco Company (BAT) was well established in China by 1900. After World War II, they were evicted when the Communists seized control of the country and nationalized the tobacco industry. "Foreign cigarettes were condemned as an evil of the capitalist West, yet remained popular; Mao Zedong was a notorious chain smoker of BAT's popular 555 State Express brand."
    Washington Post National Weekly Edition, December 16-22, 1996, p. 8

9.  The Chinese market for cigarettes was "opened" by the British American Tobacco Company between 1900 and 1910. Domestic production increased from 600 billion cigarettes in 1978 to 1400 billion in 1987.
    Tobacco Control, Spring 1994, p. 81

10. President Deng Xiaoping still smoked his Panda-brand cigarettes at age of 91; he died in early 1997 at age 92.
    New York Times, June 30, 1996, p. 12  (Travel Section)

11. 70% of all men ages 25 to 35 in China are smokers, as are 46% of health professionals.
    9th World Conference on Tobacco or Health, Paris, 1994 (H. Thai)

12. In 1989, 67.5% of male physicians in the city of Beijing smoked, higher than the national average of 57% of physicians.                                         American Medical News, October 3, 1994

13. There were 100,000 deaths from tobacco-induced disease in China in 1987. By the year 2025, these deaths will increase twenty-fold, to two million per year.                     NEJM, March 28, 1991, p. 918

14. China has expanded its tobacco production dramatically, from 18 million pounds in 1911 to 3.4 billion pounds in 1980 and 4.7 billion pounds by 1990.                     *Tobacco in History*, p. 212

15. 16 million people in China are employed in tobacco cultivation.      *Tobacco in History*, p. 8

16. The average price in China for a pack of cigarettes is 26 cents, and cigarette sales account for 12% of annual government revenue.      *Cigarettes*, (Parker-Pope), pp. 49-50

17. In 2000, tobacco taxes in China accounted for 9.05% of total government revenue.      *The Tobacco Atlas*, p. 85

18. A group of Chinese lawyers plan to sue tobacco companies on behalf of teenage smoking. China's first suit against "big tobacco" cites breaches of consumer advertising and other laws.      Financial Times, May 14, 2001, p. 1

19. The mean consumption among Chinese men was 1 cigarette a day in 1952, 4 a day in 1972, 10 a day in 1992, and 15 cigarettes a day in 1996.      *Tobacco the Growing Epidemic*, p. 13, and 10th World Conference on Tobacco or Health, Beijing, 1997.

20. "China is by far the largest cigarette manufacturer, followed by the USA. Chinese cigarette production increased from 225 billion cigarettes annually in 1960 to 1.7 trillion a year in 1995, a seven-fold increase."      *The Tobacco Atlas*, p. 48

21. The Chinese state monopoly produces 1.7 trillion cigarettes a year, three times the number sold in the United States, for the country's estimated 350 million smokers. 12% of the annual revenue of the Beijing government is from cigarette sales, even though officials estimate that they lose $2 billion a year in tax revenue, more than 10% of current cigarette taxes, because of a thriving black market in foreign cigarettes. The tax on imported cigarettes is 260%, and foreign brands hold about an estimated 3% market share, or 50 billion cigarettes per year.      Washington Post National Weekly Edition, December 16-22, 1996, pp. 8-10

22. China collects $8.5 billion a year from tobacco taxes and profits from its state-owned tobacco manufacturer.      60 Minutes, August 18, 1996

23. Farmlands planted with tobacco in China have risen 10-fold in the last 30 years to 1.6 million hectares, competing with cotton and grain. An official newspaper reports that 35% of children ages 12-15 are smokers, as are 10% of children ages 9 to 11.      *Vital Signs* 1995, Lester Brown, World Watch Institute

24. Smoking prevalence in Chinese youth is increasing by 3% each year. There are reports from China of "babies and toddlers being given puffs on lighted cigarettes to stop them from crying. Kung Mingming, a four-year-old, became so rapidly addicted that he constantly pestered his parents for cigarettes."      Tobacco Control 1993; 2:7

25. Chinese per capita cigarette consumption increased by 260% from 1972 to 1992, to 1900 cigarettes per year per capita.      Tobacco Alert, July 1996 (World Health Organization)

26. In 1994, China opened its market of 298 million smokers--more than the entire population of the United States--to American cigarettes for the first time. China has a quarter of the world's smokers and a third of its cigarette consumption.      Newsweek, March 21, 1994, p. 53, and Tobacco Control, Winter 1994, p. 303

27. In China where cigarette ads are banned, companies have circumvented the rule by creating travel and music booking agencies as promotional vehicles.      Business Week, September 9, 1996, p. 38

28. In 1984, 56% of male doctors in China were smokers. Tobacco advertising is forbidden in China, but US tobacco firms skirt the regulation. On Shanghai TV, an advertisement for Marlboro is shown with the familiar cowboy, outdoors, music and slogan, but no actual cigarette.      *Tobacco Control in the Third World*, p. 135

29. The 1992 Tobacco Monopoly Law in China bans tobacco advertising in radio, television, newspapers and magazines; students are prohibiting from smoking; smoking is banned in many public places; and health warnings are now printed on cigarette packs.      Tobacco Free Youth Reporter (STAT), Summer 1993

30. Philip Morris sponsors the twelve teams of China's national soccer league, known now as the Marlboro League. Estimates are that Philip Morris accounts for one quarter of all advertising in China. Britain's B.A.T. Industries,

makers of 555, the best known foreign brand, sponsors the annual Hong Kong to Beijing Motor Rally and gives money to schools through the B.A.T. Educational Foundation.        Wall Street Journal, December 28, 1994, p. B6

31.  The ad ban in China is circumvented by tobacco company sponsorship of broadcasts and events without actually showing cigarettes. Multinational companies have only one percent of the total market share, and with a 450% import duty, imported brands cost about US $1.75 a pack, compared with only 25 cents a pack for domestic brands.        Wall Street Journal, December 28, 1994, p. B6

32.  Every day in Shanghai, Marlboro sponsors a radio program called "The American Music Hour." As the Marlboro theme song from the movie "The Magnificent Seven" plays, the announcer says in Chinese: "Jump and fly a thousand miles. This is the world of Marlboro. Ride through the rivers and mountains with courage. Be called a hero throughout the thousand miles. This is the world of Marlboro."        New Yorker, September 13, 1993, p. 78

33.  Philip Morris is the largest single advertiser in China. In China and India, tobacco is the largest source of government revenue, and in Russia, it is second.        San Francisco Examiner, April 18, 1998, p. A1

34.  About Marlboro sales in China: "A cowboy symbolizes a strong, energetic young man...It tells teenagers that smoking Marlboros will make you fit and proud. The cowboy becomes a role model for youth."        New Yorker, September 13, 1993, p. 78

35.  Philip Morris is sponsoring the training of 15,000 physiotherapists in China.
        9th World Conference on Tobacco or Health, Paris, 1994 (Judith Mackay)

36.  The world's worst cigarette-caused fire was caused by several forestry workers in northeastern China in 1987. It burned 3.1 million acres of land, killed 300 people, and made 5000 others homeless.
        *Tobacco Control in the Third World*, p. 141

37.  In China, 300 million smokers consume 1.8 trillion cigarettes a year, and there are about half a million deaths each year from smoking.        Wall Street Journal, December 28, 1994, p. B6

38.  CNN in an August 26, 1997 broadcast in Beijing described China as a "nicotine nirvana", where 300 million men and 20 million women smoke 1.9 trillion cigarettes a year, or 15 per smoker per day. 100 million Chinese men will eventually die from smoking.

39.  In China, 1.7 trillion (1,700,000,000,000) cigarettes were smoked in 1994, and farmland planted in tobacco has increased tenfold to 1.6 million hectares in the last thirty years. Cigarette taxes account for 10% of all government revenue, but the government will pay out far more in tobacco-related medical costs than it takes in from tobacco taxes.        *Vital Signs* 1995, p. 96

40.  In China, there is a low rate of quitting (only 1.8% of men are former smokers) and a low desire to stop smoking.
        JAMA, October 18, 1995, p. 1232

41.  Total cigarette consumption in China increased from 500 billion in 1976 to 1.6 trillion in 1996. 63% of adult males (including 73% in the age group 30 to 60 years) and only 4% of females are current smokers. In the female group, 13% of women ages 60-69, 4% of women ages 40-49, and only 1% of women ages 20-29 were current smokers.
        Abstracts P 1/1 and 1/2, 10th World Conference on Tobacco or Health, Beijing, 1997

42.  In China, 55% of male and 1% of female medical workers are smokers. An estimated 50 million smoking-related deaths are expected to occur in China before 2025 among those who already smoke.
        JAMA, November 12, 1997, p. 1532

43.  In a study of tobacco-related deaths in China, of men who began smoking before the age of 25, about 47% are expected to die between the ages of 35 and 69 years, compared with only 29% of nonsmokers. Among all Chinese men, about 20% of all deaths are attributable to smoking.        JAMA, November 12, 1997, p. 1500

44. In China, foreign brands cost $1.50 a pack, and have only 2 percent of the market share. The best domestic brands are less than 50 cents a pack. Cigarette tax revenues of $8.6 billion in 1995 were the government's single greatest income source. Lung cancer deaths are increasing by 4.5 percent a year for the nation's 300 million smokers (out of 900 million adults). New York Times, March 16, 1996, p. 5

45. In a study of men in Shanghai, 36% of all cases of cancer and 21% of all deaths could be attributed to cigarette smoking. It is estimated that each year about 2 million tobacco-related deaths, including 900,000 from lung cancer, will occur in China in the year 2025 if current smoking patterns persist. JAMA, June 5, 1996, p. 1646

46. The grain yield from land devoted to tobacco cultivation in China could feed 50 million people. The amount of land for tobacco growing has doubled in the last decade.
Canadian Medical Association Journal, May 1, 1995, p. 1512

47. Smoking-related disease kills half a million Chinese each year, and deaths will increase to 2 million a year by 2025 if current smoking rates persist. Lung cancer deaths, 30,000 a year in 1975, are expected to increase to a million a year by 2025. Only 30% of Chinese, however, are aware that smoking is harmful. Cigarette consumption has tripled over the past 15 years. Canadian Medical Association Journal, May 1, 1995, p. 1513

48. The entire government antismoking effort in China includes a single physician operating on a yearly budget of $15,000. NBC News (Tom Brokaw), May 30, 1996

49. Between 1965 and 1990, the per capita cigarette consumption in China more than doubled, from 890 to 1960 per adult per year. The annual number of tobacco-related deaths, about 500,000 to 700,000 in the mid-1990's, is expected to rise to 2 million by 2025. In a district near Shanghai, 17% of total household income is used to buy cigarettes. There are also an estimated half a billion passive smokers in the country.
JAMA, April 26, 1996, p. 1221

50. In a 1989 survey, 68% of male physicians in Beijing were smokers. In 1996, Shanghai Medical University became the first medical school in China to ban smoking. In 1992, China produced 40% of the world's tobacco, 2.76 million metric tons, on 1.8 million hectares of land, and 1.65 trillion cigarettes, 31% of world production. China's state-run tobacco monopoly employs more than half a million workers in factories, 10 million in farming, and 13 million in retail trade. Tobacco taxes accounted for 10% of all government revenue, or $5 billion, in 1992, and rose to $6.6 billion in 1994. JAMA, April 26, 1996, p. 1220

51. Philip Morris has a market share in China of less than 1%. However, the company is the biggest television advertiser in the country. Dr. Judith Mackay, director of the Asian Consultancy on Tobacco control, says, "Smoking foreign cigarettes is trendy. It means you're affluent. It's become almost a mark of business success."
Canadian Medical Association Journal, May 1, 1995, p. 1512

52. At the Institute of Military Medicine in Jinan, China, 48% of the male and 4% of the female medical students were smokers. At the Guangxi Medical University, the medical student smoking rates are somewhat lower, 32% for males and 1% for females.
Abstracts PO 266 and 299, 10th World Conference on Tobacco or Health, Beijing, 1997

53. Adult male smoking prevalence in China in 1991 was 61%, with variations in areas including over 80% in Yunnan province. The prevalence peaked at 74% at age 35 years. The knowledge of tobacco's health hazards is poor; fewer than half of Chinese were aware that smoking causes lung cancer, and only 5% were aware that smoking was associated with heart disease. 10th World Conference on Tobacco or Health, Beijing, 1997 (Yang Gonghuan)

54. Smoking prevalence was 79% in a survey of male Chinese army personnel, and 65% in air force personnel.
Abstracts 229 and 274, 10th World Conference on Tobacco or Health, Beijing, 1997

55. Estimated tobacco-attributable deaths in China are expected to increase from 700,000 in 1996 to 3 million per year in 2025 (Richard Peto data). JAMA, November 12, 1997, p. 1531

56. In China in 1952, the average man smoked one cigarette a day. This rose to 4 cigarettes in 1972, and 10 per day for each man in China in 1992. In the United States it was 1 per day in 1910, 4 in 1930, and 10 cigarettes per man per day in 1950.                    10th World Conference on Tobacco or Health, Beijing, 1997 (Richard Peto)

57. In 1996, the average Chinese male smoker started to smoke at age 20, three years younger than in 1984, and smoked an average of 15 cigarettes a day, an increase from 11 in 1984.          JAMA, November 12, 1997, p. 1531

58. Chinese tobacco companies are almost all state-owned, and provide the government with $4.9 billion each year, or about 10% of overall government revenue. These revenues are offset by government expenditures of $7.8 billion a year for smoking-related diseases and fires.          New York Times, August 27, 1997, p. A7

59. In China, direct medical costs caused by tobacco are estimated to be 71.8 billion yuan (about $9 billion U.S.) in the year 2000.          Abstract S 5/2, 10th World Conference on Tobacco or Health, Beijing, 1997

60. In China, urban per capita expenditures on cigarettes are higher than medical and health care expenditures. From 1981 to 1992, per capita cigarette consumption increased by 62.8%. 1.85 million hectares of land are used for tobacco production, a 25% increase in growing area and 93% increase in production from 1981 to 1992.
                    Tobacco Control, Summer 1997, p. 136

61. China produces four times as much tobacco as the next largest producer, the United States. In 1990, 1.8 million hectares were harvested for tobacco, or 2% of arable land. The state tobacco monopoly employs over half a million workers in industry, 10 million farmers growing tobacco, and 3 million retailers.
                    World Health Organization Regional Office for the Western Pacific

62. In 1996, tobacco created jobs for 10 million peasants in poverty-stricken Yunnan Province, and profits and taxes from tobacco accounted for about 80% of the province's fiscal income.          China Daily (Beijing), August 31, 1997

63. "In China, tobacco planting invades about 1/10 of the farmland. Every year, the economic loss caused by smoking is far greater than the tax income on it. Moreover, the ailment and life lost caused by smoking can't be measured to terms of money!"          Abstract PO 23, 10th World Conference on Tobacco or Health, Beijing, 1997

64. In 1996, the Chinese government received 83 billion yuan (U.S. $10 billion) from cigarette taxes, more than 10% of total revenue. Nearly 50 billion cigarettes are smuggled into China each year, however, and escape import duties and taxes.          China Daily (Beijing), August 31, 1997

65. Though heavily taxed foreign cigarettes comprise only 3% of the legal market, an influx of illegally smuggled cigarettes, mostly from gangs centered in Hong Kong, floods the Chinese market, and costs the Chinese government more than a billion dollars (U.S.) a year in uncollected taxes. The average initial age for smoking has dropped from 23 to 19 in the last decade, and there are 5 million Chinese teenagers who smoke.
                    Charlotte Observer, October 19, 1997

66. China loses an estimated $1.8 billion in annual import tax revenue because of cigarette smuggling, mostly via Hong Kong.          Tobacco Control, Summer 1997, p. 78

67. Officially, imported cigarettes account for 4% of sales in China, or 70 billion per year. However, the real figure is probably much higher, since foreign cigarette companies sell the vast majority of their cigarettes to dealers who smuggle them into China mainly through Hong Kong to avoid high duties of about 250% on imported brands.
                    San Francisco Examiner, August 21, 1997, p. A18 and New York Times, August 27, 1997, p. A7

68. Of the foreign cigarette brands available in China, 44% of current smokers most prefer Marlboro.
                    Abstract PO 148, 10th World Conference on Tobacco or Health, Beijing, 1997

69. In 1993, Philip Morris signed an agreement with the Chinese government tobacco monopoly so that the companies would (in the words of Philip Morris) "work together to produce and sell Marlboro cigarettes for the Chinese market as well as develop and produce other brands for both domestic and export sales. The Agreement represents an unprecedented level of cooperation and sharing of resources, including technology, people and blending

70. Chinese cigarettes sell for as little as 20 cents a pack, and carry the warning, "Smoking is harmful to health." Among the seven-man ruling politburo, there is only one known smoker, and both President Jiang Zemin and Premier Li Peng have condemned the habit.                                USA Today, August 6, 1997, p. 7D

71. Addressing the opening session of the 10th World Conference on Tobacco or Health at the Great Hall of the People in Beijing, Chinese President Jiang Zemin called for more health and environmental awareness, and lamented the 700,000 yearly deaths from tobacco in China.                                China Daily, August 31, 1997

72. On October 7, 1997, Chinese President Jiang Zemin met with Philip Morris CEO Geoffrey Bible, and praised the company's efforts to retain China's most favored nation trade status. Bible pledged increased involvement in China and cooperation with Chinese companies.                                (UK) Guardian, October 14, 1997, p. 16

73. In China, 45-50% of all tobacco-related deaths are caused by chronic obstructive pulmonary disease and emphysema, 13-15% from lung cancer, and the rest from vascular and heart disease plus other cancers. The COPD death rate is much higher, and heart disease death rate much lower, than for smokers in most other areas of the world. In developed countries, 25% of deaths are from lung cancer, 15% from COPD, 35% from vascular and heart disease, and 25% from other cancers.                  10th World Conference on Tobacco or Health, Beijing, 1997
                                                                   (Niu Shiru, Richard Peto, and Jonathan Samet)

74. Chronic obstructive pulmonary disease is the main cause of tobacco-related death in Chinese smokers, accounting for half of the total; 13% of the deaths are from lung cancer, and liver, stomach, and esophageal cancer is also common.                                10th World Conference on Tobacco or Health, Beijing, 1997 (Niu Shiru)

75. "China relies on its huge deposits of high-sulfur coal for three-quarters of its electricity. Consequently, its air is among the foulest in the world. A quarter of all deaths in China are from pulmonary disease."
                                                                   National Geographic, September 1997, p. 30

76. In contrast to most countries, lung cancer and chronic obstructive pulmonary disease and emphysema are relatively common in China in nonsmokers because of the severe air pollution.
                                                       10th World Conference on Tobacco or Health, Beijing, August 1997

77. In China, deaths attributable to air pollution total an estimated 443,000 each year. 70,000 of these are from industrial (outdoor) air pollution, and the rest is primarily from smoke from indoor heating and cooking fires.
                                                                   New York Times, November 29, 1997, p. A6

78. Antismoking campaigners at the Chinese Association on Smoking and Health receive just $24,000 a year from the Chinese government. At the same time, the state monopoly tobacco industry had pretax profits in 1996 of more than $10 billion, a 17% increase from 1995.                British Medical Journal, August 30, 1997, p. 502

79. The average smoker in China spends about 25% of personal income on cigarettes. 1.7 trillion cigarettes a year (99% produced domestically) are smoked by 300 million men (63% current smokers) and 20 million women (4% of women are current smokers). 60% of male health care professionals smoke. Only 2.3% of adults were former smokers. More than 60% of female nonsmokers between ages 25 and 50 have regular exposure to passive smoke. Lung cancer is recognized by about 40% of adults as related to smoking, but heart disease was recognized as related by only about 4%.                                JAMA, October 6, 1999, pp. 1247-1253

80. Of deaths from tobacco in China (700,000 in men and 100,000 in women in 2000), 45% are from chronic lung disease, 15% from lung cancer, and 5-8% each from esophageal cancer, liver and stomach cancers, tuberculosis, stroke, and heart disease. At present smoking rates, about 100 million of the 300 million Chinese men and boys now under age 30 will eventually be killed by tobacco.        British Medical Journal, November 21, 1998, p. 1421

81. By the middle of the 21st century, three million Chinese men will die from smoking each year. Tobacco-related death will claim at least 100 million of the over 300 million males under age 30 in China. Researcher Richard Peto has said: "The truth is a third of all the young men in China will eventually be killed by smoking... you've got 300

million smokers there, and of the young ones, half of them are going to be killed by the habit." The annual consumption of cigarettes in China increased from 100 billion in the early 1950's to 1800 billion (1.8 trillion) in 1998.                                                                                                    Reuters, November 18, 1998

82.  In 1990, smoking caused about 12% of male mortality in middle age in China. This proportion is expected to increase to about 33% by the year 2030.                    British Medical Journal, November 21, 1998, p. 1423

83.  Only 2% of Chinese men had quit and were former smokers in 1993; in 1996 in China, 61% of smokers questioned thought that tobacco did them "little or no harm."                              *Curbing the Epidemic*, pp. 3 and 18

84.  Over 50% of people in China think that smoking does little or no harm, and over 60% are unaware it can cause lung cancer.                                                                       New York Times, November 20, 1998, p. A1

85.  60% of Chinese adults do not know that smoking causes lung cancer, and 96% do not know that it causes heart disease. In 1987, about 13% of deaths in Chinese men were from tobacco use, but this figure may eventually increase to 33%. Of the deaths, only 15% were from lung cancer but 45% from chronic obstructive pulmonary disease, the reverse of the pattern in the west.                                       The Lancet, November 21, 1998, p. 1683

86.  Tobacco growing areas in China increased from 0.8 million hectares in 1978 to 2.4 million hectares in 1997 (out of a total of 154 million hectares of agricultural land).                                       1998 China statistical yearbook

87.  Philip Morris in 1998 ended its five year sponsorship of China's professional soccer league, which was called the Marlboro League. Philip Morris paid about $7 million annually as a sponsor.
                                                                                        Wall Street Journal, November 30, 1998, p. C1

88.  Pepsi is the new sponsor of the Chinese National Football League, replacing five-year sponsor Marlboro. Philip Morris has also discontinued its sponsorship of the Marlboro Open tennis tournament in Hong Kong.
                                                                                                   Adweek Asia, February 12, 1999, p. 10
                                                                                    (the article also has a table summarizing restrictions
                                                                                          on tobacco advertising in countries in Asia)

# Hong Kong

1.  In Hong Kong in 1998, tobacco use was responsible for 33% of all deaths in men 35 to 69, and will likely be followed by similar death rates in mainland China within 20 years, where widespread smoking lags that in Hong Kong by about two decades. Two thirds of all young men in China now become smokers; half of these who persist will eventually die from the habit, and with present smoking rates, about one third of all the young men in China will eventually be killed by tobacco.                                                     British Medical Journal, August 18, 2001

2.  Smoking prevalence in Hong Kong is 15% (27% for men and 3% for women), and there are 3500 deaths each year from smoking.                                                   10th World Conference on Tobacco or Health, Beijing, 1997

3.  Cigarette ads in Hong Kong were banned on TV in 1990 (Thorax 1991; 46:154). In 1991, a new tax doubled the price of a pack of cigarettes from $1.50 to $3.00. In 1991, only 16.7% of the population of 5.7 million smoked, one of the lowest rates in Asia.                                                              New York Times, April 1991 (B.Basler)

4.  More than 1000 Marlboro Classics stores dot Europe and Asia, selling leather vests and cowboy boots stamped with the brand label. Marlboro beach balls in Hong Kong sell for a dollar plus three empty Marlboro packs.
                                                                                                       INFACT Update, Fall/Winter 1996-97

5.  Although based in countries with long-established television advertising bans, the British and American cigarette companies strenuously fought against Hong Kong's proposed (and successful) ban on television tobacco advertising by orchestrating a sophisticated political lobbying and disinformation campaign, which:
    • denied the health evidence
    • denied any effect of advertising on consumption

- warned that world democracy would collapse if tobacco advertisements were banned from Hong Kong television. "One strike at freedom and you have a dangerous domino effect in which freedoms go one by one" (conveniently overlooking the fact that it is the world's democracies that have enacted the most stringent tobacco control legislation)
- warned that the television stations would be severely compromised. They took out full-page newspaper advertisements showing, for example, a heavy hand across the front of the television obliterating the screen with the heading, "Soon your favorite programs could be missing from television," failing to mention that this had not happened anywhere else in the world where advertising bans had been implemented.

quote from Judith Mackay, Preventive Medicine 1994; 23:536

6. In Hong Kong, the tobacco industry attacked journalists who wrote articles on smoking, claiming to their editors "the use of pictures of cancerous lungs clearly attempts to suggest, without any foundation, that the disease was caused by smoking, and is highly irresponsible in its appeal to emotional and sensational instincts."

*The Doctor-Activist*, Ellen Bassuk, Plenum Press, 1996, p. 43

7. Philip Morris in Hong Kong in opposing advertising restrictions maintained that "tobacco advertising is the cornerstone of any free democracy."     9th World Conference on Tobacco or Health, Paris, 1994 (Judith Mackay)

8. "Smoking by teen-agers and children is soaring all over Asia, especially among girls. In Hong Kong, where American tobacco blends make up 94 percent of the market, Salem sponsors tennis tournaments featuring the American player Michael Chang, an idol of Hong Kong girls. A Madonna concert from Spain was rebroadcast into Hong Kong as a Salem Madonna concert. Stores sell Camel and Marlboro caps, watches and binoculars. While the manufacturers deny they are targeting young people, the merchandise and events they offer appeal mainly to teen-agers. Cigarette advertising is banned from television and radio, but billboards and print ads showing young people having sophisticated fun are practically identical to those in the United States. These ads piggyback on the lure of American pop culture, which represents freedom and excitement for many Asian youths."     New York Times editorial "Selling Cigarettes in Asia", September 10, 1997, p. A22

9. The City University of Hong Kong, with 15,000 students and staff, has been entirely smoke-free since 1989, including all teaching, administrative, and recreational buildings, as well as university vehicles.

Judith Mackay, M.D.

10. Dr. Judith Mackay, Hong Kong and Asia's most prominent tobacco control advocate, as been described by a U.S. smokers' rights group as "an insane psychotic just like Hitler, using fatuous smarmy drivel and distortions, and diatribes full of putrid corruption, lies, conspiracy, and total censorship."

*The Doctor-Activist*, Ellen Bassuk, Plenum Press, 1996

# Taiwan

1. In 1985, Taiwan reduced its cigarette consumption by 5 percent, and in 1986, by 6 percent. But in 1987, responding to threats of US trade sanctions, Taiwan opened its market to American cigarettes. That year, sales rose by 10 percent.     JAMA, June 13, 1990, p. 2989

2. In Taiwan before US tobacco companies entered the market, only 1% of girls had ever smoked. But after only four years of advertising, that figure had climbed to 20%.

Doonesbury cartoon, Garry Trudeau, October 8, 1993 (quote from Mr. Butts)

3. The smoking rate among high school students in Taiwan jumped from 22% the year before US companies entered the market to 32% two years later. Smoking rates among male Korean teenagers rose from 18% to 30% in one year after import restrictions were removed; among female teenagers, rates increased from less than 2% to nearly 9%.     INFACT Newsletter, June 1993

4. In Taiwan, the most popular cigarette brands are Long Life, Prosperity Island, and New Paradise. The tobacco industry there has arranged for discos to grant free admission in exchange for empty cartons of cigarettes.

NEJM, March 28, 1991, p. 918

5. In Taipei Taiwan in 1988, RJ Reynolds arranged to sponsor three rock concerts for young people. The only accepted admission "ticket" was to be five empty packs of Winstons, or ten packs for a souvenir Winston sweat shirt as well. Protests forced a cancellation.
   *The Progressive, May 1991, and Health Letter "Outrage of the Month", March 12, 1989*

6. In Taiwan, smoking prevalence is 60% for men and 5% for women. Total smoking-related deaths were 15,000 in 1995. Lung cancer deaths increased by 460% from 1971 to 1995; it is estimated that smoking contributed 65% and increased air pollution 30% of the lung cancer increase. Smoking is also related to an increased risk for hepatocellular carcinoma in Taiwan.
   *Abstracts OS 4, OS 21, and OS 192, 10th World Conference on Tobacco or Health, Beijing, 1997*

7. The United States supplies 75% of Taiwan's imported cigarettes, which constitute 20% of the total market.
   *Tobacco Control in the Third World*, p. 192

# Korea

1. In South Korea, 65% of men and 5% of women are smokers.
   *The Tobacco Atlas*, 2002

2. In 1985, former Reagan aide Michael K. Deaver as a well paid lobbyist for Philip Morris met with South Korea's president Chun Doo Hwan in an effort to persuade the Korean government to liberalize its policy regarding American cigarette imports.
   *New York Times magazine, July 10, 1988, p. 62*

3. South Korea opened its markets to American cigarettes (and a blitz of advertising) in 1988. Just one year later, the smoking rate for male teens had risen from 18% to 30%, and for female teenagers from 2% to 9%.
   *New Yorker, September 13, 1993, p. 85*

4. After American cigarettes were first introduced into Korea, the number of teenage girls who smoked jumped 450% in one year.
   *Doonesbury cartoon, Garry Trudeau, October 5, 1993*

5. Since American cigarettes and advertising were introduced in South Korea in 1986, smoking rates among adolescent boys have doubled, and among adolescent girls have quadrupled.
   *Wall Street Journal, September 27, 1990, p. A13*

6. In a 1998 survey in Korea, 42% of doctors were current smokers, compared with 49% in 1992.
   *11th World Conference on Tobacco or Health, Chicago, 2000, Abstract PO 205*

7. In late 2002, Philip Morris became the first foreign cigarette company to begin manufacture in South Korea, the world's eight largest market.
   *San Francisco Chronicle, October 23, 2002, p. D1*

8. Smoking on the golf course is now prohibited at the 138 member clubs in South Korea's Golf Business Association.
   *Golf World, March 15, 2002, p. 13*

9. A letter from the commercial counselor at the U.S. Embassy in Seoul to the public affairs manager of Philip Morris Asia read in part: "I want to emphasize that the embassy and the various U.S. government agencies in Washington will keep the interests of Philip Morris and the other American cigarette manufacturers in the forefront of our daily concerns."
   *Washington Post National Weekly Edition, November 25-December 1, 1996, p. 6*

10. South Korea has an annual per capita cigarette consumption rate of 4,153, the highest in the world.
    *USA Today, October 22, 1997*

# Thailand

1. As of November 2002, smoking is prohibited in almost all indoor places in Thailand. From 1986 to 1999 in Thailand, smoking prevalence for men declined from 48.8% to 38.9%, and in women, from 4.1% to 2.4%.
   *New York Times, December 19, 2002, p. A9*

2.  In Thailand, cigarette advertising and promotion is banned, as is smoking in most public places. Adult yearly per capita cigarette consumption is 1050, low by Asian standards. Largely because of the ad ban, American companies were denied the tools that they traditionally use to attract new customers, and imported cigarettes in 1995 had only 3% of the market share, compared to 21% in Japan, 22% in Taiwan, and 6% in South Korea.

    The Washington Post National Weekly Edition, December 2-8, 1996, p. 12

3.  Tobacco companies are waging a major battle against the Thailand Ministry of Public Health over proposed regulations requiring companies to reveal the identity and amount of additives in each brand of cigarette and cigar. Some in the Ministry plan to make the information public--a first for any nation that would make previously secret information available worldwide. Protesting vehemently, manufacturers have been persuading US, British, and Japanese Embassy officials in Bangkok to write to the Ministry of Foreign Affairs suggesting that the regulations may conflict with international trade agreements that protect trade secrets. One US Embassy letter attached to a 12-page document from Philip Morris (Thailand) Ltd encapsulated other industry complaints, including that technical standards in the regulations are "vague and ambiguous . . . contain factual errors . . . and unfairly discriminate against international manufacturers of cigarettes". If the US Trade Representative Office decides that tobacco ingredients are trade secrets rather than health hazards, the USA could threaten to impose trade sanctions on Thailand.                                    Quote from the British Medical Journal, January 13, 1996, p. 112

4.  The smoking rate for monks in Thailand (97% of the population is Buddhist) dropped from 53% in 1990 to 32% in 1996.                                    Abstract PO 92, 10th World Conference on Tobacco or Health, Beijing, 1997

5.  In Thailand for adults age 15 and older, smoking prevalence was 60% for men and 4% for women in 1986. In 1996, rates had dropped to 49% for men and 2.7% for women (23% overall). 45% of cigarettes are hand rolled, and 55% are manufactured commercially. 96% of brands are domestic, and 4% are imported.

    10th World Conference on Tobacco or Health, Beijing, 1997 (Bung-on Ritthiphakdee)

6.  The Thailand Tobacco Monopoly in 1996 proposed a plan to produce a new brand of cigarette designed for women, at a time when only 2.8% of the country's women were smokers. However, the plan was dropped after intense lobbying by public health groups.

    Abstract PO 90, 10th World Conference on Tobacco or Health, Beijing, 1997

7.  When Thailand banned cigarette ads, ads for Kent, a Lorillard brand, disappeared. But suddenly a related company was promoting "Kent Leisure Holidays." An advertising ban in Hong Kong yielded a "Marlboro Red Hot Hits" music promotion in magazines and a "Salem Attitude" clothing line. The FDA rules seek to ban such maneuvers, but industry observers expect cigarette makers to invent new ones.

    Quote from Business Week, September 9, 1996, p 37

# Singapore

1.  In Singapore, cigarettes have a limit of 1.3 milligrams of nicotine and 15mg of tar. Smoking prevalence decreased from 20% in 1984 to 17% in 1995, including only 2% of women.

    10th World Conference on Tobacco or Health, Beijing, 1997 (Chng Chee Yeong)

2.  About 15% of Singapore's 4 million people are smokers.                                    Associated Press, June 1, 2001

3.  In an aggressive campaign to make Singapore smoke-free, the government has prohibited smoking in restaurants, stores, sports arenas, subways, buses, offices, and hospitals.                                    Wall Street Journal, November 2, 1989

4.  In Singapore, the fine (strictly enforced) for smoking in a restaurant is US $310.

    New Yorker, January 13, 1992, p. 40

5.  In Singapore, fines are imposed on anyone younger than 18 carrying cigarettes in public, whether or not actually smoking. Merchants caught selling tobacco to minors face a $6300 fine.

    American Medical News, January 24, 1994

6. In Singapore, there is no smoking allowed in any air conditioned building or in any public space. The fine for offenders is US $321.

*Fodor's Exploring Singapore and Malaysia, 1994*

# Philippines

1. Smoking prevalence in the Philippines is 32.4% (53.8% of men, and 11% of women).
*The Tobacco Atlas*, 2002

2. In the Philippines, 63% of male and 37% of female doctors were smokers in the early 1990's, and 38% smoked regularly in front of their patients.

*Smoke and Mirrors*, p. 229

3. In the Philippines, the number of smokers almost doubled between 1985 and 1995. A WHO study from 1994-1995 showed that 73% of adults and 56% of children ages 7 to 17 are "regular" smokers.

British Medical Journal, July 26, 1997, p. 209

4. American cigarettes exported to the Philippines have 50% more tar and often twice as much nicotine as comparable brands consumed in the United States.

NEJM, March 28, 1991, p. 918

5. RJR's Winston brand is advertised in the Philippines as "the Taste of the USA."

New York Times, May 14, 1991, p. E16

6. In the Philippines, a calendar poster featuring the Virgin Mary has below a picture of an assortment of American cigarette packs.

San Francisco Chronicle, April 18, 1998, p. A12

7. 57% of the population in the Philippines in 1990 was unaware that cigarettes cause cancer.

Tobacco Control, Fall 1994, p. 200

8. Philip Morris plans in 2003 to complete a new $300 million cigarette manufacturing plant in the Philippines.
2002 AMA Annual Tobacco Report

# Asia – Other Countries

1. Since 1985 and under the threat of imposition of retaliatory trade sanctions, American tobacco companies have opened up markets for American cigarettes and advertising in Japan, South Korea, Taiwan, and Thailand.

NEJM, March 21, 1991, p. 917

2. Unlike in the West, where women's smoking rates often rival or surpass those of men, smoking by women in many developing countries is uncommon, thus representing a vast, untapped potential market for the tobacco industry. The industry's Tobacco Reporter observed: "The Asian market--the lucrative and elusive Asian market. There are not many places left in the world that make US cigarette manufacturers wring their hands in anticipation, and pat their wallets in hope."

*Tobacco Control in the Third World*, p. 4

3. All smokeless tobacco products are banned in Hong Kong, Singapore, Australia, Ireland, and the United Kingdom.

Journal of the National Cancer Institute Monographs 1992; 12:32

4. The Asian tobacco market will grow by 33% in the decade of the 1990's.

9th World Conference on Tobacco or Health, Paris, 1994 (T.Lam)

5. Paula Abdul appeared in Seoul in a concert sponsored by Salem, Madonna in Hong Kong also sponsored by Salem cigarettes, and Dire Straits in Malaysia in a Kent-sponsored concert.

Reader's Digest, April 1993, p. 54

6. Asian-American tennis star Michael Chang – who is idolized by the region's teen-age girls – plays regularly in Marlboro and Salem tournaments in China, Japan, South Korea and Hong Kong. The Marlboro Music Hour of American pop music is heard daily in China. American singer Roberta Flack has appeared at Mild Seven music festivals sponsored by Japan Tobacco International.

American Medical News, January 1, 1996

7. Tennis stars Pat Cash, Michael Chang, Jimmy Connors and John McEnroe have appeared in matches in Malaysia sponsored by RJR. Washington Post National Weekly Edition, November 25-December 1, 1996, p. 8

8. Multinational tobacco companies are forging aggressively into Asia looking to the region's vast young population and booming economies to offset the loss of business in the West. Over the criticism of health activists, the companies are making their products known to young people by sponsoring numerous sports, music and cultural events that effectively elude bans on direct advertising. Associated Press, February 14, 1996

9. From 1972 to 1992, cigarettes smoked yearly per person age 15 or older increased in China from 730 to 1900. In Bangladesh, the increase was from 510 to 990; in South Korea, from 2370 to 3010; in India, from 1010 to 1370; in Japan, from 2950 to 3240; and in Thailand, from 810 per capita in 1972 to 1050 in 1992. During the same period, consumption in Singapore dropped from 2510 to 1610, typical for a more developed country. Washington Post National Weekly Edition, December 2-8, 1996, p. 12

10. In Malaysia, where 41% of men and 5% of women smoked in 1987, Dunhill has promised $62.5 million to sponsor the Malaysian Cup national football competition over the next ten years, and Marlboro spent $1 million to sponsor the Thomas Cup badminton championship. *Tobacco Control in the Third World*, p. 164

11. Smoking prevalence in Malaysia is now 49.2% in men and 3.5% in women (26.4% overall). *The Tobacco Atlas*, 2002

12. In Indonesia between 1970 and 1985, per capita tobacco consumption increased by 119%. Smoking prevalence is estimated at 75% of men and 5% of women. A newly introduced cigarette brand is Remaja Jaya, or Successful Youth. *Tobacco Control in the Third World*, p. 152

13. In Indonesia, 31.4% of the adult population smokes (59% of men, and 3.7% of women). *The Tobacco Atlas*, 2002

14. The Kretek, a cigarette infused with clove oil and sweetened with sugar, accounted for 88% of the 168.5 billion cigarettes smoked in Indonesia in 1996. Business Week, April 18, 1997

15. 140 billion Kretek (clove and tobacco) cigarettes are smoked each year in Indonesia. They are very high in nicotine and tar, and are often made with corn husks as opposed to paper wrappings. Globe Trekker: Indonesia (Lonely Planet film), 2002

16. Kreteks are one third clove and two thirds tobacco. Indonesia's 210 million people, mostly its men, smoked 200 billion kreteks in 2000. Only one smoker in ten prefers standard cigarettes, called whites. Kreteks are often flavored with saccharine, cinnamon, licorice, pineapple, coffee, coriander or strawberry. New York Times, September 3, 2001, p. A4

17. Philip Morris sponsored a recent Marlboro "cyclo" taxi race in Phnom Penh, Cambodia, complete with young women in cowgirl costumes handing out free Marlboros. 9th World Conference on Tobacco or Health, Paris, 1994 (INFACT Newsletter)

18. In Phnom Penh, Cambodia, a giant billboard advertising Lucky Strikes sits across the street from King Sihanouk's palace. 66% of men and 8% of women in Cambodia are smokers. New York Times, May 14, 1994, p. E1 and *The Tobacco Atlas*, 2002

19. 46% of the 36,000 street signs in Phnom Penh, Cambodia, advertise cigarettes, and 47% of billboards advertise tobacco products. *Tobacco: the Growing Epidemic*, p. 451

20. Deep in the rural countryside of Laos, large Marlboro cowboy posters dominate village stores. Rural people use cigarette smoke to repel mosquitoes (this in a country where malaria is the leading cause of death). Tobacco Control, Spring 1994, p. 10

21. Vietnam has the highest reported male smoking prevalence in the world, 72.8%, compared to 4.3% among women. In the age group 35 to 44 years, 84% of men were smokers. Domestic brands cost 14 cents to 55 cents a pack, and

more-expensive imported brands account for only 16% of the market. On average, smokers spent $49 on cigarettes each year, an amount 1.5 times their annual per capita expense for education ($30.82), 5 times their annual per capita household expense for health care ($9.65), and about a third of their annual per capita household expense for food ($143). A new domestic brand, Boy Boy Boy, "features packaging with images of a Vietnamese Marlboro Man, complete with cowboy hat," and the transnational tobacco companies promote their products aggressively.

JAMA, June 4, 1997, pp. 1726-1731

22. Vietnamese tobacco companies are after the local teenage market with cigarettes called Titanic, Rave, and Boy Boy Boy. The Titanic brand shows on the pack Leonardo DiCaprio and Kate Winslet in a scene from the film Titanic. The picture is almost certainly being used without their permission, since Vietnam leads the world in illegally copying designer goods.                    British Medical Journal, February 12, 2000, p. 399

23. In Vietnam, cigarette expenditures amount to one third of the money spent for food, and five times the amount spent for health care. The ministry of health has a $7000 per year budget for tobacco control activities.
     Anthony So, Rockefeller Foundation, World Conference on Tobacco or Health, Chicago, August 10, 2000

24. In Vietnam on average, cigarette smokers spent about 1.5 times as much on cigarettes as on education and fives times as much as on health care. Cigarette expenditures represented about one third that for food.

*Tobacco: the Growing Epidemic*, p. 34

25. Senator Jesse Helms boasts that he intends to use his chairmanship of the Senate Foreign Relations Committee to bring the world's most lucrative emerging tobacco markets to North Carolina. He and RJR on March 30, 1996 hosted a dinner for Vietnam's ambassador-designate to Washington, along with six other envoys from Southeast Asia. RJ Reynolds has invested $21 million in a joint-venture cigarette factory in Da Nang. "At a moment when tobacco executives are fending off Federal grand juries and corporate whistleblowers armed with embarrassing internal documents, Mr. Helms is doing what he can to make sure that North Carolina tobacco gains opportunities in Vietnam, Indonesia, Malaysia and Thailand."                    New York Times, April 2, 1996, p. A2

26. Ho Chi Minh (1890-1969) chain-smoked Salem cigarettes (Dan Rather, CBS news, People of the Century program, April 6, 1998). Another account by Stanley Karnow (Time, April 13, 1998) stated that Ho preferred Camels or Lucky Strikes. He began smoking American cigarettes when he lived in Paris during World War One.

27. A Vietnam travel description of Ho Chi Minh City, the former Saigon, mentioned two minivans with "Marlboro" written on the outside pulling up on the street, and "out popped a small army who handed out free cigarettes."

Contra Costa (Calif.) Times, June 7, 1998, p. E2

# CHAPTER 28
# ADVERTISING

## Historical

1.  The first American tobacco advertisement dates from 1789, and showed an Indian smoking a long clay pipe.
    San Francisco Chronicle, May 23, 1998, p. 10

2.  The dominating force in cigarette promotion up until the age of radio advertising had been the premiums. A 1901 catalog of premium merchandise redeemable from a Richmond, Virginia, tobacco distributor contains a wide variety of items--including handguns. For one thousand coupons, you could get an "Iver Johnson .32 Special Safety Hammer Automatic Revolver."
    Quote from Cigarette Confidential, p. 128

3.  A rapid rise in per capita cigarette consumption that began around 1910 provided one of the first demonstrations that advertising and mass marketing could create demand for a product where no previous demand existed.

4.  "Shortly after the court-ordered break-up of the tobacco industry monopoly in 1911, the R. J. Reynolds Tobacco Company introduced the Camel brand of cigarettes, which contained a sweeter blend of tobaccos than other brands of the time. The marketing campaign that launched this brand was undertaken with an expensive town-by-town promotional approach. The teaser ('Camels are Coming!') was followed by unprecedented advertising of the brand in print and billboard media. In 1913, the R. J. Reynolds Tobacco Company spent nearly $800,000 on advertising and promotion; this amount increased to $2.2 million by 1916 and to $8.7 million by 1921. The money spent on marketing leveled off at about 60% of total profits. From 1913 to 1921, the R. J. Reynolds Tobacco Company's market share rose from 0.2%, representing the sale of 1.5 million Camel cigarettes, to 50% of all cigarette sales, or 18.3 billion Camel cigarettes.
    "In 1915, Reynolds was interviewed on how he came by his strong beliefs in advertising. He responded that he started with a small advertising budget for plug tobacco in 1894 and observed that his sales rose considerably. A fourfold increase in his advertising budget in the following year was associated with a doubling of his sales. According to the Winston-Salem Journal in 1915, he said that, after that, he did not need any more proof of the power of advertising."
    Health Psychology 1995; 14:505 (John Pierce)

5.  R. J. Reynolds introduced Camel in 1913 as the first national brand, and sold it for 10 cents a pack, two thirds of the price of competing brands, which were primarily Chesterfield and Lucky Strike. By 1927, more than half the tobacco consumed in the United States was in the form of cigarettes.
    The Tobacco Epidemic, p. 7

6.  In 1912, the American Tobacco Company recruited opera singer Enrico Caruso and baseball stars Ty Cobb, John McGraw, and Christy Mathewson to endorse Tuxedo smoking tobacco.
    Tobacco Advertising, p. 104

7.  "Sweet as a Nut--Clean as a Whistle."
    1915 Slogan for Beechnut Chewing Tobacco
    (Tobacco Advertising, p. 119)

8.  During World War One, an advertising campaign featured an American soldier in France leaning wearily against the side of a trench as he smoked a cigarette. The message beneath the picture read, "After the Battle, the Most Refreshing Smoke is Murad. 20 cents for 20."
    They Satisfy, p. 83

9.  In 1921, RJR spent $8 million on advertising, mostly on Camel, and inaugurated the famous "I'd Walk a Mile for a Camel" slogan. By 1923, Camel had 45% of the U.S. cigarette market share.
    www.uchsc.edu

10. A law passed in Utah in the 1920's banned all outdoor billboards, including those for cigarettes. It is still in force today.

11. The first aerial tobacco ad was in New York in 1923, when the name "Lucky Strike" was formed in letters a mile high and six miles long.
    Tobacco Advertising, p. 254

12. In 1926, Liggett and Myers ran a Chesterfield ad showing a man and woman seated in a romantic setting by a riverbank at dusk. The man is lighting up and the woman looks at him with admiration mixed with wistful envy. "Blow some my way," she coaxes, as the gender taboo begins to be broken. *They Satisfy*, p. 99

13. In 1928, the advertising expert Albert Lasker developed the slogan "Reach for a Lucky instead of a Sweet." He began the association of cigarettes with the attribute of slimness, with the principal selling idea of smoking as an aid to dieting and weight control.
*Preventing Tobacco Use Among Young People*, 1994 Surgeon General report, p. 165

14. The Lucky Strike "Reach for a Lucky instead of a Sweet" campaign resulted in a rise in sales from 13.7 billion cigarettes in 1925, when it was the third ranked brand, to over 40 billion in 1930, when it became the top-ranked brand. New York Times, January 1, 1996, p. 21

15. In the late 1920's, a Lucky Strike ad had a slim model saying, "Non, non sweets for me--I smoke a Lucky to keep petite." *Tobacco and the Clinician*, p. v

16. "The throat is a delicate instrument which all singers protect with utmost care. To avoid irritation, I smoke Lucky Strikes. They are not only kind to my throat but have the finest flavor."
"Pleasing Stage Star" Fiske O'Hara commentary on Luckies in ad, Time magazine, 1927

17. Red Grange, National Football Star writes: "While at college I learned that the condition of the throat is most important to an athlete. Coaches and captains know that throat irritation may even keep a player out of an important game. For this reason, I insist that my New York Yankees smoke only Luckies, when they smoke. I know that Luckies are smooth and mellow and can not irritate the throat."
Lucky Strike ad in Time magazine, December 7, 1927

18. Ads for Lucky Strike in 1928 and 1929: "It's toasted. No Throat Irritation--No Cough." and "20,679 physicians have confirmed the fact that Lucky Strike is less irritating to the throat than other cigarettes."
*The Cigarette Papers*, p. 28

19. Amelia Earhart and Helen Hayes endorsed Luckies during the "Reach for a Lucky instead of a Sweet" campaign of the late 1920's. New York Times, April 20, 1997, p. E3

20. "For digestion's sake, smoke Camels--that's what I do. I'm a great believer in the way Camels help ease strain and tension. Camels give me an invigorating 'lift' when I need it most."
Statement from Glenn Hardin, Olympic Champion and world record holder in the hurdles, from Time magazine ad, 1928

21. Presenting Babe Ruth in the Blindfold Cigarette test. "Old Gold's mildness and smoothness marked it 'right off the bat' as the best." Babe Ruth. "Not a cough in a carload". 1920's ad for Old Gold cigarettes

22. "20,679 physicians have confirmed the fact that Lucky Strike is less irritating in the throat than other cigarettes."
"Many prominent athletes smoke Luckies all day long with no harmful effects to wind or physical condition."
"It's toasted." "Your throat protection – against irritation – against cough."
1929 and 1930 ads for Lucky Strike (*Clearing the Smoke*, p. 62)

23. A 1930 ad showed a pot bellied gentleman struggling at golf. "Before it's too late," the ad began, "when tempted to overindulge, reach for a Lucky." Journal of National Cancer Institute, July 20, 1994, p. 1048

24. The August 11, 1930 edition of Time depicts a distinguished senior physician handing over his practice to his handsome son. "The old doctor handed over to his son a family tradition of high ideals and devoted service," the ad reads. "And another tradition has survived, too...Fatima Cigarettes."
Journal of National Cancer Institute, July 20, 1994, p. 1048

25. In the late 1920's and early 1930's, Camels stressed how they "increase your flow of energy," and famous athletes affirmed that Camels "don't get your wind...you can smoke all you want!" Old Gold Cigarettes promised "not a cough in a carload," and Philip Morris instructed the smoker, "Sure you inhale, so play it safe with your throat...scientifically proved less irritating..."    *Tobacco and the Clinician*, p. 19

26. "Do You Inhale? What's there to be afraid of? Make sure, absolutely sure, your cigarette smoke is pure, is clean, that certain impurities have been removed!"
                                Ad for Lucky Strikes, 1932 (*Smoking and the Public Interest*, Ruth Brecher, Consumers Union, 1963, p. 142)

27. "Put Sir Walter Smoking Tobacco in the Bowl, Romeo--and slip your arm around those slim shoulders. You'll fill the air with an aroma that positively encourages romance."    Ad in Time magazine, July 2, 1934

28. "Everyday, more and more people discover the Philip Morris paradox: a cigarette mild enough to smoke as often as you please, yet so robustly full-flavored as to satisfy your strongest smoke desire..."
                                Ad in Time magazine, July 9, 1934, p. 43

29. "They don't get your wind."    1935 ads for Camels (*Clearing the Smoke*, p. 63)

30. "The marketing concept of redeemable cigarette premium coupons reached an all-time low when, in 1936, a German cigarette manufacturer, Cigaretten Bildendienst, used this coupon-redemption scheme to promote the early propaganda of Adolf Hitler. The way it worked was smokers collected coupons from packages of cigarettes to exchange for a coffee-table book on Hitler... The photo book was an important part of the Nazi war machine, intended to show Hitler in a sympathetic light at a crucial time for him politically. The fact that it was sponsored by a cigarette company is ironic because of the Fuhrer's fevered loathing of smokers and anything to do with cigarettes."    *Cigarette Confidential*, p. 128

31. "When I need a 'lift' in energy, Camels is the cigarette for me."Joe DiMaggio, earning a few hundred dollars for this ad during his 1936 rookie season    (US News and World Report, March 22, 1999, p. 20)

32. In a 1937 ad for Camels, Yankee baseball star Lou Gehrig attributed part of his success to smoking. "For a sense of deep-down contentment, just give me Camels after a good, man-sized meal. That little phrase 'Camels set you right' covers the way I feel. Camels set *me* right, whether I'm batting, working, or enjoying life."
                                *Nicotine*, p. 66

33. "Camels set me right, whether I'm eating, working--or just enjoying life. All the years I've been playing, I've been careful about my physical condition. Smoke? I smoke and enjoy it. My cigarette is Camel."
                                Lou Gehrig, The Saturday Evening Post, April 24, 1937

34. "No old-hat medical claims...for a Treat instead of a Treatment, smoke Old Gold."
                                1930's ad for Old Gold cigarettes (Tobacco Control, Autumn 1997 supplement cover)

35. The Lucky Strike Hit Parade was a popular radio music show. In 1938, a sweepstakes promotion offered free cartons of "Luckies" for correctly guessing each week's most popular tunes, and drew nearly seven million entries per week.    1994 Surgeon General Report, p. 167

36. A single hour of the Review radio show in the 1930's contained 70 promotional references to Raleigh cigarettes.    1994 Surgeon General report, p. 167

37. From the 1930's until the mid-1950's, full-page color ads in magazines depicted prosperous middle-aged physicians proclaiming: "More doctors smoke Camels than any other cigarette", or "L&M filters are just what the doctor ordered."    Journal of the National Cancer Institute, July 20, 1994, p. 1048

38. "Tests showed three out of every four cases of smokers' cough cleared on changing to Philip Morris. Why not observe the results for yourself?"    1943 Philip Morris ad in the National Medical Journal

39. A series of ads for Philip Morris cigarettes in the New England Journal of Medicine in 1944 stated: "Doctor, have *you* ever suffered from throat irritation due to smoking?", and "Clinical tests showed that when smokers changed to Philip Morris cigarettes, *every* case of irritation of the nose and throat due to smoking *cleared completely* or *definitely improved*."

40. A Camel man in Times Square, New York City, blew giant smoke rings (steam actually), one every four seconds, from 1941 until 1966 when it was torn down.                    Smithsonian, February 1998, p. 41

41. "I've smoked Camels for 8 years. They have the **mildness** that counts with me."
                                                    Joe DiMaggio, advertising Camels in the late 1940's (*Cigars*, p. 15)

42. Henry Fonda touted in 1940's ads for Camels that there was "not one single case of throat irritation from smoking Camels."                                                    Dean Ornish, M.D.

43. Chesterfields were endorsed by Joe Louis in 1947 as "the champ of cigarettes." In 1946, Philip Morris was touted as "the throat-tested cigarette," claiming that scientific studies showed that the irritant effects of the four leading brands were, on average, four times as high and lasted more than three times as long as Philip Morris cigarettes.                                                    New York Times, April 20, 1997, p. E3

44. "My cigarette is the *mild* cigarette...that's why Chesterfield is my favorite."
                                                    Ronald Reagan appearing in a Chesterfield ad in 1948.

45. C.H. Long was "just another cowboy" in the Texas panhandle until a picture of him smoking a cigarette appeared on the cover of Life magazine on August 22, 1949. "Advertising mogul Leo Burnett saw the picture and was inspired to create a mythic hero who could be used to sell cigarettes: the Marlboro Man. Advertising changed a cowboy into the cowboy, a noble archetype into a sales pitch."
                                                    Life magazine 60th Anniversary issue, October 1996, p. 132

46. Model Janet Sackman was the 1949 Lucky Strike girl, did Chesterfield ads on TV, and appeared on the covers of Life and Look. She began smoking after a tobacco executive said, "It would be a good idea for you to learn how to smoke. That way you'll look authentic." In 1983, she had a cancerous larynx removed, and in 1990 part of one lung.                    New York Times, November 30, 1994, p. A19 (Anna Quindlen)

47. In 1950 the Federal Trade Commission moved to prohibit R.J. Reynolds from claiming that Camels aided digestion, did not impair the wind or physical condition of athletes, would never harm or irritate the throat, and were soothing and comforting to the nerves.    *Reducing the Health Consequences of Tobacco*, p. 510

48. "In 1950, Luckies sponsored a teenage orientated music series named *Your Hit Parade*, which ran for seven years. Its advertisements, which were played in commercial breaks, chose wholesome youth as their refrain. Lucky Strike's 'Be Happy, Go Lucky' won the newly established *TV Guide's* commercial of the year. Its champion advert showed nubile cheerleaders singing: 'Yes, Luckies get our loudest cheers on campus and on dates. With college gals and college guys a Lucky really rates.' Lucky Strike's rivals were quick to follow. In 1951, Philip Morris sponsored a new show called *I Love Lucy*, a black-and-white series about a redhead. It was the top-rated show for four of its six full seasons, during which its characters smoked a prodigious amount of cigarettes."                                                    *Tobacco* (Gately), p. 277

49. Chesterfield ads in the 1940's and 1950's featured full-page color photos of (among others): Ronald Reagan, Bob Hope, Gregory Peck, Kirk Douglas, Bing Crosby, Ben Hogan, Barbara Stanwyck, Gene Tierney, Rhonda Fleming, Lucille Ball, and Jack Webb. In 1993, the Liggett Group with a new ad campaign "reintroduced" a filtered Chesterfield, whose market share had fallen below 1%.        New York Times, November 28, 1992

50. "Right now--*Today*, man!" Jackie Robinson says: "For a treat instead of a treatment… I recommend Old Gold cigarettes."                                                    Early 1950's ad (*Cigars*, p. 15)

51. "Coughs due to smoking disappear!"        from TV ad in the 1950's advising smokers to switch to Philip Morris cigarettes.

52. A 1950 editorial in the tobacco industry trade journal U.S. Tobacco Journal stated: "...it is an historically demonstrated certainty that the more people are subjected to intelligent advertising, the more people will buy the product advertised."  
1994 Surgeon General report, p. 167

53.     When Marlboro was introduced in the US, it was promoted as a woman's cigarette: "Mild as May...red tips to match your pretty lips." A typical magazine advertisement from the 1940's featured a baby saying, "Gee, Mommy, you sure enjoy your Marlboros!"  
    In the early 1950's, the Chicago advertising agency Leo Burnett was awarded the Marlboro account. At the time, veterans of the Korean War were not welcomed home as heroes, unlike the experience of returning military personnel following World War II. Burnett redesigned the Marlboro pack as a war medallion, highlighted by a red chevron. Print advertisements showed a man's tattooed hand gripping Marlboro's new flip-top box. Literally overnight, Marlboro became a man's brand.  
Quote from *Tobacco and Health*, p. 655 (Alan Blum)

54. In the 1950's, singer Julie London warbled on TV, "Where there's a man, there's a Marlboro."  
USA Today, November 16, 1995, p. 28

55. In the early 1950's Marlboro was a brand aimed at women, much like Virginia Slims today. Marlboro sales were one quarter of one percent of the American market, and Philip Morris was last among US cigarette makers. In 1954, the brand's packaging and image were redesigned to appeal to men. The cowboy was introduced in newspaper ads, and the slogan was "Delivers the goods on flavor." The next year, the campaign featured a Marlboro man with tattoos and the slogan: "Filter, flavor, flip-top box--you get a lot to like." Sales jumped to 5 billion, a 3241 percent increase over 1954. By 1957, sales had increased to 20 billion for that year, which meant that Marlboro sold three times as many cigarettes every day as it did in the entire year of 1954.  
New York Times, August 27, 1995, p. F11

56. Marlboro had long been sold as a woman's cigarette, with lipstick-colored filters and a "Mild as May" slogan. Beginning in 1956, Marlboro was changed from a female to masculine cigarette in an enormously successful ad campaign. This success with Marlboro led Philip Morris in 1968 to launch another brand, Virginia Slims, with stereotyped female characteristics. An ad executive stated: "We try to tap the emerging independence and self-fulfillment of women, to make smoking a badge to express that."  
1994 Surgeon General report, pp. 172 and 178

57. Leo Burnett was the creator of Marlboro man in 1954. The following year, Marlboro sales increased 32-fold, and by 1972 it was the world's best-selling brand.    US News and World Report, December 27, 1999, p. 62

58. Ads for Viceroy in 1952: "New Health-Guard Filter makes Viceroy better for your Health than any other Leading Cigarette!" and "Although most filters help to remove tobacco tars, laboratory analysis *proved* that smoke from other leading filter-tip cigarettes contain up to 110.5% *more nicotine* than Viceroy!"  
*The Cigarette Papers*, p. 29

59. In the 1950's, "Chesterfield for some time printed up high school football programs for the game, free in return for a two-page centerfold Chesterfield ad which also contained the game score card. Old Gold gave textbook covers with school names and logos on the front and an Old Gold ad on the back; they provided this service for 1,800 colleges and more than 8,000 of the nation's 25,000 high schools."    *Smokescreen*, p. 66

60. Featured in full-page Camel ads in the 1950's were Charlton Heston, Henry Fonda, Tyrone Power, Eva Gabor, and Alan Ladd.    British Medical Journal, July 13, 1996, p. 98

61. Lucille Ball and Desi Arnaz promoted Philip Morris cigarettes on TV in the 1950's, and both later died from tobacco induced disease.    *Smoking*, Ambrose video/HBO, 1988  
and *Dying for a Smoke*, Pyramid Video, 1993

62. The British Medical Journal in 1957 stopped carrying cigarette ads. [The Journal of the American Medical Association had discontinued cigarette ads in 1953 – editor]    *Faber Book of Smoking*, p. 90

63. "Viceroy... the thinking man's filter, and the smoking man's cigarette."     Steve McQueen in a 1960's TV ad

64. Jesse Owens promoted Chesterfields on TV ads in the 1960's.     Cancer Wars, PBS television, 1998

65. Charlton Heston was a Camel spokesman on TV ads in the 1960's. After cigarettes were responsible for the deaths of his father and sister, he appeared in the 1993 videotape *Dying for a Smoke* and condemned smoking.

66. In the 1960's, Arnold Palmer advertised L&M's, and Willie Mays proclaimed "Smoke Chesterfields" in Sports Illustrated.     JAMA, July 17, 1987, p. 314

67. "Steady increases in sales of cigarettes offer the classic example of what advertising can do . . . advertising pays off."     US Tobacco Journal, 1960, p. 4

68. The National Football League Player of the Year, Paul Hornung of the Green Bay Packers, was featured in a 1961 Marlboro ad with him smoking and the logo: "Why don't you settle back and have a full-flavored smoke? Marlboro--the filter cigarette with the unfiltered taste."     U.S. News and World Report, May 4, 1998, p. 30

69. Former Masters golf champion Dr. Cary Middlecoff, a dentist, appeared as the Viceroy spokesman in TV ads in the 1960's.     CBS Evening News, April 4, 1998

70. The CBS television network, selling itself to advertisers in 1962, once proudly proclaimed the television set as the "greatest cigarette vending machine ever devised."     Tobacco Control, Summer 1994, p. 130

71. A 1963 Lucky Strike slogan was: "Luckies separate the men from the boys, but not from the girls." A young man in one ad looked longingly at an accomplished, mature race car driver who was enjoying a cigarette while receiving a winning trophy, and being admired by an attractive woman. One critic called ads such as this attractive to teens "by means of allusions to athletic prowess, popularity, and sexual allure...it is basically a narcotic dream with an inexcusable dosage of dishonesty."     1994 Surgeon General report, p. 169

72. In 1963, R.J. Reynolds sponsored The Beverly Hillbillies, McHale's Navy, and 77 Sunset Strip, each with more than a third of children and teen viewers.     1994 Surgeon General report, p. 169

73. In 1963, the average American teenager saw 1,350 cigarette commercials on TV, and younger children, 845 cigarette commercials during the year.     1994 Surgeon General report, p. 169

74. "It seems safe to say that no advertiser, no agency man, and no media would want to continue advertising cigarettes if it were clear that they pose a serious and positive danger to the health of the ordinary smoker."     Advertising Age, 1964 (Tobacco Control, Summer 1964, p. 138)

75.     "In 1964, following the release of the first Surgeon General's report on smoking, the nation's largest tobacco companies created a much-publicized cigarette advertising code that would bar advertisements aimed at young people. The code was to be administered by a former Governor of New Jersey, Robert Meyner, who was empowered to fine violators up to $100,000.
    "No record exists of a fine being levied, and by the early 1970's, the position of the administrator was terminated, ending even the pretext of enforcement of the code.
    "However, the code does still exist, containing weak and vague provisions, useless except as a public relations tool for tobacco companies. Because the code contains no provision to measure its outcome or success, even though a number of studies correlate cigarette advertising with youth smoking, the cigarette companies can say they don't advertise to children because their code says they don't."
    Supporting FDA: Fact Sheet #6 (Advocacy Institute), August 2, 1995

76. Kent cigarettes sponsored the famous Ed Sullivan Show in 1965 marking the American television debut of the Beatles.     1994 Surgeon General report, p. 169

77. In the 1960's, tobacco ads were not allowed on TV programs whose audiences were 45% or more under age 21; however, R.J.Reynolds sponsored "The Beverly Hillbillies" despite the fact that two successive episodes had 50% and 45% of its audience under 21.                    Tobacco Control, Summer 1994, p. 139

78. In 1963, New York Giants football star Frank Gifford promoted Lucky Strikes as "the brand to start with."
                                                                                1994 Surgeon General report

79. In the 1960's, popular television shows such as the "Ben Casey, M.D." and "Dr. Kildare" medical dramas were brought into millions of homes each week via cigarette sponsorship, and health protection was a commonly implied theme.                                                        *Tobacco and the Clinician*, p. vi

80. In the 1960's and 1970's, Lorillard tried unsuccessfully to find a counterpart to Marlboro, a full-flavored smoke with a western motif. It marketed Maverick, Redford, Luke, and Zach, all of which failed.
                                                                                *They Satisfy*, p. 227

81. A huge Winston man on a downtown Chicago billboard blew a perfect smoke ring every 20 seconds for five years in the 1970's. There were similar giant "puffers" on cigarette billboards in Times Square, New York City
                                                                                *Nicotine*, p. 60

82. The 1971 federal law banning broadcast tobacco advertising also pre-empted states from regulating tobacco advertising for health-related reasons.     *Reducing the Health Consequences of Tobacco Use*, p. 512

83. The 1971 congressional ban on broadcast cigarette advertising "effectively froze out potential new competitors by denying them the broadcast platform and put an end to the devastating anti-smoking ads then being broadcast under the fairness doctrine."                          New Yorker, May 13, 1996, p. 43

84. Details of the Virginia Slims marketing story can be found in *Women and Smoking*, 2001 Surgeon General report, pp. 502-503

85. "Considering all I'd heard, I decided to either quit or smoke True. I smoke True."
                                                                1976 ad (New York Times, April 20, 1997, p. E3)

86. A 1984 Kool Jazz Festival advertising blitz in movie theaters throughout the U.S. backfired because of bad publicity when the Kool ads ran prior to screenings of Walt Disney's *Snow White and the Seven Dwarfs*.
                                                                                *The Cigarette Papers*, p. 363

# General

1. "Advertising does not increase smoking. It only encourages current smokers to switch brands... Cigarette advertising is designed to prompt smokers to switch brands. It does not cause smoking."
                The Tobacco Institute's Horace Korengay in testimony to Congress, August 1, 1986
                                        (*The Passionate Non Smoker's Bill of Rights*, p. 27)

2. Emerson Foote, former chairman of the board of the McCann Erickson advertising firm, commented on tobacco advertising. "Isn't the only purpose of tobacco advertising to urge existing smokers to change brands? This is the public position of the tobacco industry, but I don't think anyone really believes this...Creating a positive climate of social acceptability for smoking...is of greater importance. The implied message is if it is all right to advertise, the product can't be that bad."                    JAMA, April 24, 1981, p. 1667

3. "Does tobacco advertising increase consumption? In recent years, the cigarette industry has been artfully maintaining that cigarette advertising has nothing to do with total sales. Take my word for it, this is complete and utter nonsense. I am always amused by the suggestion that advertising, a function that has been shown to increase consumption of virtually every other product, somehow miraculously fails to work for tobacco products."                                        JAMA, April 24, 1981, p. 1668 (Emerson Foote)

4. Fewer than 10% of smokers change brands each year. The average smoker spends $880 per year for cigarette purchases, and many of the "switchers" change to another brand made by the same company, or to discount brands that reduce the company's profit margin.      American Review of Respiratory Disease 1990; 142:705

5. "The tobacco industry says its advertising is designed merely to persuade existing smokers to switch brands, not to encourage nonsmokers to start. If so, why not simply ban all tobacco advertising and promotion? Surely Congress would agree to do so if the industry asked it to. And look what would happen: brand switching would largely stop, leaving market shares essentially 'frozen'. And the $4 billion the industry currently spends on U.S. advertising would fall straight to the bottom line! Pure profit! You'd think the tobacco industry would be begging for this."                                    Time, October 12, 1996, p. 76 (Andrew Tobias)

6. "Advertising is an integral part of the corporate expansion of the tobacco industry. The industry claims that advertising is not designed to increase consumption but only to maintain market share, prevent brand switching or maintain brand loyalty, and promote low-tar and low-nicotine cigarettes. But this is clearly false, as fewer than 10% of smokers change brands in any one year, much brand switching is between brands of a single company, and nearly all 250 brands marketed in the U.S are made by only six companies. Thus, brand switching cannot explain the billions spent on advertising because, with 10% of 55 million U.S. smokers switching, that would mean an expenditure of about $345 per switcher in the U.S. alone. In Hong Kong, the launching of Virginia Slims for women at a time when only 1% of women under 40 smoked was clearly not designed to foster brand switching, but to create a market among women. Further evidence of the spuriousness of the industry's claim is the fact that, even in a country where a tobacco company holds a monopoly position, its advertising activity is intensive."      *Legislative Action to Combat the World Tobacco Epidemic*, p.24 (In 2000, the total advertising budget was $9.57 billion, and the number of U.S. smokers 46 million. If 10%, or 4.6 million, switched brands, this would mean an expenditure of $2,124 per switcher--editor.)

7. Smokers are extremely brand-loyal, with fewer than 10% switching brands annually. An estimated 9.5% of smokers switched cigarette brands and 7.6% switched companies each year. Most of those who did switch brands changed from a premium brand to a discount or generic brand. Over 50% of market losses were from smokers either quitting or dying.                          Tobacco Control, Winter 1997, pp. S31 and S38

8. If the only purpose of advertising were brand switching, which the industry claims, they would make much more money if they discontinued advertising. They spend far more on advertising than they make by acquiring new smokers from their competition.                          *Tobacco Use: An American Crisis*, p. 67

9. In an April 14, 1994 congressional hearing, Rep. Mike Synar (D-Okla) estimated that 5% of the nation's 50 million smokers switch brands each year. With a yearly advertising and promotion budget of $6 billion, this would amount to a tobacco company expenditure of $2400 for each "switcher".

10. The tobacco companies say that their advertising is not aimed at attracting new smokers, but only to get established smokers to switch to their brand. In 1984, Virginia Slims was introduced to Hong Kong, where only 1% of women smoked. It was clearly targeted at young women, with the usual images of beauty, slimness, and desirability, combined with clear messages of emancipation. But because so few women in Hong Kong smoked, the number who could brand switch was negligible, and the expensive advertising blitz seemed to be a clear attempt to create a new market. The same type of promotion aimed at women is seen in many developing countries, where currently only an average of 5% of women are smokers.      Thorax 1991; 46:153

11. In 1991, the tobacco industry spent $4.65 billion--more than $12.7 million a day, $8,847 a minute--on advertising and promoting cigarette consumption, and over $100 million promoting smokeless tobacco products. These expenditures were almost four times the amount ($1.22 billion) invested in 1980.
*Growing Up Tobacco Free*, p. 107

12. $5.3 billion was spent in the U.S. on advertising and promotion in 1992. This was an increase of $582 million, or 12.5%, from the $4.65 billion spent in 1991. This amounts to $21 for every man, woman, and child in the U.S., or $115 per smoker. It is $14.33 million per day, or $9,951 per minute.
Tobacco Control, Fall 1994, p. 288

13. For advertising and promotional expenses, the tobacco companies spent: $80 million in 1954; $250 million in 1968; $491 million in 1975; $1.58 billion in 1981; $3.99 billion in 1990; $5.3 billion in 1992, and $6.035 billion in 1993. These tax deductible expenditures have increased at more than triple the rate of inflation. The tobacco industry domestic advertising and promotion budget dropped to $4.83 billion in 1994.

   *San Francisco Examiner, April 20, 1997, p. A5*

14. The U.S. tobacco industry spends about $2 billion each year for the raw material, tobacco, used in its product, much less than its expense for advertising and promotion.

15. Tobacco company specialty item advertising expenses increased by 84% from 1991 to 1992, from $185 million to $340 million. Specialty item advertising is the practice of branding items such as T-shirts, caps, sporting goods, lighters, and calendars with a brand's logo, and then giving them away or selling them to consumers.

   *Tobacco Control, Fall 1994, p. 288*

16. The National Cancer Institute spent $47 million in 1991 to develop and disseminate effective smoking intervention technologies. The same year, the major cigarette manufacturers spent $4.6 billion ($4600 million) in an effort to convince people that smoking is necessary for social acceptance, that it makes one attractive to the opposite sex, and that it enhances self-image. For every $1 that the NCI spends on research to combat smoking, the tobacco industry spends $98 to promote the addiction. *Strategies to Control Tobacco Use, p. v*

17. The billions of dollars in advertising by tobacco companies has both promoted tobacco use and effectively censored information on the adverse health consequences of tobacco use in most print media. Tobacco companies have withheld advertising from magazines and newspapers that contained information on the negative health effects of smoking.

   NEJM 1985; 312:384

18. Former Playmate of the Year and actress model Anna Nicole Smith was featured in a full page ad in the October 1992 issue of Esquire. She posed seductively in a tight dress half unzipped in front, and prominently displayed a cigarette in her right hand. The ad was not for cigarettes or dresses; it was for Guess Jeans.

19. A million of the 3 million billboards in the U.S. advertise tobacco and alcohol products. The tobacco industry is the number one spender for outdoor advertising. The intensity of cigarette billboard advertising is 2.6 times greater in black than in white neighborhoods in Columbia, S.C. and 3.8 times greater in Baltimore. Billboard ads expose children repeatedly to pro-tobacco messages and give the erroneous impression that smoking is pervasive and normative. (Billboard tobacco ads were banned in April 1999 – editor)

   *Growing Up Tobacco Free, p. 112*

20. In one 19-block stretch of a poor black area in Philadelphia, there were 73 billboards counted, all but seven of which advertised tobacco or alcohol. *American Medical News, November 15, 1993, p. 18*

21. "...pervasive tobacco promotion has two major effects. It creates the perception that more people smoke than actually do, and it provides a conduit between actual self-image and ideal self-image--in other words, smoking is made to look cool." 1994 Surgeon General report, p. iii

22. The tobacco industry's voluntary cigarette advertising code reads: "Cigarette advertising shall not show any smoker participating in, or obviously just having participated in, a physical activity requiring stamina or athletic conditioning beyond that of normal recreation." The code also specifies that firms agree not to use models under 25 and not to associate smoking with health, sophistication, or celebrities and athletes.

   American Medical News, August 15, 1992

23. "Cigarette advertising shall not suggest that smoking is essential to social prominence, distinction, success, or sexual attraction." Item No. 3 of the tobacco industry's principles covering cigarette advertising and sampling.

   *Reducing the Health Consequences of Tobacco, p. 511*

24. David Goerlitz, a model who became known as the "Winston Man", reported during a photo session that he was surprised when he found out that none of the R.J.Reynolds executives attending were smokers. "Are you kidding?" one of the executives said. "We reserve that right for the poor, the young, the black, and the stupid."

After Goerlitz quit smoking himself, he apologized to a group of school children for pushing what he called "the deadliest drug of all". He said, "The image that I projected is nothing but a bunch of lies made up by executives and the tobacco industry."                New York Times, November 28, 1993 (Bob Herbert column)

25. David Goerlitz for six years was the Winston Man, a model in newspaper and magazine ads. At the time, he smoked 3 packs a day and was paid $75,000 a year. When he gave up smoking, he also gave up the modeling job.                                                                                                              *The Last Puff*, p. 69

26. Five out of the first six cowboys hired as the "Marlboro Man" have died of lung cancer, emphysema, or heart disease.                                                                           International Journal of Health Sciences 1986; 16:280

27. Wayne McLaren, a former "Marlboro Man", died in 1992 of lung cancer at age 51. Philip Morris denied that he was ever employed by them.                                                                        Associated Press, August 1992

28. On October 12, 1995, David McLean, the longtime Marlboro Man in TV commercials, died of lung cancer.
                                                                                                          Newsweek, October 30, 1995, p. 74

29. One of the more outrageous advertising gimmicks comes from Newport cigarettes (manufactured by Lorillard): their "Alive with Pleasure" theme. This is clearly an effort to undermine the Surgeon General's warning on each pack. Truth in advertising should require those ads to read not "Alive with Pleasure," but "Dying in Agony."                                                                                            Quote from C. Everett Koop, M.D.

30. "With all the desperation it once used to deny the casual links between cigarettes and cancer, the tobacco industry is now denying the links between advertising and smoking."        Editorial, The Lancet, November 1991

31. More than 4 million people sent in cigarette pack coupons for "Marlboro Adventure Team" gear. In a similar hugely successful ad campaign, Camel's Cash Catalog contains "the smoothest stuff Camel Cash (coupons) can buy", and the Virginia Slims catalogue has the image "the fashion collection with a streetwise attitude."
                                                                                            Washington Post magazine, February 20, 1994, p. 11

32. "Last year smokers were able to exchange empty packs for racy Marlboro Adventure Team gear. This spring there's a new promotion: the mail-order Marlboro Country Store, offering cowboy boots, belt buckles, and denim jackets stenciled with logos to turn millions of Americans into walking billboards."
                                                                                                          Newsweek, March 21, 1994, p. 52

33. A "Camel Cash" promotion allows smokers to mail in coupons for a wide variety of merchandise. Likewise, "Marlboro Adventure Team" catalogs have generated 2.2 million orders for 6.5 million "Adventure Gear" items. As an example, coupons from 360 packs, or about $900 worth of Marlboros, is redeemable for a two-person kayak. 9.35 million Americans are participating in this Marlboro promotion.
                                                                                                    San Francisco Chronicle, August 17, 1993

34. The "Winston Weekends" catalog promotion offers a leather jacket in exchange for 980 Winston pack seals, which would require smoking 19,600 cigarettes. At a price of $2.50 a pack, this would be a $2,450 jacket.
                                                                                                        Tobacco Free Youth Reporter, Summer 1993

35. An issue of People magazine in March 1993 had an offer of a free black leather jacket in exchange for 350 coupons from Virginia Slims cigarette packs.

36. Brown and Williamson is test marketing a new hip cartoon mascot, Willy the Penguin, for their flagship Kool brand. Willy has Hulk Hogan biceps, a Vanilla Ice hairdo, Spike Lee high top sneakers, and a Bart Simpson attitude. From a Brown and Williamson executive: "We hope the spokes-symbol will strengthen the appeal of this brand for young smokers." Critics complain that this is a blatant appeal to children and teenagers, and an attempt to ride the coattails of RJR's Joe Camel.                                                    Tobacco Control 1992; 1:133

37. The Time-Warner magazine conglomerate, which includes Time, Life, People, Money, and Sports Illustrated, collects yearly revenues of $100 million from tobacco companies, accounting for 25% of its total ad revenues.

Washington Post, April 21, 1991, p. B7

38. The "top three" magazines for tobacco ad revenue in 1991 were Sports Illustrated ($25 million), TV Guide ($24 million), and People ($22 million). Tobacco companies spent $290 million for magazine ads in 1991, down from $373 million in 1981.

Canadian Medical Association Journal, April 1993, p. 1189

39. A "billboard bandit" has defaced 45 tobacco billboards in the San Diego area, including the huge stadium Marlboro billboard during a San Diego Padres game. In 1985, 22 of the 24 major league baseball teams had either a Marlboro or Winston logo on their scoreboards.

*Minorities and Cancer*, p. 157

40. "Through sponsorship of sporting and cultural events--ranging from soccer teams to symphony orchestras, from automobile races to traveling art exhibits--the industry attempts to create an aura of legitimacy and wholesomeness: they're gaining innocence by association." The public is encouraged to believe that there is still some question as to whether cigarettes cause illness.

Journal of Health Politics, Policy and Law, Fall 1986, p. 369

41. RJR Nabisco is the leading sponsor of automobile and motorcycle racing in the United States, including the Camel Motorcross. Philip Morris has the Marlboro Grand Prix. Motor racing ranks as the second largest spectator sport in the United States behind football.

NEJM, April 7, 1994, p. 976

42. The publicity for a racing car bearing a tobacco logo, which has the pole position at the Indianapolis 500, is worth about $3 million.

*Nicotine Addiction*, p. 266

43. International Grand Prix motor racing events are "unregulated orgies of tobacco advertising. For hundreds of millions of racing fans, particularly young men, the opposition of tobacco advertising with these thrilling icons of power, excitement, speed, glamour, and success makes an unequivocal statement: cigarette smoking is all these things too."

Tobacco Control 1993; 2:159

44. Tobacco advertising is banned on television; however, during a 1991 telecast of the Marlboro Grand Prix car racing event, Marlboro was mentioned or seen a total of 5,933 times, and appeared on screen for 49% of the 90 minute telecast.

NEJM, March 28, 1991, p. 913

45. Tobacco companies spend an estimated $250 million each year on sponsorship of stock car racing and other motor sports.

New York Times, August 29, 1996, p. B6

46. In 1996, R.J. Reynolds paid more than $70 million in prize money to stock car drivers. There are 33 Winston Cup races each year, all televised and each attended by more than 100,000 spectators, making the Winston Cup the most popular sports series in the country.

Contra Costa (CA) Times, July 27, 1997, pp. B1 and B8

47. In a "monster truck" rally in 1990, one of the drivers chose to decorate her truck with no-smoking symbols. But because the event was sponsored by a tobacco company, she was prevented from driving her decorated truck.

*Strategies to Control Tobacco Use*, p. 273

48. "The sponsorship of major sporting events by cigarette companies provides further publicity and legitimacy to their products and allows the industry to reach large numbers of children."

Committee on Substance Abuse, American Academy of Pediatrics, May 1994, p. 867

49. In a letter to the editor of the New York Times, Billie Jean King defended Philip Morris' sponsorship of the Virginia Slims tennis tournament and called PM executives "enlightened people who understand and acknowledge the possible hazards of smoking."

*Tobacco Industry Strategies and Tactics*, p. 37

50. Magazines with the highest percentage of cigarette advertising revenue are the least likely to publish articles on the dangers of smoking.

Washington Post magazine, February 20, 1994, p. 24

51. The more a magazine relies on tobacco companies for advertising revenue, the less likely it is to publish articles on the dangers of smoking. This is particularly true for women's magazines.

San Francisco Chronicle, December 4, 1992, p. D6

52. Playboy has both the largest number of cigarette ads per issue and the lowest median audience age of any "adult" magazine.

1994 Surgeon General report, p. 182

53. A survey of six large-circulation women's magazines that regularly report on women's health issues found that, from 1983 to 1987, not one of them published a full-length feature, column, review, or editorial on any aspect of tobacco addiction. During the same five-year period, lung cancer surpassed breast cancer as the number one cancer killer of women. Not one of these magazines (five of which carried tobacco advertising) mentioned it. The survey found 34 articles on breast cancer, but none on lung cancer.

University of California Wellness Letter, December 1990

54. Magazine coverage of tobacco and health issues tends to be inversely proportional to the advertising revenue that they receive from tobacco companies, and cigarette advertising in magazines is associated with diminished coverage of the hazards of smoking. Women's magazines that did not carry cigarette ads were 2.3 times more likely to cover the risks of smoking than were women's magazines that did accept cigarette ads.

NEJM, January 30, 1992, p.305 and *Reducing the Health Consequences of Smoking*, p. 509

55. "Health professionals have charged that magazines that depend on revenues from cigarette advertising are less likely to publish articles on the dangers of smoking for fear of offending cigarette manufacturers. The probability of publishing an article on the risks of smoking in a given year was 11.9 percent for magazines that did not carry cigarette advertisements, as compared with 8.3 percent for those that did publish such advertisements. For women's magazines alone, the probabilities were 11.7 percent and 5.0 percent, respectively. This study provides strong statistical evidence that cigarette advertising in magazines is associated with diminished coverage of the hazards of smoking. This is particularly true for magazines directed to women." In summary, magazines that refused to carry cigarette ads were 40% more likely to discuss the dangers of cigarettes, and women's magazines that did not print cigarette ads were more than twice as likely to publish stories on smoking and health.

NEJM, January 30, 1992, p. 305 (Kenneth Warner)

56. In a 1989 survey, two-thirds of all magazines refused ads for smoking cessation clinics. This is presumably because they were afraid to offend their tobacco company sponsors.

World Smoking and Health, Spring 1990, p. 5

57. RJR/Nabisco in 1988 canceled an $80 million annual contract with Saatchi and Saatchi for advertising food products, after that agency prepared advertisements touting the no-smoking policy of another client, Northwest Airlines.

*Passionate Nonsmoker's Bill of Rights*, p. 28

58. There are numerous items for sale with Marlboro brand names, including a Marlboro first aid kit. Philip Morris donates Marlboro Handicap Parking placards to shopping mall storeowners.    JAMA, March 17, 1993, p. 1354

59. Philip Morris spent $2,210,000,000 in 1990 on advertising in the U.S., more than the budgets of the World Health Organization and UNICEF combined. All of this was tax deductible as a business expense.

NEJM, April 7, 1994, p. 976

60. In 1993, Philip Morris spent nearly $8.8 billion on advertising and promotion for its tobacco, food, and beer products around the world, including over $2 billion in the U.S.    INFACT Newsletter, April 1994

61. 82% of ads in taxicabs and bus shelters in New York are for cigarettes. A federal appeals court has ruled that New York cannot enact a city law requiring at least one anti-smoking message for every four tobacco ads. The appeals court said that the local law was pre-empted by the 1965 federal law, the Cigarette Labeling and Advertising Act.    New York Times, August 27, 1994, p. A10

62. Nick Price, the world's number one ranked golfer at the time, played at a tournament in South Africa in 1994 wearing a shirt and carrying a golf bag both bearing the Camel cigarette logo. His endorsement fee was not

disclosed. Golf magazine, February 1995, p. 36

63. Philip Morris has begun a cigarette ad campaign in Genre, a fashion magazine for gay men. Lesbians and gays in San Francisco smoke at a rate that is 61% higher than adults in the city as a whole.
Advocacy Institute, October 8, 1992

64. A billboard between two gay bars in San Francisco showed only a denim-clad male crotch with a carton of Marlboros posed at a suggestive angle. Tobacco Control, Spring 1994, p. 67

65. An ad for Montclair cigarettes may be directed toward gay men. The ad has been described as follows: "...a mug shot of what looked to many like an aging, effeminate homosexual--Captain's cap on head, pinky ring (no marriage ring), dapper ascot--shrieking in pleasure over his cigarettes." Detroit News, July 7, 1992

66. Bert Neuborne, former legal director of the American Civil Liberties Union, represented the Tobacco Institute in a congressional hearing on a proposed advertising ban. Philip Morris gave $500,000 to the ACLU between 1987 and 1992. *Tobacco Industry Strategies*, p. 33 and 36

67. Brown and Williamson was assessed a $95,000 civil penalty by the state of Minnesota for running a cigarette giveaway promotion. State law prohibits free distribution of tobacco products.
Tobacco Free Youth Reporter, Summer 1994, p. 6

68. Discounts on turkeys, milk, and soft drinks have been used as promotions for Marlboro and other Philip Morris brands. Tobacco Control, Spring 1994, p. 72

69. The Marlboro cowboy has been the most successful advertising campaign in the history of commerce.
Good Morning America (ABC), January 18, 1995

70. Philip Morris sponsored a Russian art exhibit at the Metropolitan Museum in New York as well as the Bolshoi Ballet in Honolulu. Journal of National Cancer Institute Monographs No. 12, 1992, p. 32

71. "The values that are promoted in tobacco advertising are clear. They are images and symbols of success, elegance, power, sexual conquest, the macho role, and an enhanced ability to be sociable, self-assured, confident, daring, adventurous, and mature. The cruel irony, of course, is that the people who are all of those things do not smoke cigarettes. You declare your own inadequacy by smoking, and the tobacco companies laugh all the way to the bank." Journal of the National Medical Association, November 1989, p. 1120

72. In the U.K., Marlboro promotes the Midnite Lights Disco Tour and sponsors the Marlboro Lights Disc Jockey of the Year. Philip Morris has sponsored televised rock concerts in Budapest, Hungary, where young women in Marlboro suits gave out free Marlboro samples, while those who attended the concert and smoked the samples received a complimentary pair of "designer Marlboro sunglasses."
UICC Tobacco Control Fact Sheet 1, International Union Against Cancer, 1996

73. After winning the Salem Open, Australian tennis player Pat Cash remarked, "I'd like to thank the sponsors, even though I think it's a disgrace to smoke cigarettes." Los Angeles Times, December 18, 1997

74. In 1992, about half of adolescent smokers and a quarter of nonsmokers owned at least one tobacco promotional item such as clothing and hats, an estimated 7.4 million adolescents in all.
Tobacco Control, Autumn 1995, p. 210

75. Cigarette advertisers pulled ads from Newsweek in 1983 after the magazine ran an article entitled "The Uncivil War on Smoking." Joel Dunnington, M.D.

76. The tobacco industry saturates the annual Sports Illustrated swimsuit issue--guaranteed to be scrutinized by millions of adolescent males--with cigarette ads, many linking sexual success with smoking.
Tobacco Free Youth Reporter, Fall 1995

77. A tobacco industry document subpoenaed by the FTC recommends:

"Thus, an attempt to reach young smokers, starters, should be based, among others, on the following major parameters: present the cigarette as one of the few initiations into the adult world; present the cigarette as part of the illicit pleasure category of products and activities; in your ads, create a situation taken from the day-to-day life of the young smoker, but in an elegant manner have this situation touch on the basic symbols of the growing-up, maturity process; to the best of your ability (considering some legal constraints), relate the cigarette to 'pot', wine, beer, sex, etc.; don't communicate health or health-related points."

Examination of current cigarette advertisements shows that these recommendations apply to almost all tobacco advertisements. Cigarette smoking is presented as a way for children to exert independence from their parents and be grown-up. The tobacco industry's protestations that it doesn't want kids to smoke because smoking is an adult "custom" is an extension of this advertising theme.

*Tobacco Biology and Politics*, Stanton Glantz, p. 37

78. Joe Camel, his face fashioned after a set of male genitals. "Before the birth of Joe Camel in 1988, an estimated 3% of teenage smokers and 4% of adult smokers picked Camel cigarettes as their brand of choice. Five years later, the percentage of adult smokers favoring Camels remained the same, but among smokers age 12 to 18, Camel's market share had more than tripled to 13%." The Oregonian, August 23, 1995, p. A21

79. Marlboro ad spending increased by 27% from 1993 to 1994 and another 40% in 1995 from 1994 levels.

USA Today, November 10, 1995, p. 28

80. "Now there are 'microcigs', custom-blended smokes that, these days, are the coolest thing since the Marlboro Man." Gunsmoke's rugged Western blend appeals to smokers in the heartland, and American Spirit "sells to (believe it or not) health-conscious smokers who like their smokes 'all natural', even though they contain more tar and nicotine than Marlboros." Newsweek, November 13, 1995, p. 60

81. The tobacco industry was one of the biggest outdoor advertisers before billboards were prohibited in 1999. In 1989, of the approximately three million billboards in the U.S., thirty percent advertised tobacco and alcohol products. Inner city neighborhoods, in particular, are plastered with tobacco billboards portraying beautiful young smokers engaged in glamorous activities and lifestyles. Studies reveal that the intensity of cigarette billboard advertising in some states is two to three times greater in African-American neighborhoods than in white neighborhoods. These billboards expose children over and over again to pro tobacco messages, giving young people the impression that smoking is the social norm in this country.

*No Sale: Youth, Tobacco and Responsible Retailing*, Working Group of State Attorneys General, 1995, p. 7

82. Tobacco advertising in 1996 accounted for about $180 million in billboard ad revenue, or 10% of the national total. Associated Press, April 24, 1997

83. The billboard industry's own marketing material proclaims: "Outdoor (billboard) advertising is right up there. Day and night, lurking, waiting for another ambush." Of the 3 million billboards in the country, 30% carried ads for tobacco and alcohol products before the 1999 tobacco billboard ad ban.

Journal of Pediatrics, April 1997, p. 519

84. A study by the Centers for Disease Control shows that the three most heavily advertised cigarette brands -- the ones represented by Joe Camel, the Marlboro Man, and young Newport couples -- have captured eighty-six percent of the illegal teen market. These same brands, however, account for only thirty-five percent of overall tobacco sales, having far less appeal in the adult market.

Mortality and Morbidity Weekly Report, August 19, 1994

85. Over 100 countries in 1995 had restrictions or bans on tobacco advertising.

British Medical Journal, July 13, 1996, p. 98

86. Rolling Stone and other magazines in 1996 had a two-page Joe Camel pop-up ad offering a $25 discount for Ticketmaster tickets in exchange for Camel Cash certificates. Wall Street Journal, April 16, 1996, p. B1

87. The following is from an article "How Cigarette Makers Target Viet Community" in the San Francisco Chronicle, October 14, 1996, p. A25:

    A number of Vietnamese magazines in California have printed the glossy, full-page ads for the "555" cigarette brand. It is manufactured by the British American Tobacco Co. (BAT) and affiliated with Brown and Williamson...

    Marketing practices by 555 in the Vietnamese and Chinese communities are despicable. The company's print ads and promotional items appear in Vietnamese and Chinese. But the U.S. Surgeon General's warnings on smoking are printed in English...

    Articles sponsored by 555 promoting tobacco events are printed in the Vietnamese press. Events such as a "5.5 ounces of gold" sweepstakes and "celebrate 555 day on May 5th" parties at Vietnamese nightclubs can hardly be considered newsworthy. They flaunt the tobacco industry's arrogance when their propaganda states: "Events 555 sponsors in the Vietnamese community demonstrates its commitment to advancing the welfare of the Vietnamese community."

    The Vietnamese Lunar New Year TET Festival Organizing Committee in Northern California adopted a new policy this year banning all tobacco promotions and advertising. The tobacco industry, unhappy with the decision, apparently threatened legal action. During the festival, they put on a giant advertising blitz.

88. Philip Morris will flood stores with millions of copies of a new CD series in pop, country, and rhythm and blues music showcasing undiscovered women artists. The series will be called "Virginia Slims Women Thing Music," and the CD's will not be for sale, but will come free with the purchase of a special package of two packs of Virginia Slims.                                    Wall Street Journal, January 15, 1997, p. B1

89. In a 1995 survey in Boston, 40.4% of all taxicabs carried cigarette ads, with over half of these being for Marlboro.                                    Tobacco Control, Summer 1997, p. 128

90. USA Today awarded tobacco ads the best and worst honors for 1997. One of the best was the California Department of Health Services anti-smoking ad with Debbie Austin, who lost her larynx to cancer, speaking and smoking through a tracheostomy, or hole in her neck. An award for one of the worst ads went to a Camel Lights new campaign featuring a vamp with faint images of a Camel silhouetted in the background.
                                    USA Today, December 15, 1997, p. B3

91. In Europe, Philip Morris and other cigarette companies buy advertising space on the nozzles of gas pumps; an estimated two million people see a nozzle ad each day.                                    Tobacco Control, Winter 1997, p. 359

92. In the Whitbread yacht race, three of the nine boats, Merit Cup, Silkcut, and Swedish Match are sponsored by tobacco companies.                                    Australian Council on Smoking and Health Newsletter, December 1997

93. "The inter-relationship of tobacco advertising and tobacco consumption was examined in thirty-three countries. Overall, the study found that the greater a government's degree of control over tobacco promotion, the greater the annual average fall in tobacco consumption and in the rate of decrease of smoking among young people. In total ban countries compared with the group of countries without controls, tobacco consumption fell more rapidly, and this effect could not be explained away by tobacco price or income per capita trends. The elimination of tobacco advertising, other factors being equal, more likely than not causes tobacco consumption to decrease."                                    *Health or tobacco. An End to Tobacco Advertising and Promotion*, Toxic Substances Board, Wellington, New Zealand, May 1989, pp. xxiii-xxv

94. In 1998, 17 of the 21 largest circulation women's magazines carried tobacco advertising
                                    Journal of the National Cancer Institute, September 2, 1998, p. 1257

95. The first issue of Tina Brown's new magazine "Talk" had two pages of ads for Marlboro and one for Capri.
                                    Globalink, August 9, 1999

96. The New York Times in May 1999 joined more than a dozen other American newspapers in banning cigarette ads from its pages. Other papers include the Seattle Times, Los Angeles Times, the Christian Science Monitor, and the Boston Globe.                                    New York Times, April 28, 1999, p. C2

97. Under the national tobacco settlement, all billboards were free of tobacco ads after April 1999. The tobacco industry had been the third largest user of billboards and accounted for $200 million, or 9% of the billboard business.                                                                          USA Today, December 28, 1998, p. A1

98. "Is Philip Morris serious about protecting kids from its own products? Then prove it. Get rid of the Marlboro Man – for good."
Ad from the Campaign for Tobacco-Free Kids running in the New York Times on January 26, 1999

99. "If Philip Morris really didn't want kids to smoke... it would dump the Marlboro man."
New York Times editorial, January 26, 1999, p. A27

100. Tobacco industry incentives to retail stores far exceed those paid by other industries. These include payments for prime shelf space and in-store displays. An average retail store participating in a retailer incentive program received $3157 each year from all products, of which $2462 (78%) came from tobacco companies. In 1996, 47% of the industry's $5.1 billion total advertising budget, or $2.4 billion, went to retailer incentive programs.
American Journal of Public Health, October 1999, p. 1564

101. An ad for Naples, Italy, and Alitalia Airlines in the November 2001 issue of National Geographic Traveler features a model on a motorcycle prominently displaying a cigarette.

102. Charlie Sheen has advertised Philip Morris' Parliament cigarettes in Japan, and Antonio Banderas has done the same in Argentina. Leonardo DiCaprio and Kate Winslet both smoked in *Titanic*, "...equating cigarettes with romance and rebellion for 75 million ticket buyers in the U.S. and tens of millions more overseas."
Ad for Smokefree Movies, New York Times, June 18, 2001, p. A23

103. "Every Marlboro ad needs to be judged on the following criteria: Story value, authenticity, masculinity, while communicating those enduring core values of freedom, limitless opportunities, self-sufficiency, mastery of destiny and harmony with nature."
Philip Morris (from 2001 publication "How do you sell Death" from Campaign for Tobacco-Free Kids)

104. Half of British smokers believe that since the government allows advertising, smoking can't be all that dangerous.                                                                                 Sir Richard Peto, New Scientist, August 30, 2001

105. In 1999, advertising expenditures were $8.24 billion, an increase of 22.3% from 1998. When the industry stopped outdoor billboard advertising in 1998 to comply with the Master Settlement Agreement, they increased spending the next year in newspapers by 73%, magazines by 34%, and direct mail by 64%.
JAMA, June 12, 2002, p. 2991

106. The six largest cigarette manufacturers spent $9.57 billion on advertising and promotion in 2000, a 16% increase from the $8.24 billion spent in 1999. The largest category (41% of total industry spending) was for promotional allowances, which include payments to retailers for shelf space. Spending on retail "value-added," including promotions ("buy one, get one free") and items such as free hats or lighters, increased by 37.4% from $2.56 billion in 1999 to $3.52 billion in 2000.                  FTC Report summary released May 24, 2002

107. In the United States, annual marketing expenditures are over $200 per smoker, or 46 cents for every pack sold.
*The Tobacco Atlas*, p. 58

108. Magazine spending by the tobacco industry has dropped dramatically over the last 20 years. In 1981, tobacco companies were the biggest group placing ads in magazines in the U.S. – last year, that #1 ranking had fallen to #21. Magazine ad spending for 2001 was $237 million nationally.          2003 AMA Annual Tobacco Report

109. A comprehensive set of advertising bans leads to an average 6.3% reduction in smoking.
*The Tobacco Atlas*, p. 77

110. Billions of dollars were spent on the Marlboro Gear and Camel Cash promotional campaigns during the early 1990s.                                                                        CA-A Cancer Journal for Clinicians, March-April 2003, p. 114

111. Domestic cigarette companies spent $113.6 million on sponsoring sports and sporting events in 1999. Worldwide, auto racing relies on an estimated $350 million a year in tobacco sponsorship and advertising. The International Olympic Committee has had a smoking ban since 1988.

New York Times, November 23, 2001, p. A8

112. "Grand Prix motor racing is the most watched event after the Olympics and the Soccer Word Cup, with each race broadcast to a potential viewing audience of 350 million. Its major sponsors over the last 20 years have been tobacco companies."

Tobacco Control, September 2002

113. Philip Morris in its partnership with Ferrari spends about $23 million a year toward German Formula One racer Michael Schumacher's salary and another $65 million for Marlboro product placements on his and his teammates' cars, clothing, and helmets. The tobacco industry spends $250 million each year on Formula One racing.

Tobacco Control, June 2002, p. 146

114. Michael Schumacher, world champion of Formula One auto racing, is the world's highest paid athlete, earning $59 million a year, ahead of other elite sports figures such as Tiger Woods and Michael Jordan. Formula One racing, which is viewed on TV by 350 million people in 150 countries, relies heavily on tobacco money. Schumacher's car is a rolling billboard for Marlboro, which uses racing to sidestep Europe's strict laws against cigarette ads. In the United States, tobacco companies have used racing as a prime means of subverting the longstanding ban on televised cigarette advertising.

2002 AMA Annual Tobacco Report

115. A study published in the New England Journal of Medicine concludes that tobacco companies have broken a promise, made in their 1998 settlement with state governments, to cut back on advertising aimed at minors. Camel, Marlboro and Newport – brands favored by teens – have actually increased budgets for advertising in magazines like *People*, *Rolling Stone* and *Sports Illustrated* that have significant young audiences.

Quote from Time, August 27, 2001

116. A San Diego judge fined R.J.Reynolds Tobacco Co. $20 million for violating a 1998 agreement not to run tobacco ads in magazines intended to reach teenagers. RJR had heavy advertising for its Camel and Winston brands in magazines including *Rolling Stone*, *Sports Illustrated*, *Vibe*, and *Spin* with large under-18 readerships.

San Francisco Chronicle, June 7, 2002, p. A5

117. Following a June 2002 report from the Massachusetts Department of Health that found US Smokeless Tobacco to be targeting youth in its magazine ads, the company pulled its ads from *Sports Illustrated*, *Hot Rod*, and *Motor Trend* magazines. The company denied the charges, but said it would "be responsive to the concerns raised" and suspend the advertising in question.

2003 AMA Annual Tobacco Report

# Advertising and Children

1. "For all its pious rhetoric about being disinterested in the youth market, the tobacco industry must know the considerable effect that advertising has on children. Young people represent its commercial future. It has gone into paroxysms over proposals to have all cigarettes sold in plain, generic packs following research showing that children find such packs unappealing." British Medical Journal, October 8, 1994, p. 891 (Simon Chapman)

2. Former Surgeon General Jocelyn Elders has said that tobacco advertising aims to convince children "that they're slim, they're sexy, they're sociable, they're sophisticated, and they're successful. The teenager gets an image, and the tobacco companies get an addict." Associated Press, February 25, 1994

3. In the six years following the introduction of Virginia Slims in 1968, the number of teenage girls who smoke more than doubled, while smoking among adult women remained relatively constant.

*Strategies to Control Tobacco Use*, p. 233

4. Teenage smokers are much more likely than adults to pick the most-advertised brands. The three most advertised brands, the Marlboro Man, Joe Camel, and the Newport fun couples, had 35% of overall sales, but

86% of the teen market. Marlboro accounted for 60% of teen sales and Camel and Newport 13% each.
Associated Press, August 20, 1994 and British Medical Journal, September 10, 1994, p. 629

5.  Teenagers are three times as likely as adults to respond to cigarette advertisements, and 79% of teenage smokers prefer brands depicted by the Marlboro Man, Joe Camel, or the Newport fun couples. Whenever a brand increased its advertising budget by 10%, its share of the adult smoking market grew 3%, but its share of teenage smokers increased by 9%.                                                        Associated Press, April 3, 1996

6.  A 1998 study found that teenagers still choose to smoke the most advertised cigarette brands. 88% of 12th grade smokers, 86% of tenth grade smokers, and 82% of eighth grade smokers choose Marlboro, Newport, or Camel, the three most heavily advertised brands.                                      USA Today, April 14, 1999, p. A8

7.  Most people smoke only one to three cigarette brands in their lifetimes, making cigarettes the most "brand loyal" consumer product in the United States. Only about 18% of smokers begin to smoke at age 18 years and older, and only 5% begin at age 21 years and older.
Archives of Pediatric and Adolescent Medicine, September 1999, pp. 935-936

8.  When cigarette advertising intensity doubles, it has three times the impact on teens' choices as on those of adults, an April 1996 report in the Journal of Marketing concludes. According to the author, "If I am a cigarette manufacturer, it means that if I double my advertising, adolescents will flock to me three times faster than adults; adults are brand loyal."                                          JAMA, April 24, 1996, p. 1223

9.  Recent research not only confirms that advertising affects smoking rates, but in addition indicates that this effect is three times greater for teenagers than adults.                  JAMA, February 19, 1997, p. 532

10. Half of all adolescent smokers and a quarter of adolescent non-smokers own at least one promotional item from a tobacco company (examples are T-shirts, caps, calendars, and sporting goods).
*Growing Up Tobacco Free*, p. 110

11. After a study in the Journal of the American Medical Association showing that Joe Camel promotes smoking by children, R.J. Reynolds hired consultants to try to discredit the research, and went to court to try to force the authors to turn over their research documents.
American Medical News, July 27, 1992 and DOC News and Views, Spring 1992

12. R.J. Reynolds increased its ad spending on Joe Camel by 75% in 1993 and added female Camels in its cartoons. "I'll be damned if I'll pull the ads," R.J. Reynolds' CEO told Business Week.
9th World Conference on Tobacco or Health, Paris, 1994 (INFACT Newsletter, Summer 1994)

13. The magazine Advertising Age, which is committed to advertising and to first amendment free speech rights, has nonetheless editorialized that Joe Camel encourages children to smoke, and recommended that R.J. Reynolds drop the ad campaign.                                                        Advertising Age, January 1992

14. Comments on Camel Joe and his proboscis. "The abiding mystery is how that rude cartoon character with the testicular chin could sell...It's unclear why RJR would want to promote a scrotum." (Marketing Week, 1991) "Grossed out," the worst ad of 1990 (Forbes magazine).

15. A controversial four-page Camel ad featured a sexy blonde and Old Joe's tips on how to impress someone at the beach. "Run into the water...and drag her back to shore as if you've saved her from drowning. The more she kicks and screams, the better." The ad included a coupon for a free pack of cigarettes, and urged readers to "ask a kind-looking stranger to redeem it."                  Washington Post magazine, February 2, 1994, p. 24

16. The "Old Joe" Camel campaign's appeal to youth is so blatant that Advertising Age has editorialized that it "crossed the divide between a company's legal right to advertise and its unique social responsibility to the general public."                                                            *Tobacco Use: An American Crisis*, p. 65

17. A prominent advertising executive, Emerson Foote, ridiculed industry claims that its advertising is only for brand switching and has no effect whatsoever on recruitment: "Creating a positive climate of social acceptability for smoking, which encourages new smokers to join the market, is of greater importance to the industry...In recent years, the cigarette industry has been artfully maintaining that cigarette advertising has nothing to do with total sales. Take my word for it, this is complete and utter nonsense."

*1994 Surgeon General report, p. 173*

18. "As an argument [that tobacco advertising is only aimed at brand-switching and not at attracting new consumers] it is so preposterous it is insulting...to claim cigarette advertising does not encourage smoking flies in the face of all advertising knowledge and experience."

An Australian advertising executive (*Legislative Action to Combat the World Tobacco Epidemic*, p. 25)

19. About two thirds of advertising executives feel that a goal of cigarette ads is to persuade teenagers to smoke, and the executives also support restricting tobacco ads. These findings contrast with the tobacco industry's long-held position that its ads are designed to get adult smokers to switch brands rather than to get people of any age to smoke.

*Associated Press, December 18, 1996*

20. In 1948, Liggett and Myers Tobacco Company provided high schools with free football programs; a scorecard at the center of the program was in effect a two-page advertisement for Chesterfield cigarettes.

*1994 Surgeon General report, p. 167*

21. In 1953, plastic-coated book covers featuring school logos on the front and cigarette ads on the back were being used to promote Old Gold cigarettes to students in most of the country's 1800 colleges and in more than a third of its 25,000 high schools.

*1994 Surgeon General report, p. 167*

22. In the 1950's, cigarette companies spent about $5 million per year on college promotions. Philip Morris paid 166 student "representatives" $50 a month to distribute free cigarettes, and cigarette ads accounted for about 40 percent of the advertising income of college newspapers.

*1994 Surgeon General report, p. 168*

23. R.J. Reynolds introduced the "Joe Camel" cartoon character to promote Camels in 1988. Three years later, Camel's share of the adult cigarette market was unchanged at 4%; however, Camel sales to children under age 18 increased from 0.5% to a 33% market share, and the $6 million in sales to children increased to $478 million in the same time period. One quarter of the Camel market in 1991 consisted of illegal sales to children.

*JAMA, December 11, 1991, p. 3149*

24. 30% of three year olds and more than 80% of six year olds in a 1991 survey were able to associate a picture of Joe Camel with a pack of cigarettes. Joe Camel was as recognizable as Mickey Mouse with six year olds.

*JAMA, December 11, 1991, p. 3149*

25. "R.J. Reynolds and its industry colleagues...want us to believe that their advertising campaigns don't appeal to children. Cigarette advertising is the moral equivalent of a national campaign to 'Drive Drunk--Just for the Fun of It'."

*JAMA, December 11, 1991, p. 3185 (Henry Waxman)*

26. In 1993, the AMA and Surgeon General sponsored a nationwide "Say No to Cancer Joe" contest aimed at increasing children's awareness of the risks of tobacco. 175,000 entries from children were received. "The tobacco industry is attempting to enslave a new generation of cancer and emphysema victims--children," said John Clowe, M.D., AMA president.

*American Medical News, June 21, 1993, p. 14*

27. The March 1996 issue of the teen magazine Rolling Stone had a cardboard Joe Camel holding concert tickets in his hand that popped out of the center of the magazine.

28. Since the Joe Camel advertising campaign began, the proportion of smoking teenagers who smoke Camels rose from 4% to 13%, while the proportion of adults who smoke Camels remained unchanged at 4%.

*Journal of National Cancer Institute, April 19, 1995, p. 565*

29. In Joe Camel's nine-year U.S. lifespan from 1988 to 1997, its share of the total market went from 4.4% to 4.6%; however, among underage smokers, the market share increased from less than 1% in 1986 to 13% in 1993. USA Today, July 15, 1997

30. The Federal Trade Commission reported that the Camel market share in children under 18 increased from less than 3% in 1988, when Joe Camel was introduced, to between 13% and 16% in 1993. "Arguing that the Joe Camel campaign illegally entices children and adolescents to smoke, the FTC last week charged R.J. Reynolds with violating federal fair trade practices and asked an administrative law judge to order the company to ban the cartoon icon from ads aimed at youngsters." San Francisco Chronicle, June 2, 1997, p. A16

31. After the 1968 introduction of Virginia Slims, smoking prevalence among underage adolescent females nearly doubled, from 8% in 1968 to 15% in 1974. 1994 Surgeon General report, p. 1974

32. 71% of white adolescents who smoke choose Marlboro, versus only 9% of blacks. 61% of black adolescent smokers choose Newport, versus only 6% of whites who prefer this menthol brand. Camels are more popular among adolescents in the western states than in other areas of the country. 1994 Surgeon General report, p. 71

33. Marlboro accounted for nearly 70% of the market among 12 to 17-year-olds in 1989 (compared with about 25% of the overall market). In California, Camel has 23% of the teen market compared with less than 5% of the overall market. "These remarkable patterns are a tribute to the power of the extensive and clever advertising campaigns for the Marlboro and Camel brands. To a large extent, the teenage smoking problem is not so much a 'cigarette' problem as it is a Marlboro and Camel problem."
Adolescent Medicine, June 1993, p. 309 (John Slade)

34. "Why haven't teen smoking rates fallen in parallel with adult smoking prevalence? Probably because during the 1980's, the amount of money spent by the tobacco industry to promote smoking more than tripled, and most of the new ads were designed to encourage teens to smoke." World Watch magazine, 1992

35. "In presenting attractive images of smokers, cigarette advertisements appear to stimulate some adolescents who have relatively low self images to adopt smoking as a way to improve their own self image."
1994 Surgeon General report, p. 8

36. A 1992 study reported that a Tobacco Institute campaign aimed at retail stores and called "It's the Law" did almost nothing to discourage stores from selling cigarettes to children. A second report came to the conclusion that another Tobacco Institute program called "Tobacco: Helping Youth Say No" is "clearly designed to encourage tobacco use" by making smoking appear to be for adults only and, therefore, a desirable "forbidden fruit." American Journal of Public Health, September 1992, p. 1271

37. R.J. Reynolds is sponsoring a "Support the Law" campaign about youth smoking, with Danny Glover as spokesman. Nowhere in the ads does RJR mention anything about the health hazards of smoking, and their "Kids Should Be Kids--Help Keep Them That Way" theme actually encourages youngsters to smoke so that they can be more like adults. Tobacco Free Youth Reporter, Spring 1993

38. A RJR booklet "How to Talk to Your Kids About Not Smoking Even if You Do" says: "A natural question your child may ask is, 'Why do you smoke?' If you smoke because you enjoy smoking--as most smokers do-- say so. Then tell them that there are a lot of things adults do that kids can't."
Washington Post magazine, February 20, 1994, p. 13

39. The 1991 Tobacco Institute pamphlet "Helping Youth Say No", presented as a "public service" says: "Young people are all aware of the alleged risks associated with smoking" with no mention of addiction or health problems.

40. "By portraying smoking as an adult custom, the tobacco industry can be said to have hit upon an ideal reverse psychology. The most effective way to get children to smoke is to say, 'You're too young to smoke'."
JAMA, February 28, 1986, p.1050 (Alan Blum)

41. Philip Morris has 26 million people on its mailing lists, including an estimated 1.6 million teenagers.
*Growing Up Tobacco Free*, p. 113

42. Cigarette advertising contributes to the perception that smoking is more prevalent, less hazardous, and more socially acceptable than it really is.                                    1994 Surgeon General Report

43. Cigarette ads predominate in youth oriented magazines. The less likely that a magazine will have teenage readers, the less likely it will have cigarette ads. Penthouse, Playboy, Rolling Stone, and Cosmopolitan average 14 pages of cigarette ads and 3 packs of free cigarettes that readers could obtain by mailing in coupons. By contrast, Forbes, Business Week, Fortune, and the New Republic had not a single tobacco ad, even though these magazines accept them. Penthouse derives 25% of its ad revenue from tobacco companies, and Playboy has a million dollars worth of tobacco ads in each issue.                                    Joel Dunnington, M.D.

44. "Cigarette advertisements attempt to allay anxieties about the hazards of smoking. Ads associate smoking with good health, athletic vigor, and social and professional success. The cigarette is portrayed as an integral part of youth, happiness, attractiveness, personal success, and an active, vigorous, strenuous lifestyle."
Committee on Adolescence, American Academy of Pediatrics (Pediatrics, March 1987, p. 480)

45. Sports Illustrated, one of the magazines most heavily inundated with tobacco advertisements, has a readership one-third of which is boys under age 18.                                    NEJM, March 19, 1987, p. 730

46. The 1996 and 1998 Sports Illustrated swimsuit issues each had eight full page tobacco ads.

47. The 1997 swimsuit issue had nine pages of cigarette ads (for Marlboro, Camel, and Newport, the most popular teen brands), plus another page of cigar ads. It also had an ad for Nicoderm, a brand of nicotine patch.

48. In a study of adolescent viewing of tobacco advertisements, only 8% of the viewing time was looking at the Surgeon General's health warning, and in 44% of cases, the warning was not viewed at all. The study concluded that the federally mandated warning was completely ineffective.      JAMA, January 6, 1989, p. 84

49. The University of Vermont spent $2 million on a four-year TV and radio ad campaign with children in commercials saying that smoking is not cool. Children exposed were 35% less likely to smoke than those in areas where the campaign did not air.                                    American Medical News, August 15, 1994, p. 18

50. As an advertising columnist said, advertising is not a rifle; it is a shotgun, and children can't help but get caught in its spray. The burden of proof needs to shift: tobacco marketers need to prove that their advertising will NOT affect children.          Supporting FDA: Fact Sheet #10, August 18, 1995 (Advocacy Institute)

51. "The ad message...was always the same: smoking makes you beautiful, adventurous, and sexy, provides pleasure without penalty or pain, and turns kids into grown-ups."                                    *Ashes to Ashes*, p. 701

52. "A significant portion of tobacco marketing resources are directed at venues with widespread youth appeal such as coupons and specialty-item distribution, value-added offers, free sampling, and sponsorship of sports and music events. One study reported that 30% of teen-aged smokers had purchased a particular brand of cigarettes to obtain a free promotional item such as a T-shirt or a lighter. Another study of ninth graders found that 65% of regular smokers, 48% of occasional smokers, and 28% of nonsmokers reported they owned clothing with a cigarette brand logo. One recent national telephone survey study found that 35% of minors had actively participated in a tobacco brand promotion, leading the authors to estimate that nationwide, 7.4 million minors participated in such campaigns."                                    JAMA, February 5, 1997, p. 416

53. "More than $84 million was spent on sponsorship of sporting, musical, and other public entertainment events in 1993 in which the name of the company or brand of cigarettes is displayed. A number of studies have found that youths associate sporting events with tobacco brands. One study found that tobacco-sponsored auto races broadcast on network television in 1993 included as viewers 2.6 million children and 2.2 million teenagers."
JAMA, February 5, 1997, p. 416

54. Advertising expenditures for promotional items appealing to teens (caps, T-shirts, key chains) increased from $5.6 million in 1970 to $756 million in 1993.                    Washington Post, May 11, 1997, p. C2

55. A third of students in grades 6 through 12 in rural Vermont and New Hampshire own cigarette promotional items. The students who own these items were four times more likely to be smokers; 58% of high school seniors who owned a promotional item smoked. T-shirts and hats were the most common items, and Camel and Marlboro the most popular brands.                    New York Times, December 15, 1997, p. A18
(from December 1997 Archives of Pediatrics and Adolescent Medicine)

56. A 1973 RJR memo said that a "comic-strip type copy might get a much higher readership among younger people." And a top RJR marketing official wrote to the board of directors in 1974 that "This young adult market, the 14-to-24 age group...represent(s) tomorrow's cigarette business." He recommended a "direct advertising appeal to the younger smokers."                    San Francisco Chronicle, January 16, 1998, p. A20

57. R.J. Reynolds Tobacco Company, internal documents reveal, for decades sought to develop aggressive marketing proposals to reach adolescents as young as age 14, despite public pronouncements that it did not market to children. It determined that its financial future depended on recruiting a new generation of smokers, and launched the Joe Camel campaign in 1988 with these goals in mind. "Starting around 1980, as anti-tobacco lawsuits mounted, RJR officials stopped referring, even internally, to any interest in marketing to anyone younger than 18."                    Washington Post National Weekly Edition, January 19, 1998, p. 29

58. A 1975 report to Brown and Williamson's ad agency suggests that the company should play to the smoker's understanding that smoking is "part of the illicit pleasure category" and "falls into the same category with wine, beer, shaving, wearing a bra (or purposefully not wearing one)...to the best of your ability (considering some legal constraints) relate the cigarette to 'pot', wine, beer, sex, etc."                    Associated Press, February 6, 1998

59. "To ensure increased and longer-term growth for Camel Filter, the brand must increase its share penetration among the 14-24 age group which have a new set of more liberal values and which represent tomorrow's cigarette business."                    1975 memo stamped "RJR Secret" by company official J.W. Hind
(Time magazine, January 26, 1998, p. 50)

# Anti-tobacco Advertising

1. Tobacco counter-advertising can de-glamorize smoking through images and slogans that mock the themes of power, attractiveness, escape, popularity, and pleasure that are used now to promote cigarettes.
*Strategies to Control Tobacco Use*, p. 284

2. An antismoking commercial on TV in 1968 was a takeoff on the Marlboro man. A tough-looking Westerner in a Western saloon is unable to draw his gun on a clean-cut nonsmoker because he is overcome by a coughing fit, as a slogan reads "Cigarettes--they're killers."                    *They Satisfy*, p. 213

3. Between 1967 and 1970, the Federal Trade Commission required anti-smoking TV and radio messages to balance cigarette ads; at the peak, about a minute of anti-smoking messages appeared for every three minutes of cigarette ads. During each year of the campaign, per capita consumption fell, but rose again when the mandated messages were discontinued.                    *Smoke and Mirrors*, p. 257

4. A large freeway billboard in different California locations has two Marlboro-mimicking cowboys pictured with the caption, "Bob, I've got emphysema." It is produced by the California Department of Health Services and funded by the State Tobacco Tax Initiative.

5. David Goerlitz and David Stevens, former "Winston Man" models, have quit smoking, and now make public service anti-smoking appearances.
From *Dying for a Smoke*, Pyramid Video 1993 (*Smoking*, Ambrose video/HBO, 1988)

6. Author Andrew Tobias relates that during the summer at a Long Island beach, a plane flew by trailing the banner, "Newport, Alive with Pleasure." Perturbed, Tobias hired a plane to trail the Newport one; its banner read, "Larry Tisch sells cancer sticks." From that point on, the Newport plane was grounded by Lorillard. On another occasion, a banner with "Parliament, the perfect recess" he countered with "Parliament, the PERMANENT recess" and again, the ad plane no longer was flown.

> Interview with Ronn Owens on KGO radio, San Francisco, October 30, 1997,
> and New York Times, December 9, 1997

7. The Barfmobile, a van carrying the Barfboro Barfing team, spent much of 1993 shadowing Marlboro Adventure Team vans around the country. According to DOC, the van's sponsor, Barfboro's mission is "to laugh the pushers out of town." The organization is preparing a new line of official barfing team gear.

> Tobacco Free Youth Reporter, Fall 1993, p. 14

8. The organization Doctors Ought to Care (DOC) ridicules specific cigarette brands on a Mad magazine level, examples being "Barfboro," "Wimpston," "Virginia Slime," and "Newcorpse, Dead with Pleasure." DOC also sponsors the Emphysema Slims tennis tournament. JAMA, September 26, 1990, p. 1506

9. DOC has sponsored activities such as the Dead Man Chew softball tournament, the Emphysema Slims tennis circuit (with Billie Jean Butthead, Monica Sell-Out, and Martina Nosmokanova), and the Barfboro Barfing Team (instead of the Marlboro Adventure Team). North Carolina Medical Journal, January 1995, p. 38

10. A poster by a 5th grade girl won the New York City Smokefree Ad Contest. It showed a skeleton with a cowboy hat sitting on a horse riding through a cemetery and the logo "Come to Where the Cancer Is."

> *Kids Say Don't Smoke*, Andrew Tobias, Workman, 1991

11. The organization Women and Girls Against Tobacco contracted to place an ad in Essence magazine, a publication for African American women. It featured pictures of three now-deceased Motown legends, Mary Wells, Sarah Vaughn and Eddie Kendricks, and the logo "Cigarettes made them history." Even though a contract had been approved, the magazine reneged and would not run the ad, citing it as "too controversial."

> Tobacco Control, Summer 1994, p. 103

12. A poster from the organization DOC has a macho model posing with a cigarette stuck up his nose with the caption, "I smoke for smell."

13. A highway billboard sponsored by Tobacco-Free Washington has a bald, pale, sickly camel in a hospital bed with IVs in his arm and the caption "Joe Chemo."

14. A centerpiece of a 1997 $30 million tobacco education and cessation program in Arizona is the slogan "Tobacco. Tumor causing, teeth staining, smelly puking habit."

> Washington Post National Weekly Edition, November 10, 1997, p. 31

15. In an ad produced in Spain in 1993, a horse is running through the wild and wide western-type spaces with western-type music. A health warning appears on the screen when the horse is shown with no rider; the industry depicts tobacco as the symbol of the wild west, but it is only the symbol of death.

> European Antitobacco Videocenter, European Union Against Cancer, Geneva

16. A 1994 campaign in Sweden against smoking featured billboards showing a graveyard with the slogan imposed "Welcome to Marlboro Country." Tobacco Control, Summer 1995, p. 123

17. California is unloading on the tobacco industry with a new $22 million ad campaign that takes aim at smokers – directly below the belt. A centerpiece of the latest batch of billboards, radio ads and television spots unveiled yesterday is a theme that
smoking can play havoc with a guy's sex life.

With special effects that make cigarettes suddenly sag and dangle from a young man's lips when a sexy woman steps into the     picture – the message is that smoking is linked to impotence…

A woman in a low-cut gown walks majestically into what appears to be a swanky restaurant. Across the bar, a tuxedo-clad man taps a cigarette on his ornate cigarette case.

The man and woman's eyes lock. He lights up the cigarette.

It goes limp.

"Cigarettes. Still think they're sexy?" the ad concludes.

Quote from San Francisco Chronicle, June 2, 1998, p. A17

18. A poster collection called "the Joy of Smoking…A Spoof on Cigarette Advertising" is produced by Bonnie Vierthaler (the Badvertising Institute, RD1, Box 83, Harpursville, New York 13787; 607-693-3400). One example shows the "Merit Crush-Proof Box" – a pack of Merits lying in a coffin.

19. Researchers from the University of California, San Francisco, analyzed the effectiveness of different antismoking messages. They concluded that to compete with tobacco industry advertising, antitobacco ads "need to be ambitions, hard-hitting, explicit, and in-your-face." For children and teens, messages dealing with long term health effects, short term effects, youth access, and romantic rejection had limited effectiveness. Two strategies were highly effective in reaching all audiences: industry manipulation advertisements exposing predatory business practices, and second hand smoke advertisements to denormalize smoking. Strategies emphasizing the addictive nature of nicotine can also be effective.     JAMA, March 11, 1998, pp. 772-777

20. In September 1995, counterads created by children mocking Marlboro and Virginia Slims began appearing on New York city taxis. One depicts a skeleton on a horse in front of the word "cancer" rendered in the Marlboro typeface. Another spoofs Virginia Slims as "Virginia Slime" and shows a crone smoking and the parody slogan "You've come the wrong way, baby!"     New York Times, August 27, 1995, p. F11

21. As a beautiful woman smoking a cigarette becomes covered with gloppy tar, an American Cancer Society ad poses the question, "If what happened on your insides happened on your outside, would you still smoke?"

JAMA, September 26, 1990, p. 1505

22. The March 21, 1999 Marlboro Grand Prix marked the debut of the NicoDerm CQ-Nicorette Ford sponsored by Smith Kline Beecham, becoming the lone antismoking entry in a world of cars named for cigarette brands.

Newsweek magazine

23. A large billboard along Interstate 64 near Louisville, Kentucky reads: "Birth defects come in all shapes and sizes" above pictures of six different tobacco products.     Associated Press, November 20, 1999

24. A 65 foot high Marlboro cowboy who occupied a site on Sunset Boulevard in Los Angeles for 16 years has been replaced by a cowboy with a flaccid cigarette and the caption "Smoking causes impotence."

Tobacco Control, Summer 1999, p. 136

25. Houston's mayor in 1991 proclaimed the first "Throw Tobacco Out of Sports Day" in honor of the Emphysema Slims Celebrity Tennis Tournament. Making guest appearances were Martina Nosmokanova, the Barfboro man, Filipe Morris, and the Dakota DaCough DaCancer girls.

The Journal of Medical Activism (DOC News and Views)

26. An antismoking group in Australia uses spray paint to modify cigarette billboards. Their name is BUGAUP, or Billboard Utilizing Graffitists Against Unhealthy Promotions.     *Passionate Nonsmoker's Bill of Rights*, p, 70

27. When Philip Morris sponsored an essay competition on the first amendment as part of its "Bill of Rights" promotion DOC (Doctors Ought to Care) sponsored its own essay contest with $1000 prize for the best answer to the question: "Are tobacco company executives responsible for the death, disease, and fires that their products cause?"     *Passionate Nonsmoker's Bill of Rights*, p. 207

28. In 1984, Philip Morris created the Marlboro Adventure Team as a means of promoting its flagship cigarette brand in West Germany. This promotion marked a departure from the cowboy theme, depicting instead a variety of wilderness activities such as off-road motorcycling, white-water rafting, and mountaineering. In addition to a chance to join the team, consumers were able to purchase "Adventure Gear" equipment and souvenirs with Marlboro proof-of-purchase coupons. By 1992, the promotion had appeared in Belgium, Switzerland, Italy and Turkey.

DOC, an international organization of health professionals, was founded in 1977 to counteract the promotion of lethal lifestyles, especially tobacco advertising, by means of paid satirical counter-advertising. Between 1988 and 1992, DOC achieved modest successes in Colorado and Wyoming in ending a tobacco promotion known as the Marlboro Ski challenge, by means of the purchase of advertisements promoting the "Barfboro Ski Challenge" ("barfing" is American slang for "vomiting" and is frequently used on popular TV shows). In 1993, in an effort to undermine the Marlboro Adventure Team's US debut in the western states, DOC repainted a Volkswagen van as the Barfmobile, hired a handsome comedian as the Barf Man, printed thousands of Barfboro Barf Bags, and created the Barfboro Barfing Team. Canvassing six western states in 1993 and six northeastern states in 1994, the Barfing Team coordinated dozens of community activities designed to get young people to laugh at the Marlboro Adventure Team.

The growing popularity of the Barfboro Barfing Team – a low-cost, newsworthy, easily replicated, and readily updated promotion – highlights the importance of shifting the focus of anti-smoking efforts from generic campaigns that emphasize the dangers and the ugliness of smoking, and instead onto brand name-ridicule aimed at changing the attitudes of young users toward Marlboro.

Quote from *Tobacco and Health*, p. 656 (Alan Blum)

29.  The American Legacy Foundation spends $100 million a year on their antismoking campaign, compared to the $8 billion a year for the tobacco companies' ads and promotion.   New York Times, February 14, 2002, p. A21

30.  The American Legacy Foundation's "truth" national tobacco counter-marketing campaign has been consistently associated with an increase in anti-tobacco attitudes and beliefs among youths. In contrast, the "Think. Don't Smoke" campaign of Philip Morris to discourage teenagers from smoking is actually having the opposite effect, making children more likely to be open to the idea of smoking. "This… lends support to the assertion… that the purpose of the Philip Morris campaign is to buy respectability and not to prevent youth smoking."

American Journal of Public Health, June 2002, pp. 901-907
and Associated Press, May 30, 2002

NEJM is New England Journal of Medicine
JAMA is Journal of the American Medical Association

# CHAPTER 29
# THE TOBACCO INDUSTRY

## General

1. "I'll tell you why I like the cigarette business. It costs a penny to make, it sells for a dollar, it's addictive, and there's fantastic brand loyalty."          Warren Buffett, Salomon Brothers (The Economist, May 16, 1992, p. 21)

2. Because of the tobacco industry's increasingly automated production, 28% of tobacco manufacturing jobs were eliminated between 1982 and 1992. (Actual US cigarette production increased in this time period).
SCARC, March 2, 1994

3. In 1992, the tobacco industry had $10 billion in profits on $47 billion in sales. Total US production remains steady at 650 billion cigarettes a year. The decline in domestic sales is compensated for by greatly increasing exports, up from 8% of production in 1984 to a third of manufactured cigarettes in 1992.
American Society of Addiction Medicine, Atlanta, November 12, 1993 (Michael Eriksen)

4. Just before tobacco advertising was banned from radio and television in 1971, the Brown and Williamson Tobacco Company designed a response to its antismoking opponents, code-named Project Truth. A presentation of the project included the statements: "Doubt is our product, since it is the best means of competing with the 'body of fact' that exists in the mind of the general public...If we are successful in establishing a controversy at the public level, then there is an opportunity to put across the real facts about smoking and health".
New York Times, June 18, 1994, p. A12

5. The Brown and Williamson Project Truth program in 1971 listed objectives, including:
"Objective No 1:  To set aside in the minds of millions the false conviction that cigarette smoking causes lung cancer and other diseases; a conviction based on fanatical assumptions, fallacious rumors, unsupported claims and the unscientific statements and conjectures of publicity-seeking opportunists."
"Objective No. 2:  To lift the cigarette from the cancer identification as quickly as possible and restore it to its proper place of dignity and acceptance in the minds of men and women in the marketplace of American free enterprise."
"Objective No. 3:  To expose the incredible, unprecedented and nefarious attack against the cigarette, constituting the greatest libel and slander ever perpetrated against any product in the history of free enterprise; a criminal libel of such major proportions and implications that one wonders how such a crusade of calumny can be reconciled and under the Constitution can be so flouted and violated."
"Objective No. 6:  To establish--once and for all--that no scientific evidence has ever been produced, presented or submitted to prove conclusively that cigarette smoking causes cancer."   New York Times, June 18, 1994, p. A12

6. "If cigarette companies were held to the same standards of conduct as other companies, we would see mass demonstrations in front of the Park Avenue headquarters of Philip Morris, thundering denunciations from media pundits, and heavy pressure for stricter legislation. People who profit from the cigarette trade would be social pariahs."          *Merchants of Death: the American Tobacco Industry*, Larry C. White

7. In 1993, several members of Congress urged Attorney General Janet Reno to launch criminal investigations into tobacco companies, charging that company executives had been aware of the health hazards of cigarette smoking and of the addictive power of nicotine since the early 1960's but have conspired to suppress the information. Among the crimes that the congressmen listed were perjury and racketeering, mail fraud, wire fraud, restraint of trade, and conspiracy to defraud the public and obstruct Congress.          The Lancet, July 2, 1994, p. 49

8. Brown and Williamson Tobacco Co. has secretly developed a super potent tobacco hybrid in Brazil, call Y-1, which contains nearly twice the amount of nicotine found in standard tobacco. There are several million pounds of the leaf stored in US warehouses, and the hybrid has been used to boost the nicotine content (and thus addictive properties) of five US brands.          The Lancet, July 2, 1994, p. 49

9.  In testimony before a congressional subcommittee, FDA Commissioner David Kessler reported that FDA investigators had discovered that the Brown & Williamson Tobacco Corp., a US subsidiary of London-based BAT Industries, PLC, had secretly developed a super potent tobacco hybrid in Brazil called Y-1 that contains nearly twice the amount of nicotine found in standard flue-cured tobacco. Kessler said that Brown & Williamson has used the hybrid tobacco to boost the nicotine content of five domestic US brands and now has several million pounds of the leaf stored in US warehouses. Kessler said that Brown & Williamson had sought to conceal the existence of Y-1 and had told FDA investigators that it had not engaged in any breeding of tobacco to attain higher nicotine levels. The company admitted to the project only when confronted with evidence that the FDA had gathered about its Y-1 program.                    The Lancet, July 2, 1994, p. 49

10. An internal Brown and Williamson Tobacco Company memorandum in 1990 showed that the company had stockpiled two million pounds of the Y-1 tobacco it had developed with very high nicotine levels, and was planning to test it on smokers. In 1994, the company denied to Federal investigators that it had developed high nicotine tobacco, but later in the year admitted that it had imported five million pounds of Y-1 tobacco into the United States and used some of it in five cigarette brands.
                    New York Times, January 9, 1998, p. A12, and January 8, 1998, p. A17

11. A California biotechnology company has agreed to plead guilty to conspiring with a major cigarette producer (unofficially identified as Brown and Williamson) to increase the nicotine content of tobacco plants. The research project by DNA Plant Technology tried to produce high nicotine varieties of tobacco by using types of biotechnology such as gene splicing and advanced plant breeding. A tobacco plant was developed called "Y-1" whose leaves yielded 6% nicotine, twice the normal level. Because it is illegal to grow these high nicotine plants in the United States, company executives "were portrayed as having spent most of the past decade boarding airplanes carrying secret stashes of designer tobacco seeds" to places such as Brazil.
                    San Francisco Chronicle, January 8, 1998, p. 1

12. The Brown and Williamson Y-1 high nicotine "fumo loco" tobacco grown in Brazil was prohibited in Brazilian cigarettes, so all 8 million pounds was exported back to the United States for blending with domestic tobacco. Three million pounds was shipped in the spring of 1994; the company denied at the time that it was growing high nicotine tobacco to make a product sort of like "cigarettes on steroids." Brown and Williamson says that all Y-1 stocks, plants, and seeds have now been destroyed, and that Y-1 was only a breeding experiment.
                    CBS evening news, March 10 and 11, 1998

13. Brown and Williamson has admitted that it continues to use genetically altered high nicotine tobacco, despite the company's assurances to the federal government that it stopped the practice four years ago.
                    Wall Street Journal, February 11, 1998, p. A8

14. "Philip Morris and British-American Tobacco, the world's two biggest tobacco companies, secretly joined forces to fix cigarette prices and divide markets in Argentina, Venezuela and other Latin American countries, according to internal documents that explicitly describe the deals and the involvement of some of the companies' most senior executives."      San Francisco Chronicle, September 17, 1998, p. A7 (Myron Levin, Los Angeles Times)

15. Major recipients of donations from tobacco companies include the ACLU (American Civil Liberties Union), the Partnership for a Drug-Free America, the Gay Men's Health Crisis, the Boy Scouts, the Coalition for the Homeless, the NAACP, and the National Women's Political Caucus.

16. In the early 1990's, 55% of US medical schools accepted research money from the tobacco industry.
                    American Medical News, February 14, 1994, p. 14

17. Alvan Feinstein MD, epidemiologist and professor of medicine at Yale University Medical School, received at least $700,000 from the tobacco industry's Council for Tobacco Research.    ASH Review, November 1994, p. 3

18. The Yale Divinity School accepted a $280,000 grant from US Tobacco Company, the nation's largest manufacturer of smokeless tobacco.                    Yale alumni magazine, December 1993, p. 10

19. The National Archives, where the Bill of Rights is on display, received $600,000 from Philip Morris to help pay for the Bill of Rights' two hundredth anniversary celebration. In return, Philip Morris received permission to use the Bill of Rights in a major advertising campaign. *No Stranger to Tears*, p. 324

20. Philip Morris spends an estimated $15 million annually to support museums and the performing arts.
*Tobacco Industry Strategies*, p. 36

21. Information from tobacco industry documents indicates that for ten years beginning in 1982, the companies "used coercion and economic intimidation to muffle aggressive anti-smoking messages by the makers of cessation products such as the nicotine patch or gum." In 1984 when Merrell Dow (a subsidiary of Dow Chemical) introduced Nicorette gum and prepared material urging smokers to quit, Philip Morris canceled all purchases from Dow Chemical. The company later had the Philip Morris account reinstated, but only after it assured Philip Morris that it was "committed to avoiding contribution to the anti-cigarette effort." The Merrell Dow president agreed that he would "screen advertising and promotional materials to eliminate any inflammatory anti-industry statements." Los Angeles Times, February 14, 1999

22. The American Tobacco position from 1954 to 1980 was that cigarettes are not injurious to health. Some scientists "will tell you that this whole statistical machine is a reprehensible propaganda campaign that is based on spurious statistics and is socially irresponsible."
From a 1986 deposition by Robert Heiman, CEO of American Tobacco Company
(from Tobacco on Trial, court TV on video, Landmark cases, 1997)

23. "When the tobacco industry fights something, you almost always know it's good for public health."
C. Everett Koop, M.D.

24. Because many people find it difficult to believe that the industry still denies that smoking causes any harm to health, a few examples are worth citing. In 1987, Jean-Louis Mercier, then President of Imperial Tobacco, appeared before a House of Commons Committee and was asked whether he believed that any Canadians die of smoking-related diseases. He replied "No, I do not." He also stated that the "role, if any, that tobacco or smoking plays in the initiation and the development of these diseases is still very uncertain. The issue is still unresolved." Patrick Fennell, the President of Rothmans, Benson & Hedges Inc., asserted that "science has not established that there is a causal relationship between smoking and illness." Quote from *Smoke and Mirrors*, p. 13

25. In testimony to Congress in March 1994, a tobacco industry spokesman said: "I deny that cigarettes cause cancer and cause death." Dean Edell M.D., ABC radio, March 28, 1994

26. "We have looked at the data and the data that we have been able to see has all been statistical data that has not convinced me that smoking causes death."
Andrew W. Tisch, Chairman and Chief Executive, Lorillard Tobacco Company, in Congressional testimony, April 14, 1994 (New York Times, June 17, 1994, p. A22)

27. In April 1994, leading executives from the seven major tobacco companies testified to Congress under oath they did not believe nicotine to be addictive, that cigarettes have not been proven to cause disease in humans, and that their companies do not manipulate the levels of nicotine in their products.
Tobacco Free Youth Reporter, Fall 1995

28. "The only difference between the scientific views of the tobacco industry and the Flat Earth Society is that the former has billions of dollars to promote its position." Smoking & Health Review, June 1990

29. "I am dumbfounded to be here today. I am struck that arguing about the deadly effects of passive smoke is like discussing whether the world is round...I am flabbergasted by all the lies and distortion, and the immoral attitude of our fellow Americans in the tobacco industry."
AMA Trustee Randolph Smoak, M.D. (American Medical News, August 15, 1994)

30. When he was US Surgeon General, Dr. C. Everett Koop said, "One of the things that keeps me motivated is that the tobacco industry does such sleazy things". Tobacco Control, Fall 1993, p. 239

31. "Q: You have never explored or studied the issue of whether or not cigarettes cause disease?

"A: That is absolutely correct.

"Q: If I asked you, does smoking cause lung cancer...

"A: I don't know."     Bennett S. LeBow, Liggett Tobacco Company (Washington Monthly, February 1994, p. 6)

32. "The tobacco industry paid 13 scientists more than $156,000 for writing letters and manuscripts to discredit studies linking secondhand smoke to lung cancer," including the 1993 EPA report. Associated Press, August 5, 1998

33. An "Ex-Smoker Hall of Fame" exhibit has been developed by Roswell Park Cancer Institute in Buffalo, NY. The most unlikely ex-smokers in the display are Michael Miles, Chairman of Philip Morris, and Charles "Mike" Harper, CEO of RJR Nabisco.                    Tobacco Control, Fall 1993, p. 194

34. In 1992, Philip Morris controlled 41.4% of the US cigarette market, and RJ Reynolds, 26.6%. Each smoker contributes an average of $13,000 in profits over a lifetime to the "parent company", smoking an average of half a million cigarettes in all.                    American Journal of Public Health, September 1993, p. 1211

35. In 1993, Philip Morris (42.2%) and RJ Reynolds (30.6%) both had market share increases and controlled almost three quarters of the US cigarette market.                    New York Times, June 17, 1994, p. A22

36. In 1992, Philip Morris and RJR had combined profits of $9.9 billion.
North Carolina Medical Journal, January 1995, p. 31

37. Profit margins for name brand cigarettes are often in excess of 40%, the largest profit of any consumer product. It costs less than twenty cents to manufacture a pack of cigarettes.
Third National Conference on Nicotine Dependence,
San Diego, September 1990 (John Slade and Alan Blum)

38. Discount cigarette brands and generics such as Misty, Doral, and Cambridge accounted in 1993 for almost 40% of the US market share, up from 11% as recently as 1988. Profit margins on these brands are 30 to 50% lower than on "premium" brands. Discount brands were first introduced in 1980, and in 1982 controlled only 3% of the US market.                    American Journal of Public Health, September 1993, p. 1212

39. A 1956 memo by RJR chemist Alan Rodgman indicated his recognition that smoking causes cancer. He wrote: "Since it is now well-established that cigarette smoke does contain several polycyclic aromatic hydrocarbons and, considering the... carcinogenic activity of a number of these compounds, a method of...removal of these compounds from cigarette smoke is required."                    Los Angeles Times, August 3, 1997, p. A37

40. In 1961, three years before the first Surgeon General's report on smoking, the head of research at Philip Morris identified cancer-causing compounds in cigarettes and urged the company to develop a "medically acceptable low-carcinogen" cigarette. In 1964, Brown and Williamson "seeks patients for a reduced-risk cigarette that heats rather than burns tobacco, but the project, known as Ariel, is never brought to market." In 1996, RJR Nabisco began test marketing of Eclipse in Chattanooga, Tenn., "but is finding few takers."
Washington Post, May 11, 1997, p. C2

41. In 1961, three years before the first Surgeon General's report on smoking, the Philip Morris head of research identified carcinogens in cigarettes and urged the company to develop a "medically acceptable low-carcinogen" cigarette. In 1964, Brown and Williamson in its Project Ariel applied for patents for a safer cigarette, but the cigarette was never developed or marketed.                    New York Times, July 3, 1997, p. A16

42. Brown and Williamson in the 1960's developed a cigarette called Ariel which would have cut down greatly on cancer-causing substances in smoke, as well as the amount of secondhand smoke coming from the cigarette. It also would have reduced its potential fire hazard. The company decided not to market Ariel because it would imply that its other products were hazardous and would make them "look bad" by comparison.
New York Times, May 13, 1994, p. A10

43. Liggett "spent twenty years and millions of dollars on the 'safer' cigarette, only to keep it off the market out of fear of liability claims against the company based on the inference that the rest of the product line was therefore unsafe."
*Ashes to Ashes*, p. 657

44. The tobacco industry had a total of 57 patents approved in the United States for modifications in cigarette manufacture that could have reduced the toxic ingredients in smoke that cause disease. A report concluded that the industry never followed these patents because producing safer cigarettes "would have been expensive and an admission that existing cigarettes were unsafe."
Reuters, March 4, 1999

45. In the late 1960's and 1970's, the tobacco industry intensively tried to design a "safer" cigarette. By 1975, five companies had tested successful "safer" cigarettes, including one with a catalyst made of palladium inserted in the filter that would absorb carcinogens, and another that would deliver nicotine in warm air. However, after the late 1970's the industry strategy changed; because of legal concerns the companies began to dismantle their scientific infrastructure and laboratories and destroy or bury the data that had been collected.
*Smokescreen*, pp. 39-40

46. "We accept an interest in people's health as a basic responsibility, paramount to every other consideration in our business… We always have and always will cooperate closely with those whose task it is to safeguard the public health."
Tobacco industry advertisement, New York Times, January 1954

47. In national news magazines in 1984, RJ Reynolds published ads emphatically stating, "Studies which conclude that smoking causes disease have regularly ignored significant evidence to the contrary."
*Tobacco and the Clinician*, p. viii

48. In April 1997, Andrew Schindler, president of R.J. Reynolds, testified in a sworn deposition that cigarettes are no more addictive than coffee or carrots. Four days later, his million-dollar North Carolina vacation home burned down, the victim of a construction worker's "careless toss of a lighted cigarette butt." In the same class action suit, Alexander Spears, chairman of Lorillard, said under oath that he didn't think Americans "die of diseases caused by cigarette smoking."
New York Times, April 24, 1997, p. A29 (Frank Rich column)

49. "After three decades of investigation and millions of dollars invested…the smoking and health controversy remains unresolved. The net result of all of this effort has been that no casual link between smoking and disease has been established. This is scientific fact readily available to anyone willing to make an objective unemotional study of the existing evidence." Statement of Edward A. Horrigan, Jr. on behalf of the Tobacco Institute before the House Energy and Commerce Committee, March 12, 1982

50. The tobacco industry's Council for Tobacco Research was cited on ABC News (Peter Jennings) on September 25, 1995 as an example of "corporate welfare" and corporate tax loopholes. It received $25 million from tobacco companies in one year, paid its top executive $340,000, and paid zero in corporate tax thanks to a so-called "business league" exemption.

51. A grand jury is studying whether the Council for Tobacco Research, an industry sponsored group that finances research, is legitimately a nonprofit scientific institution or whether it has fraudulently claimed nonprofit status while defending the industry.
New York Times, March 18, 1996, p. A12

52. "The research arm of the tobacco industry was created as and has been successfully used as a public relations ploy."
Addiction 1997; 92:521 (Richard Hurt)

53. "By the 1960's, B&W and BAT had proven in their own laboratories that cigarette tar causes cancer in animals. In addition, by the early 1960's, BAT's scientists (and B&W's lawyers) were acting on the assumption that nicotine is addictive. BAT responded by secretly attempting to create a 'safe' cigarette that would minimize dangerous ingredients and the associated damage to health, but would still deliver nicotine. Publicly, however, it maintained that cigarettes are neither dangerous nor addictive…the active role lawyers had, not just as advisers, but as managers, selecting which research would be done or not done, who would be funded, and what public relations and political actions would be pursued."
JAMA, July 19, 1995, p. 223 (Stanton Glantz)

54. The involvement of tobacco industry lawyers in the selection of scientific projects to be funded is sharp contrast to the industry's public statements about its review process for its external research program. Scientific merit played little role in the selection of research projects. The results of the projects were used to generate good publicity for the industry, and to deflect attention away from tobacco use as a health danger.

JAMA, July 19, 1995, p. 241

55. In an analysis of tobacco industry smokers' rights publications, it was concluded that objectives were "to shift the focus away from smoking as a health issue and to elevate smoking to an issue of personal liberty and choice…Messages are…that the tobacco control movement is a threat to the ideals of personal freedom. Increasingly, tobacco control agencies and individuals are portrayed as liars who ignore the truth and manipulate the public to impose their lifestyle choices on others." Attempts to refute scientific evidence concerning smoking and environmental tobacco smoke serve to convince readers that there is no rationale for smoking restrictions.

American Journal of Public Health, September 1995, p. 1215

56. "In 20 years there won't be any cigarette manufacturing in North Carolina (and other tobacco states). It'll be done offshore, where it's cheaper and where the markets are."

lobbyist for Philip Morris (Coalition on Smoking or Health)

57. Health insurance companies hold large amounts of tobacco company stock, including Prudential with $248 million, Travelers with $88 million, and CIGNA with $77 million.  American Medical News, July 24, 1995, p. 16

58. Australia now has required bold pack warnings such as SMOKING KILLS. A new brand called Freedom by Rothmans is fighting back with large quotations also on the pack "Those who deny freedom to others deserve it not for themselves – Abraham Lincoln, 1859," and on the other side "If we don't stand up for our rights we may lose them altogether."                                    Tobacco Control, Autumn 1995, p. 289

59. "Now adults are being sold the tobacco party line in politics:  smoking as freedom. But the cigarette makes a perverse icon to liberty. The freedom to get hooked? The right to addiction? The issue isn't 'Health Nazis.' It's still health. The only 'Freedom-Loving Individualists' that the tobacco industry cares about are the ones in need of another fix."                                    Ellen Goodman column, March 2, 1995

60. Philip Morris has taken out full page advertisements in newspapers in Europe arguing that measures to restrict smoking indoors to protect the health of nonsmokers are an infringement of personal liberty.

The Lancet, December 9, 1995, p. 1549

61. The International Agency for Research on Cancer, a research branch of the World Health Organization, undertook a large European study on the epidemiology of passive smoking and lung cancer, finding a 16% increase in risk for nonsmoking spouses of smokers, and a 17% increase for exposure in the workplace. Philip Morris feared that the study would lead to increased restrictions in Europe, and spent $2 million in one year alone to spearhead a strategy to try to discredit the work of the research organization. Philip Morris employed a public relations company and a firm of lawyers to "stimulate controversy" about the study. "… the tobacco industry continues to conduct a sophisticated campaign against conclusions that second-hand smoke causes lung cancer and other diseases, subverting normal scientific processes."                                    The Lancet, April 18, 2000, pp. 1197-1253

62. In California and other states, the tobacco industry has used "freedom of information" laws to force "government agencies which have taken, or even contemplated, tobacco control actions to bare their internal records to the tobacco industry. Government bureaucrats who take actions displeasing to the tobacco industry face a level of hassles, hostile scrutiny, and possible public ridicule of difficult-to-explain decisions."

   The article on this practice (Tobacco Control, Autumn 1995, pp. 222 – 230) concluded: "Access to public records is every citizen's right. Unfortunately, it appears that the tobacco industry is abusing this right and turning it into a weapon to complicate and discourage public health activities." And an accompanying editorial (p. 209) commented: "Unfortunately, there is a fine line (at best) between appropriate use of legal process to defend one's rights, and the abuse of the legal process to intimidate one's opponents."

63. "The industry **intimidates** advocates, the media, and public officials through legal, economic, personal, and political attack; the tobacco companies subsidize and exaggerate **alliances** with captive advertising agencies,

restaurant associations, the ACLU (American Civil Liberties Union), and farmers; the industry underwrites **smokers' rights** and other **front groups** to masquerade as spontaneous grassroots organizations; the industry uses **political funding** to court votes and legislative favors from lawmakers; the industry hires cadres of **lobbyists** to overwhelm lawmakers and other public officials, the industry **buys science and other expertise** to produce 'independent' experts critical of tobacco control policies; the industry abuses **philanthropy** to buy organizations; and the industry uses **advertising and public relations** to blitz the public consciousness with deceptive messages full of half-truths."   *Tobacco and Health*, p. 379

64. In private depositions in April 1997 in a Florida lawsuit, executives of the nation's top four tobacco companies "clung to long-held industry dogma" that tobacco is not conclusively linked to any illness or is addictive. The depositions came a month after the Liggett Group admitted that smoking is addictive and causes cancer.
   Associated Press, April 21, 1997

65. James Morgan, president of Philip Morris, "said in a sworn statement that tobacco is no more addictive than Gummi Bears candy."   Associated Press, May 3, 1997

66. "It is not acceptable that, together, the five largest multinational tobacco companies have annual revenues from their tobacco operations that are more than 60 times higher than the entire annual budget of WHO. Even more alarming is the fact that this revenue represents more than 10 times the gross domestic product of a country like Bolivia. Indeed the gross revenue of the largest of these companies, from its international operations, is equal to the gross domestic product of Bangladesh, a country of 115 million people. It represents 100 times the total health budget of Ecuador. Equally unacceptable is the fact that the advertising budget of one company in the United States alone is equal to 50 times the total budget of the WHO tobacco or health program."
   World Smoking and Health, No. 1, 1992, p. 6

67. "Microsmokes," a takeoff on microbreweries, are the new smoke on the streets advertised as homegrown, all organic and attracting first time smokers skeptical of large corporations. American Spirit is sold in health food stores as all natural and additive and chemical-free. Another brand is Dave's, supposedly from an antiestablishment farmer in North Carolina and Dave's Tobacco Company. The only catch is that Philip Morris invented Dave.   CBS evening news, May 16, 1996

68. "Natural Smokes for a Health-Conscious Market." All-natural cigarettes, free of chemical additives, are increasingly popular. They include Born Free, American Spirit, Buz, and Sherman's. RJR and Philip Morris are marketing new brands aimed at "young, urban smokers who distrust mainstream, mass-produced products." Philip Morris has Dave's, and RJR is selling Red Kamel, Politix, B's, and Metro.
   San Francisco Chronicle, May 17, 1996, p. A1

69. "The tobacco industry should be respected and studied much like the human immunodeficiency virus, which alters its antigenic structure to outwit the host organism."Journal of Family Practice, June 1992, p. 698 (Alan Blum)

70. "The tobacco industry is the disease vector for heart disease and cancer. To control any disease you need to understand how it is spread. The difference between the tobacco industry and malaria is that mosquitoes don't make campaign contributions and hire public relations firms."
   USA Today, October 10, 1995, p. D4 (Stanton Glantz)

71. "If you want to do something about malaria, you have to study mosquitoes. And if you want to do something about lung cancer, you have to study the tobacco industry."
   Professor Stanton Glantz defending his National Cancer Institute grant on
   research into the tobacco industry (Wall Street Journal, August 7, 1995)

72. The book *The Cigarette Papers* by Stanton Glantz about Brown and Williamson files was rejected by more than two dozen publishers before being published by the University of California Press in 1996. Editors were initially enthusiastic, and several called it "the Pentagon Papers of tobacco." However, legal departments advised against it, afraid of being sued. One editor said, "If you anger a tobacco company and get into what amounts to a financial war with it, you're going to lose."   The Nation, January 1, 1996, p. 14

73. The Washington Times published an ad in March 1995 denouncing the National Cancer Institute for funding the work of Stanton Glantz, declaring that "the dismal record of the NCI to control cancer is forcing it to desperate measures." The ad was paid for by the National Smokers Alliance, which was established by Philip Morris.

*The Nation, January 1, 1996, p. 17*

74. "As Glantz began to score points against the tobacco industry, a political campaign was started to shut him up. Articles and letters ran in various right-wing publications and newsletters asking why research unfavorable to personal freedom – the right to smoke! – was getting federal support....Like the Soviet leadership did in the 1950's, members of Congress are trying to silence someone whose valid scientific findings do not suit their political tastes." St. Paul (Minn.) Pioneer Press, October 18, 1995, p. A17 (A. Caplan)

75. In November 1997, a California Superior Court dismissed a case by the tobacco industry against Dr. Stanton Glantz of University of California San Francisco, regarding his tobacco research.

76. ...the industry began promoting filter and reduced-tar cigarettes during the 1950s primarily to calm public fears about the health effects of smoking. Although the advertisements of the era suggested that the new cigarettes were "healthier," there was no real evidence that this was so. When the evidence finally began to come in (beginning only twenty years later, in 1977), the verdict was that lowering tar with filters had only a very modest effect in lowering the enormous risk of lung cancer caused by cigarettes and no effect in protecting the consumer from the more common threat, fatal heart disease.

Today the tobacco industry claims that it markets filter and "low-tar" cigarettes because of public demand, and not because it believes that these products are "safer". For instance, R.J. Reynolds--in its monograph about , a novel nicotine delivery system--refers to the development of filter and "low-tar" cigarettes as manufacturer responses to consumer demand. However, the industry itself, through its advertising campaigns, has helped create the illusion that these products are safer. *Quote from The Cigarette Papers, p. 30*

77. "The tobacco industry has used three primary arguments to prevent government regulation of its products and to defend itself in product liability lawsuits. First, tobacco companies have consistently claimed that there is no conclusive proof that smoking causes diseases such as cancer and heart disease. Second, tobacco companies have claimed that smoking is not addictive and that anyone who smokes makes a free choice to do so. And, finally, tobacco companies have claimed that they are committed to determining the scientific truth about the health effects of tobacco, both by conducting internal research and by funding external research."

*The Cigarette Papers, p. 199*

78. In 1994, the Council for Tobacco Research, funded by the tobacco industry, distributed more than $19.5 million to scientists. Canadian Medical Association Journal, January 15, 1996

79. "The tobacco industry's public relations efforts during the 'safe' cigarette era consisted largely of an attempt to confuse the public about the scientific evidence on the dangers of smoking. Whether those efforts involved in-house handbooks, books and magazine articles written on behalf of the industry, or advertising campaigns, the thrust of the material was the same: create doubt in the public mind about what the scientific evidence really says and then attack the notion that the government should meddle in the tobacco industry's business without having definitive proof of harmful effects of smoking. To this end, the industry enlisted the support of powerful friends in the political world as well as in the media, and sometimes failed to disclose the fact that certain people expressing a viewpoint sympathetic to the industry had direct financial ties to the industry." *The Cigarette Papers, p. 199*

80. A single cigarette manufacturing machine can now produce 14,000 cigarettes per minute.

*Tobacco Control, Winter 1995, p. 395*

81. The total amount of tobacco that it takes to make a cigarette dropped from 2.6 pounds per thousand cigarettes in 1955 to 1.7 pounds in 1982. Today's cigarette is only about 60% shredded tobacco leaves. The remainder is added "junk" to lower the cost, including wasted stems that are colored and reflavored and dust that is swept off the floor. *Smokescreen, p. 62*

82. "The companies are crowding out both farmers and the government in getting their share. Between 1980 and 1991, for example, the farmers' take on each cigarette is down from 7 cents to 3 cents per dollar. The

government's take is down from 34 cents to 25 cents per dollar. At the same time, the companies' take is rising rapidly, from 37 to 50 cents per dollar." *Smokescreen*, p. 62

83. Four life insurance companies are owned by tobacco companies.
*Smoking Policy: Law, Politics and Culture*, p. 206

84. "These cigarette companies, they are ruining the American reputation around the world--I repeat, around the world. They were condemned everywhere, the way they behave, the way they market, the way they sabotage or undermine other countries' efforts to control smoking. And the one who finally will be blamed is the American, because this company, the headquarters is in America." Dr. Parkit Vateesatokit, public health official in Thailand, on the American cigarette invasion (Mother Jones, May-June 1996, p. 67)

85. "Conservative defenders of the tobacco industry are put in the untenable position of arguing that when a school gives a condom to a teen, it sends a pro-promiscuity message; when Hollywood makes a slasher movie, it glorifies violence; but when cigarette companies promote their products as hip, cool, macho, etc. ...and give away gear with obvious adolescent appeal—it has zero impact. Bit of a consistency problem, no?"
Boston Herald, October 25, 1995, p. 27 (Don Feder)

86. "The irony is that while the tobacco industry spouts 'local control' rhetoric, it is cynically using front groups and statewide pre-emption laws to snuff out genuine grassroots initiatives to control smoking...In all, 28 states have now passed pre-emption laws." Mother Jones, May-June 1996, p. 55

87. "We would accept money from the Mafia if they offered it."
Statement from the manager of the Ailey dance troupe, commenting on accepting money from Philip Morris (*Ashes to Ashes*, p. 621)

88. The Council for Tobacco Research, formerly TIRC, or Tobacco Industry Research Committee, was formed by the industry ostensibly for research, but more than 50% of its budget was devoted to public relations.
*Smokescreen*, p. 15

89. The tobacco industry "disinformation machine" was created in 1953, and it might be the largest and most expensive public – issue campaign ever, expending over a billion dollars so far. The campaign began with 38 public relations experts, and the industry found scientists who said that cigarettes probably did not cause cancer. An example of a prominent scientist was Dr. Clarence Cook Little, a founder of the National Cancer Institute and former head of the organization that became the American Cancer Society. He believed in genetic susceptibility to cancer and discounted environmental influences such as tobacco smoke. "And so, he was hired on as the first chief of the Scientific Advisory Board of the newly-formed Tobacco Industry Research Committee."
*Smokescreen*, pp. 8-9

90. Dr. Little appeared on the Edward R. Murrow television show in the 1950's, where the following dialogue took place:
Question: Dr. Little, have any cancer-causing agents been identified in cigarettes?
CLARENCE LITTLE: No. None whatever, either in cigarettes or in any product of smoking.
Question: Suppose the tremendous amount of research going on, including that of the Tobacco Industry Research Committee, were to reveal that there is a cancer-causing agent in cigarettes. What then?
DR. LITTLE: Well, if it was found by somebody working under a tobacco industry research grant, it would be made publicimmediately and just as broadly as we could make it, and then efforts would be taken to remove that substance or substances.
The TIRC funded a great deal of work, and public relations executives and lawyers would screen the scientific reports before permitted them to be released. "All of this was done by the TIRC. But there was more research being done quietly--without each company knowing what the others were doing--within the company labs themselves. We now have the documents showing the results of that work, and it has proved to be not only good work, but advanced far beyond that of the top university scientists of the time. It was in these tobacco company labs, in less than eight years after Dr. Little's remarks, that company researchers found not just one cancer-causing substance in smoke, but numerous compounds that caused cancer and arrays of others which encouraged

cancer growth. The discoveries of these effects were also not made public by the companies; again they emerged only when company documents were obtained 25 years after the events." *Smokescreen*, pp. 10-11

91. Brown and Williamson has avoided "legal discovery proceedings by funneling the most damaging material in its files to legal departments, where company lawyers claimed the material was protected from disclosure by the attorney-client privilege and as attorney work product. That is fraud." The Nation, January 1, 1996, p. 18

92. "...the tobacco industry is unique among American and worldwide industries in its ability to forestall effective government regulation and to hold effective public health action at bay while marketing its lethal products. The industry manages this, despite the overwhelming scientific evidence that tobacco products kill, through a combination of skilled legal, political, and public relations strategies designed to confuse the public and to allow it to avoid having to take responsibility for the death and disease it inflicts." *The Cigarette Papers*, p. xvii

93. Carl Seltzer, a retired professor of public health from Harvard, received a total of $750,000 in grants from the industry-funded Council for Tobacco Research. His work focused on countering the evidence that smoking causes heart disease. Newspaper clippings on his work included titles "Doctor Slams Link between Smoking and Heart Disease" and "Smoking does Not Cause Heart Disease," not disclosing his link to the industry. This demonstrates how the industry was quietly paying for scientists to publicize its position that tobacco is not dangerous. *The Cigarette Papers*, p. 177

94. An editorial in Barron's in October 1967 criticized the 1964 Surgeon General's report and attacked government efforts to control tobacco. "What began a few years ago as a seemingly well-intentioned, if disturbing, effort to brainwash the citizenry into kicking the habit thus has spiraled into a crusade as menacing and ugly as Prohibition." The tobacco industry reprinted the editorial in a series of newspaper ads. *The Cigarette Papers*, p. 177

95. Stanley Frank, a well-known sports writer, wrote an article "To Smoke or Not to Smoke--That Is Still the Question" in the January 1968 issue of True magazine, concluding that "the hazards of cigarette smoking may not be so real as we have been led to believe." He later wrote another piece for the National Enquirer entitled, "Cigarette Cancer Link is Bunk." Frank did not disclose that he worked for Hill and Knowlton, the public relations firm that created the Tobacco Industry Research Committee and the Tobacco Institute; that he had been paid on behalf of the tobacco industry to write the article; or that tobacco interests had reviewed the article prior to publication. *The Cigarette Papers*, p. 179

96. "No clinical or biological evidence has been produced which demonstrates how cigarettes relate to cancer or any other disease in human beings." Statement from American Tobacco Co. at its 1967 annual meeting (*Ashes to Ashes*, p. 325)

97. "...today's scare tactics surrounding cigarettes. Because no one has been able to produce conclusive proof that cigarette smoking causes cancer. Scientific, biological, clinical, or any other kind. It's more than cigarettes being challenged here. It's freedom." From Brown and Williamson's Project Truth campaign, 1970 (*The Cigarette Papers*, p. 186)

98. "A widespread anti-tobacco industry is out to harass sixty million Americans who smoke and to prohibit the manufacture and use of tobacco products. . . . Outrageous and medically unsubstantiated assertions made by well-financed and highly organized groups opposed to smoking are disputed by many men and women of science." Statement from William Dwyer, Tobacco Institute spokesman, in 1979 (*Ashes to Ashes*, p. 468)

99. 1985 BAT (British American Tobacco) argument about the health effects of smoking:
"There is a lot of evidence which links smoking statistically with certain diseases. . . . Statistics alone cannot prove cause and effect. . . . Research is needed to clarify the situation." *The Cigarette Papers*, p. 341

100. The tobacco industry "attempts to instill in the public mind the notion that there is a controversy surrounding the scientific evidence about cigarettes and health...B&W merely has to sell a sufficient amount of doubt about the scientific evidence to establish a controversy; it can then disseminate a sufficient amount of 'truth' to sustain a controversy." *The Cigarette Papers*, p. 191

101. A tobacco company executive commented on the industry's strategy. "The object . . . is not to win. The object is to lose very slowly, to delay the day of reckoning as long as possible." Time, May 10, 1996, p. 46

102. The British equivalent of the Council for Tobacco Research is the Tobacco Research Council, which in the 1970's had its own laboratory with over 250 scientists and staff. *Cancer Wars*, p. 294

103. After a jury in Jacksonville awarded smoker Grady Carter $750,000 in damages in August 1996, the stock prices of Philip Morris and RJR dropped 14% and 13%, respectively, in one day, even though these tobacco companies were not directly involved in the litigation. NEJM, January 23, 1997, p. 306

104. Documents from Brown and Williamson demonstrated that as long ago as the 1960's, the tobacco industry knew nicotine was an addictive drug and smoking caused cancer and other disease, and that it developed a sophisticated legal and public relations strategy to keep this information away from the public, public health authorities, and the courts. JAMA, March 5, 1997, p. 751

105. A quote from *Cancer Wars* (pp. 129-130) about a tobacco industry strategy:
    *Evidence of toxic hazards is ambiguous, inconclusive, or incomplete; we therefore need "more research" to clarify ambiguities, improve estimates of risk, elucidate the mechanisms, and so forth.* This has become one of the more effective industry arguments in recent years. The tobacco industry, for example, has long used this tactic to convince consumers that it is premature to conclude that cigarettes cause cancer. The Tobacco Institute's paper on "The Cigarette Controversy" thus calls for more research" (or "far more research" and the like) half a dozen times in as many pages, the purported goal being to resolve a smoking and health "debate" or "controversy." Internal tobacco industry documents brag about the success of this "brilliantly conceived and executed" strategy to create "doubt about the health charge without actually denying it."
    Given the inherent uncertainties of the scientific process, it is always possible to delve ever deeper into the mechanisms of pharmacokinetic action, to elucidate risks with ever greater precision, to demand ever larger animal or human epidemiological studies. The call for more research often translates into a call for "less action"—and, specifically, less regulation.

106. Tobacco-industry-supported Trojan Horse "Tobacco Control" bills have similar features. These include preemption, meaning enacting state laws preventing local communities from passing ordinances more restrictive than the state law, weak and ineffective restrictions on cigarette vending machines, prohibiting youth compliance check "sting" operations, and penalizing children rather than merchants for illegal sales.
    *Stop the Sale, Prevent the Addiction*

107. The president of the Council for Tobacco Research is James Glenn, a urologist and former dean of the Emory and Mount Sinai medical schools. He has testified, "no one has been able to demonstrate that smoking, per se, causes any diseases." Science, April 26, 1996, p. 492

108. According to internal company documents, R.J. Reynolds knew as early as early as 1953 that there was a link between smoking and lung cancer. Associated Press, April 16, 1997

109. Tobacco company U.S. market shares as of December 1997 were Philip Morris 47.8%, RJR Nabisco 25.4%, Brown and Williamson/B.A.T. 15.8%, Lorillard 8.1%, and Liggett and Meyers 2%.
    Washington Post National Weekly Edition, March 9, 1998, p. 18

110. The cigarette industry through their outside law firms bankrolled Dr. Gary Huber's Texas Nutrition Institute and his Health Center for a total of $7.5 million. He became a leading critic of other scientists who were labeling tobacco smoke hazardous, but he has switched allegiance, and now may be a key witness in Texas' lawsuit against tobacco companies. When they discovered that Dr. Huber would testify for the state of Texas, tobacco company lawyers asked him to destroy some of his files and threatened him.
    Huber, a lung specialist, first worked with tobacco companies in 1972 at Harvard, when the industry funded a study of why some smokers eventually develop illnesses while other do not. The researchers were close to finding a link between cigarette smoke and emphysema when the industry cut funding for the project. Later, Huber discovered that R.J. Reynolds withheld evidence of other studies linking smoking and emphysema in animals. Huber believes that the industry paid scientists to replicate the same research to give the appearance that they

were legitimately researching the effects of smoking. Huber said, "They let us blindly chase rabbits. We got snookered."                                                              Dallas Morning News, October 25 and December 21, 1997

111. Tobacco industry lawyers contributed millions of dollars toward the work of a scientist known for poking holes in theories linking secondhand smoke to disease, according to a published report Saturday. Two law firms which represent Philip Morris and R.J. Reynolds have paid more than $7.5 million over 25 years to finance some of Dr. Gary L. Huber's work at three universities, the Dallas Morning News said. One hospital, the University of Texas Health center, hid the work Huber did for the tobacco lawyers and the $1.68 million they sent the hospital between 1985 and 1996, records show. Documents show that money was routed through an outside account with a Greek code name to keep it off hospital books.
Quote from Contra Costa (CA) Times, November 15, 1997, p. A11

112. The House Commerce Committee has released more than 800 previously secret tobacco industry documents that the industry had argued were protected by attorney-client privilege. The documents provide new details about how industry lawyers were involved in directing research projects that were not designed to find a relationship between smoking and cancer. Industry-funded lawyers in 1971 proposed paying $70,000 to a scientist who was "convinced that smoking has been given far too much consideration and air pollution too little." A Minnesota judge ruled that these documents showed that the industry and their lawyers had a long-running "conspiracy of silence and suppression of scientific research" about the health effects of smoking.
New York Times, December 19, 1997, p. A19

113. You've got to give them credit for audacity. With the noose of federal regulations and state lawsuits beginning to tighten around them, tobacco companies continue to find new, sneaky ways to promote their products-- particularly to kids. In some of their most immoral marketing initiatives to date, conglomerates such as Philip Morris and U.S. Tobacco have recently teamed up with singers and alternative rock groups to promote cigarettes and smokeless tobacco to teenagers. The slate of concert tours could not be more aggressively aimed at the youth market: from creating a slick Web page, to advertising in youthful magazines, to offering interactive games, Big Tobacco has impressionable 12- to 18-year-olds squarely in its cross hairs.

The latest outrage is the ROAR tour, a 40-city rock show that is being underwritten by U.S. Tobacco's Skoal brand of moist snuff--the most popular form of smokeless tobacco, a product whose use by teenage boys and young men has exploded in recent years. U.S. Tobacco sells a carefully graduated line of products intended to bring their young users all the way from cherry-flavored to full-blown addiction.

The ROAR (Revelation of Alternative Rhythms) tour includes '70s throwback Iggy Pop, and alternative rock groups like the Rev. Horton Heat, Sponge, Tonic, the Bloodhound Gang and others. It is being advertised on a Web site and in national magazines such as Details and Rolling Stone.

While it is illegal to sell tobacco products to anyone under the age of 18, the appeal of these bands to youth is unmistakable. Those under the age of 20 are the biggest purchasers of rock music. The companies are using the universal teen language of music to create the impression that tobacco is stylish, cool and acceptable.
Quote from Washington Post, May 11, 1997, p. C2 (William Novelli, Campaign for Tobacco-Free Kids)

114. The tobacco industry had $27.4 million in lobbying expenditures in 1996, led by Philip Morris with $19.6 million and the Tobacco Institute with $3.3 million.                              USA Today, June 24, 1997, p. 7A

115. The nation's five major tobacco companies will have spent more than $30 million on lobbying in 1997; in the first half of the year, they paid $5 million to Washington law firm for the services of political heavyweights as former Texas governor Ann Richards and former Senate Majority leader George Mitchell. The industry also retained former Republican Party chairman Haley Barbour, paying $800,000 to his law firm.
San Francisco Chronicle, December 15, 1997, p. A8 (from the New York Times)

116. The tobacco industry paid the Washington law firm of Verner, Liipfert, Benhard, McPherson and Hand a total of $4.7 million in the first half of 1997 for lobbying. The firm "has taken on a roster of senior stars--people like Bob Dole, Lloyd Bentsen, George Mitchell, and Ann Richards--whose names and influence are meant to attract big clients."                                                                       The Washington Monthly, November 1997, p. 5

117. In late 1997, the tobacco industry over several months quadrupled its expenses on lobbyists. Former Texas governor Ann Richards, an ex-smoker who implemented tough antismoking measures while in office, is

employed by Brown and Williamson, R.J. Reynolds, and Philip Morris; former senator and White House chief of staff Howard Baker is a lobbyist for these three companies plus U.S. Tobacco. He resigned his chairmanship of the board of trustees at Mayo Clinic after this apparent conflict was revealed. Ironically, Baker's first wife Joy, a heavy smoker, died of lung cancer and was treated at the Mayo Clinic. Other lobbyists on the payroll are former Senate Majority leader George Mitchell, former Republican National Committee chairman Haley Barbour, and seven former members of Congress.     CBS evening news, Dan Rather, December 1, 1997 (reporter Jim Stewart)

118. The worldwide revenues of tobacco companies exceed $120 billion each year, a larger amount than the gross domestic products of 180 of the world's 205 countries.     JAMA, May 28, 1997, p. 1652

119. In 1986, international cigarette sales for Philip Morris and R.J.R. combined were $6.8 billion, compared with $11.7 billion for domestic sales. In 1996, international sales had increased to $27.7 billion, and domestic sales to $17 billion.     USA Today, August 6, 1997, p. 7D

120. Does it matter whether the supplier of cigarettes in a country is the national government-owned monopoly or a Transnational Tobacco Company (TTC)? Absolutely. A government-owned monopoly may acknowledge the health consequences of smoking and may cooperate with government health initiatives. For example, in China all tobacco stores close on World No-Tobacco Day, to the agony of some desperate smokers. A monopoly might not advertise at all, but if it does, its ads will likely be amateurish. Product quality is typically poor, with a harsh, unflavoured taste. Lack of competition means that prices are higher and retail outlets are fewer than would otherwise be the case. Packages may be unalluring. Wholesale distribution may be inefficient.

In contrast, TTCs deny the health consequences of smoking, ruthlessly market cigarettes, vigorously fight against regulatory efforts, and if there is regulation, capitalize on loopholes in the laws. TTCs use attractive packaging, push for an expanded number of retail outlets, and sell flavoured cigarettes that are easier to smoke.     Quote from *Smoke and Mirrors*, p. 13

121. One additional point of market share for a premium cigarette brand can mean $450 million a year in additional U.S. sales. Since four companies control 98% of the market, there is little incentive to try to steal market share through price cutting; heavy discounting would only lower everyone's profits.     Washington Post National Weekly Edition, March 9, 1998, p. 19

122. "We will never produce and market a product shown to be the cause of any serious ailment."     Passage from the first draft of "A Frank Statement to Cigarette Smokers" which was left out of the final version (*Faber Book of Smoking*, p. 110)

123. Health economist Kenneth Warner, Ph.D., advocates the measures that tobacco companies could take if, as they profess, "...improving the public's health were truly their paramount interest and if they truly wanted to gain the public health community's trust and cooperation."

They are:
1. End all forms of tobacco advertising and promotion.
2. Cooperate to raise cigarette prices substantially.
3. Get serious about youth tobacco prevention programs.
4. Get out of the way of state and local government initiatives to protect nonsmokers from exposure to tobacco smoke.
5. Immediately cease all hard- and soft-money political contributions.
6. Handsomely fund an organization assisting smokers to quit.
7. Stop trying to buy the loyalty – or at least the silence – of researchers by setting up company-funded research programs.
8. Adopt plain packaging with graphic Canadian-style warning labels occupying half of the front and back of each pack.
9. Voluntarily comply with all of the marketing, manufacturing, and sales restrictions that the Justice Department is seeking in its legal action against the industry.
10. Facilitate development of effective federal regulation of all nicotine and tobacco products.     American Journal of Public Health, June 2002, pp. 898-899

124. Cigarette manufacturers in the United States spent $9.57 billion on advertising and promotion in 2000, a 16.2% increase from the $8.24 billion spent in 1999. Promotional allowances, including payments to retailers for shelf space, increased to $3.91 billion, up from $3.54 billion in 1999.    Federal Trade Commission Report, May 2002

125. The British American Tobacco factory in Southampton, England, manufactures 48 billion cigarettes each year.

*Cigarettes* (Parker-Pope), pp. 62-63

126. The first Bonsack machine produced about three cigarettes each second, compared to modern machines which produce as many as 70 cigarettes a second.    *Cigarettes* (Parker-Pope), p. 63

127. Insurance companies invest heavily in tobacco stocks. In 1999, Cigna's tobacco holdings were $42.7 million; MetLife had invested $62.1 million, and Prudential, $892 million.    JAMA, August 9, 2000, p. 697

128. The five largest U.S. cigarette companies are worth $157 billion domestically; Philip Morris' global cigarette business is worth an estimated $118 billion.    Associated Press, June 7, 2000

129. The leading cigarette brand in 2000 continues to be Marlboro, with 37.7% of the U.S. market. No other brand hits double figures. Newport, the leading menthol brand, has 7.6% of the U.S. market. Winston has only 4.8% of the market share, and Camel 5.4%. The discount brands Doral (6.2%) and Basic (5.1%) are also relatively strong.

2002 AMA Annual Tobacco Report

130. According to the World Health Organization, tobacco companies have attempted to undermine tobacco control efforts by funding seemingly unbiased scientific groups; therefore "manipulating the political and scientific debate concerning tobacco and health."    British Medical Journal, March 10, 2001, p. 576

131. In 1999, RJR sold $7.56 billion worth of tobacco in the United States, an increase of 33% from the previous year. Philip Morris' 1999 domestic sales were $19.6 billion, an increase of 28% from1998.

*Cigarettes* (Parker-Pope), p. 167

132. Biggest Tobacco Companies in the World (2000)

| Company | Global Market Share (%) | |
|---|---|---|
| China National Tobacco Corp. | 32.7 | |
| Philip Morris Cos. (USA) | 17.3 | |
| British American Tobacco Co. (UK) | 16.0 | |
| Japan Tobacco (Japan) | 9.0 | |
| R.J.Reynolds Tobacco (USA) | 2.0 | |
| Reemtsma (Germany) | 2.0 | |
| Altadis (France and Spain) | 2.0 | *Cigarettes* (Parker-Pope), p. 167 |

133. World's Most Popular Cigarette Brands (2000)

| Brand and Manufacturer | Volume Sales | World Market Share | |
|---|---|---|---|
| Marlboro (Philip Morris) | 476 billion | 9.4% | |
| Mild Seven (Japan Tobacco) | 135 billion | 2.7% | |
| L&M (Philip Morris) | 91 billion | 1.8% | |
| Winston (R.J.Reynolds) | 7.1 billion | 1.4% | |
| Camel (R.J.Reynolds) | 67 billion | 1.3% | *Cigarettes* (Parker-Pope), p. 167 |

134. U.S. Tobacco Company Cigarette Volume and Market Share

| Company | Volume | Market Share |
|---|---|---|
| Philip Morris | 212 billion | 50.5% |
| R.J.Reynolds | 96 billion | 23.0% |
| B&W | 49 billion | 11.7% |
| Lorillard | 40 billion | 9.6% |
| Commonwealth | 7.5 billion | 1.8% |
| Liggett | 6.4 billion | 1.5% |
| Others | 8 billion | 1.9% |

2002 AMA Annual Tobacco Report

135. A special review of international tobacco issues was published in the industry trade publication, *Tobacco Journal International*, in December 2001. The article indicates that the "big three" tobacco producers are Philip Morris, British American Tobacco, and Japan Tobacco. For the year 2000, their market share worldwide was:

|  | *Cigarettes Sold* | *Cigarette Production* |
|---|---|---|
| Philip Morris | 887.3 billion | 16.5% of total world production |
| BAT | 807.0 billion | 15.0% of total |
| Japan Tobacco | 447.9 billion | 8.1% of total |

Philip Morris is described as the "undisputed market leader" with the world's most popular brand (Marlboro), operating in 180 markets worldwide, with 50 factories either wholly or partly owned. Marlboro has a market volume greater than the next 7 competitive brands combined. In 2000, the company generated revenues of $22.7 billion domestically, and $26.4 internationally.

BAT has over 300 brands in its stable, with 86 factories in 64 countries. It is described as the most aggressive in promoting local and regional brands, as well as building "global" ones (Benson & Hedges, Lucky Strike, Dunhill, Pall Mall, Kool). BAT is focusing on markets outside the U.S. and European Union. In May 2001, BAT became the only major tobacco company to establish a joint venture in China, at Mianyang in the Sichuan province. This allows BAT to build a factory in China, the first such outside effort. It also has plans to build new factories in South Korea and Vietnam.

Japan Tobacco International, headquartered in Geneva, was created in 1985 by privatization of the state tobacco monopoly. When it bought the RJR international tobacco section in 1999, it became a major player in the world market. The company operates in 170 countries, and is particularly active in Russia, with a 20% market share. Its factory in St. Petersburg may be the world's largest. With over 190 brands, its 4 international brands are Mild Seven, Camel, Salem, and Winston. It is concentrating its efforts in Asia, Eastern Europe, and Russia.                                        2002 AMA Annual Tobacco Report

136. A report on tobacco companies in Latin America, *Profits over People*, "reveals that tobacco companies:
   - hired scientists throughout Latin America and the Caribbean to misrepresent the science linking second-hand smoke to serious diseases, while cloaking in secrecy any connection of these scientists with the tobacco industry;
   - designed youth smoking prevention campaigns and programmes primarily as public relations exercises aimed at deterring meaningful regulation of tobacco marketing;
   - had detailed knowledge of smuggling networks and markets and actively sought to increase their share of the illegal market by structuring marketing campaigns and distribution routes around it; and
   - enjoyed access to key government officials and succeeded in weakening or killing tobacco control legislation in a number of countries."                   The Lancet, December 21-28, 2002, p. 2057

137. In 1995, the global tobacco industry produced an estimated 2.26 million kilograms of manufactured waste, and 209 million kilograms of chemical waste.                 British Medical Association (www.tobaccofactfile.org)

138. The tobacco industry earns approximately 50,000 British pounds (equal to 82,000 U.S. dollars) during the lifetime of each new smoker that they recruit.            British Medical Association (www.tobaccofactfile.org)

139. In 1998, the combined tobacco revenues were more than $88 billion for the three largest multinational tobacco companies, Philip Morris, Japan Tobacco, and British American Tobacco.
                                        British Medical Association (www.tobaccofactfile.org)

140. Modern cigarette manufacturing machines use more than six kilometers of paper per hour.
                                        British Medical Association (www.tobaccofactfile.org)

141. In 2000, the top U.S. cigarette brands and market share were Marlboro (35.4%), Doral (6.3%), Newport (6.2%), Camel (5.3%), Winston (5.2%), Basic (4.9%), GPC (4.7%), Kool (3.3%), Salem (3.2%), and Virginia Slims (2.6%).                                     The Tobacco Timeline (www.tobacco.org)

142. London-based British American Tobacco (BAT) earned $1.5 billion in profit on revenue of more than $18 billion in 2002.                                     New York Times, February 2, 2002, p.3

143. Devised in the 1950s and the 1960s, the tobacco industry's strategy was embodied in a script written by the lawyers. Every tobacco company executive in the public eye was told to learn the script backwards and forwards, no deviation allowed. The basic premise was simple – smoking had not been proved to cause cancer. Not proven, not proven, not proven – this would be stated insistently and repeatedly. Inject a thin wedge of doubt, create controversy, never deviate from the prepared lines. It was a simple plan, and it worked.

Quote from *A Queston of Intent*, David Kessler, p. xiii

# R J Reynolds

1. After the merger of Nabisco and RJ Reynolds in 1985, RJR Nabisco became the largest consumer product company in the United States.

2. For RJ Reynolds, tobacco products account for 36% of the company's total revenue, but for 64% of company profits.
*Nicotine Addiction,* p. 47

3. At the RJ Reynolds plant in Winston-Salem N.C., 8200 workers produced 142 billion cigarettes in 1993, or 546 million each working day. Sears, Roebuck & Co. has banned smoking in all of its nationwide stores, the only exception being its store in Winston-Salem. Likewise, JC Penney made an exception for its store at the Hanes Mall in Winston-Salem.
San Francisco Chronicle, April 28, 1994

4. After Henry Kravis' leveraged buyout of RJ Reynolds/Nabisco, RJR CEO Ross Johnson resigned in early 1989 and received a $53 million "golden parachute" for leaving. RJR lost nearly $500 million on the Premier smokeless cigarette, which was never marketed.
*Barbarians at the Gate*, Bryan Burrough and John Helyar, Harper and Row, 1990, p. 507 and HBO Pictures' Barbarians at the Gate, 1993

5. "One customer said R.J. Reynold's ill-fated 'smokeless' Premier brand, which lasted only five months in 1988, smelled 'as if you'd just opened a grave on a warm day.'"    Contra Costa (Calif.) Times, July 3, 1997, p. A17

6. Fewer than 5% of smokers in testing liked the taste of Premier. "In Japan, another team of researchers quickly learned to translate at least one sentence of Japanese: 'This tastes like shit.'" CEO Ross Johnson said that it smelled "like a fart."    *Barbarians at the Gate*, Bryan Burrough and John Helyar, Harper and Row, 1990, p. 112

7. "Consumer dislike also quickly snuffed out RJR Nabisco Holdings Corp's smokeless cigarette, a $325 million project first called Premier. One person who tried it immediately declared the cigarette 'tasted like (expletive).' And he was the company's chief executive. Back to the drawing board. A $100 million reformulation led to a brand- new product called Eclipse. It quickly lived up to its name and was pulled off the shelves."
Associated Press, May 29, 1999

8. "Within weeks of its unveiling, Premier had taken its place alongside the Edsel in the pantheon of American marketing catastrophes."
*Ashes to Ashes*, p. 604

9. R.J. Reynold's "smokeless" cigarette Premier bombed in 1990 after seven years of research and $325 million. It was on the market for only four months.    U.S. News and World Report, February 24, 1997, p. 15

10. RJR Nabisco in 1992 had a new chairman and CEO, Charles "Mike" Harper. A former heavy smoker, he quit in 1985 following a heart attack. Before his RJR appointment, Harper created and became the driving force behind ConAgra's Healthy Choice line of frozen foods.    Tobacco Free Youth Reporter, Summer 1993

11. RJ Reynolds Tobacco Co. sued one of its former scientists, Anthony Colucci, and requested a court order barring him from revealing confidential information he gained during 15 years as a Reynolds scientist. Colucci, who has

smoked himself for more than 30 years, said on ABC's Primetime Live that Reynolds had shut down a biological research program in 1970 because it was on the verge of proving a link between smoking and lung cancer.

*American Medical News*, March 1, 1993

12. RJ Reynolds III, 60, grandson of the founder of the tobacco company that bears his name, died in July 1994 of emphysema and congestive heart failure after a lifetime of cigarette smoking. Attendees at his memorial service were asked to forego flowers in a favor of donations to Citizens for Smokefree America, an antismoking group founded by his brother Patrick Reynolds. *Time*, July 25, 1994, p. 19

13. "If I thought in my heart of hearts that smoking was bad for one, I would resign."

Gerald Long, RJR executive (*No Stranger to Tears*, p. 327)

14. "The occasion for tobacco's return to the political stage was the revelation, via press leaks, of the R.J. Reynolds Tobacco Company's strategy for targeting two new brands of cigarettes on groups that have proved resistant to anti-tobacco health warnings—'Uptown,' aimed at blacks, of whom some 41% smoke, compared with 31% of whites; and 'Dakota,' aimed at 'virile females' aged 18-24, not educated beyond high school, keen to have a boyfriend, and happy to share with him in 'tough man competition' spectator sports, such as hot-rod racing."

*The Lancet*, March 3, 1990, p. 527

15. RJR is testing a new nearly smokeless cigarette called Eclipse which heats rather than burns tobacco, delivering nicotine on heated vapor. It is said to show reductions of 90 percent or more in secondhand smoke and in many compounds linked to cancer. This is RJR's biggest effort to introduce a safer cigarette since the $300 million marketing debacle of Premier in the late 1980's. Philip Morris in 1989 also lost $350 million in an unsuccessful attempt to market de-nicotinized cigarettes. *New York Times*, April 12, 1996, pp. D1 and D17

16. RJR is test marketing its Eclipse smokeless cigarette in Chattanooga, Tennessee. Because the tobacco and glycerol is heated and not burned, the health risk from inhaling Eclipse secondhand tobacco smoke appears to be reduced more than 90%. But the relatively high yields of nicotine and carbon monoxide suggest that the risk for cardiovascular disease is as high as it is for regular cigarettes.

*Journal of the National Cancer Institute*, October 2, 1996, p. 1341

17. A new cigarette called Jumbos is being manufactured by an RJR subsidiary called Moonlight Tobacco Company. There is an elephant on the front and back of the box, and on the side is a little man in the moon blowing smoke rings. On each individual cigarette, where the brand name usually goes, is a tiny drawing of an elephant.

Bob Herbert column, *New York Times*, November 18, 1996

18. In Bucharest, Romania, R.J. Reynolds provided a year's supply of bulbs for traffic lights in exchange for permission to add a Camel logo in silhouette to each yellow light.

*Washington Post National Weekly Edition*, December 9-15, 1996, p. 9

19. In late 1999, R.J. Reynolds debuted vanilla, citrus, and spice flavored Camel cigarettes.

*US News and World Report*, February 7, 2000, p. 15

20. RJR in 1999 planned to sell its international tobacco business to Japan Tobacco for $7.8 billion.

*U.S. News and World Report*, March 22, 1999, p. 50

21. RJR CEO Steven Goldstone was paid more than $12 million in 1998. *USA Today*, March 19, 1999, p. B1

22. Steven Goldstone, the chief executive officer of RJR Nabisco, gave up cigarette smoking 17 years ago at this physician's insistence. But commenting on the risks of tobacco, he has said, "Not to be too red-white-and-blue about it, but taking risks is what this country is about." *NEJM*, January 23, 1997, p. 307

23. RJR is test marketing an "all-natural" version of its Winston brand in Florida. The company proclaims in ads running in Sports Illustrated, People and Rolling Stone that it has taken out the additives and flavorings and left "100 percent tobacco," branded across each ad are the words "No Bull." Health officials say the campaign is an attempt to make smokers perceive the cigarette as safer and healthier, and they fear that as a result, fewer people

will quit. Ironically, the tobacco industry says that its additives, lists of which are protected as trade secrets, are completely safe.                                                                   American Medical News, October 28, 1996

24.    The November 1997 UC Berkeley Wellness Letter contained an article entitled "It's the 94% that'll kill you." It is quoted below:

    R.J. Reynolds has launched a big ad campaign boasting that its Winston cigarettes are "100% tobacco", while other brands are "94% tobacco, 6% additives." Claims that cigarette brands are "natural" or "additive-free" are ridiculous, since tobacco naturally contains so many toxic chemicals, and there's no way of really knowing what's in any brand. Under attack by leading health groups, Reynolds denies that it is implying that Winstons are safer or that it's making any sort of health claim. We can't help wondering why, then, this Winston ad was the only tobacco ad in the September issue of *Self*, a health magazine for young women. In any case, many of the known additives have been approved for use in food. So the 6% additives may be the safest part of the cigarettes.

25.    R.J. Reynolds was one of the 1997 recipients of the Harlan Page Hubbard Lemon Award for "misleading, unfair and irresponsible" advertising. The company won for its Winston "No Bull" campaign that implies that its "additive-free" cigarettes are safer than other brands.                                    USA Today, December 5, 1997, p. B6

# Philip Morris

1.    In the 1850's a London tobacconist named Philip Morris began to manufacture handmade cigarettes on a special order basis.    *Cigarette Confidential*, p. 84

2.    "Among those catering to the new fashion in smoking was a Bond street tobacconist named Philip Morris, about whom little is known personally other than that he died at a relatively young age in 1873 and the business was carried on for a time by his widow, Margaret, and brother Leopold. In his early days Morris discreetly sold fine Havana 'seegars' and Virginia pipe tobacco to the carriage trade, but when returning Crimean veterans began asking for cigarettes, he quickly accommodated. Stressing to his select clientele that he had the cleanest factory and used the best paper, the purest aromatic tobaccos, and the finest cork tipping to keep the cigarette from sticking to the lips, Philip Morris helped lend to the product a cachet it had not previously enjoyed. He called his brands Oxford and Cambridge Blues, later adding Oxford Ovals."                                    *Ashes to Ashes*, p. 13

3.    "Philip Morris, the man, was a London tobacco merchant who was among the earliest purveyors of hand-rolled cigarettes under the brand names Oxford and Cambridge Blues. Morris dies in 1873, but the company continued without him. In 1902, the tiny firm opened a New York office, and by World War II the company was prospering and traded on the New York Stock Exchange. Today Philip Morris is the world's biggest commercial tobacco company (not counting China's state-controlled tobacco monopoly), and its famous Marlboro brand is the world's best-selling cigarette, with an 8.4 percent share of the world market."                                    *Cigarettes* (Parker-Pope), p. 31

4.    "The firm of Philip Morris, which had moved across the Atlantic and was now a New York niche manufacturer, was first into the market. It revived one of its English trademarks, named after the Duke of Marlborough, which it abbreviated to 'Marlboro'. The new brand – slogan: 'Mild as May' (1924) – began life as one for the ladies, targeting 'decent, respectable' women. Initial advertising copy adopted a softly softly approach –as if there was still a need to justify women smoking: 'Has smoking any more to do with a woman's morals than has the color of her hair?… Women – when they smoke at all – quickly develop discerning taste. That is why Marlboros now ride in so many limousines, attend so many bridge parties, and repose in so many handbags.' Marlboros were not only branded but engineered for women, incorporating an ivory tip of greaseproof paper to prevent them adhering to lipstick."                                    *Tobacco* (Gately), p. 244

5.    "Women--when they smoke at all – quickly develop discerning taste. That is why Marlboros ride in so many limousines, attend so many bridge parties, repose in so many hand bags." 1927 advertisement (*Ashes to Ashes*, p. 74)

6.    In 1960, Marlboro had only a 4% market share, and 3% of the 18-year-old market. Sales began to increase rapidly in 1963, when Philip Morris "launched a big-budget television ad campaign with the Marlboro cowboy riding along through the sagebrush."                                    Washington Post National Weekly Edition, March 9, 1998, p. 19

7. Philip Morris in 1965 began to use ammonia in Marlboro cigarettes. The chemical boosted the brand's nicotine "kick" as well as improved the taste. Ammonia makes the smoke less acidic, which increases the amount of "free nicotine," which is more readily absorbed in the lungs. RJ Reynolds, makers of the Winston competing brand, called ammonia "the secret of Marlboro." Associated Press, February 9, 1998

8. The 1.6-million-square-foot Philip Morris plant in Richmond, VA, is being expanded to produce between 580 and 600 million cigarettes each day. This is 410,000 cigarettes every minute, or about a third of domestic consumption. And the company's plant in Cabarrus County, N.C., is undergoing a $400 million expansion.
New York Times magazine, March 20, 1994

9. The Philip Morris plant in Richmond VA produces half a billion cigarettes each day. The factory tour for visitors and the gift shop were closed in late 1993, and visitors are no longer permitted to enter the plant, ostensibly as a cost-cutting measure. New York Times, March 8, 1994, A14

10. Marlboro cigarettes are the best-selling packaged product in the world, and the Marlboro cowboy is the most widely recognized advertising image in the world. Marlboro sales were $15 billion worldwide in 1993.
New York Times magazine, March 20, 1994, p. 36
and Washington Post National Weekly Edition, July 11, 1994, p. 19

11. On April 2, 1993, Philip Morris cut the retail price of a pack of Marlboros by 40 cents. The move cost the company $2 billion at the time, but a year later, the Marlboro market share had risen from 22 to 27 percent, its highest point ever. New York Times magazine, March 20, 1994, p. 73

12. Philip Morris cut Marlboro prices by 40 cents a pack in April 1993. One comment was: "Virtually all new users of Marlboro start as teenagers or younger. It's that market that they're trying to expand and addict before the Federal Government increases the tax" (New York Times, April 3, 1993, p. A1). Another media comment was: "Philip Morris' new motto should be, 'sell'em cheap, hook'em young.'" SCARC, April 28, 1993

13. Philip Morris stock was up by 48% from May 1994 to May 1995. The Philip Morris decision to cut prices of their premium brands by 20% on April 2, 1993 is now seen as a brilliant decision. That day has now become known as Marlboro Friday, when the company got back a lot of smokers who had switched to cheaper discount brands. Marlboro's market share increased from 22 percent in April 1993 to 30 percent in April 1995, a market share more than for all of RJR's brands combined. San Francisco Chronicle, May 1995

14. "In pushing its cigarettes, Philip Morris acts just like a shelf drug dealer selling cocaine or heroin. Standard operating procedure for a dealer is to give away the drugs free or at low cost to get the kids addicted. Once hooked, the dealer starts charging as much as he can. As cigarette sales of the Philip Morris flagship brand Marlboro slipped, the cigarette merchant lowered the price sharply to make a pack easier to purchase by those with fewer dollars, such as the young and the poor. Lured by the low prices, thousands got hooked on Marlboros."
*Radical Surgery*, Joseph A. Califano, Times Books, 1994, p. 106

15. Marlboro is not only the leading cigarette in the US and in the world, it is the number one consumer product in the world, slightly ahead of Coca-Cola. INFACT, April 1994 (9th World Conference on Tobacco or Health, Paris, 1994)

16. 340 billion Marlboros were smoked worldwide in 1991. 26% of adult Americans choose Marlboro as their brand, but the Marlboro market share in adolescents is well over 50%. Journal of Family Practice, June 1992, p. 698

17. "Cigarette companies are adjusting to the changing marketplace by introducing new products. Next up: Marlboro Express, a shorter cigarette with the same amount of tar and nicotine. It's aimed at those hurried folks who now must suck down whole cigarettes as they huddle outside their smoke-free office buildings."
Newsweek, March 21, 1994, p. 53

18. The president of Philip Morris denied reports that the company is developing a new shorter high-nicotine cigarette called "Marlboro Express" for people who want to get their nicotine "fix" quickly on smoke breaks.
April 14, 1994, testimony to Congress (CSPAN)

19. At the 1992 Philip Morris annual meeting, a video montage of company products was shown as actor James Earl Jones intoned: "Consumers choose our brands with confidence." Against images of Marlboro cowboys and Virginia Slims tennis players, the actor boasted that such advertising "rises above barriers of language and geography--dynamic brands generating unforgettable excitement."

20. Philip Morris in 1992 had a 50% profit margin on its premium brands and $59 billion in revenues.

American Medical News, November 14, 1994, p. 16

21. Philip Morris paid $4.5 billion in taxes in 1992 on revenues of $59 billion. It employs 161,000 people (92,000 in the US), spends $2 billion a year on advertising (including $50 million for the introduction of Marlboro Medium in 1991), and contributes $50 million a year to charitable organizations. Some of the latter include the NAACP, the United Negro College Fund, and the National Association on Drug Abuse.

New York Times magazine, March 20, 1994, p. 36

22. The 1996 Marlboro US market share increased to 32.1%, the highest ever. Philip Morris now has 46.1% of the domestic market, while RJR continues to decline, now controlling 25.7%.

Wall Street Journal, April 16, 1996, p. B1

23. Marlboro is the first tobacco product to be named to the marketing Hall of Fame, and now has a 30% market share, more than five times the market share of Winston, the No. 2 brand.    New York Times, April 10, 1996, p. D6

24. The United States accounts for less than half of Philip Morris's $23.8 billion in tobacco sales, but nearly 75% of its $6.5 billion in tobacco profits.    San Francisco Chronicle, January 12, 1993, p. C1

25. In 1996 Philip Morris sold 891 billion cigarettes worldwide, a record, up 9.3% over 1995. Total revenue was $69.2 billion with profits of $6.3 billion, and its domestic market share was 49%. For the first time, the company produced more than 400 billion cigarettes in its United States facilities. Overseas, its Eastern European market share grew from 22% to 28% in a single year. The company's market value was $94 billion in 1996, and it was the third most profitable American company, after Exxon and General Electric.

New York Times, January 30, 1997, p. D2, and Time, March 31, 1997, p. 33

26. About half of the $69 billion Philip Morris annual revenue comes from cigarettes.

Associated Press, August 21, 1997

27. Philip Morris annual revenues are greater than the $52 billion gross domestic product of the country of Chile.

Sierra magazine, May-June 1998, p. 17

28. In 1997, Philip Morris had 51% of the United States cigarette market, led by Marlboro, with a 35.2% market share.

New York Times, July 23, 1997, p. D2

29. In the 1980's, Philip Morris acquired General Foods (Miller, Lowenbrau and Sharp's beer, Tang, Kool-Aid, Breyers ice cream, Birds Eye Vegetables, Post cereals, Oscar Meyer hot dogs, Stove Top, Log Cabin, Jello, Maxwell House coffee) and Kraft (Miracle Whip, Parkay margarine, Velveeta cheese, Cheezwhiz). RJR acquired Nabisco (Ritz crackers, Oreo cookies, Life Saver candies) and Del Monte.

US News and World Report, February 15, 1993, p. 86

30. After Kraft Foods was taken over by Philip Morris, the company was forced to change its smokefree policy, and "no smoking" signs were replaced by ashtrays.    Tobacco Free Youth Reporter, Fall 1993, p. 9

31. Philip Morris stock climbed from $22 per share in mid-1988 to $87 in 1992, quadrupling an investor's money if reinvested dividends are included. 65% of the company's profits and 42% of revenues come from cigarette sales, primarily the Marlboro brand. The share price had been $10 in 1984, and increased at a 35% annualized rate of return to 1991.    Kiplinger magazine, July 1992, p. 28

32. John S. Reed, the chairman of Citicorp, sits on the board of directors of both Philip Morris (for a yearly fee of $40,000) and the Memorial Sloan-Kettering Cancer Center.    New York Times magazine, March 20, 1994, p. 37

33. Joseph Cullman, former president of Philip Morris, characterized his company as "one of the most socially responsible corporations in the world" in response to criticism by former Surgeon General C. Everett Koop.

Yale magazine, March 1991, p. 10

34. Hamish Maxwell served as chairman of Philip Morris from 1983 to 1991. During this time, the company's stock multiplied nearly eight-fold, and he was given a $46 million bonus on his retirement. This was more than the entire combined annual income of all of Virginia's tobacco farmers, and more than the annual amount of tobacco taxes that the state of Virginia collects each year.

35. In May 1995, Philip Morris had a $200 million recall of eight billion cigarettes with filters contaminated with methyl isothiocyanate, a chemical used as a commercial pesticide. The affected cigarettes had a foul odor and metallic taste, and caused eye, nose, and throat irritation, dizziness, coughing, and wheezing.

Tobacco Control, Autumn 1995, p. 215

36. After the recall, Philip Morris stock held steady as investors determined that a $200 million recall was of little consequence for a company so large and profitable.                San Francisco Chronicle, May 27, 1995, p. E1

37. In May 1995 when Philip Morris recalled 8 billion cigarettes because of methyl isothiocyanate in the filters, most of the health complaints from persons smoking the cigarettes came from cigarette smoke itself, not the contaminant.

JAMA, April 26, 1996, p. 1225

38. One observer commented about the 'voluntary" recall of Philip Morris cigarettes with defective filters in the spring of 1995: "They've taken a product that kills you and have recalled it because it makes you dizzy."

NEJM, September 26, 2996, p. 981

39. Philip Morris has sponsored the Bolshoi Ballet in Hawaii and a Russian art exhibit at the Metropolitan Museum of Art in New York.                Journal of the National Cancer Institute Monograph No. 12, 1992, p. 32

40. "I'll tell you what I like about the business. First, there are no surprises. There is nothing more to be said or discovered about the cigarette business or the industry...Second, no new company wants to get into the tobacco business. That's great. Third, we have the best partners in the world: the governments."

David Dangoor, Executive Vice President, Philip Morris International (INFACT, April 1994)

41. Philip Morris gave $75,000 to Strive, an East Harlem job-training program for disadvantaged young people. However, they then spent an equal amount to buy a two page ad in the New York Times magazine touting this contribution.                *Ashes to Ashes*, p. 620

42. Philip Morris ran a full page ad in the New York Times (March 3, 1998, p. A11) touting its financial support of New York's meals on wheels program. The company promised to match all donors' gifts to the meals program, and said: "It's more than food. It's comfort, dignity, and knowing that someone cares...sharing the commitment. Building the solution. Philip Morris Companies Inc."

43. An estimated 19 million T-shirts, caps, jackets and other items with Marlboro logos were sent out in 1994, making Philip Morris the nation's third largest mail order house.                New York Times, August 27, 1995, p. F11

44. According to one study, Marlboro cigarette's sponsorship of an automobile racing team in the 1989 season gave Marlboro nearly 3 ½ hours of television exposure and 146 mentions of the brand name. This exposure had a value of $8.4 million. In the Indianapolis 500, Marlboro received more than $2.6 million in advertising exposure. In the Marlboro Grand Prix, race officials wore Marlboro Grand Prix shirts and caps, and the Marlboro logo or game appeared 5,933 times during the broadcast.                Federal Register, August 11, 1995, p. 41337

45. In 1972, Marlboro became the world's No. 1 cigarette, and now has a brand name (valued at $39.5 billion in 1993 by Financial World magazine) that vies with Coca Cola for the title of the world's most valuable trademark. Its US

market share is now 30 percent, the highest ever, and outsells the brands ranked second through sixth combined.

New York Times, August 27, 1995, p. F11

46. Margaret Thatcher accepted a $1 million retainer from Philip Morris to act as a global consultant and to advise the company on "penetration of tobacco markets in Eastern Europe and Third World countries." She does not smoke, although her husband is a heavy smoker.

Canadian Medical Association Journal, January 15, 1993, p. 243, and The Lancet, August 1, 1992, p. 294

47. The industry has hired big guns to help it expand internationally. Philip Morris hired former British Prime Minister Margaret Thatcher as a consultant on "geopolitical affairs," reportedly paying her US $1 million over 3 years. A 1992 company memo listing issues on which she "may be able to offer guidance and assistance" included "China Entry Strategy," "Vietnam Entry Strategy," and "Singapore Anti-Tobacco Programs." Clayton Yeutter, US Trade Representative from 1985 to 1989, has since jointed BAT's Board of Directors. To help break into South Korea, R.J. Reynolds hired Richard Allen, one-time national security adviser to US President Ronald Reagan; Philip Morris hired Michael Deaver, a former White House aide to Reagan. A Philip Morris memo would later boast that Deaver "was given a welcome ordinarily reserved for the highest foreign dignitaries" when he visited South Korea on behalf of the company.

Quote from Smoke and Mirrors, p. 214

48. A Philip Morris internal report concedes that nicotine is chemically similar to cocaine and that people smoke primarily to get nicotine into their bodies. A Philip Morris spokesman said that the report did not reflect the view of the company.

Associated Press, December 9, 1995

49. "The number one cause of death in our society is not drugs, alcohol, or tobacco. It is not heart disease, lung cancer, or emphysema. It's Marlboro."

Journal of Medical Activism, 1994 (Alan Blum)

50. "...health care professionals would do well to view the leading preventable cause of death as Marlboro rather than as heart disease, lung cancer, or emphysema."

Journal of Family Practice, June 1992, p. 698 (Alan Blum)

51. Billie Jean King in a letter to the editor of the New York Times in December 1993 wrote defending Virginia Slims tennis, "The Philip Morris executives I know...are enlightened people who understand and acknowledge the possible hazards of smoking."

Ashes to Ashes, p. 390

52. Billie Jean King has been nominated to the Philip Morris Board of Directors. The former world champion tennis player has a 30-year relationship with the company since her participation in the first Virginia Slims tennis matches.

Alan Blum. M.D.

53. Time, January 8, 1996, commented on a Philip Morris promotion. "Philip Morris has the ticket. To Marlboro Country. This August the Marlboro Unlimited--a multimillion-dollar, 20-car, specially built train sporting high glass-domed passenger cars, a cinema, a dance club, hot tubs, staterooms with private baths and, everywhere, the Marlboro logo--embarks from Denver for the first of 20 five-day treks through the West. One hundred winners of a sweepstakes drawing, who must testify they are smokers over 21, will be flown to the train with their guests and receive $1,000 mad money. They will take side trips on horseback, white-water raft and hot-air balloon. They will see private shows by country singers and rodeo stars and savor a guilty pleasure few trains now offer: smoking catarrhs--sorry, smoking cars--galore. There will also be a few smoke-free areas."

54. In 1984, Philip Morris created the Marlboro Adventure Team as a means of promoting its flagship cigarette brand in West Germany. This promotion marked a departure from the cowboy theme, depicting instead a variety of wilderness activities such as off-road motorcycling, white-water rafting, and mountaineering. In addition to a chance to join the team, consumers were able to purchase "Adventure Gear" equipment and souvenirs with Marlboro proof-of-purchase coupons. By 1992, the promotion had appeared in Belgium, Switzerland, Italy and Turkey. DOC, an international organization of health professionals, was founded in 1977 to counteract the promotion of lethal lifestyles, especially tobacco advertising, by means of paid satirical counter-advertising. Between 1988 and 1992, DOC achieved modest successes in Colorado and Wyoming in ending a tobacco promotion known as the Marlboro Ski challenge, by means of the purchase of advertisements promoting the "Barfboro Ski Challenge" ("barfing" is American slang for "vomiting" and is frequently used on popular TV shows). In 1993, in an effort to undermine the Marlboro Adventure Team's US debut in the western states, DOC

repainted a Volkswagen van as the Barfmobile, hired a handsome comedian as the Barf Man, printed thousands of Barfboro Barf Bags, and created the Barfboro Barfing Team. Canvassing six western states in 1993 and six northeastern states in 1994, the Barfing Team coordinated dozens of community activities designed to get young people to laugh at the Marlboro Adventure Team. The growing popularity of the Barfboro Barfing Team--a low-cost, newsworthy, easily replicated, and readily updated promotion--highlights the importance of shifting the focus of anti-smoking efforts from generic campaigns that emphasize the dangers and ugliness of smoking, and instead onto brandname-ridicule aimed at changing the attitudes of young users toward Marlboro.

Quote from *Tobacco and Health*, p. 656 (Alan Blum)

55. Philip Morris magazine is sent out free six times a year to 13 million people on the company's mailing list.
*Ashes to Ashes*, p. 626

56. Philip Morris is producing a new quarterly magazine called Unlimited: Action, Adventure, Good Times. About 2 million free copies will be mailed out at a cost of up to $3 million an issue. "Marlboro marketers probably hope the magazine makes readers feel smoking fits well with an adventurous lifestyle and that tobacco opponents are wimps." Associated Press, October 9, 1996

57. Philip Morris claims that more than 200,000 U.S. retailers receive merchandising benefits as part of its retail incentive programs. There are 1.5 million U.S. cigarette retailers in all.     Stop Tobacco Access for Minors Project

58. Marlboro passed Winston as the best-selling U.S. cigarette at the end of 1975. In 1977, Financial World named PM CEO Joseph Cullman as U.S. executive of the year.     *Ashes to Ashes*, pp. 397 and 407

59. The San Diego Museum of Art rejected a Philip Morris-sponsored exhibition, reportedly worth $1 million, and the Del Mar fair (San Diego County) has rejected $175,000 from Philip Morris to conduct tobacco promotions at the fair.     ANR Update, Summer 1996

60. The Molecular Sciences Institute of La Jolla, California is the beneficiary of the largest single grant a tobacco company has ever offered for scientific research: a $225 million commitment from Philip Morris.
Science, April 26, 1996, p. 489

61. A Philip Morris ad campaign in Europe suggests that inhaling secondhand smoke is less dangerous than eating cookies or drinking milk. But the campaign backfired and has been discontinued. The fiasco has become the butt of jokes among European Union lobbyists. "Do you mind if I smoke?" asked a lobbyist. "Not at all," came the reply, "now that I know it won't do me as much damage as a glass of water."     Wall Street Journal, July 1, 1996, p. B1

62. In late August 1999, eight Philip Morris insiders sold over 750,000 shares of company stock for $36-38 a share. (The CEO, Geoffrey Bible, sold about 315,000 shares.) Within two months, the stock had fallen to $21 after adverse court rulings in lawsuits against the company. Professor Richard Daynard, a tobacco liability expert at Northeastern University in Boston, said: "The natural suspicion is that they knew in August that their stock would 'tank' once the investment community understood the implications of the August 2 ruling."
British Medical Journal, October 30, 1999, p. 1153

63. Philip Morris profits from domestic tobacco sales were $5.19 billion in 1998 and $5.12 billion (est.) for 1999. However, company stock price per share dropped from a high of $59.50 in November 1998 to as low as $21.25 in October 1999.     Associated Press, November 20, 1999

64. Philip Morris spent $7.6 billion in 1999 in dividends and stock buybacks; the dividend yield was 9.7%. Despite this, Philip Morris stock fell from $60 a share at the end of 1998 to $19 in February 2000.
Time, February 21, 2000, p. 137

65. Philip Morris in late 1999 unveiled a new internet site (www.philipmorris.com) where it admitted the addictiveness of nicotine and the association of smoking with lung cancer, heart disease, and emphysema. This was part of a $100 million corporate image campaign, and "by making more disclosures about smoking risks, producers also went to make it harder for those who start smoking now to sue by claiming they were unaware of the dangers."
New York Times, October 13, 1999

66. Philip Morris 1998 revenue was $74 billion, with market cap $130 billion. Its domestic share cigarette sales have grown to 52% in the United States and 14% worldwide. RJR Nabisco revenue was $17 billion, with market cap $9.5 billion.                                    Money magazine, February 1999, p. 40A

67. Tobacco accounted for 68% of Philip Morris's $15.4 billion operating income in 1998. The company's marketing budget for domestic tobacco is $3 billion, and its domestic market share is almost 50%, up from 45% in 1995.
                                    Forbes, August 9, 1999, p. 98

68. William Campbell, president of Philip Morris USA, testified to Congress in 1994 that his company "does not manipulate nor independently control the level of nicotine in our cigarettes." However, three former PM officials have declared that the company was preoccupied with manipulating the nicotine level in cigarettes to hook smokers. Ian Uydess said that nicotine levels were routinely targeted and adjusted, and Jerome Rivers, a shift manager at the PM Richmond plant, stated that tobacco nicotine levels were measured "approximately once per hour." If levels fell, they were boosted. Company management was acutely aware of nicotine's addictive powers, euphemistically termed "impact."
                Time, April 1, 1996, p. 50 and USA Today and Los Angeles Times, March 19, 1996

69. Scientists working for Philip Morris in the 1980s informed the company's president during a visit to the laboratory that rats in their experiment were self-administering nicotine out of physiological need, giving credence to the claims that nicotine is a reinforcing drug, one that carries with it an abuse liability. The lab was shut down a short time later. According to the researcher's testimony: "It was April 5, the first Thursday, in 1984. It was at three in the afternoon, and Dr. Charles—Jim—called me to his office and was telling me what a great job we had done for the company. ...and he said, 'However, we are discontinuing animal research beginning now.' And I was basically to shut the equipment off; terminate the experiments, even if they were ongoing; to kill all the animals the following day; and that was the end. Our badges were discontinued access to the research center. By the following Monday, we couldn't get back in."                         Quote from *Cigarette Confidential*, pp. 54-55

70. Philip Morris researchers wrote of destroying documents and the need to "bury" unfavorable nicotine research in the 1970's. The company also used a research lab in Germany to conduct work the company was "reluctant to do in this country," and a research director had a note in his files that said all important documents should be sent to his home, where "I will act on these and destroy." The state of Minnesota in a lawsuit contends that the German research lab was part of "mounting evidence...of purposefully using third parties to maintain their documents, apparently to preclude discovery."                         Associated Press, September 18, 1996

71. Steven Parrish, 46, vice president for corporate affairs at Philip Morris, took up smoking at the age of 40. Almost no one begins to smoke so late in life.         Washington Post National Weekly Edition, January 13, 1997, p. 9

72. David McLean, one of the original Marlboro men who appeared in the TV ad blitz of the 1960's, died of lung cancer in 1995. His widow is suing Philip Morris.                         CBS evening news, December 30, 1996

73. "Tobacco will kill you, and I am living proof of it." Some of the last words from Marlboro Man model turned anti-smoking crusader Wayne McLaren, as he lay dying of lung cancer at age 51.     The Guardian, July 25, 1992

74. We intervened with the White House, OMB and HHS to urge that [Surgeon General] Dr. Novello take no position on any pending anti-tobacco legislation. We stressed to her handlers and to interested parties that we were interested in making sure she focused on non-tobacco health problems. We were successful in that both of our objectives were met."         Philip Morris memo from Tim Dyer dated 8 March 1990,
                                    Washington Post magazine, December 3, 1995, p. 20

75. In 1996, Philip Morris had $12.5 billion in domestic and $24.1 billion in international tobacco revenues. R.J. Reynolds had $4.6 billion in domestic and $3.6 billion in overseas tobacco revenues.
                                    USA Today, June 23, 1997, p. 3B

76. Philip Morris had a 33.8% profit margin in 1996, and RJR Nabisco, 31.9%. New York Times, April 23, 1997, p. D8

77. Philip Morris is China's biggest spender on advertising. Marlboro billboards do not show or mention cigarettes, circumventing China's partial ban on tobacco advertising.                *Smoke and Mirrors*, p. 221

78. From 1990 to 1997, sales of Philip Morris cigarettes rose by 4.7% in the United States, but by 80% overseas.
New York Times, September 10, 1997, p. A22

79. Philip Morris has adopted the slogan, "It takes art to make a company great." The tobacco industry "has fostered close ties to the Metropolitan Museum of Art, the Lincoln Center for the Performing Arts, the Joffrey Ballet, the Folger Shakespeare Library, and hundreds of other acting troupes, orchestras, opera companies, art associations, museums, and historical associations."
Abstract PO9, 10th World Conference on Tobacco or Health, Beijing, 1997 (Alan Blum)

80. Since 1981, Philip Morris has contributed $27 million to American dance companies, and since 1990, more than $115 million to hunger relief.                Tobacco Reporter, November 1997, p. 51

81. Philip Morris spent $77 million on Formula One races in 1997; overall, tobacco companies contribute over $200 million of the $790 million that Formula One receives for sponsorships and prize money.
New York Times, December 4, 1997, p. D1

82. Philip Morris was the number one corporate donor in America in 1997, up from number 25 in 1984. Rupert Murdoch has been on the Philip Morris board of directors since 1989.
10th World Conference on Tobacco or Health, Beijing, 1997 (Jennie Cook)

83. Philip Morris was the number one contributor to political parties and candidates in the 1995-96 election cycle, with $4.2 million for political action committees, individual gifts to campaigns, and "soft money" to political parties. 79% was to Republicans, and 21% to Democrats. RJR Nabisco contributed $2.3 million (80% to Republicans), and U.S. Tobacco $1.46 million (83% to Republicans).                Washington Post, December 2, 1997, p. A25

84. "Philip Morris, the #1 campaign contributor in the 1995-96 US election cycle, has increased its pressure on the international front to ensure expansion. International sales for Philip Morris have quadrupled over the last 10 years. Philip Morris has over 60% of the cigarette market in Argentina; over 50% in Hong Kong and Italy; and over 40% in Singapore, Germany, and Switzerland. The tobacco giant is one of the top ten advertisers in Hong Kong, Austria, Belgium, Poland, Romania, Sweden, Switzerland, Puerto Rico, Venezuela, Kuwait, Oman, and Saudi Arabia. Philip Morris has also challenged tobacco control laws of Australia, Canada, and Thailand."        INFACT Update, Fall 1997

85. In 1996, Philip Morris had at least 240 registered lobbyists at the state and federal levels.
INFACT Update, Fall 1997

86. LOOK MA, NO SMOKE! If Philip Morris' new smokeless cigarette system is the future of nicotine, concerned parents can rest easy. The battery-powered gadget may trap and eliminate secondhand smoke in its portable 4 oz. case, but the clumsy looking, pager-size puffing device seems sure to turn more kids away from smoking

87. than the most morbid public-service campaign. One look at the Accord, which uses special low-tar cigarettes and will be tested in the U.S. and Japan next month, and image-conscious youngsters seduced by a Camel's cool allure are liable to say, "What a drag!"                Quote from Time, November 3, 1997, p. 39

88. Philip Morris has launched a promotional campaign in Beijing, China, to offer Marlboro Sportswear and other items in exchange for empty Marlboro cigarette packs.                Advocacy Institute news item, January 21, 1998

89. Marlboro market share increased to 36% in 1999, and Philip Morris U.S. cigarette revenues were $19.6 billion.
Associated Press, May 21, 2000

90. The New York City Victim's Services organization has a 24-hour hotline for women in crisis. The biggest corporate sponsor, contributing $200,000 a year, is Philip Morris.                CBS evening news, February 23, 1998

91. Philip Morris has nearly half of its profits and two thirds of its sales from overseas markets.
San Francisco Chronicle, November 20, 2002, p. A23

92. "It takes art to make a company great." Philip Morris has sponsored the arts since 1955, the first American company to do so, and is the world's leading sponsor of dance.

Alan Blum, M.D., World Conference on Tobacco or Health, Chicago, August 10, 2000

93. Philip Morris spends $60 a year on philanthropy, but $100 million a year on ads to tout these charitable contributions. Charyn Sutton, World Conference on Tobacco or Health, Chicago, August 10, 2000

94. "Philip Morris wants you to think it's a good corporate citizen…it spent $2 million on domestic violence programs, $60 million on other charities – and $108 million in public relations campaigns to tell us all about it."

San Francisco Chronicle, November 27, 2000, p. A22

95. And the industry, led by a $100 million Philip Morris public relations campaign, has sought skillfully to reposition itself in the public mind as a chastened, reformed sinner. The essence of their message: "Oh, that was then; this is now. Those were bad guys that ran the companies back then; we're reformers. We've paid our debt to society. And now, we really don't want kids to smoke, and we're funding programs – approved by public health authorities – to help keep them from smoking." Quote from *Smoke in Their Eyes*, p.247

96. "The recent, well-publicized Philip Morris campaign to remake the company's image (even renaming the entire Philip Morris parent corporation Altria in an attempt to shed its tobacco associations) demonstrates the importance of public relations and public opinion to corporate legitimacy and, in turn, the importance of legitimacy to the tobacco industry's survival and growth. …the tobacco industry needs 'respectability' to buttress its political power and avoid regulatory attention." American Journal of Public Health, June 2002, p. 959

97. Former Philip Morris CEO Geoffrey Bible retired in 2002. He gave up smoking in 2000, and in 1999 received $21.2 million plus stock options worth $8.1 million on the days that they were granted. He owns a chalet in Switzerland and a house in Bermuda. Tobacco Control, December 2002, p. 289

98. Philip Morris retired CEO Geoffrey Bible receives $3.5 million per year for his pension, a car and driver, an office and secretary, use of the company plane for life, and many other benefits. CBS Evening News, May 7, 2002

99. Claiming that it comes with "no strings attached," the National 4-H Council has announced that it is accepting $4.3 million from tobacco giant Philip Morris. The money is to be used to develop and disseminate a nationwide youth tobacco prevention program. Not surprisingly, the "design team" for the program includes four representatives from Philip Morris. Quote from ANR Update (Americans for Nonsmokers Rights), Spring 1999

100. Philip Morris in November 2002 put 17-page booklets with its positions on smoking risks and policies into major U.S. newspapers that reached 16 million readers. The newspapers included the New York Times, Washington Post, USA Today, and the San Francisco Chronicle. Associated Press/Newsday, November 13, 2002

101. Marlboro has been the most popular cigarette since 1972. *Cigarettes* (Parker-Pope), p. 91

102. Philip Morris stock chare price increased by 80% from January to December 2000 in an otherwise down market. The price of cigarettes rose by an average $1.15 a pack from 1997 to 2000. Bloomberg News, December 19, 2000

103. Philip Morris is a $112 billion company. Medical Economics, May 10, 2002, p. 40

104. Philip Morris uses women as cowgirls in German movie ads, and states that "The values Marlboro stands for, such as freedom and adventure, self-confidence, and self-determination are today just as true for women as they are for men." 2002 AMA Annual Tobacco Report

105. Louis Camilleri, 47. took over as Philip Morris president and CEO in April 2002, replacing Geoffrey Bible.

106. In 1992, Financial World ranked Marlboro as the world's most valuable brand and consumer product, with a worth of $31.2 billion; by 1993, the value had increased to $39.5 billion. The Tobacco Timeline (www.tobacco.org)

107. Altria Group, Inc. is the new official name of the parent company of Kraft Foods and its tobacco subsidiaries, Philip Morris USA and Philip Morris International.                    Business Wire, January 29, 2003

108. "Former FDA head David Kessler, in his book *A Question of Intent*, writes about 'Saint', a former chemical engineer for Philip Morris who discovered cancer-causing ingredients could be stripped from tobacco by the same process used to decaffeinate coffee. 'If it's that easy,' Kessler asks, 'why wouldn't the company pursue it?' Philip Morris refused to confirm or deny the report."                    U.S. News and World Report, January 15, 2002, p. 22

# CHAPTER 30
# TOBACCO FARMERS

1. Farm cash receipts for tobacco were $2.34 billion in 1990, 90% from the six states of North Carolina, Tennessee, Kentucky, Virginia, South Carolina, and Georgia.           *Tobacco Use: An American Crisis*, p. 84

2. In 1990, about 137,000 farms (down from 179,000 in 1987) grew tobacco on an estimated 763,000 acres.
   *Tobacco Use: An American Crisis*, p. 84

3. The county's 125,000 tobacco farms face a worldwide glut of tobacco. Large and expanding exporters, including China, Brazil, Argentina, and Zimbabwe, sell tobacco for prices that are one half to two thirds of American prices. Foreign competition has contributed to a 10% decline in prices for American flue-cured tobacco and a 25% decline in the number of tobacco farms in the last decade.
   New York Times, August 28, 1994, p. 1

4. There are 62,000 tobacco farmers in the US, including 15,000 in North Carolina, a decline of 40% in the last 15 years. Administrative costs for all tobacco programs, including price supports and crop insurance, are $20 to $40 million in most years, but were $103,000,000 in 1988 because of drought. The US tobacco industry now imports a great deal of cheaper foreign tobacco from countries such as Brazil and Zimbabwe, and because of a new law requiring domestic cigarettes to use 75% US grown tobacco, American companies are increasingly building manufacturing plants overseas.           San Francisco Examiner, May 1, 1994, p. A15

5. "Farmers and workers are suffering hard times because tobacco companies are now importing more than one third of the tobacco used in US-made cigarettes, producing more cigarettes overseas and automating production to eliminate manufacturing jobs. While encouraging American farmers to fight tobacco taxes, major tobacco companies are teaching growers in other countries how to produce tobacco for the US market. These actions by tobacco manufacturers have caused more job losses among farmers and workers than a tobacco tax ever will."
   Former President Jimmy Carter (Washington Post, February 9, 1994, p. A23)

6. The U.S. tobacco subsidy takes the form of a price support system, which guarantees a minimum price for the crop. The system was established during the 1930's, when a period of market instability threatened to put many farmers out of business. One could argue that it still offers at least one public benefit; it tends to inflate prices, which may help discourage consumption. But the security that the system confers on tobacco farmers also offers a huge benefit to the cigarette companies. It does more than effectively guarantee them a crop. It has allowed them to build a powerful political base: a farm constituency.

   To understand the value of this constituency, you have to see it in action, providing political cover for the manufacturers. Whenever Congress threatens to raise tobacco taxes, the companies bring a few tobacco farmers and their families to Washington--to display at a press conference, or to testify before the appropriate congressional subcommittee. Voting for a tax increase that might put family farmers like these out of work is not a politically appealing prospect. The industry is spared the extra taxes, and the tobacco companies score PR points by portraying themselves as representatives of rural America.
   Quote from World Watch magazine, July-August 1997, p. 26 (Anne Platt McGinn)

7. Most politicians from the southern tobacco states have used their clout to blindly back the tobacco industry's agenda instead of truly helping the tobacco farmer. They mistakenly assume that if the manufacturers prosper, as they have been with rapid growth in sales and profits, the struggling farmers will also.
   *Tobacco Use: An American Crisis*, p. 85

8. The government guarantees tobacco farmers a minimum price for their crop, and when the free market doesn't meet that price, taxpayers make up the difference. Ever some staunch defenders of tobacco criticize the public cost. "The American taxpayer got stuck for $800 million," says Rep. Charlie Rose (D-NC), former chairman of the House subcommittee on tobacco.           Common Cause magazine, April 1991, p. 9

9. The "tobacco subsidy" is a system of federally mandated tobacco price supports that assures farmers a buyer for their crop at guaranteed minimum price. In 1986, there was a major bailout of farmers that will eventually cost

about $1 billion, or $5,000 of taxpayer money for each of the nation's 200,000 tobacco farms.
Journal of the National Cancer Institute, March 16, 1988, p. 82

10. Shunned by tobacco companies who are now buying most of their tobacco from foreign growers, tobacco farmers in Kentucky, the Carolinas, and other tobacco-growing states are turning to anti-smoking advocates for help in getting aid for growing other crops, the New York Times reported March 4. "I've been in these wars since 1990," said Anthony J. DeLucia, a professor at East Tennessee State University who is the chairman of the American Lung Association. "It used to be the health groups would parade up somebody with emphysema or cancer, and the tobacco industry would have the farmer. We'd use these human shields in our arguments, as symbols. But the tobacco industry can't jerk the chain on the tobacco farmers like they used to, because the farmers have realized that the industry would love to just move everything overseas, where they can pay a next-to-nothing wage and spray any pesticide they want." One group helping farmers obtain a federal buyout is the Campaign for Tobacco-Free Kids. The public health group is lobbying Congress for a $16-billion buyout for tobacco farmers in exchange for the growers' support of tobacco regulation by the Food and Drug Administration. Quote from tobaccofreekids.org Tobacco News, March 5, 2003: "Tobacco Farmers Aligning with Anti-Smoking Advocates"

11. In 1986, the 137,000 tobacco farms in the US were less than a quarter of their 1950 number. Manufacturers of cigarettes and other tobacco products in 1950 employed 87,340 workers in 900 factories; by 1987, there were only 137 factories with 44,740 workers. American Medical News, November 14, 1994, p. 14

12. In North Carolina, where 56% of America's cigarettes are made, the number of tobacco farms fell from 100,000 to 41,800 between 1985 and 1991, and poultry is now a bigger business. From 1972 to 1992, tobacco's share of farm receipts in North Carolina fell from 37% to 20%. George Will column, February 10, 1992 and Coalition on Smoking or Health 1995 newsletter on tobacco growers

13. Tobacco farmers received much less of each dollar spent on cigarettes in 1991 as compared to 1967 (from 9 cents to only 3 cents), while the share for tobacco manufacturers increased from 19 cents to 53 cents in the same period. North Carolina Medical Journal, January 1995, p. 6

14. The share that tobacco farmers earned for every retail dollar of sales dropped from 16 cents in 1957 to only 3 cents in 1993, compared that year for 63 cents of every dollar to manufacturers, 5 cents for retailers, and 29 cents for excise taxes. World Watch, July-August 1997, p. 26

15. During flue curing, the green tobacco leaf is kept at high temperatures for about a week. Affluent nations use oil or gas as fuel, but third world nations use wood. Worldwide, about 2.5 million tons of tobacco are flue cured each year with wood. Tobacco growing thus requires the destruction of forests and results in adverse environmental impact in some developing countries where tobacco production is encouraged, often at the expense of staple food crops. AMA Fact Sheet on Smoking

16. The cost of tobacco constitutes only about 8% of the retail price of each pack of cigarettes. This translates to a total cost of about $2 billion per year for the 24 billion packs of cigarettes made for domestic consumption, much less than the $5.3 billion "overhead" for advertising and promotion.
Journal of the National Cancer Institute, March 16, 1988, p. 83

17. In 1952, US tobacco manufacturers bought 1.6 billion pounds of tobacco from US farmers. By 1994, this had dropped to 0.8 billion pounds. In the same period, imported tobacco increased from 10% to 40% in American cigarettes despite 150 million pounds of surplus stockpiled tobacco that was bought up at double the price of imported tobacco. Videotape "The Tobacco Trap"

18. More people work on tobacco farms than in cigarette plants, but the manufacturing jobs are year-round and better paying. The average yearly salary of a tobacco farmer in North Carolina is 5,600 U.S. dollars. The salary of those employed in the tobacco manufacturing industry is 43,750 U.S. dollars per annum, or 8 times more. While tobacco farmers have to pray for a couple of pennies annual increase in the price of a pound of tobacco, the tobacco industry makes billions of dollars in profit.
When profits for BAT totaled 1 billion pounds in 1992, the chairman Sir Patrick Sheehy got a 54% annual

salary increase to 980,000 pounds. The retiring chairman of Philip Morris did even better. He received a bonus of $26 million.

Quote from *Tobacco and Health*, p. 69

19.     The American tobacco producers have no problem with the kind of variety that they grow, nor with the quality of their leaf. The problem of the American growers is the price, which is twice as high as comparable leaf from Zimbabwe or Brazil. In 1993, U.S. cigarette companies used an estimated 45% of imported tobacco. That was up from 30% just three years earlier. American tobacco growers were alarmed by this development and asked their members of Congress to limit the imports of foreign tobacco.

    Effective lobbying by the farmers resulted in the domestic content law that, from 1st January 1994, severely penalizes any U.S. cigarette manufacturer whose cigarettes contain more than 25% foreign leaf. The immediate result of the law was that the import of tobacco leaf in the U.S. decreased in 1994 by 44%.

    The long term effect of the law is probably that it will do more damage than good to American growers. A report from the U.S. Department of Agriculture predicted that some U.S. manufacturers may shift cigarette manufacture abroad (to Mexico for instance) in an effort to continue using cheaper foreign tobacco.

    This law appears to be incredibly hypocritical, protectionist and a clear contravention of the Gatt Agreement.

Quote from *Tobacco and Health*, p. 68 (Luk Joossens)

20. In global terms, tobacco is considered to be the most widely grown non-food crop, although it accounts for only 0.3% of cultivated land (but over 1% in China). This compares to 13% for grain, 2% for cotton, and 0.7% for coffee. About 87% of the tobacco crop ends up in cigarettes.     *Tobacco in History*, p. 7

21. A 1986 report estimated that tobacco usurps the place of food crops and uses land that could otherwise grow food to feed 10 to 20 million people.     *Smoke and Mirrors*, p. 223

22. If the 5 million hectares (12.35 million acres) of cropland now used to grow tobacco were turned over to growing grain, it would provide enough grain to support the world's population for 6 months.

World Watch, December 1995, p. 19

23. 1997 world tobacco production was 7.3 million metric tons, led by China with 3.3 million tons, the United States, 668,000 tons, India, 544,000, Brazil, 497,000, and Turkey, 245,000 tons.

Tobacco Control, Spring 1998, p. 77

24. 16 states grow tobacco. 1993 production figures in millions of pounds by state were North Carolina, 596, Kentucky, 472, Tennessee, 129, South Carolina, 110, Virginia, 110, Georgia, 96, Pennsylvania, 20, Ohio, 19, Florida, 19, Indiana, 17, Maryland, 13, Wisconsin, 9, Missouri, 6, West Virginia, 4, Connecticut, 2, and Massachusetts, 0.6 million pounds.     Economic Research Service, U.S. Department of Agriculture

25. The top ten tobacco producing states in 1995 by cash receipts (in millions) were North Carolina $871, Kentucky $615, South Carolina $187, Tennessee $178, Virginia $147, Georgia $133, Florida $31, Ohio $28, Indiana $25, and Pennsylvania $22. In 1996, 674,300 acres of tobacco were harvested in the United States, producing 1.32 billion pounds, down nearly 16% from 1994.     USA Today, June 23, 1997, p. 3B

26. U.S. tobacco farmers harvested 797,000 acres in 1997, led by North Carolina with 314,000 acres and Kentucky with 221,000 acres. The gross per-acre profit in 1996 was $3,800 (1980 pounds at $1.92 per pound), and the net per-acre profit was $1,844. (In 1993, net per-acre profit for soybeans was $73, and for corn, $30.)

Wall Street Journal, July 16, 1997, p. A24

27. The gross value of an acre of flue-cured tobacco is $3916, compared to $107 for an acre of soybeans.

Wall Street Journal, February 15, 2000, p. A28

28. The 1995 U.S. tobacco crop was worth $2.3 billion, the seventh largest cash crop behind corn, soybeans, hay, wheat, cotton, and potatoes. However, tobacco was the most economically productive on a per acre basis, averaging $4,191 per acre, compared to $136 for wheat, $190 for hay, $228 for soybeans, $306 for corn, $478 for cotton, and $760 for peanuts.     *The Tobacco Epidemic*, p. 34

29. Tobacco is the most profitable crop in the US, fetching about $4000 an acre gross, while the next closest, peanuts, bring $800 to $900.                    American Medical News, November 11, 1994, p. 17

30. In 1993, Americans smoked 485 billion cigarettes. Leaf sales generated about $3 billion for farmers, about $3,782 per acre. This compared to $352 per acre for cotton, $208 for soybeans, and $176 for wheat.
                                                            USA Today, August 12, 1995, p. 6

31. Tobacco farming yields a revenue to farmers of around $4,000 per acre; tobacco sells at around $1.80 per pound but costs only a dollar to produce. A single acre can yield as much as 2,500 pounds. In 1994, each acre of U.S. tobacco grown for domestic use brought in $43,000 in state and federal excise taxes at the retail level.
                                                            New York Times magazine, August 25, 1996, p. 43

32. North Carolina produces 52% of all domestically grown tobacco.
                                                            Los Angeles Times magazine, August 10, 1997, p. 9

33. Tobacco farms in North Carolina have declined from 300,000 fifty years ago to 58,000 now.
                                                            New York Times magazine, August 25, 1996, p. 45

34. There are 60,000 tobacco farmers in Kentucky.                    New York Times, September 14, 1996, p. 8

35. Tobacco is Virginia's largest cash crop, worth $180 million to the state's 8500 tobacco farmers.
                                                            Washington Post, December 6, 1996, p. A21

36. The state of Virginia has 8,400 tobacco farmers, 120,000 tobacco related jobs, and $186 million in 1996 tobacco cash receipts.                    Wall Street Journal, April 25, 1997, p. A16

37. Before World War II, Maryland was a major tobacco-producing state, with 300,000 acres cultivated. By 1995, only 7000 acres were still devoted to tobacco growing.        San Francisco Chronicle, March 5, 1994, p. A4

38. Two hurricanes striking North Carolina in the summer of 1996 caused tobacco crop losses of $335 million, leading to prices in the Georgia-Florida market of $1.92 per pound, the highest since 1984.
                                                            American Medical News, November 4, 1996, p. 18

39. Worldwide tobacco production increased to 7.17 million tons in 1996, up from 6.51 million tons in 1995.
                                                            Tobacco Control, Autumn 1996, p. 177

40. In Malaysia, the profit margin for tobacco farmers is only 2%. It is 79% for manufacturers of cigarettes.
                                                            UICC Tobacco Control Fact Sheet 5, International Union Against Cancer, 1996

41. The World Bank between 1974 and 1988 gave $1.5 billion in loans to support tobacco growing and processing. This policy was changed in 1992, and such loans are no longer made.        *Smoke and Mirrors*, p. 232

42. About $1.6 billion for tobacco subsidies were spent by the European Commission in 1992, an amount 800 times more than the budget that was provided for smoking prevention. There are half a million tobacco-related deaths every year in the European Union.        Journal of the National Cancer Institute, September 4, 1996, p. 1188

43. Pesticide poisonings in the tobacco field workers are not uncommon, particularly in developing countries where worker safety regulations and precautions are often lax or non-existent. Tobacco cultivation is very chemical intensive. During the early tobacco growing stages, up to 16 applications of pesticides in a three month period are recommended. Some of the pesticides used are parathion, methyl bromide, carbofuran, and aldicarb.
                                                            Panos Briefing, September 1994, and Yenyen Chan, Pesticide Action Network, San Francisco

44. The top new tobacco producing countries in 1997 were China (42% of world total production), the United States (9.3%), India (7.8%), Brazil (7.2%), and Turkey (3.7%).        *Curbing the Epidemic*, p. 59

45. The tobacco industry estimates that 33 million people are engaged in tobacco farming worldwide, including 15 million in China, 3.5 million in India, and 100,000 in Zimbabwe. The United States has 120,000 tobacco farms, and the European Union has 135,000.
*Curbing the Epidemic*, p. 68

46. The four major U.S. tobacco companies have agreed to establish a $5.15 billion trust fund for tobacco farmers to help compensate them for losses incurred as a result of the tobacco settlement with the states.
New York Times, January 22, 1999, p. A20

47. Since the 1960s, the bulk of production has moved from the Americas to Africa and Asia: land devoted to tobacco growing has been halved in the USA, Canada and Mexico, but has almost doubled in China, Malawi and United Republic of Tanzania. The production of tobacco leaves has more than doubled since the 1960s, totaling nearly 7 million metric tons in 2000. The greater use of fertilizers and pesticides, as well as the increased mechanization, that have produced these higher yields are environmentally damaging. The problem does not end with growing tobacco: the processes used in curing tobacco leaves cause massive deforestation. There are millions of tobacco farmers worldwide. The tobacco industry exploits them by contributing to their debt burden, while using their economic plight to argue against efforts to control tobacco.
Quote from *The Tobacco Atlas*. p. 46

48. Seeds for low-nicotine tobacco were essentially banned by the USDA in 1963. To this day, in order to be eligible for full government price supports, farmers must certify each year that they are not growing any low-nicotine varieties. The USDA's Minimum Standards Program, which requires nicotine levels in tobacco to fall within a prescribed range, was instituted at the urging of Big Tobacco. High nicotine makes American tobacco attractive around the world. It has a desirable flavor and, more important, it carries the satisfying chemical kick that smokers crave.
Quote from San Francisco Chronicle, December 1, 2002, p. D4 (Joan Ryan column)

49. The 1996 "Freedom to Farm" Act phased out federal subsidies for most crops, but peanuts, sugar and tobacco were exempted because of the influence of the powerful southern agricultural lobby.
*Cigarettes* (Parker-Pope), p. 57

50. It costs just 18 cents to manufacture a pack of cigarettes, "including leaf, labor, packaging and transportation. The cash outlay to farmers is only 3 cents for each pack sold."
*Cigarettes* (Parker-Pope), p. 26-27

51. In 1996, the European Union paid 684.5 million British pounds in tobacco subsidies to farmers, which is sixty times the amount spent (10.3 million pounds) for programs designed to reduce smoking.
British Medical Association (www.tobaccofactfile.org)

52. Half of the tobacco in U.S. manufactured cigarettes was imported in 2001 from countries such as Brazil, Argentina, and Zimbabwe, an increase from about a third imported in 1990.
New York Times, March 4, 2003, p. A21 (USDA graph)

53. Taxpayers may be stuck paying $637 million for 224 million pounds of surplus tobacco – enough to fill a 40-mile convoy of truck trailers. The federal government already is spending more than $280,000 a month in warehouse fees to store the tobacco, harvested in 1999 and unsold because much of it is weather-beaten. Hurricane Floyd damaged about 81 million pounds of this flue-cured tobacco while drought afflicted 143 pounds of cooler-climate burley. Three tobacco grower co-operatives in Kentucky, North Carolina, and Tennessee used $637 million in government loans to buy the leaf from growers two years ago. The co-ops planned eventually to sell the leaf and repay the government as they do every year under the 60-year-old tobacco price-support program. That never happened. The last time the government took control of a surplus tobacco crop was in 1986, when $376 million was written off at taxpayers' expense for the 1983 burley crop.
Quote from Richmond Times-Dispatch, August 17, 2001

# Tobacco and Deforestation

1. Tobacco-caused deforestation is a major problem in parts of the developing world, particularly in Brazil and in the tobacco-growing countries of East Africa.
Tobacco Control, Fall 1994, pp. 192-92

2.  Brazil, the world's fourth largest tobacco producer, dries or cures its crop by burning wood, as does most of Africa and much of India, Thailand, and the Philippines. More affluent countries flue-cure their tobacco with coal, gas, or oil. One report claims that fuelwood curing requires about one tree per 300 cigarettes, and another that the crop from each acre of tobacco requires the felling of one acre of the adjacent woodland each year.
    *Tobacco Control in the Third World*, p. 57 and JAMA, June 20, 1986, p. 3244

3.  With flue curing of tobacco, the green leaf must be kept at high temperatures by circulated heat for about a week. Brazil and most African and Third World tobacco producing countries cure their crop by burning wood.
    Tobacco Control, Fall 1994, p. 191

4.  About half of the tobacco output of the countries of the developing world is cured with wood. An average of 7.8 pounds of wood is needed to cure one pound of tobacco, and trees from one acre of land may be needed to cure one acre of tobacco.
    Panos Briefing, September 1994

5.  The proportion of flue-cured tobacco (in contrast to air- and sun-cured tobacco) continues to rise, accounting for 54% of world output in the late 1980s. Unlike the other methods of curing, flue-curing is capital- and resource-intensive, particularly in its use of wood.
    *Tobacco in History*, p. 215

6.  2.5 million tons of tobacco worldwide is flue-cured using wood each year. This requires 6.2 million acres of forest to be cut yearly to meet this need. Pakistan consumes 1.5 million cubic meters of wood for tobacco curing; Tanzania consumes 1.3 million cubic meters of wood fuel.  *Tobacco Control in the Third World*, p. 57

7.  In terms of the use of wood in curing tobacco, different studies give different results on deforestation, and the subject is controversial. The following data are reported: one tree is felled for every 300 cigarettes, one hectare of tobacco requires between 0.5 and 1 hectare of forest for curing; one in twelve trees felled worldwide is used in curing tobacco; or, each kilo of tobacco demands about 160 kilos of wood; however, another report downgrades the environmental impact and estimates lower ratios of wood usage for tobacco curing. Unfortunately, facts about trees cut and deforestation have been uncritically repeated many times, and are not proven.
    *Tobacco in History*, p. 243

8.  Dr. Helmut Geist from Nuess, Germany, published a detailed review article "Global assessment of deforestation related to tobacco farming" in Tobacco Control, Spring 1999, pp. 18-28. An estimated 200,000 hectares of forests are lost from tobacco farming and flue curing each year. The deforestation occurs mainly in southern Africa, South and East Asia, South America, and the Caribbean. This accounts for about 1.7% of global net losses of forest cover, but nearly 5% of the total deforestation in the developing countries of the world. An estimated 11.4 million tons of wood, much taken from native forests in the developing world, is consumed each year for flue curing of tobacco. 93% of tobacco-related deforestation occurs in developing countries, and 90% of all land cultivated for tobacco is in developing countries. In Tanzania, wood is used for 100% of flue-cured tobacco that is produced.

9.  The environmental damage is considerable in developing countries from the cultivation of tobacco, where it is flue cured by wood. In Tanzania, 12% of all trees felled annually are used for tobacco curing, and neighboring Malawi has already cut down one third of its forested land for this purpose.    NEJM, March 28, 1991, p. 918

10. About half the tobacco grown in the world is flue cured over wood fires, significantly contributing to deforestation.
    *The Real Cost*, Richard North, p. 99

11. Since 5 to 7 acres of forest are needed to flue cure one ton of tobacco, tobacco cultivation has substantially contributed to deforestation in many Third World countries. Other estimates are one to two acres of forest to cure one ton of tobacco.
    International Journal of Health Sciences 1986; 16:288
    And NEJM, March 28, 1991, p. 918

12. Selected countries and the proportion of total annual deforestation in 1999 attributable to tobacco growing: Korea, 45%; Uruguay, 41%; Bangladesh, 31%; Malawi, 26%; Jordan, 25%; Pakistan, 19%; China and Syria, 18%; and Zimbabwe, 16%.

*The Tobacco Atlas*, p. 46

13. The economy of Malawi, in central Africa, depends heavily on tobacco, which accounts for 75% of the country's total export earnings. 93% of all fuel used in Malawi is wood, with 23% of the total (420,000 cubic meters a year) consumed by the tobacco industry, mostly to dry and cure burley tobacco leaves.

Panoscope, October 1994, p. 16

14. During flue curing, the green tobacco leaf is kept at high temperatures for about a week. Affluent nations use oil or gas as fuel, but third world nations use wood. Worldwide, about 2.5 million tons of tobacco are flue cured each year with wood. Tobacco growing thus requires the destruction of forests and results in adverse environmental impact in some developing countries where tobacco production is encouraged, often at the expense of staple food crops.

AMA Fact Sheet on Smoking

15. Pesticide poisonings in the tobacco field workers are not uncommon, particularly in developing countries where worker safety regulations and precautions are often lax or non-existent. Tobacco cultivation is very chemical intensive. During the early tobacco growing stages, up to 16 applications of pesticides in a three month period are recommended. Some of the pesticides used are parathion, methyl bromide, carbofuran, and aldicarb.

Panos Briefing, September 1994, and Yenyen Chan, Pesticide Action Network, San Francisco

# CHAPTER 31
# TOBACCO IMPORTS AND EXPORTS

1.  "Tobacco exports should be expanded aggressively, because Americans are smoking less."
    Vice President Dan Quayle, 1990 (The Progressive, May 1991, p. 28)

2.  "The tobacco industry demonstrates that by responding to the great challenges of global marketing with energy and enthusiasm, US industry can regain its leadership role in international trade."
    Donald S. Harris, Philip Morris International (New York Times magazine, July 19, 1988, p. 62)

3.  In 1982, 25% of world markets were open to US tobacco products. By 1992, 90% of world markets were open.
    9th World Conference on Tobacco or Health, Paris, 1994

4.  American trade negotiators opened up markets in the Far East for US brands in the late 1980's. Along with market access, they also demanded exemptions from local tobacco advertising bans that had long been in force.
    American Medical News, November 16, 1990, p. 15

5.  "In one of the most disgraceful examples of private enterprise gone amok, the cigarette industry is focusing its high-powered marketing attention on the unprotected citizens of Third World countries... As Surgeon General, I am appalled by this corporate behavior of American companies, and further, I am shocked by our own government's support of such behavior."
    C. Everett Koop, Godkin Lecture at Harvard, 1989 (The Progressive, May 1991, p. 29)

6.  Asia's tobacco monopolies are mainly government departments that admit the health evidence, do not promote cigarettes, and cooperate at least in part with government health measures. In contrast, the transnational tobacco companies now invading Asia deny the health evidence, aggressively promote their products, and try to prevent tobacco control measures. Their profits return primarily to stockholders in the North America and Europe
    9th World Conference on Tobacco or Health, Paris, 1994 (Judith Mackay)

7.  In April 1990, Dr. James Mason of the Department of Health and Human Services called it "unconscionable" for tobacco companies to be "peddling their poison abroad." A month later, the White House prevented him from testifying on the Hill about the health consequences of US tobacco exports.
    Wall Street Journal, September 27, 1990, p. A13

8.  The cigarette companies "play our free-trade laws like a Stradivarius violin."
    Dr. James Mason, Bush administration health official (New Yorker, September 13, 1993, p. 84)

9.  The tobacco industry projected a worldwide goal of exporting one trillion cigarettes by 1996. The industry saw the decade of the 1990's as "a time of unprecedented opportunity," claiming that "the good days for US products on the world market may be just beginning. Our future is particularly bright in developing areas."
    Social Science and Medicine 1993; 38:106

10. During the 1970's, the US exported over $1 billion in tobacco leaf to the developing world as part of the Food for Peace program. The inclusion of tobacco in this program ended in 1982.
    Journal of the National Cancer Institute Monograph 1992; 12:32

11. The United States is "sending Asians a message that their lungs are somehow more expendable than American lungs" by not requiring warning labels on exported cigarettes. Rep. Chet Atkins, D-Massachusetts (New York Times magazine, July 10, 1988, p. 62) In 1992, US manufacturers did add the warning labels to exported cigarettes. (Associated Press, February 6, 1992).

12. In 1992 the US Agriculture Department spent $3.5 million to help promote US tobacco overseas exports. The House later voted to end this practice. In studies comparing the tar content of similar brands of cigarettes sold in the United States and the Philippines, the Philippine cigarettes had a 50% higher tar content, and sometimes

twice as much nicotine. World Smoking and Health No. 1, 1993, p. 13

13. US tobacco exports, mostly to Asia and Eastern Europe, increased from $2.7 billion in 1985 to $4 billion in 1988 and $7 billion in 1990, an annual growth rate of 25%. Prevention File, Summer, 1991, p. 10

14. US smokers consumed 524 billion cigarettes in 1990, a 3% decline from 1989, and an 18% drop from the record high of 1981. But the declining domestic sales are more than compensated for by the booming export market. In 1990, the US exported 164.3 billion cigarettes worth $4.2 billion, up 41% from the previous year, and the US is now the world's leading exporter of cigarettes. These exports if placed end to end would circle the equator 347 times, or the equivalent of 18 round trips to the moon. Social Science and Medicine 1993; 38:106

15. US cigarette exports increased from 56 billion in 1984 (8% of total production) to 194 billion in 1991 (25% of all cigarettes manufactured). From 1987 to 1988 alone, the tobacco export trade surplus increased by 40%, from $2.5 to $3.5 billion. NEJM, April 7, 1994, p. 977

16. Cigarette exports, less than 60 billion in 1985, increased to 188 billion cigarettes in 1992 (San Francisco Chronicle, December 31, 1992), 195.5 billion in 1993 (USA Today, May 18, 1994), and 215 billion in 1994.
*Tobacco Situation and Outlook*, USDA, December 1994

17. $180 million worth of cigarettes were sold overseas in 1930, making tobacco the country's third leading export at the time. *Tobacco Advertising*, p. 263

18. The US exported 188 billion cigarettes worth $3.9 billion, and another $1.8 billion of other tobacco products in 1992. This accounted for a substantial portion of the overall agricultural trade surplus of $18 billion in 1992. 29% of the cigarette exports were to Japan.
San Francisco Chronicle, December 31, 1992, and Discovery Journal, June 1993

19. 31% of US-made cigarettes are now exported, a total of 243.9 billion in 1996, and tobacco and tobacco products are now the leading US agricultural export.
USA Today, April 18, 1997, p. 4B, and NEJM, March 28, 1991, p. 917

20. From 1975 to 1994, US cigarette exports soared 340% to 220 billion cigarettes, or 30% of all domestic production. American success in removing trade barriers has not simply let US companies gain market share, but substantially increased the total number of Asian smokers.San Francisco Chronicle, September 30, 1996, p. E1

21. In 1992, Philip Morris reported a 19% increase in overseas sales from the previous year, with 421.1 billion "units" sold. PM has been issued a business license for Vietnam, and RJR Nabisco was represented in a US delegation that visited Vietnam in late 1993. Americans for Nonsmoker's Rights Update, Spring 1994, p. 3

22. In 1984, about 640 billion cigarettes were manufactured in the United States for domestic use, the most ever, and overseas exports were another 52 billion. By 1993 manufactured cigarettes for domestic consumption had declined to below 500 billion, but overseas sales of American cigarettes had increased to 195.5 billion per year.
Newsweek, July 4, 1994, p. 45, and USA Today, May 18, 1994

23. Between 1983 and 1993, combined Philip Morris and RJ Reynolds international cigarette sales increased from 329 billion to 634 billion "units." In the same time period, domestic US sales from these two companies decreased from 493 to 335 billion cigarettes.
9th World Conference on Tobacco or Health, Paris, 1994 (Greg Connolly)

24. US cigarettes now have 17.5% of the Japanese market. In 1993, 55.5 billion US cigarettes were exported to Japan. Time, April 18, 1994, p. 63 and US News, April 18, 1994, p. 35

25. Between 1985 and 1995, the market share of imported cigarettes increased from 2% to 6% in South Korea, 2% to 21% in Japan, and zero to 22% in Taiwan. World Watch, July-August 1997, p. 22

26. Overall US cigarette exports increased 275% from 1985 to 1993. Exports to Japan increased from 6.5 billion in 1985 to 56 billion in 1993; to South Korea from 1.3 billion in 1987 to 4 billion in 1993; and to the former Soviet Union countries from 4.6 billion in 1991 to 13.6 billion in 1993.

    Cancer Facts and Figures, 1994 (American Cancer Society)

27. American cigarette sales to Japan grew from $76 million in 1985 to $606 million in 1988. In the same period, sales to Taiwan rose from $4.6 million to $119 million, and to South Korea, from $2.1 to $5.6 million. Most of the increase came from US threats to invoke retaliatory trade sanctions against countries that were considering excluding American cigarettes.

    The Lancet, March 3, 1990, p. 528

28. Philip Morris and RJ Reynolds exported 37 billion cigarettes to the Soviet Union in 1990. After full death rates from smoking appear in a country, there are about 1000 smokers who die from their habit for every billion cigarettes consumed.

    Wall Street Journal, September 27, 1990, p. A13

29. "In Mexico and Argentina, sales of Marlboro and other US brands over the past five years have jumped by more than 700 percent. Philip Morris earns 30 percent of its profits on exports, and has opened plants in El Salvador, Guatemala and Costa Rica."

    San Francisco Chronicle, December 26, 1994, p. A17

30. In 1969 the US imported nine million pounds of tobacco. By 1983, this had risen nineteen-fold to 240,000 metric tons.

    *Tobacco Use: An American Crisis*, p. 85

31. The amount of tobacco leaf used per 1000 cigarettes has decreased by more than half since the 1950's. Tobacco imports have increased 75% since 1986, and now account for 25% of leaf used in US cigarettes.

    American Medical News, November 14, 1994, p. 16

32. A 1993 law requiring 75% domestic tobacco content in US-made cigarettes has been ruled in violation of GATT trade agreements, and is being replaced by a less restrictive tariff rate quota.

    American Medical News, January 16, 1995, p. 15

33. "The same US government that threatens countries that export cocaine to our shores also threatens countries that attempt to maintain barriers to our own deadly drug pushing: the exportation and aggressive marketing of American cigarettes and smokeless tobacco products."

    Kenneth E. Warner, Ph. D

34. "It is the height of hypocrisy for the United States, in our war against drugs, to demand that foreign nations take steps to stop the export of cocaine to our country while at the same time we export nicotine, a drug just as addictive as cocaine, to the rest of the world."

    C. Everett Koop, M.D., NEJM, March 28, 1991

35. More Colombians die today from diseases caused by tobacco products exported to their country by American tobacco companies than do Americans from Colombian cocaine.

    Social Science and Medicine 1993; 38:113

36. Marlboro is sold in 170 countries, and in 1993 was the only foreign cigarette manufactured and sold in the Soviet Union, where 418 billion cigarettes are consumed each year.

    Social Science and Medicine 1993; 38:113

37. American tobacco companies sell $17 billion worth of cigarettes a year domestically, but $26 billion overseas.

    60 Minutes, August 18, 1996

38. 1995 Philip Morris sales in the European Union were $11.4 billion.

    Wall Street Journal, July 1, 1996, p. B1

39. In 1994, 260 billion Marlboros were consumed outside the US market (some of these were manufactured abroad). In 1995, domestic US cigarette consumption was 490 billion, and another 230 billion (or $4 billion worth) US made cigarettes were exported, as contrasted with 585 billion consumed and about 60 billion exported in 1986.

    Washington Post National Weekly Edition, November 25--December 1, 1996, p. 7

40. The United States exported 244 billion cigarettes in 1996, up from 50 billion in 1975. 38% of the exports are to Asia, and the US share of the Japanese market has increased from 2% to 23% in the last 10 years.
10th World Conference on Tobacco or Health, Beijing, 1997 (Luk Joossens and Frank Chaloupka)

41. In the last decade, domestic tobacco consumption has dropped by 17%, while exports rose by 259%. Philip Morris and RJR now sell more than two thirds of their manufactured cigarettes overseas.
Contra Costa (Calif.) Times, June 8, 1997, p. F3 (from a Los Angeles Times commentary by Ralph Nader)

42. Some public health officials have asked whether it is any less morally offensive for the United States to export hundreds of billions of cigarettes overseas to lessen the trade deficit than it was for England in the 1830's to export opium to China to balance the imports of silk and tea, leading to the so-called "opium wars."
NEJM, April 7, 1994, p. 977

43. In the early 1800's, British merchants smuggled opium into China and made a fortune; Americans and other Europeans were involved too, but to a lesser extent. Although opium was completely illegal, addictive, and terrible for health, caused all kinds of other social problems, and drained China of vast quantities of silver, the merchants aggressively pushed their product. Apologists for the merchants denied that opium was bad for health. The British argued that if they didn't sell opium, trade would be lost to merchants from other countries. In 1839, after a decade of escalating problems with opium, the Chinese tried to stop the trade by confiscating opium stored by British merchants. This led to the Opium War (1839-42). The British won, and the opium trade continued to flow.

In the 1980's, the American tobacco companies spearheaded a modern-day opium war in the Far East. At the time, Taiwan, Thailand, South Korea, and Japan each had a closed market dominated by government-owned monopoly. American tobacco companies had no access to these markets. American tobacco companies do not like to be told "No," so they pressured Yeutter, the US Trade Representative, to take action to open the markets. By 1985, the USTR agreed. He warned the four governments that if they didn't open up their markets, the United States would impose severe trade sanctions. Here was the US government, with its health warnings and advertising restrictions to discourage smoking at home, turning around and using threats in order to increase sales abroad. The US government pushed much harder to open the foreign markets for cigarettes than for other American products, no doubt a reflection of the powerful tobacco lobby.
Quote from "The Modern Opium War," *Smoke and Mirrors*, p. 217 (Rob Cunningham)

44. A rural development task force headed by former White House chief of staff Erskine Bowles has recommended to North Carolina state officials that they pressure the U.S. government to make acceptance of American cigarettes a condition of China's admission to the World Trade Organization.
Reported in Raleigh, North Carolina, March 9, 2000

45. U.S. cigarette exports reached a record 243 billion in 1996, and have since declined to 217 billion in 1997, 201 billion in 1998, and 151 billion in 1999.
Associated Press, May 22, 2000

46. The Campaign for Tobacco-Free kids (www.tobaccofreekids.org/global) in 2002 published two booklets on public health and international trade. Liberalization of trade in tobacco products stimulates consumption and "has a significant negative impact on public health in low and middle-income nations."

47. U.S. cigarette exports increased from 110 billion in 1988 to a peak of 250 billion cigarettes in 1996, then declined to 200 billion in 1998. Domestic consumption decreased from 575 billion cigarettes in 1988 to approximately 470 billion in 1998.
Newsweek, July 31, 2000, p. 38

# CHAPTER 32
# SMUGGLING

1. An August 25, 1997 New York Times front page article was entitled "Cigarette Makers are Seen as Aiding Rise in Smuggling. Tobacco Giants Deny Role in Illegal Trade; Inquiries Show There May Be One." The estimated number of cigarettes smuggled worldwide has increased from 100 billion in 1989 to 280 billion in 1995, or 28% of the one trillion cigarettes exported each year by all countries manufacturing cigarettes. The manufacturers benefit because they receive the same price for cigarettes even in contraband markets; the smuggling costs governments $16 billion a year in lost tax revenue, and the cheaper cigarettes undermine initiatives to reduce smoking. Companies commonly sell "huge quantities of top brands to traders and dealers who are little more than pipelines to the smugglers." As well, industry employees have at times had a significant role in stimulating the smuggling. Two organized crime groups in Italy make $500 million a year by smuggling in Marlboro cigarettes that they buy from Swiss dealers.

2. The difference between global cigarette exports and imports increased from 137 billion in 1989 to 324 billion in 1994. Most of these "missing" cigarettes are smuggled.
    UICC Tobacco Control Fact Sheet: Cigarette Smuggling. International Union Against Cancer, 1996

3. "Smuggling helps the multinational companies because it creates a kind of illegal introductory price for their brands – far below what the legal products are selling for. This helps 'soften' the market up for a bigger sales assault… WHO estimates that about one-third of the cigarettes produced in 1994 were moved from the legal market into the smuggling economy – a 300% increase since 1989. Cigarette smuggling is now thought to be costing governments some $16.2 billion annually."                    World Watch, July-August 1997, p. 24

4. It is clear that governments are the main losers of tax revenue. But it is interesting to look at who benefits from smuggling. Given the magnitude of the gap between world cigarette exports and imports, it is intriguing to speculate what might be the attitude and role of the chief beneficiaries of this illegal trade: companies that manufacture the cigarettes. They benefit from smuggling in several ways. First they gain their normal profit by selling the cigarettes (legally) to distributors. The cigarettes then find their way on to the streets where they sell at greatly reduced prices, stimulating demand. This puts pressure on governments not to increase tax because of the loss of revenue, which may also result in lower prices and higher consumption. Then the industry uses this to urge governments to reduce, or not to increase, taxes. Finally, contraband cigarettes that are intercepted by customs have then to be replaced – yet more sales.          Quote from UICC Tobacco Control Fact Sheet, Cigarette
                                                                                    Smuggling. International Union Against Cancer, 1996

5. In 1995, world cigarette exports were 963 billion cigarettes, and imports were 689 billion. The "missing" 274 billion cigarettes were smuggled, often with the collusion of tobacco companies. In the European Union, 50 billion cigarettes were smuggled, resulting in $6 billion in lost tax revenue; one smuggled truck load can evade $1.2 million in taxes. Contrary to the claims of the tobacco industry, high taxes do not encourage smuggling. Spain, with the lowest price, has high smuggling rates, as does Italy. Sweden has the highest price and only ½% smuggled; the UK has only 1% of cigarettes smuggled, and France, 2%.
                                    10th World Conference on Tobacco or Health, Beijing, 1997 (Luk Joossens)

6. Contraband cigarette market shares in European Union countries are Spain and Austria 15%, Italy 11.5%, Germany 10%, Greece 8%, Ireland 4%, France, Sweden, and Norway 2%, and the United Kingdom, 1.5%. Countries with the highest prices tend to have the lowest rates of smuggling.
                                                                                    Tobacco Control, Spring 1998, p. 67

7. There has been a steady increase in the number of missing cigarettes. In 1994, 910,000 million cigarettes were exported but only 586,000 million imported, a difference of 324,000 million. After deducting 45,000 million for legitimate duty free sales, there are still almost 280,000 million cigarettes missing. The only plausible explanation is smuggling. At a conservatively estimated average duty on these cigarettes of only US$1/pack (and it is much, much higher in most developed countries), it represents revenue of more than US$16,200 million being lost annually by governments. Quote from UICC Tobacco Control Fact Sheet, Cigarette Smuggling

8. Antwerp, Belgium, is one of the main distribution points for American cigarettes. In Spain, Winston is the most popular foreign brand, and 60% of its sales there are contraband. In 1996, 2.3 billion Winston cigarettes worth $200 million were smuggled into Spain. A cargo ship from Antwerp with 160 million Winstons was seized by Spanish police in January 1997; it went to Spain despite shipping documents indicating that the cigarettes were bound for Senegal in West Africa.                    New York Times, August 25, 1997, p. B2

9. In the European Union, the market for contraband cigarettes is about 60 billion per year, resulting in about $6 billion per year in lost tax revenue.
                    Abstract S13/2, 10th World Conference on Tobacco or Health, Beijing, 1997

10. By 1993 between a quarter and a third of all cigarettes consumed in Canada were smuggled in from the United States to avoid Canada's high taxes. There was strong evidence that the tobacco manufacturers promoted the smuggling. In 1994, taxes were rolled back, and smoking rates began to increase for the first time in decades; in Quebec and Ontario, retail prices plummeted from $47 to $23 a carton.          JAMA, May 28, 1997, p. 1652

11. The European Union is investigating smuggling activities by RJ Reynolds and whether the company is selling cigarettes to traders and dealers who immediately resell them in the black markets to avoid foreign taxes. The director of the EU's anti-fraud unit commented, "As Reynolds has previously refused any cooperation whatsoever, we intend to take up this issue with US authorities." Cigarette smuggling is a major organized crime activity in addition to costing European governments $1.5 billion in lost taxes in 1997.
                    New York Times, May 8, 1998, p. A1

12. A single case in the Hong Kong courts involves $1.2 billion worth of Brown and Williamson cigarettes that were smuggled into China. When asked whether she blamed foreign companies for the smuggling problem, Dr. Judith Mackay, executive director of the Asian Consultancy on Tobacco Control, responded: "It would be libelous to suggest that the foreign tobacco companies are actually smuggling their own cigarettes. But it is the case that approximately one third of all cigarettes are smuggled and unaccounted for in company ledgers..."
                    Multinational Monitor, July-August 1997, p. 23

13. Former British-American Tobacco Ltd. executive Jerry Lui Kin-Hong was sentenced in Hong Kong to three years and eight months in prison for plotting to accept $23 million in bribes and a corrupt $10 million loan from cigarette distributors. The justice in the case said that major companies were assisting international criminals, and that the highly lucrative smuggling encouraged crime and undermined efforts to persuade youngsters in Hong Kong not to smoke by providing them with cheap black market cigarettes. The justice also said that there is evidence that the companies knew that vast quantities of the cigarettes were being sold to smugglers.
                    South China Morning Post, June 25, 1998

14. An RJR executive has plead guilty to helping smugglers sell $700 million worth of cigarettes on the Canadian black market.                    Associated Press, March 26, 1999

15. Cigarettes are being smuggled by the truckload from Virginia, where the cigarette tax of 2.5 cents a pack is the lowest in the country, to New York, where the tax is $1.19, the highest in the United States. New York is losing hundreds of millions of dollars a year in unpaid taxes, estimated one distributor. A van holding 4500 cartons can reap a profit of $52,425 per trip, and discount stores along I-95 in Virginia are dotted with cars and vans with New York license plates. "Each customer loads shopping carts with as many cigarettes as he can buy for under $10,000, the cash limit that triggers a report to federal authorities." New York authorities believe that tobacco companies knowingly oversupply Virginia stores in order to get the excess cigarettes to New York.
                    Washington Post National Weekly Edition, March 13, 2000, pp. 30-31

16. In December 1999, the government of Canada sued RJ Reynolds for $1 billion, alleging that the company set up an elaborate network of smugglers and shell companies to flood Canada with cheap cigarettes after steep tax increases in 1991. Most of the smuggling was via the Mohawk Indian reservation in northern New York State into Ontario. In 1984, 40% of all cigarettes sold in Canada were smuggled and sold on the black market. The lawsuit contends that Reynolds worked hard to conceal its links to the alleged scheme.
                    Associated Press, December 22, 1999

17. Northern Brands International, an RJR International affiliate, pleaded guilty to charges that it smuggled cigarettes into Canada to avoid paying $2.5 million in U.S. excise taxes. The company agreed to pay a $15 million fine for its role in a scheme to transfer cigarettes out of Canada ostensibly for export to Eastern Europe, then smuggling them back into Canada through an Indian reservation in New York state to avoid U.S. excise taxes. US Attorney Thomas Maroney accused RJR of setting up Northern Brands specifically for smuggling.

New York Times, December 23, 1999, p. A1

18. About 30% of internationally exported cigarettes, 355 billion in all, are lost to smuggling, a far higher percentage than most internationally traded consumer products.          *Curbing the Epidemic*, p. 63

19. About 30% of cigarettes smoked in Canada in the early 1990's were smuggled in, including contraband cigarettes accounting for up to 75% of the market in Quebec. Because of this, Prime Minister Jean Chretien slashed federal tobacco taxes by $11 per carton in February 1994.          JAMA, March 2, 1994, p. 647

20. By early 1994, two-thirds of the cigarettes sold in Quebec and one-third of those sold in Ontario were contraband. In February, the federal government in Ottawa cut the tax, and the price of a "legal" carton of 200 cigarettes sold in Quebec fell from $47 to $22.73 overnight. Public health authorities warn that despite cutting smuggling from the United States, the price decreases will induce additional 245,000 Canadian teenagers to begin smoking.          Canadian Medical Association Journal, April 15, 1994, p. 1295

21. In 1994, five eastern provinces in Canada lowered cigarette taxes, dropping the price from (Canadian) $47 a carton to $26 or less. The provinces in western Canada, British Columbia, Alberta, Saskatchewan, and Manitoba, kept their taxes high, and a carton still costs from $45 to $46. This results in smuggling and contraband sales; an estimated 20% of cigarettes sold in British Columbia are contraband, resulting in a tax revenue loss of up to $125 million each year.          Canadian Medical Association Journal, January 13, 1998, p. 97

22. "...price is only one of many factors that influence smuggling rates. Other more important factors include: the tobacco industry's own role in facilitating smuggling; the lack of appropriate controls on tobacco products in international trade; and the existence of entrenched smuggling networks, unlicensed distribution, lax anti-smuggling laws, weak enforcement and official corruption."

World Health Organization, 2000 (*The Tobacco Atlas*, p. 54)

23. Between 300 and 400 billion cigarettes were smuggled in 1995, equal to about one third of all the legally imported cigarettes. Cigarettes are the world's most widely smuggled legal consumer product. They are smuggled across almost every national border by constantly changing routes. Cigarette smuggling causes immeasurable harm. International brands become affordable to low-income consumers and to image-conscious young people in developing countries. Illegal cigarettes evade legal restrictions and health regulations and, while the tobacco companies reap their profits, governments lose tax revenue.quote from *The Tobacco Atlas*, p. 54

24. One third of cigarettes traded worldwide, about 350 billion a year, are illegally sold without paying duty; about 20% of cigarettes smoked in the United Kingdom are smuggled. In the European Union alone, governments are losing 10 to 12 billion Eurodollars each year in lost taxes.          The Lancet, February 16, 2002, p. 586

25. The European Union loses about 6 billion British pounds in tax revenue each year because of smuggling.

British Medical Association (www.tobaccofactfile.org)

26. "Federal Judge Lewis A. Kaplan was part of the 2-1 majority that gave the tobacco industry one of its biggest legal victories in recent years – a ruling upholding dismissal of Canada's cigarette smuggling case against R.J. Reynolds Tobacco Holdings, Inc. The ruling last October by the U.S. 2nd Circuit Court of Appeals not only derailed Canada's billion-dollar claim, but also led to dismissal of similar suits against cigarette makers by the European Union and Colombia. Internal documents disclosed in tobacco litigation show that Kaplan had represented Brown & Williamson Tobacco Corp. as a private attorney during the 1970s and 1980s. The documents show that as part of Kaplan's work for Brown & Williamson, he participated in meetings of the Committee of Counsel, the inner sanctum of top tobacco lawyers that mapped the companies' joint legal and political strategies – including how to temper government action on tobacco smuggling. Kaplan did not disclose his former ties with the industry to lawyers for the government of Canada, though legal experts say he didn't

have to. Nonetheless, tobacco industry foes, who said the ruling was of immeasurable benefit to the entire industry, not just R.J. Reynolds, reacted with surprise and anger."

quote from Los Angeles Times (Myron Levin), September 9, 2002

27. "Tobacco giant R.J. Reynolds smuggled cigarettes into Iraq in a scheme that violated U.S. sanctions and enriched both Saddam Hussein's regime and a Kurdish separatist group accused of terrorism, the European Union alleges in a lawsuit...It said the scheme cheated the EU out of billions of dollars in tax revenues." RJR is alleged to have supplied a billion cigarettes to an Iraqi distributor, and Saddam's son Uday oversees and profits from this illegal importation. (A Los Angeles Times article reported that in 1999-2001, RJR sold almost 8 billion cigarettes to Iraq.)

Associated Press, November 1, 2002

28. Saddam Hussein's son, Uday, is thought to supervise a massive cigarette smuggling operation in Iraq.

U.S. News and World Report, November 4, 2002, p. 46

29. One-quarter of all the tobacco distributed around the world is illegal contraband, according to research done by the World Health Organization expert Luk Joossens. Industry figures show a worldwide smuggling system is at work, he says. The American-based multi-national cigarette industry manufactures and exports about 100 billion cigarettes very year, but statistics of worldwide imports show only 75 billion cigarettes imported. The difference, 25 billion cigarettes, find their way into contraband, unauthorized markets. Joossens has been following the pattern of contraband distribution for many years. He says the channels used to be through Belgium, but they were closed off. Spain then became the major route through the world, but those ports were closed to undocumented tobacco containers. Now, Iraq is the main supply line between U.S. tobacco manufacturers and the clients, says Joossens. The irony is that Saddam Hussein's son controls Iraq's tobacco industry, so American tobacco companies are helping keep Hussein's family rich. The losers in this pattern of commerce are the governments, deprived of tobacco taxes and the health of people who can get cigarettes more cheaply than they would if they were controlled and taxed the legal way.

Quote from Tracey Madigan, Online News Journalist CBC Montreal, September 16, 2002

30. In less than a two-year period, RJR has sent 8 billion cigarettes into Iraq. "You've heard of all the shortages sanctions have brought to Iraq: food, medicine, spare parts, but cigarettes? No problem. The best-known American brands are piled high in very marketplace. How do Winstons find their way to Iraq? R.J. Reynolds says it doesn't know, but the company is being taken to court right now by people who say RJR knows perfectly well and is totally complicit."

60 Minutes II transcript, CBS News, February 12, 2003

31. Saddam's sons Uday and Qusay, "have also masterminded cigarette-smuggling deals, which are worth as much as several hundred million dollars. The European Union is currently suing R.J. Reynolds, charging it with violation of the Racketeer Influenced and Corrupt Organizations (RICO) Act because the company has allegedly allowed its products to be smuggled into Iraq, depriving the EU of millions of dollars in tax revenue. The company has strenuously denied the EU charges, which include a court filing that says 'Uday oversees and personally profits from the illegal importation of cigarettes into Iraq.'"

Time, March 10, 2003, p. 37

32. According to the World Health Organization, 25% of exported cigarettes are smuggled. Smuggling has enabled multinational tobacco companies to increase sales volume dramatically by evading taxes and competing with domestic brands, thereby helping to establish internationally recognizable brands.

The Nation, April 18, 2002, via tobacco.org

33. About 20 billion packs of cigarettes are smuggled worldwide every year, cheating governments of $25 to $30 billion in tax revenue.

Associated Press, July 31, 2002

34. Imposing taxes at the point of production/importation instead of at the point of sale can reduce tobacco smuggling.

*Tobacco: The Growing Epidemic*, p. 392

35. The true beneficiaries of smuggling are the tobacco companies; the industry has lobbied governments to reduce tobacco taxes, arguing that this would solve the smuggling problem, but this notion has proven to be untrue.

British Medical Journal 2000; 321:947-950

36. "...large volumes of cigarettes manufactured in Brazil for export to Paraguay are smuggled back and consumed as tax-free contraband in Brazil."2002 National Conference on Tobacco or Health, Abstract EVAL-264-105 and
World Trade and Smuggling, pp. 379-395 in *Tobacco: The Growing Epidemic*, 2000 Surgeon General report

37. In Brazil, 58 billion smuggled contraband cigarettes constituted 37% of the domestic cigarette market in 1998 and deprived the government of an estimated $500 million in tax revenue. Large volumes of cigarettes manufactured in Brazil for export to Paraguay are smuggled back and consumed as tax-free contraband in Brazil. In 1988, less than 1% of Brazil's domestic cigarette production was exported; by 1998, exports had risen to 51% of production. These exports fell sharply when Brazil imposed a 150% export tax on cigarettes at the end of 1999.
Tobacco Control, September 2002, pp. 215-219

38. The duty free kingdom of Andorra in the Pyrenees clears huge numbers of cigarettes imported from other European countries, a total of 24,000 cigarettes per capita each year. Most are presumed to be smuggled elsewhere to avoid taxation.
*Tobacco* (Gately), p. 358

39. At Felixstowe, a port on England's North Sea coast, 1.6 billion contraband cigarettes were seized in 1999.
Newsweek, July 31, 2000, p. 39

40. A Hezbollah terrorist organization cell of Arabic men in Charlotte, North Carolina, operated a multi-million dollar smuggling ring transporting truck loads of North Carolina cigarettes, taxed at only 50 cents a carton, to Michigan, where the tax was $7.50 a carton, and pocketed the difference.
U.S. News and World Report, March 10, 2003, p. 30

41. In North Carolina, a low-tax state, a smuggling ring was broken up which was reselling cigarettes in Michigan, where taxes are much higher. The profits were allegedly used to fund the terrorist group Hezbollah. No tobacco companies were implicated in the scheme.
Newsweek, July 31, 2000, p. 38

42. "The Canadian government files criminal charges Friday against affiliates of tobacco giant R.J. Reynolds, accusing them of helping to flood that country with cheap contraband cigarettes during the 1990s. Also charged with fraud and conspiracy were eight current or former senior executives who allegedly took part in a scheme that authorities said robbed the federal government and the provinces of Ontario and Quebec of more than $800 million in cigarette taxes. Several observers called it the biggest corporate fraud case ever filed in Canada. The charges stemmed from a 4½-year investigation by the Royal Canadian Mounted Police of the smuggling boom that prompted Canada to rescind a steep cigarette tax meant to curb smoking. Investigators said the probe was continuing and could result in charges against more tobacco companies or executives."
Los Angeles Times, March 1, 2003

43. "A European Union lawsuit maintains that Reynolds, the world's second-largest tobacco company, has been complicit for years in a worldwide money-laundering system in which cigarettes are as important a currency as the U.S. greenback.
"The notion that black-market cigarettes can cause big problems isn't new. According to some health and law enforcement officials, as many as a third of all cigarette exports wind up being sold on the black market, cheating governments of tax revenue and encouraging smoking by keeping cheap cigarettes available.
"But the EU suit adds a fresh twist to the concept of cigarette smuggling that goes way beyond simple tax evasion. The allegations, say money-laundering experts here and abroad, underscore the role that cigarettes – ubiquitous, easily transportable commodities usually bought and sold for cash – have come to play in lubricating the movement of capital for drug traffickers, tax evaders, terrorists and others who need to conceal the sources of their funding . . .
In copious detail, the suit describes stratagems RJR allegedly employed to distance itself from criminal partners, including eradicating identification numbers from illicit shipments, using secret bank accounts and third-party checks and establishing intermediary companies through which to do business...
"If the allegations are true, they would raise serious questions for U.S. officials. 'If RJR cigarettes really are the currency of international money-laundering rings, how did this escape the attention of the U.S. government?'

"Other instructions included orders that the master cases – containers of 10,000 cigarettes each – should be 'neutralized and decoded', meaning that marks and numbers allowing the containers to be traced and tracked should be removed, the suit alleges.

"The suit also contends that RJR and its co-conspirators used 'an organized group of money couriers whose function was to receive criminal proceeds in Italy and other parts of the European Union and to illegally ferry those proceeds out of Italy and the European Community to Switzerland, where the couriers would hand the cash proceeds' to Swiss money-laundering organizations."

Quote from Los Angeles Times (Michael Hiltzik), November 5, 2002

# CHAPTER 33
# WORLD HEALTH ORGANIZATION and
# THE FRAMEWORK CONVENTION TREATY (FCTC)

1. Representatives from 160 countries have met three times to negotiate a treaty called the Framework Convention on Tobacco Control (FCTC) to be ready for ratification by individual nations in 2003. The agreement could be used "to establish standards for international tobacco control, assist governments in developing effective domestic legislation, and create a global mechanism to counter the political influence of the tobacco industry." At the first negotiating session in October 2000, the U.S. delegation supported strong tobacco-control positions; however, at two 2001 meetings, the new U.S. delegation appointed by the Bush administration reversed previous positions, now opposing increased taxation and a ban on advertising and promotion. The new delegation also opposed mandatory restrictions on passive smoke exposure, a proposal that public health concerns can take priority over trade rules, and another proposal banning the misleading labeling of cigarettes as "mild" or "light." The prognosis for the treaty is unclear, and "without improvements in the U.S. position, a unique opportunity to control the enormous worldwide toll of tobacco consumption may be lost."

New England Journal of Medicine (Rep. Henry Waxman), March 21, 2002, pp. 936-938

2. The United States was once the world leader in tobacco control. It had pioneered the science and the research to label tobacco use a deadly addictive habit. It had produced a series of Surgeon General's reports detailing the science. Its federal and state agencies had implemented many novel tobacco control measures, such as youth prevention, secondhand smoke restrictions, and documented their success. But now it lags behind the rest of the world in tobacco control. Canada and Brazil have full color picture and graphic health warning labels on all tobacco packages that shock and educate. The European Union and Brazil have banned the use of deceptive terms such as "low tar" and "light," terms that mislead consumers to believe that one product is less hazardous than another. And Thailand and South Africa have sweeping and all-inclusive advertising bans. What happened to the U.C. commitment to tobacco control at home and is this lack of commitment guiding the U.S. response to the negotiations on the Framework Convention on Tobacco Control?"

Quote from Abstract POLI-202 "United States: A Straggler in Tobacco Control"
presented at the 2002 National Conference on Tobacco or Health, San Francisco, November 20, 2002

3. The United States has "turned its back on the world community" by its attempts to weaken the International Tobacco Control Treaty. Unlike the well-publicized U.S. repudiation of the Kyoto treaty to ameliorate global warming, this story went virtually unreported in the American media. The World Health Organization convened the tobacco summit, called the Framework Convention on Tobacco Control (FCTC), in Geneva. Former Surgeon General C. Everett Koop told the conference, "If the U.S. government fails to actively support a strong FCTC, we will be doing the entire world a disservice." The chair of the conference, Brazilian diplomat Celso Amorim, expressed outrage at the U.S. delaying tactics. Clive Bates, director of the United Kingdom-based Action on Smoking and Health (ASH) stated: "The U.S. contribution has been entirely negative--weakening, delaying, and deleting anything that might have substance. It would be best if the U.S. delegation goes home…, adopts its increasingly familiar ostrich stance and stays out altogether."Earth Island Journal, Autumn 2001, p. 33

4. The U.S. tobacco industry, facing declining opportunities at home, is looking to addict new customers overseas. The Clinton administration, recognizing the lives and economies that could be wrecked as a result, was working with other nations on a treaty to control tobacco use and advertising. Now the Bush administration seems to be backing away from this sensible U.S. commitment. The tobacco giants must be delighted.

Among much else, the administration is reported to have tried during recent negotiations on the treaty to delete a provision calling on governments to tax up the price of tobacco to discourage use, and another urging them to ban marketing terms like "light" or "mild" that convey a false impression of reduced risks. The administration likewise sought to ease provisions calling for the licensing of retailers as a way or reducing sales to minors, and for bans on smoking in places of work and public buildings.

The head of the U.S. delegation to the talks was quoted as saying that the administration "really is committed to making this an effective agreement," but its apparent efforts to weaken the text point in the opposite direction. Quote from editorial, Washington Post National Weekly Edition, May 21-27, 2001, p. 24

5. "The United States…stands accused of being more concerned with the health of corporations like Philip Morris and British-American Tobacco than with public health in other countries."
*Christian Science Monitor*, commenting on the Framework Convention on Tobacco Control
(ASH Smoking and Health Review, May-June 2001)

6. "We are outraged at the Bush Administration's apparent reversal of the United States' International tobacco policy during ongoing negotiations in Geneva on the proposed Framework Convention on Tobacco Control, the world's first treaty on tobacco. If implemented domestically in the United States, these proposals would give the tobacco industry the weak and ineffective approach to tobacco regulation that it seeks. These proposals sound more like those of the tobacco industry than of a world leader in international health."
American Lung Association and Campaign for Tobacco-Free Kids
(reported in ASH Smoking and Health Review, May-June 2001)

7. "Unfortunately, the Bush administration is kowtowing to the powerful tobacco industry by blocking progress in negotiations [at the World Health Organization] to create an international treaty against smoking." Representatives Nancy Pelosi D-Calif. commented: "The Marlboro Man is not a suitable ambassador for the United States, but he may be the most visible representative we are presenting to young people all over the world. We can and must set a better example."        Editorial, San Francisco Chronicle, May 19, 2002, p. D4

8. The global convention that would restrict tobacco marketing would commit countries "to banning all tobacco advertising and sponsorships to the extent allowed by their constitutions, requires that at least 30% of a tobacco product's package be devoted to health warnings and either urges or mandates tobacco taxes, measures to protect against secondhand smoke, a crackdown on smuggling and steps to block sales to minors."
New York Times, March 8, 2003, p. A33

9. "The administration has also sought to water down an international treaty on tobacco. A draft urged governments to tax up the price of tobacco to discourage its use. The Bush folks don't like tax increases; nor did they like some of the regulatory suggestions in the draft…His policy thus far has been to do nothing, but not to acknowledge the inaction. That pleases the cigarette makers, who invested heavily in his election."
Editorial, Washington Post National Weekly Edition, July 2-8, 2001, p. 25

10. The world's first international treaty designed to reduce world smoking – the W.H.O.-sponsored Framework Convention on Tobacco Control – is in trouble, in large part because the Administration is trying to kill it. Here are some examples from an analysis by the Wall Street Journal:
    - "The U.S. opposed licensing of retailers, a provision designed to curb smuggling," saying it might be too expensive.
    - "The U.S. delegates in Geneva, reflecting the Bush administration's wishes, also backtracked on crackdowns on advertising aimed at children and on mandating tobacco taxes (which undoubtedly reduce…consumption).
    "And again, in opposition to most other countries, the delegation reversed this country's position on curbing the effects of passive smoking."
    Apparently as a result, the U.S.'s chief negotiator, Thomas E. Novotny, quit. The Washington Post reported that "he had privately expressed frustration over the administration's decision to soften the U.S. positions on key issues, including restrictions on secondhand smoke and the advertising and marketing of cigarettes."        quote from ASH Smoking and Health Review, May-June 2001

11. After two weeks of debate, nearly all the 171 nations at the World Health Organization conference in Geneva last week had agreed on a way to help put an end to the 4 million tobacco-related deaths that occur worldwide annually. But the United States, home to the world's most powerful tobacco lobby, is one of two nations to "give explicit statements that they will have difficulty coming onboard," says Derek Yach, a WHO official. The United States opposes a treaty ban on tobacco advertising. But most public health advocates dismiss this logic, pointing to a disclaimer that allows countries to ignore elements of the treaty that violate their own constitutions. "The Bush administration has done everything that they can to weaken the tobacco treaty," said Matt Myers, president of the Campaign for Tobacco-Free Kids.
Quote from Newsweek, March 10, 2003, p. 10

25. The tobacco industry spent more than $15 million in the first six months of 1996 in lobbying Congress, federal agencies, and the White House in an effort to thwart federal plans to restrict teenage access to tobacco, grant the FDA regulatory authority over tobacco, and restrict advertising. Philip Morris alone spent $11.3 million. The above amounts did not include campaign donations; the industry from 1995 to mid-1996 gave $4 million in unregulated "soft money" to the GOP and $750,000 to the Democrats.    Associated Press, September 9, 1996

26. The FDA proposed rule would have yielded substantial health-related benefits ranging from $28 to $43 billion each year.                                                        NEJM, September 26, 1996, p. 993

27. The FDA received more than 700,000 comments on its proposed regulations restricting the sale and distribution of cigarettes and smokeless tobacco to children and adolescents, including 2,500 pages of text and nearly 50,000 pages of exhibits from the cigarette and smokeless tobacco industries alone.
                                                        NEJM, September 26, 1996, p. 988

28. The FDA was created in 1906, and had a 1997 budget of $980 million. In 1994, House Speaker Newt Gingrich called the FDA "the leading job killer in America."         New York Times, August 3, 1997, p. 24

29. "The FDA regulations constitute an important change in the regulatory approach to tobacco. Cigarettes have traditionally been one of the most underregulated products in American life. Congress typically excluded cigarettes from major food and drug legislation, often as a result of tobacco company lobbying. In 1905, tobacco was removed from the Pharmacopoeia, thus avoiding regulation in the Pure Food and Drug Act of 1906.
Defined as neither food nor drug, tobacco fell outside the aegis of subsequent regulatory legislation. Tobacco, for example, has been specifically excluded from drug abuse, public health prevention, and consumer product safety legislation."                                                        JAMA, February 5, 1997, p. 411

30. The record before the agency showed that several methods of enhancing nicotine delivery are commonly used in the manufacture of commercial cigarettes. Tobacco blending to raise the nicotine concentration in low-tar cigarettes is common. According to the vice chairman and chief operating officer of Lorillard Tobacco Co., for instance, "the lowest 'tar' segment is composed of cigarettes utilizing a tobacco blend which is significantly higher in nicotine." Another common technique for enhancing nicotine delivery in low-tar cigarettes is the use of filter and ventilation systems that by design remove a higher percentage of tar than nicotine. Yet a third type of nicotine manipulation is the addition of ammonia compounds that increase the delivery of "free" nicotine to smokers by raising the alkalinity or pH of tobacco smoke. These ammonia technologies are widely used within the industry.                                                        Quote from JAMA, February 5, 1997, p. 407

31. The day that FDA commissioner David Kessler announced his resignation, Philip Morris and US Tobacco stock rose by 3%, RJR by 1.5%, and Loews Corp. by 4%.         San Francisco Chronicle, November 26, 1996, p. A11

32. "We know that prohibition won't work. But we should try to phase out tobacco use over the next several decades. There are three ways to do this: Prevent young people from smoking, help adults break their habit and manufacture the products so that they are not addictive."
                                C. Everett Koop and David Kessler (New York Times, June 4, 1997, p. A24)

33. An economic analysis estimated that the proposed $368 billion tobacco industry settlement of June 1997 would have resulted in a 62 cent a pack increase per pack to cover the cost. The eventual 15 cent federal tax increase would bring the total increase to 77 cents. At this price, at least 10 million fewer Americans would smoke by 2002 (falling from 50.2 million to 39.5 million) and teenage smoking would be 28% lower, dropping from 3.5 million in 1997 to 2.7 million in 2002.    Washington Post National Weekly Edition, August 25, 1997, p. 35

34. "Americans can be counted upon to do the right thing—after trying everything else."
                                                        Winston Churchill (JAMA, February 18, 1998, p.550)

35. The tobacco industry spent $40 million to defeat the 1998 McCain bill to regulate tobacco, and House Whip Tom Delay scorned it in an op-ed piece: "Limousine Liberals, by forcing their vision of a healthy lifestyle on American workers, will cost them billions of dollars."                         *Smoke in Their Eyes*, pp. 225-226

36. In 1995, with the strong endorsement of President Bill Clinton and Vice President Al Gore, the commissioner of the Food and Drug Administration (FDA), Dr. David Kessler, announced that the agency had jurisdiction over tobacco and would regulate cigarettes as "drug-delivery devices." The tobacco companies objected and sued the FDA, arguing that Congress had not given the FDA jurisdiction over their product. The Supreme Court, in a five-to-four opinion issued in March 2000, agreed with the tobacco companies.

Quote from New England Journal of Medicine, December 14, 2000, p. 1802

37. Senate Majority Leader Trent Lott, speaking of C. Everett Koop and David Kessler, "launched into an unprovoked tirade," deriding them as "Dr. Kook and Dr. Crazy."  *Smoke in Their Eyes*, p. 201

38. On March 21, 2000, in a 5 to 4 decision, the United States Supreme Court held that the FDA lacks jurisdiction under the Federal Food, Drug, and Cosmetic Act to regulate tobacco products. "As a result of this decision, the FDA's August 1996 assertion of jurisdiction over cigarettes and smokeless tobacco and regulations restricting the sale and distribution of cigarettes and smokeless tobacco to protect and adolescents . . . are invalid."

*Reducing Tobacco Use*, 2000 Surgeon General report, p. 16

39. "Tobacco use, particularly among children and adolescents, poses perhaps the single most significant threat to public health in the United States…It is plain that Congress has not given the FDA the authority it seeks to exercise here."  Majority decision of the U.S. Supreme Court, March 21, 2000 (reported in INFACT newsletter)

40. Attempts to ban tobacco advertising in the United States have run afoul of the Supreme Court's new interpretation of the First Amendment. Prior courts having ruled that commercial speech could be banned if the government provided a compelling justification in terms of the public good. However, a more conservative Supreme Court has recently reversed this legal precedent by placing the First Amendment value of cigarette advertising above the value of protecting the public from the promotion of a product that is responsible for 20 percent of all deaths in the United States. This decision places the U.S. Supreme Court's interpretation of freedom of speech at odds with those operating in the vast majority of constitutional democracies in the free world. In 2002, the European Parliament approved a total ban on tobacco advertising in the European Economic Community.  Quote from CA-A Cancer Journal for Clinicians, March-April 2003, p. 114

# State Lawsuits

1. The state of Mississippi joined Florida, Minnesota, and West Virginia in filing suit against the tobacco industry to pay for the medical bills of the state's Medicaid patients who have required care for tobacco-related illnesses. "For decades, the tobacco cartel has conspired intentionally, fraudulently, and maliciously to mislead the public in order to peddle defective products they know are addictive and deadly," said Mississippi Attorney General Mike Moore. "This lawsuit is based on a simple notion: you caused the health crisis; you pay for it. The free ride is over. It's time these billionaire tobacco companies start paying what they rightfully owe to Mississippi taxpayers."  The Lancet, July 23, 1994, p. 253, New York Times, May 24, 1994, p. A12, and San Francisco Chronicle, December 21, 1995

2. Philip Morris admitted that it organized Mississippi businesses to fund Governor Kirk Fordice's legal fight to block the state's Medicaid lawsuit, which was settled out of court in 1997.  ANR Update, Spring 1997

3. Florida in 1994 introduced legislation, the Medicaid Third Party Recovery Act, seeking to hold the tobacco industry liable for the state's cost of treating smoking-related illnesses in Medicaid patients, a sum amounting to $1.2 billion since 1989. Governor Lawton Chiles commented, "We're going to take the Marlboro man to court. With this law, Florida sends a loud and clear message to the tobacco giants that they will be held accountable for sponsoring sickness and death."Associated Press, May 27, 1994, and Wall Street Journal, May 3, 1994, p. A3

4. In Florida, a new law allows the state to use statistical analysis to prove that the tobacco companies caused damages to the state's patients. This is a much easier legal burden than proving a direct causal relationship between tobacco use and any individual smoker's illness. The state never chose to smoke, and thus can seek damages as an "innocent party." Lawrence Tribe, Professor of Law at Harvard, stated on June 1, 1994 on the

MacNeil/Lehrer News Hour: "There's no good reason in terms of sound economics or legal principle why taxpayers should subsidize the tobacco industry by absorbing these costs. The state is an innocent third party, and it makes eminent sense to have this kind of lawsuit."                    Advocacy Institute, July 1, 1994

5.  The Texas settlement with the tobacco industry for $15.3 billion came with a lawyer contingency fee of 15%, or $2.3 billion. Calling the proposed fees outrageous, Governor George Bush has gone to federal court to block the payment to the 150 lawyers who assisted Texas in the lawsuit. San Francisco Chronicle, February 9, 1998, p. A2

6.  In the final renegotiated settlement of the Texas tobacco suit, the industry will pay the state a total of $17.6 billion over the next 25 years.                    Wall Street Journal, July 20, 1998, p. B8

7.  The state of Minnesota has filed a lawsuit against the tobacco industry to claim reimbursement for tobacco-caused Medicare expenses. The suit also changes fraud and conspiracy, deceptive advertising and trade practices, and a violation of antitrust laws. At the first hearing, the tobacco industry sent 28 attorneys, all white males in white shirts and business suits. The industry has filed innumerable motions and five appeals. It has submitted 9 million pages of documents that fill two document warehouses.
       Douglas Blanke, office of the Attorney General, state of Minnesota (address in St. Louis, July 9, 1996)

8.  Minnesota Attorney General Hubert Humphrey III has been a champion of the importance of disclosure; in preparation for his state's 1998 lawsuit with the industry, he has 500,000 top-secret industry documents totaling 33 million pages.                    Multinational Monitor, July-August 1997, p.13

9.  The Minnesota state tobacco lawsuit was settled in May 1998 for $6.6 billion over 25 years, a larger per capita settlement that the previous ones for Texas ($15.3 billion), Florida ($11 billion), and Mississippi ($3.36 billion).
                    Associated Press, May 9, 1998

# Master Settlement Agreement

1.  Three books published outline the history of state lawsuits begun in 1994 by Mississippi Attorney General Mike Moore which culminated in the 1998 $368.5 billion legal settlement with the tobacco industry. They are: *Big Tobacco at the Bar of Justice*, Peter Pringle, Henry Hold, 1998, *The People vs. Big Tobacco*, Carrick Mollenkamp et al, Bloomberg Press, 1998, and *Assuming the Risk: the Mavericks, the Lawyers, and the Whistle-Blowers Who Beat Big Tobacco*, Michael Orey, Little, Brown and Company, 1999.

2.  The Master Settlement Agreement (with the tobacco industry) was reached in 1998 for a total of $368.5 billion over 25 years. In 2001, the average state received $28.35 per capita from this agreement, yet allocated just 6% for tobacco control and 4% for research. The states with the highest rates of lung cancer tended to spend the least on tobacco control, including Pennsylvania (only 10 cents per capita), Kentucky, with the nation's highest lung cancer rates (84 cents per capita), and Louisiana, 37 cents per capita.    PR Newswire, November 20, 2002

3.  An article by Richard Daynard, JD, PhD, discussed the implications for tobacco control of the 1998 master settlement agreement between major tobacco manufacturers and the U.S. states.
                    American Journal of Public Health, December 2001, pp. 1967-1971

4.  With only a few exceptions, the states are failing to invest even the minimum amounts recommended by the Centers for Disease Control to prevent and reduce tobacco use and related health care costs and harm. 2001 state tobacco prevention spending was $768 million. At the same time, the tobacco industry has dramatically increased its marketing expenditures, from $6.73 billion in 1998 to $8.24 billion in 1999 and $9.57 billion in 2000. (This is cigarette company advertising and marketing, not including smokeless tobacco and cigars.)
                    National Center for Tobacco Free Kids (Eric Lindblom), May 24, 2002

5.  In the closing weeks of the 1997 session, a torrent of public outrage…had forced Congress, with near unanimity, to overturn a provision, stealthily inserted by Senate Majority Leader Trent Lott and House Speaker Newt Gingrich in July into the Senate-House conference report of a tax bill, that would have granted the

tobacco companies a $50 billion tax credit to offset the $368 billion settlement payment the industry had agreed to. The odor hung in the air throughout the fall. *Quote from Smoke in Their Eyes*, p. 195

6. Only a small fraction of the multi billion tobacco settlement money to the states is being used to try to deny young replacement smokers to the tobacco companies. Only 5% is going into smoking prevention. Mississippi attorney general, Michael Moore, who began the original huge state lawsuit, commented: "The tobacco guys are sitting there laughing at us." *Boston Globe*, August 12, 2001

7. Only 5% of the $21 billion that the tobacco industry paid out to the states between 2000 and 2002 went toward antismoking efforts, which was the original intent of the master settlement. *Newsweek*, August 19, 2002, p. 33

8. "But perhaps no state has been quite so brazen in distorting the purpose of the settlement money as tobacco-producing North Carolina, which has directed only 1.2% of tobacco revenues to smoking prevention."
*Time*, July 1, 2002, p. 16

9. Tobacco settlement money has been used for flood protection projects in North Dakota and building harbors in Alaska. In North Carolina, $40 million has been spent, money going to help a new tobacco processing plant, and helping 6700 tobacco farmers stay in business by direct grants to upgrade furnaces in their curing barns.
*CBS evening news (Dan Rather)*, December 30, 2002

10. AMA President Richard Corlin, M.D., had several nominees for the "Golden Butt Award" for the most egregious misuses of tobacco settlement money. They included Stanislaus County, California, who used $4 million in settlement money for street repairs, and the state of North Dakota, spending 45% of their share on water reclamation projects. *American Medical News*, August 20, 2001, p. 32

11. The American Legacy Foundation, funded by the settlement, is broadcasting and publishing – in each of the five years beginning in the year 2000--$145 million worth of aggressive, national, state-of-the-art paid counter-advertising, targeted at young people. It has also generously funded innovative activities especially designed to broaden the reach of the tobacco control movement to youth and minority communities. It may not, under the terms of the multi-state agreement, directly attack the tobacco companies, but it has aggressively pressed the limits of its mandate, for instance, by shifting focus and unmasking the tobacco industry's massive new target marketing of college-age smokers and potential smokers. *Quote from Smoke in Their Eyes*, p. 239

12. Lorillard Tobacco has sued the American Legacy Foundation over their highly effective Truth anti-tobacco campaign. *ANR Update*, Spring 2002

13. State and Local Legislative Action to Reduce Tobacco Use, Smoking and Tobacco Control Monograph No. 11, National Cancer Institute, 2000, gives details on state and local legislative actions.

14. Regarding the tobacco industry's settlement to the states, only five states are meeting the standard of using 20% to 25% of their payments for tobacco control, as recommended by the Centers for Disease Control and Prevention. Those five states are among the fewer than 20 that meet even half the CDC standard. Several states put nothing from the settlement, or even their tobacco taxes, into smoking and tobacco use prevention.
*American Medical News*, February 18, 2002, p. 22

15. "Like Congress, none of the state legislatures are prepared to do the things necessary to make the books balance. So they are engaged in a wild dance with budget mirrors and accounting tricks – the favorite idea seems to be spending the next 30 years' worth of revenue from the tobacco settlements tomorrow."
*New York Times editorial*, May 19, 2002, commenting on the new state and federal budget deficits

16. The tobacco companies pay about $16 billion yearly to the states as part of the $246 settlement in 1998. In 2001 and 2002, just 5% of the states' share from the settlement payout and sales taxes from tobacco have been allocated to tobacco cessation or prevention programs, far less than the 25% that the CDC recommends to reduce smoking. In many states with severe budget problems, the share allocated is being reduced even further. "Tobacco Programs Wither as States Divert Settlement Revenue" stated the *Journal of the National Cancer Institute*, November 6, 2002, pp. 1598-1599.

17. Slashing of tobacco control programs in California and Massachusetts was termed "public health malpractice" by Thomas Houston, M.D., of the American Medical Association. The landmark 1998 tobacco master settlement agreement, plus state taxes, are paying the states $20.3 billion in 2003, but states are spending fewer and fewer dollars of these funds on smoking prevention efforts. Cheryl Healton, president and CEO of the American Legacy Foundation, commented, "History will view [the settlement] as a golden opportunity for public health that fell flat on its face." Overall, in fiscal year 2003, the states will spend about $700 million on tobacco prevention and cessation.                                   American Medical News, February 17, 2003

# Justice Department Lawsuit

1.  A Justice Department lawsuit against the nation's tobacco companies was originally filed in 1999. A pretrial document contained proposed tobacco control measures, including:
    - A ban on use of terms such as "light" or "low-tar."
    - Disclosure of all ingredients and additives.
    - Elimination of cigarette advertising in stores.
    - Use of graphic warning labels filling at least 50% of the space on cigarette packs and print ads.
    - A ban on lobbying against ordinances directed at secondhand smoke.
    - An end to the estimated $3.5 billion the industry spends each year on point-of-purchase advertising and promotions, including in-store signage and display racks.
    - Restriction of cigarette ads to black-and-white print format.
    - Creation of a foundation to develop, test, and promote less hazardous cigarettes, funded by cigarette makers.                                   2002 AMA Annual Tobacco Report

2.  Justice department lawyers asked Attorney General John Ashcroft**Error! Bookmark not defined.** for $57 million for the 2002 fiscal year to continue their 1999 lawsuit against the tobacco industry. Ashcroft's answer was a budget proposal of $1.8 million.                                   USA Today, June 1, 2001, p. 15A

3.  "The Justice Department is choking off a groundbreaking 1999 lawsuit against cigarette makers, which charges that the industry defrauded the public by lying about the risks of smoking. Department lawyers asked Attorney General John Ashcroft for $57 million in the coming fiscal year for staff and fact-finding, warning that without adequate funding, the lawsuit would have to be abandoned – a gift to Big Tobacco. Ashcroft's answer is a budget proposal of $1.8 million, a warning that the suit could languish and die."
                        Editorial (undated) in USA Today quoted in ASH Smoking and Health Review, May-June 2001

4.  The federal justice department lawsuit against the tobacco industry from 1999 received a boost in funding to $25 million in direct funding and $18 million through other funding sources in John Ashcroft's proposed budget for 2002-2003.                                   Wall Street Journal, March 11, 2002

5.  "The Justice Department is demanding that the nation's biggest cigarette makers be ordered to forfeit $289 billion in profits derived from a half-century of 'fraudulent' and dangerous marketing practices. Citing new evidence, the Justice Department asserts in more than 1400 pages of court documents that the major cigarette companies are running what amounts to a criminal enterprise by manipulating nicotine levels, lying to their customers about the dangers of tobacco and directing their multi-billion dollar advertising campaigns at children." The lawsuit was initiated in 1999 by President Bill Clinton and Attorney General Janet Reno.
                                   New York Times, March 18, 2003, pp. A1 and A27

# CHAPTER 35
# POLITICAL ISSUES

## General

1. "Smoking has ceased to be a health controversy, and is now primarily a political issue that must be tackled by political means."
The Lancet, November 2, 1985, p. 989

2. "Smoking...has yet to be proven to have a causal role in the development of diseases."
Walker Merryman, Tobacco Institute spokesman, 1994 (Newsweek, July 4, 1994, p. 45)

3. In testimony to Congress in April 1994, Andrew Tisch, the chairman and CEO of Lorillard, was asked whether smoking caused cancer. "I do not believe that," he answered. The tobacco executives also insisted that nicotine is no more addictive than sugar or caffeine.
San Francisco Chronicle, April 15, 1994, p. A4

4. "Eminent scientists believe that questions relating to smoking and health are unresolved." The Tobacco Institute, 1985. The industry tries to create doubt about the health charge without actually denying it, and to foster a scientific "debate" about the smoking and health "controversy." Surgeon General Koop said that the Tobacco Institute's insistence that "the jury is still out" on smoking is the result of "their lack of belief in science." He added: "Not a single smoker should be given assurance that the case against smoking is still in doubt. It is not."
Los Angeles Times, December 20, 1985

5. In 1993, the president of the Tobacco Institute received $505,786 in salary, benefits and allowances.
ASH Review, January 1995, p. 6

6. The Tobacco Institute has four speakers to travel around the country to present the tobacco viewpoint. Their speeches, primarily to civic and business organizations, stress the freedom of choice theme.   *Cigarettes*, p. 101

7. The Tobacco Institute closed in early 1999 after 40 years as the industry's lobbying group. "It gave thousands of campaign dollars to friendly lawmakers, flew them to expenses-paid golfing weekends at lavish resorts and once paid a Washington researcher $10,000 to write a letter to a medical journal."
San Francisco Chronicle, January 30, 1999

8. Text of full page tobacco company ad running in more than 400 newspapers and other publications in 1964 in "A FRANK STATEMENT TO CIGARETTE SMOKERS. Distinguished authorities point out:
That medical research indicates many possible causes of lung cancer.
That there is no agreement regarding what the cause is.
That there is no proof that cigarette smoking is one of the causes.
That statistics purporting to link cigarette smoking with the disease could apply with equal force to any one of many other aspects of modern life. Indeed, the validity of the statistics themselves is questioned by numerous scientists."
New York Times, June 16, 1994, p. D22

9. Since tobacco is not considered to be either a food or a drug, it is not subject to any regulatory control by the government.
*Koop*, p. 165

10. The 1965 Cigarette Labeling and Advertising Act mandated a conditional warning "Cigarette smoking may be hazardous to your health." State and local action that might strengthen the federal action was preempted, and a New York Times editorial called it "a shocking piece of special interest legislation." This was the primary basis of the tobacco industry's "perfect record" on more than 800 product liability lawsuits through 1994.
Tobacco Control, Summer 1994, p. 140

11. In January 1971, cigarette ads were removed from TV and radio broadcast media at the request of the tobacco companies. In return, they were granted immunity from antitrust laws. As well, antismoking media messages mandated by the 1967 Fairness Doctrine, which were leading to reduced tobacco sales, were discontinued.

Consumer Reports called the volunteering to abandon broadcast media "one of the shrewdest business decisions the cigarette industry ever made."                                                                                    Tobacco Control, Summer 1994, p. 141

12. Tobacco industry "front groups" have names such as Veterans for Freedom, Citizens Opposed to Special Taxes, Inter-Community Parent/Business Task Force on Youth Smoking, and the California Business and Restaurant Alliance. Michigan Citizens for Fair Taxes, Californians for Uniform Statewide Restrictions, and Colorado's Citizens Against Tax Abuse and Government Waste were campaigns almost entirely funded not by state citizens but by out of state tobacco companies.
*Tobacco Industry Strategies,* p. 15, and American Medical News, December 5, 1994, p. 15

13. Pierre Salinger, former press secretary to JFK and a cigar smoker, served on the advisory board of the National Smokers Alliance, a "front group" of smokers set up by Philip Morris.
Washington Post National Weekly Edition, October 24, 1991, p. 15

14. The sole financial backer for the National Coalition Against Crime and Tobacco Smuggling is RJ Reynolds. This is a front group established by the industry to fight higher federal tobacco taxes.
*Tobacco Industry Strategies,* p. 16

15. A prominent tobacco industry front group is Healthy Buildings International of Fairfax, VA, an indoor air consulting firm. The organization examines workplace ventilation systems, and theorizes that the cause of most workplace air quality problems is poor ventilation, not specific pollutants such as tobacco smoke. Three workers who made measurements that were cited as industry arguments against control of smoking in workplaces say that their data were altered to show that secondhand smoke is not a significant hazard in the workplace.
*Tobacco Industry Strategies,* p. 16, New York Times, December 21, 1994, and SCARC, July 31, 1992

16. The Council for Tobacco Research created in the 1950's "legitimized the tobacco industry's media campaign to confuse the public about the strength of the scientific evidence linking cigarette smoking and disease."
*Changes in Cigarette-Related Disease Risks,* p. 17

17. The industry-supported Council for Tobacco Research (CTR) has financed $220 million worth of research since it was founded in 1954, much of it on "sympathetic science." In May 1994, the president of CTR testified under oath to Congress that he did not believe that smoking caused cancer or that cigarettes were addictive, and that the tobacco industry exercised no control over the council's activities. A former chief executive of Lorillard wrote: "CTR is the best and cheapest insurance the tobacco industry can buy, and without it, the industry...would be dead."                                                                                    *Tobacco Industry Strategies,* p. 29

18. The Council for Tobacco Research, funded by the tobacco industry, has given out over $240 million in research grants since its inception in 1954. None of this research "has resulted in any damaging information about cigarettes coming to light."                                                       *Cigarette Confidential,* p. 44 and *Cancer Wars,* p. 106

19. The Council for Tobacco Research has never funded research on how to prevent tobacco use or to stop smoking.                                                                                                                            *Cancer Wars,* p. 109

20. The Council for Tobacco Research was formed by the tobacco companies in 1954 to promote research on whether smoking caused illness. A federal judge in a ruling stated that these research findings were "nothing but a public relations ploy- a fraud- to deflect the growing evidence against the industry, to encourage smokers to continue and non-smokers to begin, and to reassure the public. Despite some rising pretenders, the tobacco industry may be the king of concealment and disinformation."                                    American Medical News, June 24, 1988

21. The Council for Tobacco Research provided more than $1 million in research funds to Dr. Carl Seltzer, a biological anthropologist who disputes the role of smoking in causing heart disease. Similarly, CTR gave $1.1 million for research to Dr. Theodur Sterling, who believes that occupational exposure to toxic fumes is a more likely cause of illness than smoking.                                                       Tobacco Control, Winter 1994, p. 297

22. "The primary aim of tobacco industry science-as-propaganda is to produce a semblance of a need for 'balance' in the 'debate.'" Stanton Glantz has described this strategy as an attempt "to jam the scientific airways with noise."

*Cancer Wars*, p. 110

23. Harvard researchers got $5 million from the tobacco industry's Council on Tobacco Research for special projects that the council hoped would dispute links between smoking and fatal diseases. In the early 1990s, 55% of US medical schools acknowledged receipt of research funds from the tobacco industry.

American Medical News, December 21, 1992, p. 6, and August 15, 1994, p. 18

24. The Council for Tobacco Research awarded a total of $82 million in grants to 250 hospitals and medical schools between 1954 and 1979.

*Cigarettes*, p. 95

25. In 1992, 52 of 95 medical schools reported receiving tobacco money.

Science, April 26, 1996, p. 491

26. Eight scientists at the R.J. Reynolds tobacco company are also faculty members at the Bowman Gray Medical School. Wake Forest College moved its medical school to Winston-Salem, North Carolina, from Wake Forest in 1941 with $750,000 from the estate of Bowman Gray, the third president of R.J. Reynolds, and changed its name to that of its benefactor. Since 1963, the tobacco industry has provided $17 million to the school, including $3.5 million in the past five years to pay for research. The latest was a $993,000 grant from Reynolds to the Department of Pulmonary Medicine for a study comparing health effects of ordinary cigarettes to those of Reynolds' new low-smoke cigarette, Eclipse.

American Medical News, April 14, 1997

27. A quarterly journal called the American Smoker's Journal published in Kentucky in the late 1980's was skeptical of research findings of the Environmental Protection Agency (EPA), which the publisher called "Extremists Panicking America."

American Medical News, June 24, 1988

28. A common tobacco industry strategy is to depict itself as a defender of personal liberty against the "health Nazis," and to paint a scenario of prohibition and big government interference in peoples' lives. Hugh Cullman of Philip Morris talked about the "creeping intolerance of these neo-Prohibitionists and anti-smoking zealots...It's no joke when people hide behind the socially acceptable cloak of moral self-righteousness to publicly humiliate others."

*Tobacco Industry Strategies*, p. 41

29. "Critics have dismissed antismoking groups as 'health Nazis' and 'health nannies'--repressive killjoys who want to control how people live and deny them the 'freedom' to smoke."

*Cigarettes*, p. xiv

30. "Right now the anti-tobacco lobby seems intent on banning smoking completely. They are pursuing a new era of prohibition and in the process are ignoring the individual rights of not just the 45 million Americans who choose to smoke, but all Americans as well. Who knows what will be next? Alcohol? Caffeine? High-cholesterol foods? Books and movies? A cigarette ban is just the beginning."

RJ Reynolds Tobacco Co. full page ad in USA Today, New York Times, and Wall St. Journal, June 1994 (SCARC, July 1, 1994)

31. "I suppose the day will come when the last smokers on earth will be found cowering in a box canyon south of Donner Pass while tobacco agents in a helicopter overhead demand they surrender. Oh, how merciless the righteous can be in saving us all from ourselves."

Point After, Sports Illustrated, June 3, 1991

32. The Tobacco Institute of Australia was found by the courts to have engaged in misleading and deceptive advertising. It ran advertisements claiming "there is little evidence and nothing which proves scientifically that cigarette smoking causes disease in nonsmokers."

British Medical Journal, March 11, 1995, p. 620

33. "What we are witnessing in the anti-tobacco campaigns resembles the Colonial witch hunts of the 1600's. The antismoking zealots allow no discussion. They manipulate science and the facts to suit their preordained conclusions. They dismiss any attempt at reasonable discourse as tantamount to treason. For them, there is no middle ground."

Editorial, Cigar Aficionado, October 1999, p. 19

34. "The 'threatened' ban on cigarettes is a strawman that Philip Morris and RJ Reynolds are desperately seeking. No one...has been advocating any such radical move."
Michael Pertschuk, "Puffery," Washington Post, March 26, 1994

35. A billboard on Interstate 40 in Clemmons, N.C., reads: "The Time is Now to Stand Up for Tobacco Rights!" Arby's bans smoking in their company-owned stores, but the Arby's in Clemmons (a suburb of Winston-Salem) has a large sign reading "Smokers Welcome." Tobacco-Free Youth Reporter, Summer 1994, p. 8

36. Orange juice and toothpaste are more heavily regulated for health and safety reasons than is tobacco.
SCARC, April 8, 1994, and Scott Ballin, Coalition on Smoking or Health

37. "Many eminent scientists hold the view that no case against smoking has been proved."
The Tobacco Institute, 1980 (International Journal of Health Sciences 1986, 16:280)

38. "The smoking and health controversy remains unresolved." Edward A. Horrigan, CEO, RJ Reynolds
(World Smoking and Health No. 2, 1992, p. 3)

39. The tobacco industry willfully launched a massive misinformation campaign to undermine the credibility of the 1964 Surgeon General's report. It used the same energy its unsuccessful attempts to scuttle the 1993 EPA report on secondhand smoke and to vilify the reputation of the agency itself. *Tobacco Use: An American Crisis*, p. 5

40. "Cancer is a communicable disease. You get it from tobacco companies."
Joe Tye, Founder, STAT (Stop Teenage Addiction to Tobacco)

41. "The cigarette company is to the lung cancer epidemic what the mosquito is to malaria. It is the vector of disease." John Slade, MD, New Jersey College of Medicine

42. A 1991-1992 Bill of Rights tour sponsored by Philip Morris was accompanied at each stop by Nicotina, a 15-foot replica of the Statue of Liberty holding a cigarette and wrapped in the chains of addiction.
1. Journal of Medical Activism (DOC News and Views), Winter 1991 and Summer 1992

43. An ad running in 400 newspapers in 1954 read: "The tobacco industry considers their customer's health paramount to every other consideration of our business." Primetime Live, ABC News, February 1993

44. Ex-smoker and Olympic champion diver Greg Louganis was asked by the American Cancer Society to be the national chairman for the 1984 Great American Smokeout. Unfortunately, Philip Morris owned his Mission Viejo training facility and informed Greg that if he accepted the offer, both the training facility and his coach would no longer be available to him. *Merchants of Death*, Larry White, 1988, p. 215

45. 70% of smokers are unable to identify the specific theme of even one of the surgeon general's warnings on cigarette packs. JAMA, January 6, 1989, p. 45

46. Several federal appeals courts have ruled that the presence of warning labels on cigarette packs since 1965 exempts tobacco companies for any liability for the disease and death caused by smoking.
JAMA, January 6, 1989, p. 44

47. Harvard University and the City University of New York were the first educational institutions to sell all their tobacco company stock. Dr. Kenneth Kizer, the director of the California Health Department, has asked California's universities and major pension funds to sell their tobacco company stock. He was the first public health official in the country to publicly advocate divestiture. The AMA sold its tobacco stocks in 1981.
Los Angeles Times, February 1, 1991, and American Medical News, August 9, 1993, p. 14

48. Comments critical of tobacco advertising made by Dr. Jay Gordon, the staff pediatrician on ABC TV's Home show, were censored from the show's broadcast on March 9, 1994. *Tobacco Industry Strategies*, p. 10

49. When William Bennett, a smoker, was named as the nation's first "Drug Czar" by George Bush, a coalition of anti-tobacco groups issued a "Drug-Free Challenge to William Bennett" to spotlight his tobacco addiction.

Public Health Reports, November 1993, p. 722

50. George W. Bush indicated in the 2000 campaign that, if elected president, he would reverse the Clinton no-smoking policy in the White House. [He did not – editor]   San Francisco Chronicle, December 28, 1999, p. C11

51. George W. Bush's top political aide is Karl Rove, who worked from 1991 to 1996 as a consultant to Philip Morris. Bush in the late 1970's was on the board of the Midland, Texas chapter of the American Cancer Society, and signed a tough bill restricting sales of cigarettes to minors in Texas. Bush "once smoked cigarettes and chewed tobacco and is often seen with an unlit cigar in his mouth."

Washington Post National Weekly Edition, March 13, 2000, p. 14

52. The Hooters 500 auto race in November 1993 at the Atlanta Motor speedway was one of the Winston Cup NASCAR series, and was attended by 100,000 people, the largest sporting event in Georgia. This series includes 30 races in 14 states each year. The Skoal trailer had a sign that read, "Keep Government Out of Racing Sponsorships...WARNING LABELS DO NOT BELONG ON RACE CARS."        John Slade, M.D.

53. Michael Lippman, MD, had had it. Armed with a can of blood-red spray paint, he set out before dawn one winter morning to scale the billboard near his hospital "CAMEL FILTERS. It's a whole new world," the sign screamed. "OF CANCER," the Seattle family physician added, before police led him off in handcuffs.

American Medical News, August 9, 1993

54. In 1985, Philip Morris paid former Ronald Reagan aide Michael Deaver $250,000 to try to secure concessions from South Korea on tobacco imports.        The Progressive, May 1991, p. 29

55. A New York Times editorial referred to the "white collar drug pushers" in the tobacco industry.

Tobacco Free Youth Reporter, Summer 1993

56. A militant newspaper ad sponsored by STAT (Stop Teenage Addiction to Tobacco) reads: "Meet five of America's richest drug pushers." It features mug shots of middle-aged white businessmen, three of whom head tobacco companies, and two publishing moguls whose magazines are widely read by teens and carry heavy quantities of cigarette advertising. They are Rupert Murdock, Larry Tisch, Michael Miles, Henry Kravis, and Si Newhouse. Three are billionaires, and none smokes.        Washington Post magazine, February 20, 1994, p. 11

57. "Henry Kravis, prime mover behind the RJR Nabisco buyout and a man desperately in need of profits from cigarette sales to pay off the debt from this record-breaking leveraged buyout, earns a special STAT Hypocrite Award. Not only does he target children for cigarette sales, but then he hypocritically attends a fund-raising dinner for and contributes to the Center on Addiction and Substance Abuse."

Tobacco Free Youth Reporter, Summer 1993

58. In the early 1960's before the first Surgeon General's report on smoking, Brown and Williamson Tobacco Company researchers found that cigarettes caused lung cancer, contributed to heart disease, and might cause emphysema. The information in these internal documents remained suppressed until 1994, when "stolen" copies were released.        San Francisco Chronicle, May 7, 1994, p. A7

59. The Canadian government is studying plans to require plain packaging for all tobacco products sold there. US lobbyists argue that this would violate the free trade agreements that Canada has signed with the US. Lawyers for RJ Reynolds and Philip Morris swarmed into Ottawa and were compared by some critics to the soft-spoken, well-dressed characters from "The Godfather" movie.        San Francisco Chronicle, May 30, 1994, p. D1

60. After Lawrence and Preston Tisch of P. Lorillard Tobacco Company and Loews Corp. gave $30 million to New York University, its hospital was renamed for them. Larry White wrote for Newsday that it was "unique in the history of medical philanthropy that donors gave not only the hospital, but the patients as well." And thoracic surgeon William Cahan wrote in the Daily News: "Naming a hospital after tobacco men is just too ironic. Around town, the University Hospital is becoming known as Lorillard General."   *No Stranger to Tears*, p. 371

61. Dr. Will Cahan, a thoracic surgeon at Memorial Sloan-Kettering Cancer Center in New York, gave his operating room the name "Marlboro Country." *No Stranger to Tears*, p. 321

62. In November 1983, Newsweek ran a 16-page special health supplement written by the American Medical Association. The section of the manuscript dealing with tobacco and nicotine addiction was deleted. That issue of Newsweek had 12 full-page cigarette ads. Journal of Health Politics, Policy and Law, Fall 1986 p. 375

63. The following dialogue is from a transcript of depositions taken in a case brought by airline flight attendants who contend that their exposure to smoke in the cabin caused them to develop cancer and other illnesses. Andrew H. Tisch, Chairman and CEO of Lorillard, was asked:
"Q: Does cigarette smoking cause cancer?
"A: I don't believe so.
"Q:..This warning on the package which says that smoking causes lung cancer, heart disease and emphysema is inaccurate? You don't believe it's true?
"A: That's correct.
"Q: Because if you believed it were true, in good conscience you wouldn't sell this . . . ?
"A: That's correct." Washington Monthly, January/February 1994, p. 6

64. One tobacco industry method of fomenting doubt about health hazards is to arrange scientific meetings and invite well-established researchers and industry consultants as speakers. The consultants voice doubt about research findings that are repeated in letters to the editor and advertisements in the popular media. Science, April 17, 1987, p. 251

65. In an interview with Mike Wallace of 60 Minutes, former Brown and Williamson vice president Dr. Jeffrey Wigand said that B & W attempted to develop a fire-retardant and less hazardous cigarette, only to abandon these plans and alter documents to delete any reference to the aborted effort. (Safer cigarettes would be an admission that other cigarettes are dangerous). He also said that the company's CEO, Thomas Sandefur, perjured himself before Congress when he denied knowledge of how cigarettes were used to deliver nicotine. Wigand also said that coumarin was added to pipe tobacco to give it a sweeter flavor, even though it was known to be a carcinogen and was being used at a hundredfold the safety level. When Wigand recommended the coumarin no longer be used as an additive, Sandefur refused because it would adversely impact sales. The interview initially was not broadcast on 60 Minutes because of fear of B & W legal action against CBS, but a transcript was leaked to the New York Daily News, and it was aired in February 1996.
Time, November 27, 1995, p. 88 (Richard Lacayo)
and New York Daily News, November 17, 1995 (Jim Dwyer)

66. The movie *The Insider* is the story of Jeffrey Wigand, former chief scientist for Brown and Williamson, and his interview, initially suppressed, with the program "60 Minutes." New York Times, November 26, 1999

67. Victor Crawford was a former $200-an-hour lobbyist for the Tobacco Institute who turned anti-smoking activist when he developed throat cancer. His story was featured on 60 Minutes. "As tobacco kills off people like me, they need kids like you to replace me. It's too late for me, but it's not too late for you," he said before his death at age 63 from his cancer. He had smoked since age 13. USA Today, March 5, 1996, p. 7A

68. In 1990 alone, Philip Morris gave $91,800 to Citizens for a Sound Economy, a Washington, D.C., think tank that advocates less regulation and lower taxes, as well as $40,000 to the Tax Foundation, a Washington think tank that sponsors the annual "Tax Freedom Day." That year, the company also gave $20,000 to the Southern Governors Association and $12,000 to the National Governors Conference.
Washington Monthly, May 1996, pp. 21-22

69. "The embattled tobacco industry is spending more money than ever to influence the political process, but some of its largess eludes political radar. That's because the industry's record $4.1 million in donations to political candidates and parties last year represents but a portion of its contributions – the part that must be disclosed to the public. There's another, largely undisclosed, dimension to the tobacco industry's political giving. Philip Morris Cos. and R.J. Reynolds Tobacco Co., for example, also lavish donations on like-minded think tanks and

other groups that share its views – particularly an antipathy toward David Kessler's Food and Drug Administration, which wants to regulate cigarettes. These tobacco donations represent a kind of stealth spending that reinforces the industry's direct political contributions. No one knows exactly how much additional money this giving represents because the groups don't have to disclose it."

Wall Street Journal, March 25, 1996, p. A22 (T. Noah and L. McGinley)

70. Tobacco giant Philip Morris systematically wooed scientists who might help the company counter the growing consensus on the health risks of secondhand tobacco smoke and "keep the controversy alive," according to a 1988 internal tobacco-company document. The British American Tobacco Co. memo, obtained by the Washington Post, laid out in great detail Philip Morris' presentation at a February 1988 conference of its global strategy for dealing with environmental tobacco smoke (ETS). The company was "spending vast sums of money" to find scientists amenable to its cause and funding research by them, the memo said.

Quote from San Francisco Chronicle, May 9, 1997, p. A4

71. In a January 9, 1998 Washington Times op-ed, William Rusher compared the "snowballing national hysteria over smoking" with the Salem witch trials of the 1600's in Massachusetts.

72. Tobacco interests gave $4.5 million in 1997 to national political parties and federal candidates, an industry record for a non-election year. The industry also spent $53 million on lobbying in 1997.

New York Times, March 8, 1998, p. 1, and April 1,1998, p. A18

73. The National Smokers Alliance claims to be a grassroots organization supported by more than 3 million dues paying members. However, the group's 1996 report to the IRS showed that of $9 million collected in 1996, only $74,000 was from membership dues. Most of the funding is from Philip Morris, which contributed nearly $7 million in 1994, or 96% of the group's income for that year. Los Angeles Times, March 29, 1998

74. The National Smokers Alliance, a tax-exempt, nonprofit group, helped to arrange coalitions in an unsuccessful attempt to repeal the California ban on smoking in bars. The alliance received more than $42 million from the tobacco industry between 1993 and 1996. One of the world's largest public relations firms, Burson-Marsteller, which has long had close ties to the tobacco industry, has guided an intensive legislative lobbying effort in California, and received more than $4.4 million from the National Smokers Alliance between 1993 and 1996.

Washington Post National Weekly Edition, February 23, 1998, p. 32

75. The National Smokers Alliance website has information such as quotes "whole milk has a higher carcinogen rating than environmental tobacco smoke" and news stories about the health benefits of smoking for Alzheimer's sufferers. Americans for Nonsmokers' Rights newsletter, Summer 1997

76. Philip Morris announced an end to its financial support of the National Smokers Alliance after the organization filed an ethics complaint against Senator John McCain, sponsor of the failed 1998 national tobacco legislation.

Wall Street Journal, June 30, 1999, p. C13

77. Brown and Williamson spent $24.9 million, and Philip Morris $23 million, in 1998 for lobbying expenses, which included their successful effort to kill federal tobacco control legislation and the McCain bill. A B& W spokesman commented: "Drastic measures sometimes require drastic…expenditures to defend oneself."

Roll Call, April 8, 1999, p. 1

78. 1998 tobacco company lobbying expenses amounted to $67.2 million. NBC News, March 18, 2000

79. The tobacco industry spent more than $43 million on lobbying in the first half of 1998, much of it in their successful effort to kill national tobacco legislation, the $516 billion comprehensive anti-tobacco bill. $7.2 million of the amount went to a single Washington law firm, Verner, Liipfert, and Hand, where Ann Richards and George Mitchell worked on the tobacco issue. San Francisco Chronicle, October 30, 1998, p. A10

80. The respected Washington law firm of Verner Liipfert took in $18 million in fees for lobbying from 1997 to 1999 from tobacco companies looking to negotiate a legislative settlement with Congress. Members of the firm include Bob Dole, George Mitchell, Ann Richards, and Lloyd Bentsen.

Washington Monthly, October 1999, p. 26

81. "Big Tobacco Pressured Drug Companies To Soften Quit-Smoking Message." According to tobacco industry documents, from 1982 through 1992, tobacco companies used coercion and economic intimidation to muffle aggressive anti-smoking messages by the makers of cessation products, such as the nicotine patch or gum. In 1984, Philip Morris canceled chemical purchases from Dow Chemical after one of Dow's subsidiaries, Merrell Dow, introduced Nicorette and prepared literature for doctors' offices urging smokers to quit. Dow Chemical eventually got the Philip Morris account back, but only after Dow assured Philip Morris it was "committed to avoiding contribution to the anti-cigarette effort," and Merrell Dow president David Sharrock informed tobacco executives that he would personally begin to "screen advertising and promotional materials to eliminate any inflammatory anti-industry statements."          Quote from news summary regarding article "Big Tobacco Threatened Drug Manufacturers With Reprisal" by Myron Levin in Los Angeles Times, February 14, 1999

82. Nicotine replacement products "are promoted in a manner certain to minimize conflict with cigarette manufacturers... For at least a decade (from 1982 to 1992), Philip Morris sought to intimidate drug firms marketing the stop-smoking products, using the threat of economic reprisals to make them tone down their ads and refrain from supporting the anti-smoking cause, according to once-secret documents..." Internal memos showed that the cigarette industry threatened to cancel supply contracts with the corporate parents of the drug firms. The February 14, 1999 article by Myron Levin in the Los Angeles Times gives details of the tobacco industry's successful efforts to water down the anti-smoking message by Merrell Dow and Ciba-Geigy in their marketing campaigns for nicotine replacement products. The National Association of State Fire Marshals receives $50,000 a year from Philip Morris for "administrative expenses." The tobacco industry for decades has courted firefighters to weaken their support for the manufacture and regulation of fire-safe cigarettes.
Baltimore Sun, February 16, 1999

83. The tobacco industry has a strategy of claiming that federal funds have been used for "illegal lobbying" by public health professionals on policy interventions for tobacco control. The industry filed formal complaints alleging illegal lobbying activities against four ASSIST states. ASSIST (American Stop Smoking Intervention Study) was a National Cancer Institute – funded comprehensive tobacco control project. In 11 of the 17 ASSIST states, public health professionals said that fear that claims of illegal lobbying would be made against them made them self-censor their activity to some degree. The tobacco companies have also used the Freedom of Information Act as a tool to slow the implementation of tobacco control programs by requesting program-related documents, which has disrupted the work of health departments.
Quote from American Journal of Public Health, January 2001, pp. 62-67

84. "...a disturbing case study of Rice University, which has collected more than $500,000 over the past two years for hosting major tobacco-sponsored events, yet has refused to permit the subject of the university's relationship with tobacco sponsors to be discussed by the Board of Trustees. Rice has also ignored a campaign by alumni to divest considerable holdings in tobacco stocks."
11th World Conference on Tobacco or Health, Chicago, 2000, Abstract p. 440

85. "The victory of pro-business interests in the recent U.S. elections has given the tobacco industry the confidence to invest again [in constructing new plants and production facilities]."   editorial in Tobacco Reporter, July 2001

86. Information on the 1989 Philip Morris Bill of Rights Tour is in *Reducing Tobacco Use*, 2000 Surgeon General report, p. 408

# Tobacco and the American Civil Liberties Union (ACLU)

1. The American Civil Liberties Union (ACLU) has been lobbying since 1986 against restrictions on cigarette advertising on the grounds that it would violate the First Amendment. Since that time, it has received more than half a million dollars in contributions from Philip Morris, and more from other tobacco companies.
Newsweek, August 9, 1993

2. The ACLU (American Civil Liberties Union) has a longstanding financial relationship with the tobacco industry, stalling federal legislation limiting tobacco advertising and promotion to children, and lobbying against legislation limiting smoking in restaurants, workplaces, and other indoor areas.

*Advocacy Institute, August 25, 1993*

3. In Pennsylvania, the legislative director of the state ACLU chapter testified against a bill prohibiting smoking in cars carrying children. In New Jersey, the ACLU director reportedly traveled in the same caravan with tobacco industry representatives to radio stations and press events in support of a smokers' rights bill.

*Tobacco Industry Strategies,* p. 13

4. "The ACLU's clients have always been the long line of individuals whose basic rights were threatened by oppressive government action. How did Philip Morris and RJ Reynolds jump to the front of that line?"

*Advocacy Institute, August 25, 1993*

5. "How could anyone seriously believe that advertising of harmful products is protected by the First Amendment?"

*Washington Monthly, September 1993, p. 11*

6. A Philip Morris representative said, "when it comes to protecting the rights of smokers, there's virtually no limit on the amount of money we'll spend."

*Tobacco Industry Strategies,* p.17

7. The ACLU has ferociously opposed any limits on cigarette ads, or any restrictions on deceptive marking or ads aimed at minors. The ACLU also lobbied against a bill which would have disallowed the companies' tax deduction for advertising expenses. The ACLU has received $770,000 from Philip Morris and $150,000 from R.J. Reynolds in the last 10 years; its executive director, Ira Glasser, defends having accepted the money, saying that he'd take a donation from John Gotti were it offered.     The Washington Monthly, April 1996, pp. 10-11

8. ACLU executive director Ira Glasser was quoted by New York times columnist Anna Quindlen as saying, "If John Gotti wanted to give $10,000, we would take it."

*Cigarette Confidential, p. 148*

9. Comments on the ACLU from *Cigarette Confidential,* pp. 144-147:

"The ACLU has transcended lust for the contributions of cash it receives from Philip Morris and R.J. Reynolds--in fact the organization has become insidiously dependent upon them. The group is hooked. Without money from tobacco companies, a significant number of ACLU activities and departments might have to be shut down. In order to rationalize this dependency, the ACLU has placed a disproportionate emphasis on its advocacy of smokers' rights and the rights of cigarette companies to target their products through advertising and marketing programs to whomever, whenever and wherever they see fit, under the First Amendment right to freedom of speech.

"In the eyes of many longtime members and supporters, the ACLU has been responding to a civil rights 'emergency' that doesn't really exist in order to justify its continuing reliance upon the cigarette money that keeps many of its operations afloat...

"The information exposes an entrenched pattern of conflict of interest unparalleled in the history of the modern civil rights movement. Many of the ACLU's resources have been hijacked, its mission perverted to satisfy the long-range goals and short-term whims of Philip Morris and RJR executives who keep the ACLU on a tight leash with regard to the protection of their industry's interests, using cash contributions as leverage. The work the ACLU has undertaken on behalf of cigarette manufacturers has been undertaken in direct exchange for funding--a quid pro quo arrangement in direct conflict with the institution's status as a government-subsidized, tax-exempt, nonprofit institution.

"To wit, the ACLU has successfully mounted an ambitious nationwide legislative lobbying campaign on behalf of cigarette companies in the areas of employment protections for smokers, freedom of speech protections for unrestricted cigarette advertisements, national health care reform legislation favoring smokers over nonsmokers, and protection of smoker's rights in parental custody cases of asthmatic children.

"The ACLU has conducted elaborate privacy surveys using questionable methodology to sway lawmakers and public opinion, aggressively intimidated municipalities and private employers with regard to smoker's rights and actively engaged in an international public relations campaign on behalf of cigarette manufacturers and trade associations."

10. "Cigarette manufacturers have spelled out in full-page advertisements, and through their lobbying organizations in Washington, such as the ACLU and the Tobacco Institute, how a 'bureaucracy run wild' is preparing to prohibit smoking and abolish cigarettes. What will be next, goes the cigarette company line, a new prohibition on alcohol? Caffeine? Fatty foods? Sweets and candy? In fact the FDA already regulates candy, caffeine and fatty foods under the Federal Food, Drug and Cosmetic Act. Traditionally, cigarettes have not been subject to even the same scrutiny as a cup of coffee."  *Cigarette Confidential*, p. 19

11. "In at least one instance, Philip Morris's in-house advertising and graphic art department designed, wrote copy for, produced and sent out an entire direct-mail campaign concerning smokers' rights that used the ACLU name and logo."  *Cigarette Confidential*, p. 158

12. Lew Maltby is director of the ACLU's Workplace Rights Project. In 1992, he traveled to Copenhagen at the expense of the Tobacco Institute to address a conference on smoking restrictions, and in his speech stated "many of the claims made about the health effects of smoking are exaggerated."  *Cigarette Confidential*, p. 158

# Federal and Congress

1. "Congress has been paid to do nothing. The tobacco lobby distributes hush money to the legislators, not to buy action, but to buy inaction. The fact that tobacco money buys pro-tobacco results is clear, consistent, and irrefutable."  Public Citizen, October 1993

2. The federal cigarette labeling law prohibits states from regulating tobacco advertising for health reasons.  *Nicotine Addiction*, p. 138

3. There were at least 26 tobacco control bills at the federal level stuck in committee and not passed in 1994, including bills that would eliminate tax breaks for tobacco advertising, force disclosure of chemical additives in cigarettes, end tobacco price supports, prohibit handing out free samples, require new Surgeon General's warnings on cigarette packs, and ban smoking in all public buildings.  *Tobacco Industry Strategies*, p. 27

4. In 1905, tobacco state congressmen had the word tobacco removed from that year's edition of the US Pharmacopoeia where it had been listed at the turn of the century. This was significant because the Food and Drug Administration, which was created in 1906, could only regulate drugs that appeared in the US Pharmacopoeia.  Annual Review of Public Health 1986; 7:130

5. The Cigarette Labeling and Advertising Act of 1965 created the first warning label stating "cigarettes may be hazardous to your health." This was a minor defeat in a large victory for the tobacco industry; the Act made for federal pre-emption of state and local regulation of advertising. This meant that no state or local government could pass a more restrictive advertising ban than the federal government's advertising restrictions.

6. Dr. Jesse Steinfeld was labeled "Public Enemy Number One" by the tobacco industry in 1971 when as Surgeon General he proposed a "Nonsmoker's Bill of Rights." In 1972, President Nixon received a letter from the president of R.J. Reynolds reminding him of their generous contribution to his recent campaign, and urging that he fire his Surgeon General because of overzealous antismoking activity.

7. Former U.S. Surgeon General Jesse Steinfeld was named to a four year term as surgeon general by President Nixon in late 1969. However, he was asked for his resignation a year before his term was over. RJR president David People wrote repeatedly to Nixon in 1972 to complain about Steinfeld's anti-tobacco activism and his 1971 proposal to curb smoking in public places because of concerns that nonsmokers were being harmed by secondhand smoke.  Reuters, August 8, 1997

8. In a 1980 North Carolina campaign appearance, Ronald Reagan promised to "end what has become an increasingly antagonistic relationship between the federal government and the tobacco industry. I can

guarantee that my own cabinet members will be far too busy with substantive matters to waste their time proselytizing against the dangers of cigarette smoking."  Washington Monthly, March 1987, p. 18
and New York State Journal of Medicine, December 1983, p. 1278

9.  In 1981, the new Reagan Administration moved to cut the budget for Department of Health and Human Services anti-smoking programs, and also planned to block any increase in cigarette taxes.

New York Times, June 18, 1994, p. A12

10.  In 1987, the Federal Trade Commission, which governs tobacco advertising and labels, ceded responsibility for measuring cigarette tar and nicotine levels to the Tobacco Institute, the industry's lobbying arm.

U.S. News and World Report, April 18, 1994, p. 35

11.  An Advocacy Institute report concludes:  "Tobacco money buys influence to oppose federal legislation to increase tobacco taxes, to restrict tobacco advertising and promotion, and to enact other laws to control the use of this deadly substance."

12.  "We should actively oppose any legislation that preempts stronger local laws, that criminalizes children for tobacco purchase, use or possession, that shields tobacco companies from product liability or elevates smoking to protected 'rights' category. These issues serve to protect the tobacco industry."

*Tobacco Use:  An American Crisis*, p. 102

13.  The preemption provision of the Cigarette Advertising and Labeling Act has served to inhibit major public health initiatives such as billboard bans, restrictions on youth-oriented marketing, and product liability suits.

*Tobacco Use:  An American Crisis*, p. 104

14.  Strong congressional influence has enabled the tobacco industry to preempt or avoid potential federal regulation under the Hazardous Substances Act, the Toxic Substance Control Act, the Consumer Product Safety Act, the Food Drug and Cosmetics Act, and the Fair Packaging and Labeling Act.*Nicotine Addiction*, p. 138

15.  Tobacco has been exempted from every major federal health and safety law enacted by Congress including the Consumer Product Safety Act, the Fair Labeling and Packaging Act, the Toxic Substances Act, and the Hazardous Substances Act. The FDA (Food and Drug Administration) regulates foods and drugs, but tobacco is not classified as either a food or a drug, so is not subject to FDA regulation. Tobacco is the least regulated consumer product in the U.S.

*Tobacco Use:  An American Crisis*, p. 53 and Washington Monthly, September 1993, p. 22

17.  The tobacco industry has gained exemptions from all key consumer safety legislation. Examples are:
THE CONSUMER PRODUCT SAFETY ACT
   The term "consumer product" does not include tobacco and tobacco products.
THE FAIR PACKAGING AND LABELING ACT
   "Consumer commodity" does not include any tobacco or tobacco product.
THE HAZARDOUS SUBSTANCES ACT
   The term "hazardous substance" shall not apply to tobacco and tobacco products.
THE TOXIC SUBSTANCES CONTROL ACT
   The term "chemical substance" does not include tobacco or any tobacco product.

Frontline (PBS television), January 3, 1995

18.  During the 1970s Congress enacted a number of statutes to protect the American consumer from a variety of potentially dangerous substances while specifically excluding the regulation of tobacco. In 1970, the Controlled Substances Act was passed, but excluded tobacco from the definition of "controlled substance." Two years later, the Consumer Product Safety Act was enacted, but it excluded tobacco and tobacco products from the definition of "consumer products." Likewise, the Toxic Substances Act passed in 1976 excluded tobacco from its definition of a "chemical substance." Also in that year, the Federal Hazardous Substances Labeling Act was specifically amended to exclude tobacco and tobacco products from the definition of "hazardous substances."

JAMA, April 24, 1996, p. 1259

19. "In the last 30 years, we've had 23 Surgeon General's reports and more than 60,000 scientific studies linking tobacco use with death and disease."                                    Scott Ballin, Coalition on Smoking or Health,
    "30-year Report Card for the Federal Government on Tobacco Control."

20. "The failure of the federal government to act quickly and decisively on tobacco 30 years ago has perpetuated one of the cruelest epidemics in US history. 30 years later we find perhaps the most lethal and addictive products in our society still manufactured, advertised and distributed virtually without regulation or adequate restrictions."                    Charles Le Maistre MD, member of the US Surgeon General's Advisory
    Committee for the 1964 report and president, M.D. Anderson Cancer Center, Houston

21. "This is the greatest human disaster of our times, and future generations will find it simply unbelievable that our governments failed to respond, knowing that they could have prevented millions of deaths."
    Public health official quoted in Social Science and Medicine 1993; 38:113

22. Between 1991 and 1994, 62 antitobacco bills were introduced in Congress, most dealing with tougher smoking regulation. Only three minor bills became law.                    NBC News, March 9, 1994

23. Congress has failed to pass more than 1000 tobacco control bills proposed since 1964, and has accepted $9.3 million in tobacco industry campaign contributions in the elections of 1988, 1990 and 1992.
    Washington Post, January 12, 1994

24. In the 1987-88 Congress, 145 anti-tobacco measures were introduced and 144 were defeated, the successful one the ban smoking on airline flights of two hours or less. In the 1991-92 Congress, a minor bill to eliminate a federal subsidy for overseas tobacco advertising was approved, the only anti-tobacco bill approved out of 29 considered.                    *Smokescreen*, p. 177

25. 174 pieces of federal public health legislation related to tobacco were introduced in Congress in the late 1980's and early 1990's; only two passed.                    1998 INFACT letter

26. Speaking of the pervasive influence of the tobacco industry on Congress, Walker Merryman of the Tobacco Institute said: "Our opponents cannot even get the (anti-tobacco) legislation out of subcommittee."
    Boston Globe, September 24, 1989, p. 1

27. "They (the tobacco industry) have friends in many high places and have managed to make certain those friends were in key decision-making positions in virtually every administration and Congress."
    Greensboro News and Record, September 28, 1992, p. A5

28. "Right now, dozens of lobbyists are on Capitol Hill, trying to cut a back room deal to kill the tobacco tax. Because the industry knows that tobacco taxes mean one thing: fewer smokers. Current smokers will quit, kids won't start."                    former Tobacco Institute lobbyist Victor Crawford,
    as broadcast in nationwide radio ads (Advocacy Institute, August 31, 1994 )

29. "The Clinton administration at one time talked about a $2 tax on cigarettes in order to help finance health care reform; today, in the Senate conference bill the tobacco industry has whittled that down to 45 cents on its deadly products. That was because...the White House needed the vote of Rep. Lewis Payne of Virginia--who not coincidentally received $30,300 from tobacco interests."                    Washington Post, August 21, 1994, p. C2

30. Many senators and representatives from tobacco-producing states have stated that they will not support any health care reform legislation if it contains significant hikes in tobacco taxes. "The industry's strategy has been to essentially hold the tobacco tax hostage for votes on health care."
    American Medical News, September 5, 1994, p. 14

31. A report entitled "Well-Heeled: Inside Lobbying for Health Care Reform" called the tobacco lobby "one of the most effective special interests in Washington threatening to sabotage health care reform" because of their opposition to an increase in excise taxes on tobacco products.                    Advocacy Institute, August 31, 1994

32. "It's not enough that their products kill 1100 Americans every day, cost our health care system a billion dollars a week and addict hundreds of thousands of our children every year. Now the tobacco lobby is threatening to kill any health care reform plan that makes tobacco pay its fair share."

> Former Surgeon General C. Everett Koop
> (Advocacy Institute, August 31, 1994)

33. There was a modest proposal in 1993 to ban smoking in buildings housing federally funded children's programs like Head Start. It passed the Senate 95 to 3, but then died in the House.   NBC News, March 9, 1994

34. The "Pro-children Act of 1994" did ban smoking in schools, day care centers, Head Start programs, and other places receiving federal funding for children's services.          ASH Review, September-October 1994

35. Two of the three clients of the lobbying firm Stanton and Associates are Philip Morris and the University Hospitals of Cleveland. "Such lobbyists, attorneys, and other consultants create a smokescreen in Congress by showing up one day representing a hospital and the next day a maker of cigarettes. They're playing both sides, and the public loses."          Journal of Medical Activism (DOC), May 1994, p. 3

36. In 1986, the State Department redecorated its elaborate Treaty Room near the Secretary of State's office with $1,400,000 in contributions from the Tobacco Heritage Committee, which consists of seven American tobacco companies.          New Yorker, September 13, 1993, p. 83

37. At the request of several members of Congress, the justice department and Attorney General Janet Reno are looking into allegations that tobacco industry executives were guilty of several criminal offenses, including conspiracy to defraud the public and perjury before Congress.

> British Medical Journal, October 8, 1994, p. 890, and American Medical News, June 27, 1994

38. When the first Surgeon General's report was issued in 1964, up to two thirds of US senators smoked. In 1994, only five of 100 senators were smokers.          Tobacco Control, Fall 1994, p. 204

39. 10% of U.S. senators in 1997 admitted to being smokers, as did 40 of the 430 House members. This included the then-number two House Republican, Dick Armey, and John Boehner, chairman of the Republican Conference.          Dean Edell, M.D. radio program, July 8, 1997,and Roll Call, June 27, 1998

40. US Senator Wendell Ford campaigned across Kentucky in 1992 with the boast that he has smoked for 50 years without harm.          *Tobacco Use: An American Crisis*, p. 20

41. Regarding tobacco PAC contributions to members of the House Subcommittee on Health and Environment, members who opposed the Smokefree Environment Act (HR 3434) received five times as much in tobacco industry campaign contributions from 1987 to 1993 as those who supported the bill.

> *Tobacco Industry Strategies*, p. 19

42. The Public Health Cigarette Smoking Act of 1969 prohibits states from enacting any regulations or prohibitions regarding cigarette advertising or promotion.          *Tobacco Use*, p. 70

43. "Cigarettes are no different than syringes. They are a drug delivery device for nicotine. They should be regulated just as we regulate morphine and heroin."

> Dr. Randolph Smoak, AMA spokesman (Reuters, June 8, 1994)

44. "...if the Government will only undo its fatal mistake of 1965 and repeal the mandated warning labels on cigarette packages...The warnings provide legal protection for the industry, minimizing the threat of successful litigation...To fully protect themselves, the companies would either devise a very detailed label or, unlikely as it seems, require a signed, informed-consent form before purchase. . . bghRemove the warning label, now."

> Elizabeth Whelan, New York Times, August 17, 1994, p. A15

45. Craig Fuller, the senior vice president for corporate affairs for Philip Morris, was chief of staff for then-Vice President George Bush from 1985 to 1988. He was chairman of the 1992 Republican National convention in

Houston, where Philip Morris was a major sponsor and maintained a hospitality suite. In 1995, he moved to California to run Governor Pete Wilson's campaign for president.

New York Times magazine, March 20, 1994, p. 41, and SCARC, August 31, 1992

46. RJR Nabisco and Philip Morris "coughed up" $318,000 for the Clinton campaign and (together with US Tobacco) over $700,000 for the Bush campaign in the 1992 election.      Common Cause, Winter 1992, p. 9

47. The tobacco lobby gave half a million dollars to the two parties during the 1988 presidential campaign. This increased five-fold to $2.5 million in the 1992 election. In addition, 1992 contributions by tobacco PAC's (political action committees) to House and Senate candidates were over $2.2 million, about twice the 1990 election amounts.      NEJM, April 7, 1994, p. 977

48. The tobacco industry became the single biggest supporter of the Republican National Committee in 1994, contributing more than $600,000 from July until the 1994 election. An RJ Reynolds lobbyist gave Newt Gingrich's political action committee more than $50,000. FDA commissioner David Kessler, who was contemplating regulation of tobacco, was called a "bully and a thug" by Gingrich.

Newsweek, November 28, 1994, p. 31

49. Republican Rep. Thomas Bliley of Richmond, VA, home of Philip Morris, has received $93,790 from tobacco interests since 1987. He has said: "I don't think we need any more legislation regulating tobacco", and "I am proud to represent thousands...who earn their livelihood producing this legal product...And I'll be damned if they are to be sacrificed on the altar of political correctness."

Washington Post National Weekly Edition, November 21-27, 1994, p. 15

50. Rep. Bliley total tobacco industry contributions were $159,416 by 1998.      New York Times, March 8, 1998

51. Rep. Thomas Bliley of Virginia received paid trips and $23,500 from tobacco interests in the 1992 election cycle, including $7,500 from Richmond-based Philip Morris. As a member of the House of Representatives so-called "Cigarette Pack," he subjected EPA staffers to extraordinary pressures and repeated inquiries, suggesting that the agency was manipulating data and withholding information, in an effort to delay or water down the 1993 EPA report on passive smoking.      San Francisco Examiner, January 3, 1993, p. A9

52. Republican representative Thomas Bliley of Virginia, who has been called the "Congressman from Philip Morris," in 1995 took over from Rep. Henry Waxman the chairmanship of the House Commerce Committee, which has jurisdiction over most issues related to cigarettes and tobacco.      ASH Review, January 1995, p. 2

53. Rep. Bliley "is an undertaker whose family has run the most prominent funeral home in Richmond for more than a century. He is so loyal to his roots in tobacco country that he keeps a framed picture with every brand of cigarette made by Philip Morris in his congressional office."      New York Times, December 20, 1994

54. "Cigarettes and conservatives are being packaged together as tightly these days as the radio and the right wing...A star of this group is Virginia's Tom Bliley, a pro-tobacco mortician who now heads a House subcommittee on health and the environment. Talk about conflict of interest."

Ellen Goodman column, February 28, 1995

55. Of the 1994 Congressional leaders, Dick Armey smokes cigarettes, and visitors to Newt Gingrich's office "walk through a thick cigarette fog created by aides. Republicans may try to clean up politics, but they will do it from inside smoke-filled rooms." Newt's father and stepfather both died from lung cancer.

Newsweek, November 28, 1994, p. 31

56. RJR Nabisco has contributed at least $50,000 to GOPAC, Newt Gingrich's secretive political action committee, and the House Speaker has been known to travel in the RJR corporate jet.

Common Cause, Spring 1995, p. 20

57. During 1992 and 1993, 60 members of Congress participated in free trips sponsored by tobacco companies.

Advocacy Institute, August 31, 1994

58. In a report on the Top Ten Sponsors of Congressional Junkets, the Tobacco Institute ranked third (with 29 sponsored trips for members of Congress), and Philip Morris ranked ninth (with 12 trips).

Time, July 4, 1994, p. 14

59. The tobacco industry donated $2.4 million to members of the US Congress in 1991 and 1992. The fact that congress in these years failed to enact a single piece of tobacco control legislation (such as a tax increase) is strongly associated with these campaign contributions.         JAMA, October 19, 1994, p. 1171

60. Tobacco money strongly influences a legislator's voting behavior, and legislators frequently voted contrary to the wishes of their constituents to help tobacco interests who had financed their campaigns.

JAMA, October 19, 1994, p. 1217

61. Philip Morris hired a Washington lobbying firm to get people to write letters against proposed federal regulations banning workplace smoking. Bonner and Associates earned at least $1.4 million for a campaign that produced 7300 letters and an additional $100 each for more than 1500 faxes to congressmen. PM also planned to bring up to 500 smokers to Washington, all expenses paid, to testify at a hearing.

Newsweek, September 12, 1994, p. 6

62. "Now adults are being sold the tobacco party line in politics:  smoking as freedom. But the cigarette makes a perverse icon to liberty. The freedom to get hooked?  The right to addiction?  The issue isn't 'Health Nazis'. It's still health. The only 'Freedom-Loving Individualists' that the tobacco industry cares about are the ones in need of another fix."         Ellen Goodman column, February 28, 1995

63. Campaign contributions from the tobacco industry buy Congressional silence and inaction, and tobacco interests are put ahead of the public interest. Industry supporters held a health care reform proposal hostage in 1994 until its key financing mechanism, a proposed increase on tobacco taxes, had been cut almost in half.

Common Cause, Spring 1995, p. 19

64. 100 members of Congress in 1993 wrote a letter to President Clinton recommending for the post of US surgeon general former Congressman from Georgia J. Roy Rowland. Rowland, a former family physician, would have been the first "pro-tobacco" surgeon general. While in Congress he voted against the commercial airline smoking ban on short flights in 1987, objected to a bill restricting smoking in public buildings, and took $35,900 in PAC contributions and at least $7000 in honoraria from the tobacco industry.

Common Cause, Spring 1995, p. 22

65. The tobacco industry contributed more than $16.6 million from 1985 to 1995 to federal candidates, PAC's and political party committees. In 1993 and 1994, the industry gave almost $2 million in unlimited "soft money" contributions to Republican party committees.         Common Cause, Spring 1995, p. 19

66. Philip Morris informed its shareholders that as a result of the 1994 elections, "new faces and new leadership on Capitol Hill (mean) tremendous opportunities to get new and unbiased hearings on the issues that concern us most."         San Francisco Chronicle, April 13, 1995

67. In 1981, the Department of Health and Human Services in the new Reagan administration canceled an advertising campaign aimed at teenagers and featuring Brooke Shields in a poster with cigarettes sticking out of her ears and the logo "Smokers are losers." One of the officials snuffing out the campaign was a former aide to Senator Jesse Helms (D-NC). The following year, the budget for the Office on Smoking and Health was cut from $2.6 to $1.9 million.         New York State Journal of Medicine, December 1983, p. 1278

68. In 1981, the Office on Smoking and Health accepted an offer by Brooke Shields for a series of antismoking television messages to counter increased smoking by teenagers, especially girls who linked smoking with slimness and sexiness. However, "higher-ups" in the Department of Health and Human Services said that Shields was an "inappropriate" role model for American teens and vetoed the idea. The director of the Office on Smoking and Health then took the Shields messages to the American Heart Association, which said that they were "too controversial," and the American Cancer Society, which also declined to air them.

*Ashes to Ashes*, p. 492

69. "IMPORTANT ALERT FOR CONSUMERS OF COPENHAGEN AND SKOAL!
Anti-tobacco activists are trying to take away your freedom to enjoy smokeless tobacco products. The time has come for consumers to take a stand!" Mass mailing from US Tobacco Company in 1994, apparently to respond to proposals for higher taxes on smokeless tobacco as part of the Clinton administration health care reform plan

70. "The Republicans' record-breaking 1995 soft money fundraising total climbed higher in March as the Republican National Committee raised $621,071 in soft money during the month." The top two donors were Philip Morris and the National Rifle Association.          Common Cause press release, May 5, 1995

71. "The tobacco lobby's use of political contributions is a classic example of the influence money scandal in Washington. Members of Congress are as addicted to large campaign contributions as smokers are to nicotine."
          Ann McBride, president of Common Cause, press release, March 24, 1995

72. "Tobacco industry contributions to members of the US Congress strongly influence the federal tobacco policy process. Unless this influence is diminished through a combination of members refusing tobacco money and campaign finance reform, this process of contributing to death by thwarting tobacco control will continue to claim hundreds of thousands of lives a year."          JAMA 1994; 272:1171

73. A group of 42 Republican academic physicians and scientists wrote to House Speaker Newt Gingrich to urge that he not cede the anti-tobacco movement to Democrats. They blasted Gingrich for meeting with industry executives and for ridiculing anti-smoking efforts. Gingrich said the FDA had lost its mind in contemplating the regulation of tobacco, and his press secretary characterized zealots in anti-tobacco ranks as "health Nazis." Gingrich was the main speaker at a New York fund raiser in June 1995 attended by the chairmen of Philip Morris, Brown and Williamson, and RJ Reynolds, each of whom donated or raised $100,000.
          Associated Press, July 23, 1995, and American Medical News, August 7, 1995

74. "You're not going to see any anti-smoking legislation come out of Congress as long as the Republicans have control…(the tobacco industry is) one of the most sophisticated, well-organized lobbying machines in the world."          Victor Crawford, former tobacco industry lobbyist (JAMA, July 19, 1995, p. 202)

75. "Living with the lie of tobacco, North Carolina has prospered, has been deformed. If you know that your major crop kills, you need big-time spin control. You need a pit-bull single-issue politician who will make a militant merit of his state's lowest common denominator xenophobia. You need somebody smart who's still willing to yuk it up with the good old boys at the tobacco warehouses. A man of preternatural energy willing-in a familiar Southern mode – to play the fool to disarm any enemy. Meet Jesse Helms."
          New York Times, August 18, 1995, p. A15 (Allan Gurganus)

76. Representative Edolphus Towns, Democrat of Brooklyn, elected in 1982 and the former head of the congressional Black Caucus, has been such an ardent supporter of the tobacco industry's causes that he is known on Capitol Hill as "the Marlboro Man," though he has never smoked. Towns grew up in North Carolina, the son of sharecroppers on a tobacco farm, and began picking tobacco when he was 10 or 11. In 1994, he voted against a bill to ban smoking in most public places in the nation, the day after he received $4,500 from the RJ Reynolds political action committee. Within a week of the vote he received another $2,000 from other tobacco political action committees. In 17 floor and committee votes on tobacco since 1987, he voted 15 times against the position supported by the Coalition on Smoking or Health.
          New York Times, November 19, 1995, p. 21

77. At the 1996 Republican convention in San Diego, a corporate beach party had surf boards with large labels saying "Thank You Phillip (misspelled) Morris."          Time, August 26, 1996, p. 21

78. "The watchdog group INFACT has identified the top nine politicians who suck-up to the smoke-peddlers. While nearly 80% of all Congressmembers pocket tobacco money…the 'Nicotine Nine' stand apart." They are (with tobacco money total): Sen. Bob Dole (R-KS), $45,900; Rep. Newt Gingrich (R-GA), $41,000; Rep. Tom Bliley (R-VA), $111,476; Rep. Charlie Rose (D-NC), $96,000; Sen. Wendell Ford (D-KY), $87,000; Sen. Jesse Helms (R-NC), $64,500; Rep. Lewis Payne (D-VA), $68,149; Rep. Dick Gephardt (D-MO), $54,260;

and Rep. Tom DeLay (R-TX), $36,700.

Earth Island Journal, Winter 1995-96, p. 30

79. In 1957, "John Blatnick, a five-term representative from Minnesota—and a devoted smoker—leads the sub-committee on government operations through hearings on the Federal Trade Commission's oversight of cigarette advertising. Blatnick bristles as the testimony, the first ever presented to federal lawmakers on the relationship of smoking to health, reveals that the new filtered brands use stronger tobaccos, and so yield about as much tar and nicotine as the old unfiltered brands—a fact never noted in the industry's advertising. In the aftermath of the hearings, Blatnick introduces a bill in the House to limit the tar and nicotine yields of cigarettes and grant the FTC injunctive powers against deceptive tobacco advertising. So powerful is the tobacco industry, however, that the House not only denies the Blatnick bill a hearing but strips its sponsor of his subcommittee chairmanship and dissolves the subcommittee itself."     Mother Jones, May-June 1996, p. 41

80. Congress in 1966 voted to send 600 million cigarettes to flood victims in India as a form of relief.

*Smokescreen*, p. 2

81. C. Everett Koop commented on Ronald Reagan:
"Before he was inaugurated, there was correspondence between the chief executive officer of R.J. Reynolds and the president, calling attention to the fact that the tobacco company would hope that this president would not be too tough on the tobacco industry. And the president wrote back—I don't know who wrote the letter for him, but I could hardly believe it when I eventually read it:  'My administration will be too busy with more important things.'"                                         Mother Jones, May-June 1996, p. 66

82. A speech by C. Everett Koop in 1984 entitled "Toward a Smoke-Free Society by 2000 A.D." led RJR's Edward Horrigan to write President Reagan to express his dismay "at the increasingly shrill preachments" of the Surgeon General "and his call for a second Prohibition," which amounted to "the most radical anti-tobacco posturing since the days of Joseph Califano."                                         *Ashes to Ashes*, p. 540

83. Of the top 10 soft money donors to the Republican Party since January 1991, three are tobacco companies. They are Philip Morris, second behind Amway with total contributions of $2,291,776, RJR Nabisco, ranked fourth with $1,626,757, and US Tobacco Co., eighth with $865,466 in contributions. These three companies also gave $453,500, $579,900, and $201,308, respectively, to the Democratic Party in "soft money" over the same time period. Since 1986, the tobacco industry has given more than $20 million to the political parties.
Common Cause magazine, Summer 1996, pp. 21 and 36

84. From 1992 to 1996, the tobacco industry gave $6,096,000 to the Republicans and $1,035,000 to the Democrats.                                         CBS Evening News, July 3, 1996

85. Philip Morris and RJ Reynolds gave $1.7 million to the Republicans and $325,000 to the Democrats in 1995. When Democrats controlled Congress, they received the bulk of tobacco money. Overall, tobacco companies gave $4.1 million to political parties in 1995, 78% to Republicans, according to Common Cause.
US News and World Report, May 20, 1996, p. 25

86. Big Tobacco's contributions to the Republican Party increased from $546,000 in "soft" donations in 1993 to $2.4 million in 1995.                                         Mother Jones, May-June 1996, p. 36

87. A cartoon in USA Today on July 10, 1996 showed a cigarette pack with a new warning label on the side: "Your congressmen have determined that tobacco campaign contributions are necessary for their political health."

88. The tobacco companies are sponsoring the Republican "get-the-government-off-our-backs" revolution.
Mother Jones, May-June 1996, p. 3

89. Haley Barbour, the Republican National Committee chairman, has intervened to try to derail anti-smoking legislation in two states, Arizona and Texas. Mark Killian, the Republican speaker of the Arizona house, received an unexpected and unwelcome phone call from Barbour at his home, urging him to consider a tobacco industry sponsored pre-emption bill. Killian refused, and accused Barbour of doing the bidding of

tobacco interests. Barbour also inquired about a similar bill in the Texas legislature, but it was vetoed by Governor George W. Bush.

New York Times, March 20, 1996, (Frank Rich)
and ABC News, March 11, 1996 (Peter Jennings)

90. In June 1995, GOP Conference chairman John Boehner distributed about half a dozen tobacco industry campaign donation checks on the House of Representatives floor to his colleagues. Although no rule or law was violated, Boehner said that he would stop the practice.　　　Associated Press, May 11, 1996

91. "The Senator from North Carolina…would never describe lung cancer patients as the victims of their own 'deliberate, disgusting, revolting conduct' even though, as a rule, they are. He should have resisted the temptation to say it about AIDS patients."　　　Jesse Helms in the Boston Globe, July 11, 1995 (Jeff Jacoby)

92. A tobacco study by Stanton Glantz at UC San Francisco funded by the National Cancer Institute was entitled "Effect of Tobacco Advocacy at the State Level." After reports of the project appeared in right-wing journals, tobacco state politicians protested the grant as a misuse of cancer research funds. In an exceedingly rare congressional intrusion into the NIH grant process, the House Appropriations Committee, in its funding bill for NCI's parent agency, the National Institutes of Health, terminated support for the remaining portion of the project.　　　The Lancet, September 23, 1995, p. 831

93. When JAMA published the five articles on the B&W documents, each of the articles by Glantz and associates carried the same note: "This work was supported in part by grant CA-61021 from the National Cancer Institute", the N.C.I. research program in "Tobacco Prevention and Control." The institute had solicited proposals that would "evaluate the effect of advocacy in the development of tobacco control policy." Glantz's proposal had been approved by a peer-review committee of the National Institutes of Health, parent of the N.C.I. Reviewers gave it a score ranking it above 90 percent of the other proposals recommended for funding.

　　Despite this careful screening, a week after the JAMA issue appeared, the Republican-controlled House Appropriations Committee took action to cancel Glantz's funding from the N.C.I. A subcommittee report declared that the grant that funded Glantz's work did "not properly fall within the boundaries of the N.C.I. portfolio," and that therefore no further funding should be provided "for this research grant." The staff director for the House Appropriations Committee is James Dyer, a former Philip Morris lobbyist. This is the only case in the history of the N.C.I. in which a grant has been singled out for defunding by Congress.

　　The tobacco companies had now broadened the fight over corporate control of information by enlisting Congress in its attempts to silence a leading critic. This marked an unprecedented political intrusion into medical research.

Quote from the Nation, January 1, 1996, p. 16

94. "House Majority Whip Tom DeLay uses a tobacco-funded operative from a firm called Ramhurst Corp. to run his political fundraising organization. Ramhurst has also hired the son of Majority Leader Dick Armey as a contractor. Last August, Speaker of the House Newt Gingrich was feted at a 'Salute to Newt' banquet that netted $100,000 apiece from the chairmen of Philip Morris, R.J. Reynolds, and Brown & Williamson."

Mother Jones, May-June 1996, p. 51

95. Edward Kennedy remarked of the Tobacco Institute, "Dollar for dollar, they're probably the most effective lobby on Capitol Hill." And, Sidney Wolfe of Public Citizen said, "They have completely paralyzed Washington in terms of any significant ability to regulate cigarettes."　　　*Ashes to Ashes*, p. 466

96. Arthur C. Upton, director of the National Cancer Institute under President Carter, was visited by half a dozen tobacco industry representatives in 1978, shortly after Health & Human Services Secretary Joseph Califano had declared smoking "public health enemy number one." The tobacco group threatened to have its friends in congress cut off N.C.I. funds unless the N.C.I. director eased up on the smoking issue. Upton's family about this time received several threatening telephone calls, which he still today attributes to the industry's effort to intimidate him.　　　*Cancer Wars*, p. 295

97. In the first Reagan administration budget of February 1981, the Surgeon General's Office on Smoking and Health was zeroed out. Funds for the office were later restored after Senator Lowell Schweiker defended it to OMB director David Stockman.　　　*Cancer Wars*, p. 292

98. In 1988, C. Everett Koop invited Dr. Judith Mackay from Hong Kong to speak on the topic "U.S. Trade Policies on Tobacco." When White House officials learned of the meeting, they forced a last-minute change of topic, told Dr. Koop not to meddle in international health, and (too late) demanded cancellation of Dr. Mackay's appearance.                          *The Doctor-Activist*, Ellen Bassuk, Plenum Press, 1996, p. 49

99. In 1989, former Senate minority leader and White House chief of staff Howard Baker joined the lobbying team of Philip Morris. He "undertook an aggressive 'entertainment schedule' that included the obligatory golf and fishing expeditions as well as wining and dining tobacco-policy decision makers and their wives."

*Cigarette Confidential*, p. 11

100. Senator Howard Baker was Senate majority leader from 1981 to 1985 and later White House Chief of Staff in the Reagan administration. After leaving government service, he worked for Philip Morris as a partner in the Washington office of a Tennessee law firm. Philip Morris lobbyist Jim Dyer wrote the following in a memo in 1989: "...Senator Baker's attachment to this company gives us an effective high level advocate of our policies. If we need a message delivered, he can do it best. If the Company needs to be publicly identified in a positive way with an issue, he can do it best. If we need to make instant input into a high level decision making process, he is best equipped to do it. Based on his experience, he knows how to exert a positive influence, not only on the process in Washington, but also on the thinking processes at the top of this Company...The Senator's relationships with the Bush Administration, Congress, the media, and the business community make him a positive asset to any public relations or public event we undertake here in D.C. I am confident the coming months will provide countless opportunities to maximize the Senator's activities on our behalf."

Washington Post magazine, December 3, 1995, p. 22

101. Former U.S. Senator Howard Baker, chairman of the Mayo Foundation's board of trustees, has been hired as lobbyist by several tobacco companies.                          Minneapolis Star Tribune, October 19, 1997

102. "...in 1985 an amendment was offered in the House of Representatives to eliminate federal price supports for tobacco—a program estimated to cost taxpayers more than $600 million. The amendment was defeated, 230 to 195. Between 1981 and 1986, the tobacco industry donated nearly $1 million to members of Congress. Forty-nine representatives got more than $5,000 each; when the price-support vote came up in 1985, 90 percent of them voted in favor of the subsidy—as opposed to only 26 percent of those who got no tobacco-industry donations. In other words, it cost the industry less than $1 million to preserve more than half a billion dollars in price supports. That's some payback. It's also a distortion of the democratic process: an issue decided not by what's best for the nation but by what's best for the constituent buying the most influence."

Editorial, Audubon, January-February 1997, p. 4 (Michael Robbins)

103. The tobacco industry spent $15 million in the first half of 1996 alone on lobbying Congress and federal agencies. In March 1996, the Senate defeated a plan to increase tobacco taxes, with the revenue targeted for health care and a program to help tobacco farmers convert to new crops. The 62 senators who voted to kill the amendment received an average of $19,003 in contributions from tobacco-industry PACs from 1991-1996; the 38 who supported it received an average of $2,436.

Center for Responsive Politics data reported in San Francisco Chronicle, March 2, 1997

104. 82% of the members of Congress in 1996 had received tobacco company contributions.

The Lancet, March 23, 1996, p. 823

105. "As Congress raced to pass a massive tax cut bill last month, Senate Majority Leader Trent Lott, R-Miss., and House Speaker Newt Gingrich, R-GA, insisted on a provision that would give tobacco companies a $50 billion credit against the sum they had pledged to settle anti-tobacco litigation." The one-sentence credit provision "was placed unobtrusively in the tax bill's 'miscellaneous provisions' section."

San Francisco Chronicle, August 17, 1997, p. A20 (John Mintz, Washington Post)

106. Former Republican National committee chairman Haley Barbour, now paid $50,000 a month as a tobacco industry lobbyist, was the apparent "mastermind behind the biggest heist of the year--the delivery of a $50 billion tax break for tobacco companies." When the details of the tax break were released, it was rescinded, but the same week, members of Congress flew to New York on a U. S. Tobacco company jet to attend a

tobacco industry fund raiser. In the past year and a half, the tobacco industry has contributed $1.9 million to Republicans and $300,000 to Democrats.    Time, September 29, 1997, p. 29 (Margaret Carlson)

107. About $220 million each year is spent in the United States each year on tobacco control at the federal level, including the tobacco control activities of the National Cancer Institute and Centers for Disease Control. State funded tobacco control efforts are $180 million per year; Massachusetts and California are the leaders, and these two states have had 30% per capita cigarette consumption declines since 1990.
10th World Conference on Tobacco or Health, Beijing, 1997 (Gregory Connolly)

108. Dozens of members of Congress and congressional aides spent three days in February 1997 at the lavish Phoenician resort in Arizona, courtesy of the Tobacco Institute. The "golf junket" was legal even though under new congressional ethics rules, legislators may not accept gifts from special interests. However, they may accept privately paid travel for educational, fact-finding events that are consistent with the interests of their constituents.    Associated Press, February 18, 1997

109. Margaret Carlson in an article "The Gravy Train Never Stops" from Time magazine (January 19, 1998, p. 14) writes the following:
"Last February, Congress Watch documented a typical outing. The Tobacco Institute flew 11 members, including Republican House leaders Tom DeLay and John Boehner, to the Phoenician, a Scottsdale, Arizona resort, for a 'legislative conference,' complete with morning seminars on the harmlessness of nicotine and afternoons free for golf and spa treatments at the Centre for Well-Being, at a cost of $62,890. There's no linkage, of course, but five months later the Republican leadership slipped a $50 billion tax break for tobacco into the budget bill."

110. Between 1984 and 1994, the cigarette industry donated $10.6 million to political candidates. The Philip Morris political action committee made 4822 separate contributions to 383 different candidates for the House and Senate between 1979 and 1994, giving them a total of $3.6 million.    *Cigarette Confidential*, p. 4

111. In the 1996 campaign cycle the Republicans received nearly $7.1 million in tobacco money, more than four times the $1.6 million given to the Democrats.    New York Times, April 22, 1997, p. A14

112. In the 1995-96 election cycle, soft money (unrestricted) political party donations totaled $262 million, triple the amount that was raised four years earlier. The leading contributor of all corporations and groups was Philip Morris with $4.2 million in soft money, 79% of the total donated to the Republican party and 21% to the Democrats.    Center for Responsive Politics data reported by the New York Times, November 25, 1997

113. Philip Morris doled out more than $2 million to sponsor events at the 1996 Republican presidential convention, and at least $100,000 to the Democratic convention.    INFACT, Update Fall/Winter 1996-97

114. Common Cause reports that tobacco interests gave more than $3 million in unregulated soft money to the national parties in 1997, 82% to Republicans. Philip Morris gave $1.9 million in soft money to the Republican Party, and $243,000 to the Democrats.    Washington Post, March 13, 1998, p. A23

115. The National Republican Congressional Committee gave $60,000 to U.S. Tobacco in February 1998 for the use of its corporate jets for trips by House speaker Newt Gingrich and other Republican leaders for fundraising purposes. In 1997, Senate Majority Leader Trent Lott (R-MS) and House Majority whip Rep. Tom DeLay (R-TX) were among politicians who received rides from R.J. Reynolds.    USA Today, April 16, 1998, p. A1

116. Tobacco companies provided their corporate jets to Republican legislators on 32 dates between January 1997 and May 1998 for as many as 84 flights. There were no reports of Democrats travelling on tobacco jets in the same time period. Lawmakers must reimburse the owners of the private jets the equivalent of first class commercial airfare to the same destination. The National Republican Congressional Committee paid tobacco companies $190,000 for travel in this period, making it the "biggest single recipient of subsidized travel from the tobacco industry." The Republican committee chair said that he sees "nothing wrong" with the travel.
Washington Post, July 20, 1998, p. A1

117. The Tobacco Institute spent $53,705 on trips for members of Congress in 1997.

Washington Post, July 21, 1998, p. A17

118. The Speaker of the House of Representatives, Rep. Dennis Hastert R-Ill, in 1994 publicly threatened then-FDA commissioner David Kessler with contempt of Congress at a hearing on the agency's probe of the tobacco industry.

Washington Post, January 5, 1999, p. A1

119. In the 1997-1998 election cycle, Philip Morris contributed $2 million in soft money to Republicans and $419,000 to the Democrats. RJR had $1 million to Republicans and $100,000 to Democrats.

Associated Press, February 23, 1999

120. In 1999 the tobacco industry gave more than $1.2 million in political contributions, 90% to Republicans and $62,000 to the Bush candidacy.

Wall Street Journal, December 2, 1999, p. A23 (Albert Hunt)

121. In 1986, Bob Dole joined Connecticut Senators Christopher Dodd and Lowell Weicker in a letter to the government of Hong Kong on behalf of Greenwich-based US Tobacco company. The letter urged Hong Kong not to ban smokeless tobacco and implied that the United States might engage in trade retaliation if it did. Dr. C. Everett Koop wrote in his memoirs, "I imagine they thought it was more important to save a Connecticut firm's profits than Asian lives."

Washington Post National Weekly Edition, May 27, 1996, p. 14

122. During the 1985 federal budget negotiations, a bipartisan bill was introduced in Congress to raise excise taxes on chewing tobacco and make it less affordable to adolescents. Dole defeated the measure (simultaneously slipping in a tobacco growers' subsidy crafted by Sen. Jesse Helms). As Common Cause magazine reported, Dole promised he would reconsider the excise tax hike if the pending surgeon general's report linked smokeless tobacco to oral cancer. The 1986 Surgeon General's report did; the Kansas senator didn't. "Dole was very loyal to the smokeless tobacco industry," a former industry representative told Common Cause. "He was someone that they could rely on in Congress to derail legislation."

Quote from Mother Jones magazine, May-June, 1996, p. 3

123. Bob Dole has total tobacco industry contributions of $477,000, and has flown 38 times aboard tobacco industry corporate jets. He commented that smoking is not necessarily addictive; former Surgeon General C. Everett Koop said that Dole's remarks "either exposed his abysmal lack of knowledge of nicotine addiction or his blind support of the tobacco industry." Dole in response to Katie Couric on the Today show suggested that "perhaps a little bit" Koop had been brainwashed by the liberal media, and also created more controversy by his statement "We know it's not good for kids. But a lot of other things aren't good…Some would say milk's not good."

Los Angeles Times, June 16, 1996, p. 16, San Francisco Chronicle, June 28, 1996, and San Francisco Examiner, July 7, 1996, p. B7

124. "Tobacco doesn't seem an obvious benefactor for a senator from Kansas, where there are plenty of wheat fields but few tobacco farms. Still, Dole has received more than $330,000 directly from RJR, Philip Morris, and U.S. Tobacco during his career, in addition to untold tobacco soft money through the Republican National Committee. Meanwhile, Dole has consistently fought tobacco tax increases—even when proposed by fellow Republicans…

"In less dramatic fashion, Elizabeth Dole has also earned Big Tobacco's appreciation. In 1987, while serving as secretary of transportation, she refused to ban smoking on airplanes, ignoring recommendations from Surgeon General C. Everett Koop and the National Academy of Sciences. Perhaps coincidentally, tobacco contributions to the American Red Cross, which she heads, have escalated. Philip Morris, Brown & Williamson, and RJR gave the charity a combined $265,530 in 1995, compared to a total over the previous five years of $321,427."

Mother Jones, May-June, 1996, p. 40

125. Bob Dole took at least 26 subsidized rides (billed at about 5 percent of their actual cost) on U.S. Tobacco Company's corporate jet. The tax breaks that Dole engineered for the company cumulatively amounted to at least $250 million.

Mother Jones, May-June, 1996, p. 5

126. "Roderick DeArment, a former Dole chief of staff, is chairman of Lawyers for Dole, a group of about 700 lawyers raising funds for Dole's campaign. DeArment is a law partner at Covington & Burling, which

represents the major tobacco companies (Philip Morris, R.J. Reynolds, Lorillard, and Brown & Williamson), as well as The Tobacco Institute. Covington & Burling spent more than $1 million in Philip Morris money to fund Healthy Buildings, an international magazine using phony science to promote the tobacco industry's idea that indoor smoking bans are unnecessary. Covington & Burling also commissioned a dubious 1996 study purporting federal tobacco restrictions could cost the nation 92,000 jobs and $7.9 billion in lost output..."

Mother Jones, May-June 1996, p. 37

127. Steve Merksamer was a senior adviser and California strategist for the 1996 Dole campaign.. His Sacramento law firm, Nielson, Merksamer, Parrinello, Mueller & Naylor, has collected $1.9 million from the tobacco industry since 1988, more than any other California firm. In 1994, Nielson, Merksamer was paid an additional $350,000 to write Proposition 188, called the Tobacco Control Act. The proposition promised tough statewide restrictions, but its language actually weakened state law by acting as a "pre-emption law" to kill dozens of tougher local restrictions throughout the state. When the media exposed Proposition 188 as a tobacco industry ploy, voters defeated it.                                 Quote from Mother Jones, May-June 1996, p. 37

128. "Must you debase our nation and threaten our children for the sake of corporate profits?"

Bob Dole in 1995, talking about Time Warner (Mother Jones, May-June 1996, p. 62)

129. Even worse, any bill must satisfy and be signed by a president who demonstrated, in Texas, little taste for regulating tobacco, and who remains within earshot of his former campaign manager, Karl Rove, now a senior White House advisor, formerly a strategic consultant to Philip Morris. The face and voice of FDA and the Bush administration on FDA legislation will be that of Health and Human Services secretary Tommy Thompson, former Wisconsin governor. One might not think of Wisconsin as a tobacco state, but it is surely a Philip Morris state – with Philip Morris subsidiaries Miller beer and Oscar Meyer meat products among its largest employers. So close was Thompson to Philip Morris that he not only received more than $70,000 in campaign contributions from the company but enjoyed its surreptitious funding of three overseas junkets.

There remains one sharp arrow in the government's quiver that could be used to prod Philip Morris and the other companies to concede McCain-strength FDA authority: the Clinton-initiated Justice Department "racketeering" lawsuit that charges the companies with a conspiracy to deceive the American public, including the government, as to the risks of tobacco use. That conspiracy, the Justice Department lawyers argue, resulted in billions of dollars in excess Medicare costs incurred in treating tobacco's misled victims, borne by American taxpayers – billions that the government now seeks to recover.

The lawsuit's outcome is uncertain. Its legal theory is novel, though it has passed initial industry challenges before an exemplary federal district court judge in Washington. The case does, once again, expose the companies to the risk, however remote, of a multibillion dollar jury award, and hence an incentive to settle. It is certainly conceivable that part of the Justice Department's price for such a settlement might be the companies' agreement to support McCain-bill FDA authority. But not under Attorney General John Ashcroft. On April 30, 1998, when Senator McCain achieved the high-water mark for his bill (the 19-1 supporting vote of the Senate Commerce Committee), the one No vote was then-senator John Ashcroft of Missouri. And Ashcroft, as soon as the Justice Department suit was filed, promptly labeled it "unwise."

Quote from *Smoke in Their Eyes*, pp. 244-245

130. As Wisconsin governor, secretary of the Department of Health and Human Services Tommy Thompson visited three continents at the expense of Philip Morris, including a trip to Australia that included a scuba diving excursion with a tobacco lobbyist.                                 Associated Press, January 11, 2001

131. In 1996, "Geoffrey Bible, CEO of Philip Morris, chairs a dinner underwritten by Philip Morris for the Republican Governors Association, and speaks to the governors about tobacco's benefits to the economy. The gala dinner pulls in an unprecedented $2.6 million."                 The Tobacco Timeline, www.tobacco.org

132. ". . . filmmaker Michael Moore published on his website...an addition to his book "Stupid White Men." In the excerpt available online, Moore pointed out that, despite forbidding objects as diverse as hockey sticks, road flares and cattle prods on planes, the Transportation Safety Administration (TSA) permitted and apparently still permits travelers to bring matches and lighters (except gun lighters) on-board. Moore sought an explanation for this aberration and ultimately obtained on from an unidentified young man, who said, "I work on the [Capitol] Hill. The butane lighters were on the original list prepared by the FAA [Federal Aviation Administration] and

sent to the White House for approval. The tobacco industry lobbied the Bush administration to have the lighters and matches removed from the banned list. Their customers (addicts) naturally are desperate to light up as soon as they land, and why should they be punished just so the skies can be safe?"

Quote from Stan Shatenstein via GLOBALink, September 11, 2002

133. "The tobacco industry, led by Philip Morris…contributed heavily to the Bush and other Republican campaigns in the last election…82% of its giving was to Republicans. The industry would be hugely disappointed if the president were to back a serious regulatory effort. The country will be the big loser if he does not."

Editorial, Washington Post National Weekly Edition, May 7-13, 2001, p. 25

134. In the 1999-2000 election cycle, Republicans received $3.75 million from tobacco companies, and Democrats, $705,790.

Center for Responsive Politics

135. The tobacco industry gave more than $8.4 million to political parties and candidates during the 1999-2000 election cycle, more than 80% to Republicans.

USA Today, June 1, 2001, p. 15A

136. In the 2000 campaign, tobacco companies contributed $7.0 million to George W. Bush and the Republicans, and $1.4 million to Democrats. Since the election, the industry gave another $2.3 million to Republicans and $400,000 to Democrats.

New England Journal of Medicine, March 21, 2002, p. 938

137. In direct contributions to presidential candidates, tobacco interest donors favored George W. Bush over Al Gore by nine to one in the 2000 presidential election.

New York Times, September 6, 2002, p. A19

138. Philip Morris was recognized in Washington in May 2001 at a Bush fundraising gala for a $250,000 donation to the Republicans.

USA Today, June 1, 2001, p. 15A

139. "It's easy to see why tobacco giant Philip Morris was recognized in Washington last month at President Bush's fundraising gala for its $250,000 GOP donation. The once-beleaguered tobacco industry has seen its fortunes flip since the Bush administration arrived in the nation's capital. Despite efforts to mask its steps, the administration is leaving footprints that mark a sharp retreat from Clinton-era anti-smoking strategies."

Editorial, USA Today (undated) quoted in ASH Smoking and Health Review, May-June 2001

140. According to a recent report issued by the National Center for Tobacco-Free Kids Action Fund and Common Cause, the tobacco industry gave more than $5.8 million in soft money and political action committee (PAC) contributions to federal candidates, political parties, and political committees from January 1, 2001 to June 30, 2002.

Since 1991, the industry has contributed more than $22 million, including $14.2 million in soft money and more than $7.8 million in PAC contributions. Since 1999, the four largest cigarette companies have spent more than $44 million on lobbying Congress.

To the industry, all this is money well spent; millions in contributions protect billions in profits. For example, the report demonstrates how industry contributions have influenced the sponsors of two competing bills relating to FDA regulation of tobacco. The 17 House members who are sponsoring an ineffective bill (H.R. 2180) supported by Philip Morris have received, on average, more than 19 times as much money from the tobacco industry as the 126 sponsors of a public health community-supported bill (H.R. 1097).

Quote from ANR (Americans for Nonsmokers Rights) Update, Fall 2002

141. From 1991 to September 2002, tobacco interests gave $23.5 million in political donations, 81% to Republicans and the remainder to Democrats.

Common Cause newsletter, October 2002

142. The federal Office on Smoking and Health's budget was increased from $20 million to $102 million during the Clinton administration; the first Bush budget called for a 5% cut.

USA Today, June 1, 2001, p. 15A

143. In 2002, seven Republican senators were flown in corporate jets, one supplied by U.S. Tobacco, to the Greenbriar resort in West Virginia "for a weekend of golf, tennis, and skeet shooting with major campaign contributors."

Washington Monthly, September 2002, p. 6

144. In the year 2000 election cycle, soft money contributions to national party committees by the tobacco industry were $4.8 million to Republicans and $558,000 to Democrats. *Meet the Press, March 18, 2001* (Total soft money contributions from all sources increased from $22 million in 1984 to $84 million in 1992, $235 million in 1996, and $463 million in 2000, before passage of the McCain-Feingold soft money ban. – editor)

145. This is a scandal of some in Congress trading public health for PAC money and believing the slick ads of the tobacco industry…this is a scandal of politics for sale and, to my dismay, some Republicans going to the highest bidder. The industry hired one lobbyist for every two members of Congress. The major manufacturers spent over $30 million in lobbying fees last year alone, a number that does not include the millions in campaign contributions or the billions spent on advertising, "grass roots," and front organizations. That, I suppose, is business as usual in defending the right to sell cancer to unknowing and immature minors.

Quote from a speech by Dr. C. Everett Koop at the National Press Club following the 1998 sinking of the McCain bill regulating tobacco (*Smoke in Their Eyes*), pp. 2-3

146. Oklahoma congressman Mike Synar was the author of the Synar amendment, "virtually the only tobacco control measure ever passed by Congress, which prods states to enforce laws against underage tobacco purchases." Synar died of brain cancer in 1996 at age 45.

*Profiles in Courage for Our Time*, Caroline Kennedy, Hyperion, 2002, pp. 113-132

# State and Local Governments

1. The so-called preemption clause of the Cigarette Smoking Act of 1969 prohibits states from regulating cigarette advertising because the federally legislated restriction "preempts" state action.

Journal of Health Politics, Policy and Law, Fall 1986, p. 386

2. Preemption bills sponsored by the tobacco industry that prohibit local governments of the ability to regulate tobacco have been introduced in almost every state legislature, and about 15 states have enacted such ordinances. Some of the bills began as tobacco control measures that the industry and legislators transformed into a pro-tobacco trojan horse. In addition, 25 states have enacted so-called "Smokers' rights laws" which prohibit employment discrimination against smokers

*Tobacco Industry Strategies,* p. 26, and Tobacco Control 1993; 2:132

3. New Jersey in 1991 with the strong support of the American Civil Liberties Union passed a smokers' rights bill that makes it illegal for an employer to make hiring or firing decisions on the basis of smoking status. In other states, the tobacco lobby has introduced and passed weak statewide no-smoking laws that contain clauses specifically pre-empting stronger city and county laws. American Medical News, October 19, 1992

4. In 1993, only 35% of bills introduced in state legislatures regarding nonsmokers' rights and youth access laws were passed. However, 88% of the local city and county anti-tobacco ordinances passed. There is currently an all out tobacco industry effort to preempt local ordinances by state legislation. Tobacco control legislation at the state level usually fails because of the industry's "clout" with state legislatures and unbeatable financial resources. However, local community efforts and local antismoking ordinances have been very successful.

ANR Update, Spring 1994, p. 8

5. The tobacco industry uses its vast wealth and resources at the state level to support watered-down legislation and laws that preempt local antismoking laws. Laws in 19 states are tobacco industry backed and have preemptive clauses that bar more strict local ordinances. About half were adopted in 1993. Another industry approach is to support laws that protect smokers' rights in the job market. Since 1990, 27 states and D.C. have passed laws protecting smokers' civil rights on the job. American Medical News, April 25, 1994, p. 31

6. "Preemption of local regulatory authority is the number one goal of the tobacco industry nationwide."

Victor Crawford, former Tobacco Institute lobbyist, September 1995

7. "In tobacco control, preemption has emerged as a major strategy of the tobacco industry to undermine, overturn, and prohibit future efforts to adopt local tobacco control policies…

"The tobacco industry exercises strong influence over the U.S. Congress and state legislatures, but has far less sway at the local level. Federal laws currently preempt certain actions by states regarding cigarette advertising. The industry has sponsored bills that would preempt local action in every state in the U.S."

*Stop the Sale, Prevent the Addiction*, Centers for Disease Control, 1995

8.  The tobacco industry commonly pushes a state pre-emption bill, "often spun as being anti-tobacco, that replaces tough local laws with weak statewide measures. Such laws have been enacted 29 states."

Business Week, November 10, 1997, p. 140

9.  By late 1995, more than 1000 communities had enacted local tobacco control ordinances. In response, the tobacco industry has advanced legislation that in 29 states has been enacted to preempt or restrict local authority to regulate tobacco products. Only one state, Maine, has yet repealed a tobacco preemption law.

"The tobacco industry has responded to the rapidly increasing diffusion of community-based tobacco control policy interventions by using its political influence at the state level to promote the passage of state laws that preempt local regulation of tobacco. These preemption laws eliminate the authority of local jurisdictions to enact their own legislation to control the tobacco epidemic. Often, these laws repeal strong local ordinances. Almost uniformly, state preemption laws establish policies that do not provide adequate public health protection; for example, most preemptive state clean indoor air laws merely require separate sections for smokers and nonsmokers in workplaces and restaurants…The promotion of state legislation that preempts the authority of local government to enact and enforce tobacco control ordinances is an important tobacco industry strategy that undermines the public's health. One of the Healthy People 2000 objectives set by the Department of Health and Human Services is to 'reduce to zero the number of states that have clean indoor air laws preempting stronger clean indoor air laws on the local level." JAMA, September 10, 1997, pp. 858-863

10. One of the national health objectives for the year 2000 is (was) to reduce to zero the number of state with preemptive smoke free indoor air laws. However, in 1999, 30 states had preemptive tobacco control laws, which are considered undesirable by public health advocates.

Morbidity and Mortality Weekly Report, January 8, 1999, p. 1112

11. The Tobacco Institute had a budget of $38 million in 1993. In Minnesota, one legislator estimated that the industry maintains at least 60 lobbyists. In New York, the tobacco industry spent $1.1 million on lobbying in 1993. And to fight a bill to reduce youth access in Washington state, the industry hired nine outside lobbyists at a cost of $200,000. *Tobacco Industry Strategies,* p. 22

12. New York City considered a new workplace and restaurant smoking ban in 1994. Philip Morris told the mayor that if the law passed, they would consider moving their corporate headquarters and its 2000 jobs out of the city, and stop donations for New York cultural activities and the arts. (Nevertheless, Mayor Giuliani signed the ordinance in January 1995.)      New York Times, September 26, 1994, p. A1, and Reuters, January 11, 1995

13. In November 1994, a proposed tobacco tax increase in Colorado was defeated after a $5.1 million campaign by tobacco companies. This amounted to an investment of $7.43 for every vote against the measure. "Pro-health" advocates had only about one per cent as much to spend.      American Medical News, December 5, 1994, p. 15

14. The tobacco industry contributed $3 million to its front group "Coloradans Against Tax Abuse and Government Waste"  to challenge a tobacco excise tax increase proposal. Health groups were able to raise only $18,000 (a ratio of 167 to 1). The industry was successful, and the tax was defeated.

ASH Review, September-October 1994

15. In 1994, Colorado earned the dubious distinction of becoming the first state in which Big Tobacco successfully used subterfuge to win a statewide popular vote. Until then, the industry had relied on friendly legislators to derail anti-tobacco proposals

Tobacco's success came in a battle with a coalition of state health groups that had introduced a referendum for a 50-cent cigarette tax. Early polls showed 72 percent of the public supported the tax. But the tobacco industry had a bold new strategy:  It funded a front group to capitalize on the anti-tax, anti-government sentiment buoying right-wing politics and turned a tobacco tax battle into a referendum on "big government."

During the campaign, tobacco's front group, Citizens Against Tax Abuse and Government Waste, portrayed the ballot issue as a power grab by Colorado Department of Health "bureaucrats" who wanted to pad their salaries with the $132 million the new tax would generate. (Actually, the proposal designated half of the funds to health care for the poor and half to educational activities and medical research.) The ploy worked nonetheless. An onslaught of negative advertising turned public opinion around, and the proposal lost 62 to 38 percent...

In all, the tobacco industry contributed $5 million to defeat the proposal. The coalition of health groups that launched the initiative, by contrast, raised only $300,000. "The bottom line is that it was money, money, money," says Arnold Levinson, the coalition's campaign coordinator. Citizens Against Tax Abuse and Government Waste, he says, was pure camouflage: "There was not a single citizen in it. Every dime they had was tobacco money."

Quote from Mother Jones, May-June 1996, p. 55

16. In Arizona, a local PR consulting firm hired by Philip Morris tried to disrupt a cigarette tax increase petition drive by recruiting smokers through newspaper ads to harass the petition gatherers. (The 40 cents per pack tax increase passed in November 1994.) *Tobacco Industry Strategies*, p. 10

17. In 1993, Philip Morris offered coupons for free packs of cigarettes for smokers who would call Illinois state legislators to protest a hike in the state cigarette tax. Tobacco Free Youth Reporter, Fall 1993, p. 6

18. All 50 states have tobacco industry lobbyists, a mean of nine per state and 450 total. In contrast, there are a total of only 16 health lobbyists in nine states lobbying for an organization whose primary mission is a reduction of tobacco consumption. American Journal of Public Health, August 1996, p. 1140

19. More than 300 health organizations in the United States employ on their behalf a lobbyist who also works for the tobacco industry. Almost half (220 out of 450) of the tobacco lobbyists active at the state level also lobby for a health organization.

"The potential adverse effects on public health of such conflicts of interest were demonstrated recently in Florida, where lawmakers had passed legislation in 1994 making it easier for the state to pursue its $1.4 billion lawsuit on recovering Medicaid expenses for smoking-related illnesses. A bill to repeal the legislation passed the Florida state senate in April of 1995, supported by a 53-member lobbying team assembled by the tobacco industry. Two thirds of the tobacco industry lobbyists also represented hospitals and health insurance companies. The lead lobbyist for Philip Morris at the time reported that 'we wanted to have the first team, the best people we could possibly find...We didn't care about their other clients.' By hiring health lobbyists to work for the tobacco industry, the industry assured itself of detailed information about important health care bills, thus allowing it to 'try to pass [bills] in every conceivable form at every conceivable opportunity.'"

American Journal of Public Health, August 1996, p. 1141 (Adam Goldstein)

20. "Nearly one-third of the states have passed some form of 'smoker's rights' legislation, including New Jersey, where Philip Morris lobbyists wrote the law, which included barring insurance companies from charging higher premiums to smokers." *Ashes to Ashes*, p. 682

21. Philip Morris in Texas in 1989 spent $441,000 on lobbyists and consultants, not including other outlays such as $10,000 for a "legislative buck hunt." *Ashes to Ashes*, p. 686

22. Between 1989 and 1994, the Smokeless Tobacco Council and U.S. Tobacco paid $9.2 million in fees to "state legislative consultants." The Washington Monthly, May 1996, p. 22

23. A Business Week article "Big Tobacco's Hidden War: Hardball politics at the local level" (November 10, 1997, pp. 139-140) described how "industry sponsored groups flood state health departments with Freedom of Information requests, then use the information to file suits alleging misuse of taxpayer dollars. In Colorado, this tactic helped kill a proposed tobacco tax increase."

24. Tobacco control programs have often been subject to harassment by the tobacco industry.

"Using state and federal public records laws, tobacco industry lawyers, consultants, and front groups have been making massive requests for documents from state and local health departments. In Colorado, requests for documents from the state ASSIST program totaled over 13,000 pages --but the lawyers who requested them only picked up 6,000; the cost in staff time to respond to the request was over $50,000. These requests are often followed by charges of improper use of public funds."

ANR Update, Winter 1997

25. The Tobacco Institute surreptitiously financed an expensive advertising campaign to defeat a ballot proposition in Oregon to increase the tobacco tax from 38 to 68 cents a pack. The advertisements were placed under the name of a so-called citizens group, the Fairness Matters to Oregonians Committee, but it was actually organized and 100% financed by the Tobacco Institute. The Tobacco Institute intended to spend up to $7 million, while pro-tax health groups planned to spend about half a million dollars. (New York Times, October 19, 1996) The proposition was passed by a 56% to 44% margin, despite the $2.6 million that the tobacco industry spent to try to defeat it. (ANR Update, Winter 1996)

26. For a member of the Mississippi legislature, Charlie Williams gets around. In the past two years, Mr. Williams has gone to Spain, Belgium, Australia, and Costa Rica, all courtesy of the New York Society for International Affairs. The non-profit society receives almost all of its funding from Philip Morris, and recruits its trip-goers through two political organizations, the National Governors Association and the Council of State Governments. Its president, Andrew Whist, has worked for Philip Morris since 1966, and serves as senior vice president for external affairs, advising the company on international trade issues. Back in Mississippi, Charlie Williams commented, "More people die of fat each year than from tobacco."

Quote from the Wall Street Journal, August 4, 1997, p. A20

27. Wisconsin Governor Tommy Thompson in 1995 and 1996 took three foreign trips, including one to Australia and one to Africa, which were paid for by nonprofit groups financed by Philip Morris, a large campaign donor to the governor.

Associated Press, July 30, 1997

28. Wisconsin Governor Tommy Thompson "took trips to England, Australia, and Southern Africa that were paid for by innocent-sounding foundations such as the New York Society for International Affairs, which turned out to be largely funded by Philip Morris. Not coincidentally, Philip Morris executives accompanied Thompson on these trips."

Washington Monthly, November 1997, p. 6 (Charles Peters)

29. The state of Florida has decided to divest the state's retirement fund of $825 million in tobacco stocks.

New York Times, May 29, 1997, p. B10

30. Virginia attorney general James Gilmore announced that he would not enforce FDA regulations to reduce the sale of tobacco to children. He then took a Philip Morris jet to Philip Morris headquarters in New York to raise $50,000.

CNN Capital Gang, March 29, 1997

31. New York state officials canceled a talk by Jeffrey Wigand, whose whistle-blowing was at the heart of "The Insider," at a state-sponsored conference on young people and smoking. Wigand was barred because he planned to criticize New York Governor George Pataki for vetoing a bill about cigarettes and fire safety standards. A health department spokesman told the New York Times that the remarks would have been too political.

quote from San Francisco Chronicle, June 9, 2000, p. C204

# California Political and Economic Issues

1. The June 1992 Supreme Court ruling that smokers have a right to sue tobacco companies does not apply in the state of California. The "Willie Brown Civil Liability Reform Act" of 1987 in California prohibits people from suing the manufacturers of "inherently unsafe" products such as cigarettes, and a state Court of Appeal in 1989 ruled that the law provides nearly complete immunity for manufacturers of tobacco.

San Francisco Chronicle, June 24, 1992

2. California Assembly Speaker Willie Brown (a nonsmoker) received $410,517 in campaign contributions from tobacco companies from 1980 until 1993, with $221,367 in the 1991-92 election cycle alone. This made him the largest single legislative recipient of tobacco industry contributions in the United States.

American Journal of Public Health, September 1993

3.  Willie Brown's campaign contributions, gifts and legal fees from tobacco interests now total $750,000.
    San Francisco Examiner, September 17, 1995, p. B1

4.  The $16 million yearly California anti-tobacco media campaign mandated by the state tobacco tax had an unsuccessful attempt at elimination by Governor Pete Wilson. The tobacco industry spends $433 million yearly in California to promote their products.
    JAMA, July 22, 1992, p. 524

5.  Governor Pete Wilson received a $25,000 Philip Morris contribution toward his inaugural reception in 1990, and was the guest of Philip Morris at a $5000-per couple fundraising dinner to "help elect Republicans in California."
    Advocacy Institute, June 30, 1992

6.  In February 1993, Governor Pete Wilson signed an executive order that forbids smoking in all of the 21,600 buildings owned or leased by the state, including prisons. There are 180,000 California state employees and 109,000 prisoners, who will be allowed to smoke only in outdoor prison yards. Seven other states also have smoke-free government buildings.
    San Francisco Chronicle, February 24, 1993

7.  Smoking costs California more than $10 billion each year in medical costs and lost productivity due to death and illness. Direct medical costs are $3.6 billion (or $793 per smoker per year), lost productivity costs for employers $860 million (another $230 per smoker), and a loss to the state economy of $6.4 billion because of lost productivity due to premature death from tobacco.
    San Francisco Chronicle, October 20, 1994, p. A23

8.  Smoking caused 14,292 fires in California in 1990, causing more than $31.5 million in property damage and loss.
    San Francisco Chronicle, October 20, 1994, p. A23

9.  There are 58,000 deaths caused by tobacco each year in California.
    JAMA, May 27, 1992, p. 2723

10. In 1988, the tobacco industry spent $21,242,893 in an unsuccessful campaign to defeat Proposition 99, which raised the state cigarette tax from 10 cents to 35 cents per pack. The industry also spent $1.3 million in 1983-84 in an unsuccessful referendum campaign to repeal San Francisco's workplace smoking ordinance.
    American Journal of Public Health, September 1993

11. Proposition 99, which raised the California tobacco tax in 1988, has been called "the most important public health measure since the introduction of sewers" (Stanton Glantz, Ph.D.). One million smokers have quit since the proposition was passed.
    National Public Radio, March 11, 1994

12. In 1992, 112 out of the 120 members of the California legislature received contributions from the tobacco industry.
    American Journal of Public Health, September 1993, p. 1211

13. Californians for Fair Business Policy, a statewide political action committee, was established specifically to organize and finance referenda campaigns for the tobacco industry. It is 99.5% funded by tobacco companies. Through this organization, the tobacco industry spent $1,775,379 in 1992 in an unsuccessful attempt to repeal by referendum a Sacramento city and county ordinance restricting smoking. This amounted to a remarkable $17.27 per "no" vote. The CFBP also spent $216,000 in an unsuccessful signature petition drive to overturn by referendum the 1993 Los Angeles ordinance banning smoking in the city's 7000 restaurants.
    JAMA, July 28, 1993, p. 481

14. In 1993, the tobacco industry spent nearly $3 million on political contributions, lobbying and other political activities in California.
    JAMA, May 11, 1994, p. 1390

15. California state legislators collected more than $1.2 million from the tobacco lobby in 1991-92, half as much as all of the US Congress (Senate and House of Representatives). A study found that there is a significant link between the amount of money that legislators take from tobacco interests and their tendency to vote against anti-smoking legislation, and also that tobacco industry contributions not only sway legislators' votes, but do so at variance with the attitudes of their constituents.
    San Francisco Chronicle, October 20, 1994

16. The tobacco industry now seeks out tobacco control efforts and challenges them with their high-priced lawyers. In California, RJ Reynolds threatened 22 television station with a libel lawsuit if they broadcast a Department of Health Service's tobacco control ad that used footage from congressional hearings where tobacco industry CEO's swore that nicotine was not addictive. Three stations did stop broadcasting the ad after the threat.               *Tobacco Industry Strategies*, p. 8, and ASH Review, November-December 1994

17. RJR Chairman James Johnston threatened in 1994 to sue the state of California, alleging that an anti-smoking TV commercial accused him of committing perjury. The ad was withdrawn within two months, After 190 billboards with the logo "Are you choking on tobacco industry lies? Secondhand Smoke Kills" were papered over, critics complained of a pattern of Wilson administration efforts to water down the anti-smoking media campaign.               San Francisco Chronicle, September 25, 1996, p. A10

18. California state senator Gary Hart in 1994 introduced a bill that would have eliminated the state tax deduction that tobacco companies receive for advertising and promotional expenses. Tobacco use costs California more than $7,600,000,000 a year in lost productivity and medical costs. The state's anti-smoking ad campaign is outspent by the tobacco industry by a margin of 23 to 1; the industry spends over a million dollars every day in California on advertising and promotion.               Contra Costa Times, March 13, 1994, p. 14A

19. Philip Morris in 1994 submitted a proposed state ballot initiative in California which if passed would have preempted or wiped out strong local ordinances to replace them with weak state legislation. The initiative was drafted by the Sacramento law firm, Nielsen Merksamer, which has close ties to both the tobacco industry and Governor Wilson. The campaign, bankrolled at $8 million (as a PM tax deductible business expense), was run by the California Business and Restaurant Alliance, a Philip Morris sponsored front group. Another company was paid $2 per head to collect signatures.               ANR Update, Spring 1994, p. 1

20. A Philip Morris-sponsored pro-smoking petition deliberately mislabelled as a "tobacco control" act qualified for the November 1994 California ballot. PM spent $1.8 million collecting 600,000 signatures for the initiative, which would have pre-empted or overturned 270 local bans in cities including San Francisco and Los Angeles. Many signers complained that the "Californians for Statewide Smoking Restrictions" committee misrepresented the initiative as a tough no-smoking measure, not a drive backed by the nation's largest cigarette maker.               San Francisco Chronicle, June 2, 1994, p. A1,
New York Times, May 16, 1994, p. A1, and American Medical News, November 28, 1994, p. 24

21. A Philip Morris-sponsored ballot initiative in California was certified despite the statement by Tony Miller, California Secretary of State:  "Philip Morris takes the position that misrepresenting the purpose of an initiative has nothing to do with whether it should be placed on the ballot, and that it's all right to lie about who is sponsoring a measure in order to obtain signatures. Philip Morris should be ashamed of itself."
               New York Times, June 12, 1994, p. A39

22. In lobbying for its Proposition 188, Philip Morris sent all tobacco retailers in California a letter urging them to support the pro-smoking initiative "because if it does not pass, your cigarette sales and profits will drop." It then says that a Philip Morris representative will call on your store to drop off pro-Proposition 188 brochures for display and distribution.               KGO Radio, October 25, 1994 (Ronn Owens)

23. Five tobacco companies poured more than $17 million into their unsuccessful advertising campaign for Proposition 188, including $12.5 million from Philip Morris.               Associated Press, November 1994

24. Proposition 188 received only 29% of the vote in the November 1994 election; $17 million divided by 2,284,431 votes equals $7.46 that the tobacco industry invested for each of their votes.
               San Francisco Chronicle, November 10, 1994

25. Philip Morris told stockholders that passage of Prop 188 was "of paramount importance to our consumers, our employees and you, our stockholders." Such comments contrasted with the company's public pronouncements, which portrayed the initiative as an anti-smoking measure to increase protection for children.
               American Medical News, November 28, 1994, p. 24

26. After the defeat of Prop 188, Assembly Bill 13 became effective in January 1995. It bans smoking in most indoor places of employment in California, including restaurants.　　San Francisco Chronicle, July 20, 1994

27. The 1988 Proposition 99 saved more than $1.5 billion in health care costs in the first five years since its enactment because of reduced tobacco use. In an ad financed by the state's tobacco tax, an actor playing a tobacco company executive exhorts his staff in smoke-filled room to help enlist 3100 new customers a day to replace those who quit or die from smoking-related disease. "We're not in this business for our health," he jokes in a smoke-graveled voice.　　Washington Post National Weekly Edition, July 4-10, 1994, p. 11

28. California's 1997 budget bill had a provision prohibiting disbursing any of the $60 million in tobacco research funds for "partisan political purposes." All such funding would have to be approved by a panel of political appointees. Statehouse staffers tell reporters "This is to get Stan", referring to Stanton Glantz, who published work showing the relationship between tobacco campaign contributions and lawmakers' propensity to vote with the industry. The state's top universities are refusing to accept any of the $60 million if the restrictive provisions stand.　　Washington Post National Weekly Edition, July 8-14, 1996, p. 15

29. About two-thirds of California legislators have taken tobacco money since 1997; the tobacco industry contributed $5 million to campaigns and spent $9.1 million on lobbying in California from 1997 to 2002.
Associated Press, October 11, 2002

NEJM is New England Journal of Medicine
JAMA is Journal of the American Medical Association

# CHAPTER 36
# LEGAL ISSUES

1. In more than 800 lawsuits between 1954 and 1994, the tobacco industry went to trial only 23 times, lost twice, and never spent a dime in damage payments.
The Nation, August 28, 1995, p. 193

2. In tobacco liability cases, the industry has a policy of never settling, regardless of the merits of individual cases, and of doing everything possible to run up the plaintiff's bill. One industry lawyer explained, "to paraphrase General Patton, the way we won these cases was not by spending all of Reynolds' money, but by making that other son of a bitch spend all his."
*Tobacco Use: An American Crisis*, p. 80

3. The tobacco industry is the corporate world's most ferocious litigator, an opponent that never settles. In the Cipollone case in New Jersey, the industry spent $50 million, dragged it out for ten years and finally took it to the Supreme Court. It buried the other side in paper, filing 100 motions. One witness was questioned for nine days. Rose Cipollone had 24 hours of depositions as she was dying from lung cancer. In another case, a plaintiff in a second-hand smoke lawsuit in Mississippi was lying on his bed the day before he died when a helicopter began hovering over the house. The tobacco lawyers were apparently waiting for him to die so that they could immediately make a motion for an autopsy.
The Nation, August 28, 1995, p. 194

4. In the Rose Cipollone lung cancer case in New Jersey, "the industry expended over $80 million in pretrial preparation alone. No plaintiff could match such 'scorched earth' expenditures, especially when there was to be no reward or compensation at the end of the process."
*The Tobacco Epidemic*, p.14 (Gary Huber)

5. The 1992 Supreme Court decision in the Cipollone case ruled that tobacco liability suits were allowed, but only in cases of misrepresentation or fraud. The decision disagreed with the industry's contention that such lawsuits had been pre-empted by federal laws requiring warning labels on cigarette packages.
American Medical News, July 20, 1992

6. An appeals court removed a federal judge, H. Lee Sarokin, from a cigarette-hazards lawsuit brought by the family of Rose Cipollone. The court said that the harshly critical remarks that he made about the tobacco industry made it impossible for him to be impartial, but another appeals court called a previous effort to remove Judge Sarokin "entirely without merit, and a thinly disguised effort at judge shopping." The removal of the judge from cigarette cases is part of the success of the tobacco industry for almost 40 years in defending suits by "wearing down the tobacco litigants through a seemingly inexhaustible expenditure of resources," to quote a study by Prof. Robert Rabin of Stanford Law School. Indeed, in October 1992, the Cipollone family dropped the case, which had originally ordered the Liggett Group, Inc., to pay the family $400,000. The award was overturned by a federal appeals court in 1990.
Newsweek, June 27, 1988, p. 48, American Medical News, June 24, 1988 and<br>July 6, 1992, and NEJM, November 26, 1992, p. 1604

7. It was estimated that the cigarette industry spent at least $75 million defending the Cipollone case.
*Reducing Tobacco Use*, p. 227

8. The tobacco industry's successes in court have come from a two-part strategy: blame the victim and bankrupt the victim's lawyer. The lawyers in the Cippollone case against the industry reportedly spent $650,000 in expenses and contributed $2.9 million in professional fees, but came away with nothing.
Journal of the National Cancer Institute, January 3, 1996, p. 7

9. "Despite some rising pretenders, the tobacco industry maybe the king of concealment and disinformation...The plaintiff has presented strong evidence that defendants knew of the health risks implicated by cigarettes."
Judge Lee Sarokin (World Smoking and Health, No. 1, 1992, p. 3)

10. The first outsider ever to see the tobacco papers that describe some of the unusual story of tobacco and health research was Judge H. Lee Sarokin of the U.S. District Court in New Jersey, in the spring of 1988. The papers were not allowed in open court, but were first read by the judge while they were sealed. After reading them, he

wrote that the jury could reasonably conclude that the Tobacco Industry Research Council "was nothing but a hoax created for public relations purposes with no intention of seeking the truth or publishing it...The intensity of the advertising and public relations was sufficient to create the desired doubt in the minds of the consumer, and overwhelm or undermine pronouncements as to the dangers...The magazine *Tobacco and Health* mailed free to practically every doctor in the country... was a blatant and biased account of the smoking 'controversy.'" For those remarks, the tobacco companies protested to a higher court, and Judge Sarokin was removed from the case for bias.

Quote from *Smokescreen*, p. 21

11. After Philip Morris filed a $10 billion lawsuit against ABC, the time that network news shows devoted to the tobacco industry fell by more than 75% during the second half of 1994.

New York Times, December 9, 1995, p. 15

12. A legal brief written by lawyers for ABC-TV a month before the network settled its libel suit with Philip Morris contradicts Philip Morris statements to Congress that the company does not control or manipulate the nicotine in cigarettes. "To this extent [the Philip Morris plant] is a tobacco extract factory," the brief says.

American Medical News, February 12, 1996

13. Attorney General Janet Reno and the Justice Department at the request of members of Congress began an investigation of tobacco company executives' testimony to Congress that could result in charges of perjury, conspiracy to defraud the public and conspiracy to obstruct Congress. Even if the executives lied about alleging that nicotine is not addictive, however, some legal experts believe that they may be "off the hook" because they prefaced their statements by "It is my opinion that..." and "I believe that..." (nicotine is not addictive).

American Medical News, June 27, 1994, p. 8

14. "A narrow probe of possible perjury charges against several tobacco executives for 1994 congressional testimony has been expanded into a far-reaching Justice Department investigation into whether industry officials have systematically made false or misleading statements to Congress and government agencies about the addictive nature of tobacco and about industry practices."     Washington Post, September 8, 1996, p. A1

15. Six federal judges have accepted trips in recent years at international and domestic conferences paid for by two groups funded by Philip Morris. Two of the judges later were involved in tobacco-related cases.

(Minnesota) Star Tribune, July 19, 1998

16. The display since 1965 of federally mandated warning labels has had the unintended effect of shielding tobacco manufacturers from all product liability lawsuits brought against their products.

1994 Surgeon General report, p. 261

17. Three former Food and Drug Administration (FDA) lawyers now represent the tobacco companies RJ Reynolds, Philip Morris, and Brown and Williamson. Norman Redlich, former dean of the New York University Law School, is helping to lead Philip Morris' $10 billion libel suit against ABC. Carla Hills, former US Trade Representative, is working for RJR to help fight Canada's plain packaging (tombstone) legislation. And former US Attorney General Griffin Bell has been retained by Brown and Williamson for damage control regarding the company's leaked internal documents showing that they knew of the health hazards of tobacco at least thirty years ago.     *Tobacco Industry Strategies*, p. 33

18. Philip Morris as of 1994 had won 26 tobacco liability cases without a loss.

Washington Post National Weekly Edition, July 11, 1994, p. 19

19. The tobacco industry unsuccessfully sued the Environmental Protection Agency to try to nullify its report which classified second hand smoke as a "Group A" (or known human) carcinogen. "They are masters of creating scientific controversy where there is none": Dr. Gregory Connolly, Mass. Dept. of Public Health. "It's like the Flat Earth Society suing NASA for publishing photographs showing the Earth is round": Cliff Douglas, the Advocacy Institute.     Advocacy Institute, June 30, 1993

20. Flight attendants have filed a $5 billion class action suit against a number of tobacco companies because of illnesses caused by their exposure to second-hand smoke on flights before the 1989 smoking ban. Exposure was equivalent to actively smoking about one cigarette per flight.

*New York Times, November 6, 1994, p. A11, and*
*Audio Digest Internal Medicine, November 3, 1993 (Neal Benowitz)*

21. Flight attendant Norma Broin led a lawsuit against Philip Morris alleging that second-hand smoke is responsible for the illnesses of about 60,000 nonsmoking flight attendants. "A Mormon who never smoked, drank or used caffeine, Broin contracted lung cancer after 13 years of working in airplane cabins filled with smoke. It was her testimony that helped to persuade Congress to ban smoking on domestic airplanes in 1990. Now she is one of two women leading a class action lawsuit against the tobacco giant on behalf of all nonsmoking flight attendants who believe they have been injured by environmental tobacco smoke."

*Contra Costa (California) Times, March 11, 1996*

22. A Miami judge ruled in 1994 that for the first time second-hand smoke as a cause of illness could be accepted as the grounds for a class action lawsuit. As many as 60,000 current and former flight attendants seek damages of more than $1 billion from Philip Morris and seven other cigarette makers.

*New York Times, December 13, 1994*

23. The Norma Broin and 60,000 flight attendants second hand smoke lawsuit was settled in October 1997. The tobacco industry agreed to pay $300 million over three years to create the Broin Research Foundation to study tobacco-related illnesses. The industry will also pay attorneys fees and costs of the suit, estimated at $46 million and $3 million, respectively. Robert Kline of the Tobacco Control Legal Clinic at Northeastern University in Boston contended that by agreeing such a large payout in the settlement, the tobacco industry in effect "admitted that secondhand smoke causes cancer." The door is now open for similar cases by other workers, such as employees of restaurants and bars.     *New York Times, October 11, 1997, p. A1 and A8 and*
*US World News and World Report, October 20, 1997, p. 35*

24. "While Washington awaits the results of his slow-moving Whitewater investigation, independent counsel Kenneth Starr is moonlighting as a corporate lawyer. [He is] the lead counsel for 12 tobacco companies seeking to block a massive class-action lawsuit against the industry... He'll draw about $1 million this year from his law firm, in addition to what he's billing the government for his Whitewater work."

*Newsweek, June 12, 1995, p. 6*

25. Lawyer Kenneth Starr in 1995 acting on behalf of his client Brown and Williamson was unsuccessful in his efforts to invoke attorney-client privilege and in other legal maneuvers so that the company would not have to release documents suggesting "that the company had known that nicotine was addictive since 1963 and had suppressed research linking smoking to cancer and heart disease."

*New York Times, June 6, 1998, p. A23 (Frank Rich column)*

26. Whitewater independent counsel, Kenneth Starr, and his law firm have given greater priority to tobacco client Brown and Williamson than to the Whitewater investigation. Starr argued B & W's position in a New Orleans class action suit that nicotine is not addictive and that manufacturers have no financial responsibility for the health problems caused by their product.     *New York Times, April 6, 1996, p. 15*

27. A federal judge in early 1995 ruled that the tobacco industry could be sued in a huge class action lawsuit alleging that the companies hooked smokers while concealing knowledge that nicotine is addictive. The Castano suit will have the major US tobacco companies against a consortium of 60 prominent negligent law firms, with the plaintiffs contributing $6 million per year to cover trial expenses.

*San Francisco Chronicle, February 18, 1995, p. 1*

28. In May 1996, a Federal appeals panel in New Orleans dismissed the above Castano class action lawsuit brought against the tobacco industry on behalf of millions of smokers. Within an hour of the announcement, Philip Morris stock gained $5.4 billion in value. The consortium of 60 plaintiffs' lawyers now plan to file new class action lawsuits in all 50 states, and the case itself will continue as a lawsuit on behalf of four plaintiffs, instead of an entire class of smokers.     *New York Times, May 24, 1996, p. A1*

29. Liggett Group, Inc., which makes Chesterfield and Eve cigarettes and controls 2% of the US market, agreed to settle a class action lawsuit brought on behalf of all American smokers who said they were addicted, as well as claims filed by five states seeking to recover health care costs related to smoking.

Associated Press, March 14, 1996, and The Lancet, March 23, 1996, p. 823

30. There have been six cases against Lorillard involving its asbestos filters it used in Kent cigarettes in the 1950's. The company has won five cases and is appealing the sixth, a mesothelioma victim who was awarded $2 million in a California verdict in 1995. American Medical News, January 15, 1996

31. The following is from a deposition given by Jeffrey Wigand, a PhD biochemist and former chief of research for Brown and Williamson under its president Thomas Sandefur.

Q: Let me see if I understand you correctly, sir. You learned that coumarin had been taken out of cigarettes because it was dangerous, and you learned that coumarin had been taken out of other companies' pipe tobacco because it was dangerous, and you requested that coumarin be taken out of Sir Walter Raleigh pipe tobacco, is that fair? Is that what you said?

A: Yes, I did.

Q: And what did Mr. Sandefur tell you when you asked him to take that rat poison out of that particular pipe tobacco?

A: We got into a very significant debate. I'd probably consider it an argument. And that it could not be removed because it would impact the sales of the STP business, particularly since the aromatic pipe tobacco was one of the higher selling products.

Q: What did he say to you in general in the various times you recommended a search for a safe cigarette?

A: That there can be no research on a safer cigarette. Any research on a safer cigarette would clearly expose every other product as being unsafe and, therefore, present a liability issue in terms of any type of litigation. *Smokescreen*, pp. 162-163

32. Jeffrey S. Wigand entered a tiny courthouse in Pascagoula, Miss., where about 40 attorneys were waiting to hear his sworn account of his life inside Brown & Williamson Tobacco Corp. During the next two and a half hours, the tobacco industry's highest-ranking defector showed why he may be one of the biggest threats cigarette makers have ever faced. As a lawyer for B&W objected time and again, Mr. Wigand accused his ex-boss, former Chairman Thomas E. Sandefur, of lying under oath to Congress about his views on nicotine addiction. He charged that B&W in-house lawyers repeatedly hid potentially damaging scientific research, including altering minutes of a scientific meeting. And he said top company officials insisted that a compound found in rat poison remain as an additive in pipe tobacco, even though he told them he was concerned about its safety. Mr. Wigand, who has a doctorate in biochemistry and endocrinology, was B&W's research chief until he was fired in March 1993, shortly after Mr. Sandefur was promoted from B&W president to chairman and chief executive officer. Mr. Wigand's deposition was part of the trial preparation in the state of Mississippi's lawsuit seeking to force tobacco companies to pay for the cost of smoking-related illnesses. A key allegation in the suit is that industry executives knew nicotine was addictive but didn't tell the public.

Quote from the Wall Street Journal, January 26, 1996, p. 1

33. Wigand also remembers vivid scenes of his employers' covering their tracks in anticipation of the very lawsuits they are now battling. He alleges, for instance, that with Sandefur's approval, a company lawyer deleted 12 pages from the minutes of a meeting attended by Wigand and other top scientists from B&W's affiliates in which there was discussion of developing a "safer cigarette."

Quote from Time, February 12, 1996, p. 54

34. To give an example of the crazy mismatch in the cases, one plaintiff's lawyer, Stanley Rosenblatt in Miami, has written that the average case against tobacco nowadays costs $10,000,000, lasts ten years, and does not typically end with a tobacco victory, but ends when the plaintiff is completely exhausted and can afford not another day in court even though his case is not ended. In a typical legal case, for example, an important preliminary is to take depositions from those who are likely to testify. They are a sort of dry-run for both sides to see what each witness will offer and what issues the witness will raise. It is not uncommon to take an entire day to depose one witness, or even two or three days, for the most important witnesses in the toughest cases. But like a one-team league, the tobacco companies set records just by stepping on the field. In one case, a scientist who was testifying about the hazards of cigarette smoke for a plaintiff was grilled in deposition for 22

days; when the case ended (an exhausted plaintiff again) the industry lawyers had indicated they were not finished with him. In the same case (called Haines vs. Liggett Group), the industry had taken depositions of plaintiffs' witnesses for 292 days, consuming three years of court time. The judge in that case recalled a quotation from a Reynolds attorney on the strategy being employed: "The aggressive posture we have taken regarding depositions and discovery in general continues to make these cases extremely burdensome and expensive for plaintiffs' lawyers.... To paraphrase General Patton, the way we won theses cases was not by spending all of RJR's money, but by making that other son of a bitch spend all of his." At the end of the Haines case the lawyers for the widow of the dead smoker had to quit. They had spent $6.2 million, and ten years, and were not near a conclusion. They offered to turn the whole thing over to a fresh lawyer, and not even ask for expense reimbursement. No attorney could be found to take up the case.

*Smokescreen*, pp. 196-197

35.  ". . . the involvement of tobacco industry lawyers in the industry's external scientific research programs. These lawyers encouraged scientific research to refute the scientific evidence about tobacco, to provide results that could be used to respond to adverse publicity. To this end, the lawyers selected topics for research to perpetuate controversy about the health effects of tobacco, and manipulated the publication of research results through funding mechanisms run by lawyers rather than scientists....
The decision-making process revealed in the documents is unheard of in research programs funded by other sources, such as the National Institutes of Health. The documents confirm that scientific merit played little role in the selection of special projects or consultancies. Instead, grantees were selected by tobacco industry lawyers on the basis of their potential legal or political usefulness to the tobacco industry. Projects or investigators that had the potential to produce data unfavorable to the industry were not funded."

*The Cigarette Papers*, pp. 288 and 327

36.  "...the role of lawyers in selecting research projects and methodologies and controlling the dissemination of results is perhaps the most important insight offered by the documents. The industry's increasing reliance on lawyers to manage research reveals an industry policy toward research that was adversarial and elevated advocacy over objectivity. By putting lawyers in charge of scientific research, the tobacco companies effectively adopted a research policy that had nothing to do with finding out and disseminating the truth about the health effects of tobacco or with sponsoring truly independent research on that subject. It had everything to do with protecting the political and legal position of the industry and protecting its profits."

*The Cigarette Papers*, pp. 437-438

37.  As they had decided not to make safer cigarettes, the only place the data could ultimately be used was in court against them. So the companies began the dismantling of their scientific establishment. The elaborate facilities at R.J. Reynolds in Winston-Salem, North Carolina, referred to as the "mouse house," went first. On one day in December 1970, without warning, the workers at the lab were dismissed, their notebooks were collected by lawyers, and piles of papers were shredded. One man from RJR, Joseph Burngarner, said he was told that the Surgeon General was already "slitting our throats, we don't need to do it ourselves" as well. The British tobacco industry's laboratory at Harrogate was abruptly closed in 1974; that was the end of jointly sponsored research in England. At Philip Morris, the biology labs were shut down in 1984. Victor DeNoble, a scientist a Philip Morris at the time, said that the only explanation he got was from his superior in the research department, who told him, "that the lab was generating information that the company did not want generated inside the company, that it was information that would not be favorable to the company in litigation." On the day when the ax fell, April 5, 1984, DeNoble said the department chiefs told everyone not to discuss their work, and were warned not to attempt to publish it. They were told to halt all experiments, kill the laboratory rats, turn off the lab instruments, and give back their security badges by the next morning.

Quote from *Smokescreen*, p. 40

38.  ". . . an industry which lawyerly paranoia quickly metastasized into every vital organ. Lawyers coached the executives appearing before congressional committees, oversaw the woefully self-serving 'independent' research that the industry sponsored, and made sure that all paperwork connected with studies of addiction or cancer was funneled through an outside counsel so that it could be protected under the attorney-client privilege."

New Yorker, May 13, 1996, p. 45

39. "To conceal their knowledge of harmful effects of tobacco, companies involve their legal departments in the selection, conduct, and reporting of internal research. By involving lawyers in this way, results that run contrary to industry statements about smoking and health can be with held from the public by invoking attorney-client privilege. These actions are clearly inconsistent with acceptable practices of objective scientific investigation and dissemination of findings."  Addiction 1997; 92:517 (Kenneth Perkins)

40. In the 1988 lawsuit by the relatives of Nathan Horton who had died of lung cancer after smoking Pall Malls for thirty years, the American Tobacco Company argued, "cigarette smoking is not injurious to health. Customers are justified in relying on that statement" (Robert Heimann). And a person should not "expect to get lung cancer" or "expect to get emphysema" from smoking Pall Mall cigarettes (Preston Leake). Also: "the Surgeon General's dead wrong" (Robert Heimann).  Washington Post magazine, December 8, 1996, p. 14

41. In August 1996, shares of Philip Morris lost $12 billion of market value in a single day after a Jacksonville jury awarded a $750,000 judgment against Brown and Williamson on behalf of Grady Carter, a smoker with lung cancer.  New York Times, April 6, 1997, p.22

42. After a jury in Jacksonville awarded smoker Grady Carter $750,000 in damages in August 1996, the stock prices of Philip Morris and RJR dropped 14% and 13%, respectively, in one day, even though these tobacco companies were not directly involved in the litigation.  NEJM, January 23, 1997, p. 306

43. In August 1996 in Jacksonville, a jury awarded $750,000 in damages from Brown and Williamson for the lung cancer of Grady Carter, a long-time Lucky Strike smoker. "Coming on the heels of the Liggett settlement, their verdict sent tobacco shares tumbling on Wall Street. Philip Morris, which had nothing directly to do with the Jacksonville case, saw its stock fall about 14 percent in one day."
The Washington Post magazine, December 8, 1996, p. 34

44. A Florida appeals court reversed the above verdict in 1998, saying that the lawsuit had been filed too late.
Los Angeles Times, June 23, 1998

45. Still, the industry's insistent dismissal of the hazards of smoking has not changed. Senior executives giving private depositions in a Florida liability case again denied that cigarettes were addictive or a proven health risk. According to the Miami Herald, Andrew J. Schindler, president of R.J. Reynolds Tobacco Co., acknowledged that his father, a three-pack-a-day man, died of a stroke after the doctor warned him to quit. Yet under oath Schindler insisted tobacco was no more addictive than coffee. "What they were giving me was the same old party line," says Stanley M. Rosenblatt, the Miami-based plaintiffs attorney who took the deposition. "It's like they old hard-line Communists. They know what they say is absurd, but they stick to it anyway."
Quote from Washington Post National Weekly Edition, May 5, 1997, p.7

46. In pretrial testimony in the Florida lawsuit against tobacco companies, RJR Nabisco chairman Steven Goldstone said that cigarettes play a "role in causing lung cancer." And Philip Morris chairman Goeffrey Bible conceded that about 100,000 Americans "might have" died from diseases caused by smoking.
Associated Press, August 21, 1997, and New York Times, August 23, 1997, p.3

47. A Florida jury has ordered Brown and Williamson to pay $500,000 in compensation and $450,000 in punitive damages to the daughter of a smoker who died of cancer after many years of smoking Lucky Strike cigarettes.
Wall Street Journal, June 11, 1998

48. A Massachusetts law effective in July 1997 requires tobacco companies to disclose the ingredients of their cigarette brands. The law was upheld by a federal judge in response to a lawsuit by four tobacco companies trying to block disclosure of their brand's ingredients as a trade secret.  Reuters, February 8, 1997

49. R.J. Reynolds in late 1996 faced 234 active lawsuits from individual smokers and their families, up from 54 cases two years earlier. (In March 1998, the number had increased to 540 lawsuits – editor.)
Washington Post National Weekly Edition, May 5, 1997, p.6

50. As of 1997, there were 15 class action suits against the tobacco industry for addiction and treatment, 4 for direct harm, and more than 500 individual cases. Cases involving R.J. Reynolds have increased from 60 in 1994 to 460 in 1997.                          10th World Conference on Tobacco or Health, Beijing, 1997 (Greg Connolly)

51. Israel's Health Ministry plans to sue U.S. tobacco companies to recover the costs for treating smoking-related diseases, estimated at $429 million annually.                          Washington Post, December 19, 1997, p. A43

52. The Israel Health Ministry plans to sue cigarette companies $5.88 billion for the cost of treating smoking-related illnesses. The suit resembles the U.S. multi-state action.                          The Lancet, June 14, 1997, p.1754

53. Former asbestos product maker Raymark Industries, Inc., has filed suit against the tobacco industry, seeking to recover $400 million that the company paid to asbestos victims who also smoked.
                          Wall Street Journal, October 1, 1997, p. B4

54. A jury has awarded $2 million to a man who developed mesothelioma, a type of cancer frequently caused by asbestos, after smoking Kent cigarettes made with asbestos-laced micronite filters in the 1950's.
                          Associated Press, September 4, 1995

55. Lorillard Tobacco Company has paid $1.5 million to the family of Milton Horowitz, the first American to actually collect a smoking-related judgment from a cigarette company. Horowitz had sued Lorillard after he developed mesothelioma, a rare form of asbestos-related lung cancer. He smoked Kent cigarettes at a time (1952-1956) when this brand had asbestos filters.                          San Francisco Chronicle, January 1, 1998

56. A Minnesota judge will review 150,000 pages of sensitive documents that tobacco companies sought to keep confidential under lawyer-client privilege. The judge said that there was sufficient preliminary evidence of possible fraudulent activity by the tobacco industry to justify the review.          USA Today, May 12, 1997, p.1B

57. For 42 years of litigation from 1954 to 1996, the tobacco industry had a perfect record of never paying out a penny in damages.                          British Medical Journal, January 8, 2000, p. 111

58. Only 8% of state revenues from the 1998 tobacco settlement are devoted to antismoking programs. In Texas, lawyers received 10 times as much in 1999 as went to antismoking efforts, and in Michigan, tobacco control will receive no money at all from the settlement. The majority of states "appear to view the dollars primarily as a hefty new revenue source to be spent on whatever the state needs."   Los Angeles Times, December 27, 1999

59. British Columbia in November 1998 became the first Canadian province to sue the tobacco industry to recover smoking-related health costs, which cost the province about $345 million each year.
                          Reuters, November 11, 1998

60. The tobacco industry spends $750 million a year on legal and court fees.          CBS evening news, July 8, 1999

61. Michael Orey's book *Assuming the Risk* has a detailed discussion of the Nathan Horton case.

62. More details on Merrell Williams and Brown and Williamson can be found in Michael Orey's 1999 book *Assuming the Risk.*

63. Twelve law firms representing Mississippi have been awarded $1.4 billion for their work on lawsuits against the tobacco industry, including $340 million for the firm of attorney Richard Scruggs (who coincidentally is the brother-in-law of Senate majority leader Trent Lott). Five firms in Massachusetts will share $775 million, money to be paid by the tobacco industry and which will not affect each state's settlement money.
                          Washington Post, July 30, 1999, p. E10 and Associated Press, July 30, 1999

64. The law firm of Mississippi attorney Richard Scruggs will receive $874 million of the fees awarded to lawyers who handled lawsuits in Mississippi, Florida and Texas.          Washington Post, December 20, 1998, p. A26

65. A detailed discussion of the Mississippi lawsuit can be found in Michael Orey's 1999 book *Assuming the Risk.*

66. A $206 billion settlement was announced in November 1998 between the tobacco industry and 46 states. Within a week, the companies announced a 38% wholesale price increase, which added 45 cents to each pack sold at retail.
    *Reuters, November 24, 1998*

67. Only five of the 46 states that signed the tobacco settlement have allocated a significant portion of the money that they will be receiving toward tobacco control programs.    *Wall Street Journal, August 24, 1999, p. A4*

68. Philip Morris stock declined 8.3% and then another 6.8% on consecutive days in late March 1999 "amid investor fears that recent courtroom losses for the tobacco industry signal a shift in attitude among juries."
    *New York Times, April 1, 1999, p. C9*

69. A San Francisco jury in February 1999 awarded a 52-year-old smoker with inoperable lung cancer, Patricia Henley, $1.5 million in compensatory damages plus $50 million in punitive damages from Philip Morris.
    *Associated Press, February 11, 1999*

70. A jury in March 1999 in Portland, Oregon awarded $80 million to Mayola Williams, the widow of a Marlboro smoker who died of lung cancer.    *Los Angeles Times, March 31, 1999*

71. In San Francisco, a jury awarded $1.7 million for medical care and lost wages and another $20 million in punitive damages to Leslie Whiteley, a 40 year old who smoked for 26 years and is dying of lung cancer.
    *San Francisco Chronicle, March 28, 2000, p. A1*

72. Dr. Freddy Homburger was hired to conduct smoking studies on hamsters for the Council for Tobacco Research in the early 1970's. When he found that cigarette smoke caused cancer in lab animals and submitted the results to the council, he was told that he would "never get a penny" of his payment if the paper went to press as written. They suggested that all references to cancer be deleted from the article.
    *San Francisco Chronicle News Services, December 18, 1998*

73. The Supreme Court in March 2000 ruled 5 to 4 that the FDA lacked the jurisdiction to regulate tobacco.
    *New York Times, March 21, 2000*

74. "The litigation situation in Britain has had serious setbacks... however, a legislative and policy approach is achieving results. Taxes raised on tobacco in the United Kingdom exceed the value per smoker of the U.S. master settlement agreement between the industry and the states by a factor of eight – with no payments to lawyers or risk of failure in court. Tobacco advertising is to be banned, and existing health and safety legislation will be deployed to reduce passive smoking in the workplace... In the United States, such a national strategy would, without question, be blocked by Congress. Perhaps the success of litigation in the United States is a response to the failure of the legislative and executive branches of the U.S. government to curb the excesses of the tobacco industry."    *British Medical Journal, January 8, 2000, p. 113 (Richard Daynard)*

75. Kenneth Starr was the lead counsel in 1995 for twelve tobacco companies who tried to decertify a class action suit against the tobacco industry. He invoked attorney-client privilege in 1995 before an appellate court to aid his client Brown and Williamson in their "efforts to intimidate and frustrate [Congressmen] Henry Waxman and Ron Wyden, who'd used a cache of Brown and Williamson internal documents in their House investigation of the cigarette industry." (Frank Rich, New York Times). Representative Waxman commented: "It is questionable for a special prosecutor to moonlight at all. But to front for the tobacco industry to stop the public from hearing the truth is not helpful in insuring confidence in the highly political Whitewater case." Starr's hourly rate was $390. *And the Horse He Rode In On,* James Carville, Simon and Shuster, 1998, pp. 72-74

76. The tobacco industry spends $900 million each year on lawyers and legal costs to deal with tobacco litigation.
    *Cigarettes* (Parker-Pope), p. 23

77. As of 2001, about 1500 lawsuits are pending against the tobacco industry.    *Time, July 2, 2001, p. 39*

78. The tobacco industry has issued subpoenas to ten universities, demanding more than a half century's worth of documents relating to government-financed research of smoking dating back to the 1940s. The universities include Harvard, Johns Hopkins, and four universities in the University of California system. The general counsel for Hopkins commented, "This is a serious infringement upon the academic freedom and rights of our faculty…The tobacco companies have commenced nothing short of a campaign of harassment against the academic institutions that discovered that smoking is injurious to the public health."

San Francisco Chronicle, January 20, 2002, p. A8 (from the New York Times)

79. A Miami jury in June 2002 ordered four cigarette manufacturers to pay $5.5 million in damages to Lynn French, a flight attendant, who blamed her chronic sinus infections on secondhand smoke. She inhaled secondhand smoke for the first 14 years of her career, flying for TWA, until smoking was banned on U.S. airlines in 1990. This verdict is thought to be the first time that a U.S. jury has ruled against the tobacco industry in a passive smoke case.

Miami Herald, June 19, 2002 (via tobacco.org)

80. In the largest damage award in American history, a Miami jury ordered the tobacco industry to pay $144.8 billion in punitive damages to half a million sick Florida smokers.

New York Times, July 15, 2000

81. The New South Wales Supreme Court awarded $A450,000 to a nonsmoking bartender after she developed throat cancer after years of heavy exposure to passive smoke. This was the first successful litigation of the kind in Australia.

The Lancet, May 12, 2001, p. 1511

82. In April 2002, a supreme court in Victoria, Australia ordered British American Tobacco to pay Rolah McCabe, a 51-year-old smoker dying of lung cancer, $A700,000 in damages. She is the first smoker ever in Australia to obtain a damages verdict against the tobacco industry. Justice Geoffrey Eames ruled that BAT had "subverted" the process of discovery "with the deliberate intention of denying a fair trial to the plaintiff," and struck out BAT's defense to the claim, "a truly exceptional step taken only in the most extreme circumstances." It was found that BAT deliberately destroyed thousands of documents, misled the court as to what had happened to missing documents, and "warehoused" documents with third parties to keep them from discovery, while maintaining access to them should they be helpful in the defense of a claim.

Tobacco Control, September 2002, p. 271

83. An Australian grandmother became that country's first successful plaintiff against the tobacco industry in April 2002, when she was awarded 700,000 Australian dollars. A lung cancer victim, the 51-year-old woman has only a few months to live, according to press accounts. The defendant, British American Tobacco, lost the verdict when the judge ruled that the plaintiff could not receive a fair trial because the company had engaged in systematic shredding of important internal documents as recently as 1998, hiding the destruction under the guise of innocent activities. The possibility exists for criminal action against attorneys who sanctioned the document destruction, and investigation of the company for obstruction of justice in other countries may be on the horizon.

2003 AMA Annual Tobacco Report

84. In Italy, two managers of the Paribas Bank in Milan were convicted in July 2002 of criminal manslaughter in the death of a 35-year-old female bank employee who suffered a fatal asthma attack in 1999 from workplace exposure to secondhand smoke. They were sentenced to jail and fined 50,000 Euros, reported the Italian news agency, La Stampa. Her repeated requests to be moved to a smoke-free space were ignored by her employers, even though she had provided several reports from her doctor that her health was worsening because of smoke exposure.

2003 AMA Annual Tobacco Report

85. British American Tobacco faced 4,419 lawsuits in the USA alone at the end of 2001. *The Tobacco Atlas*, p. 86

86. A Los Angeles jury awarded Betty Bullock, 64, $850,000 in compensatory damages from Philip Morris, plus $28 billion in punitive damages. She is dying of lung cancer.    San Francisco Chronicle, September 27, 2002, and People, October 21, 2002, p. 90

87. A Los Angeles judge reduced Betty Bullock's damage award from Philip Morris to $28 million from the original $28 billion.

New York Times, December 19, 2002, p. A23

88. Snuff maker UST has settled a lawsuit (for an undisclosed amount) with a former customer who contracted tongue cancer. *Associated Press, October 13, 2002*

89. In 2002, a California judge fined RJR $14.8 million for violating a state law prohibiting marketing practices aimed at children. RJR distributed more than 100,000 free packs of cigarettes at various events, including the Long Beach Jazz Festival and a hot rod race at the Pomona Raceway. *2003 AMA Annual Tobacco Report*

90. The U.S. Supreme Court ruled 5-4 in 2001 that a Massachusetts regulation on outdoor advertising of tobacco products is unconstitutional and that it violated the first amendment as it applies to commercial speech. The regulation would have kept tobacco ads from being displayed within 1000 feet of schools and playgrounds, including convenience stores. *2002 AMA Annual Tobacco Report*

91. In June 2002, RJR was fined $20 million for targeting youth in its magazine advertising. The State of California had brought the action against the company, charging that it had violated the Master Settlement Agreement's provisions. The state's courts agreed, and levied the fine. RJR will appeal. *2003 AMA Annual Tobacco Report*

92. An Oregon appeals court has upheld and reinstated a $79.5 million punitive damage verdict against Philip Morris in the case of a 1999 jury award on behalf of Jesse Williams, a Portland janitor who died of lung cancer after smoking Marlboros for 42 years. *Associated Press, June 6, 2002*

93. A Los Angeles jury awarded Richard Boeken, a smoker with lung cancer, a record verdict of $5.5 million in compensatory damages and $3 billion in punitive damages from Philip Morris. Kenneth Starr, attorney for Philip Morris, argued against the huge award for punitive damages, and a judge reduced the award to $100 million. *2002 AMA Annual Tobacco Report and Associated Press, August 10, 2001*

94. A Los Angeles jury awarded $3 billion from Philip Morris to a sick smoker, Richard Boeken, 56, who has incurable lung cancer. Philip Morris is appealing. *San Francisco Chronicle, June 7, 2001, p. A3*

95. Richard Boeken, a longtime smoker whose $100 million award from Philip Morris (reduced from $3 billion by a judge) was the largest ever won by an individual, died at age 57 of lung cancer. *Associated Press, January 19, 2002*

96. A retired Miami lawyer, John Lukacs, who is dying from oral cancer, won a $37.5 million judgment against major tobacco companies when a Miami jury found that they caused his cancer. *Miami Herald, June 12, 2002*

97. A few days after the Lukacs verdict, another Florida jury found in favor of a flight attendant who claimed that her chronic sinusitis was cased by years of exposure to ETS in airline work. The jury awarded $5 million, which the industry immediately appealed. This suit is one of hundreds expected in the aftermath of the 1997 Broin verdict that found the tobacco industry liable for damages in ETS-related suits brought by airline flight attendants. *2003 AMA Annual Tobacco Report.*

98. A judge in June 2002 ordered RJR to pay $15 million in punitive damages to David Burton, a 43-year Camel smoker, who had his legs amputated in 1993 because of vascular disease linked to smoking. Earlier, a jury had awarded him $196,000 in compensatory damages. *Associated Press, June 21, 2002*

99. A San Francisco jury's $26.5 million award to a former smoker with lung cancer, Patricia Henley, was upheld by a state appellate court, rejecting an appeal by Philip Morris. *San Francisco Chronicle, November 9, 2001*

100. Cancer patient Patricia Henley's $51.5 million award from Philip Morris in 1999 was reduced to $26.5 million. *Associated Press, August 22, 2001*

101. An Oregon jury ordered Philip Morris to pay $150 million in punitive damages for falsely representing that low tar cigarettes are not as dangerous as regular ones. The plaintiff was the estate of Michele Schwarz, who died in 1999 at age 53 after smoking low tar Merit cigarettes. There was also an award of $168,000 in compensatory damages. *Associated Press, March 23, 2002*

102. Over five years after Brown and Williamson was found liable in the tobacco suit brought by Grady Carter in Florida, the appeals process has finally stopped, and the company must pay $1.1 million in damages plus Mr. Carter's legal fees. The U.S. Supreme Court declined to hear the case. Big Tobacco faces over 1600 individual plaintiff actions nationwide.                           2002 AMA Annual Tobacco Report

103. TWA flight attendant Lynn French, awarded $5.5 million for chronic sinus disease in a secondhand smoke lawsuit, had the amount reduced to $500,000 by a Miami judge.                           Associated Press, September 13, 2002

104. In the spring of 2002, several U.S. cigarette makers were found liable in a suit in Florida, and must pay $37.5 million in compensatory damages to a sick smoker. In addition to the compensation, the six-member jury's verdict entitles John Lukacs, who lost his tongue to cancer and can no longer talk, to part of a record $145 billion in punitive damages awarded two years ago in a class-action suit by Florida smokers. Plaintiffs' lawyers say that as many as 700,000 people are eligible to share in the punitive award. The verdict may open cigarette makers to millions of dollars in additional compensatory damages, as smokers go to court to prove they're entitled to share the punitive damages. Tobacco companies, which are appealing the punitive award, say the individual suits may take decades. The jury said Liggett was 50 percent responsible for his illness, while Brown & Williamson and Philip Morris were each 22.5 percent responsible. Lukacs was 5 percent responsible, jurors said.                           2003 AMA Annual Tobacco Report

105. Engle vs. R.J. Reynolds, the Florida class action case where tobacco companies were ordered in July 2000 to pay $144.8 billion in punitive damages to a statewide class of injured smokers, remains on appeal.
                          Los Angeles Times, September 21, 2002

106. On July 14, 2000, a Florida jury ordered the tobacco industry to pay $144.8 billion in punitive damages to 500,000 sick Florida smokers. Tobacco executives called the award ridiculous.
                          New York Times, July 15, 2000

107. Class action lawsuits against the tobacco industry have been filed in 11 states; the suits contend that the companies use terms such as "light" to mislead smokers into believing that those brands are safer.
                          Associated Press, March 26, 2002

108. An Illinois judge has found Philip Morris USA guilty of fraud and ordered the company to pay $10.1 billion in a class action lawsuit for failing to inform consumers that its "light" cigarettes were not less harmful than full flavor brands.                           New York Times, March 22, 2003, p. A8

109. An Illinois judge in March 2003 ordered Philip Morris to pay $10.1 billion for misleading smokers into believing its "light" cigarettes are less harmful than regular labels. The plaintiffs said that Philip Morris "knew the light brands were just as unhealthy as regular cigarettes when it introduced them in the 1970s, but marketed them as a healthier alternative...The case was the first class action lawsuit in the nation to come to trial alleging a tobacco company committed consumer fraud in its advertising of light cigarettes."
                          Associated Press, March 22, 2003

110. An Illinois judge ordered Altria (Philip Morris) to post a $12 billion bond while the company appeals a $10.1 billion judgment for misleading smokers into believing that its light cigarettes, Marlboro and Cambridge Lights, were less harmful than regular brands. Altria said that it would be unable to post the bond, and its stock dropped to under $30 a share, below the previous 52-week low. The Illinois lawsuit was a class action suit filed on behalf of the one million Illinois smokers of the two light brands.                           Associated Press, April 1, 2003

# CHAPTER 37
# ECONOMIC ISSUES

1.  The five largest multinational tobacco companies have annual revenues from tobacco sales that are more than 60 times higher than the entire annual budget of the World Health Organization, or 10 times the gross domestic product of the country of Bolivia.                                  World Smoking and Health, No. 1, 1992, pp. 2 and 6

2.  5,450,000,000,000 (5.45 trillion) cigarettes were sold worldwide in 1991, enough to supply every person on earth with about three each day. This is a 300% total increase and 50% per capita increase since 1950.
                                                                          American Medical News, September 21, 1994, p. 22

3.  Worldwide, there are 47 million jobs provided by tobacco. 30 million of these are in growing the crop, including 15 million tobacco farmers in China.
                                    10th World Conference on Tobacco or Health, Beijing, 1997 (Kenneth Warner)

4.  American cigarette consumption peaked at 640 billion in 1981, and dropped to 500 billion in 1993. But Philip Morris now has 60% of its sales from outside the United States, and its profit margin was 27 percent in 1993.
                                                                                   Newsweek, March 21, 1994, p. 52

5.  U.S. manufacturers in 1992 produced 685 billion cigarettes, of which 173 billion were exported, leaving domestic consumption of 512 billion that year.                          *Tobacco Use: an American Crisis*, p. 84

6.  Cigarette prices quadrupled during the 1980's, with manufacturers increasing their price at more than double the inflation rate. Taxes decreased from a third to a quarter of the cost of a pack.
                                                                   American Medical News, November 14, 1994, p. 16

7.  The US tobacco industry in 1994 had annual sales of $54 billion, and tobacco contributes $13 billion in taxes to federal, state, and local governments.                            San Francisco Examiner, August 9, 1995

8.  In 2002, the average price in U.S. dollars of a pack of 20 cigarettes were Spain $1.66, Italy $1.93, Greece $1.79, the Netherlands $2.56, Austria $2.37, Belgium $2.63, Germany $2.76, France $2.76, Iceland $4.39, Denmark $3.77, the United Kingdom $6.33, Sweden $3.64, Norway $7.56, Hong Kong $3.97, Australia $4.02, and New Zealand $3.88.                                      ASH Smoking and Health Review, July-August 2002

9.  The average Marlboro retail price per pack in December 1999 was $0.70 in Russia, $0.98 in Mexico, $1.37 in Poland, $1.50 in Argentina, $2.42 in Spain, $2.75 in Japan, $3.17 in the United States and Germany, $3.19 in Italy, $3.36 in France, $3.82 in Canada, $4.08 in Australia, and $6.32 in the United Kingdom.
                            Report "Cigarette Prices Around the World," Equity Research, Global/Tobacco, January 7, 2000

10. In 1992, 68.7% of the US cigarette market was for so-called low tar (15mg or less of tar) and nicotine brands (up from 54% in 1988). 71% of all advertising and promotional dollars were spent on these brands in 1992. The market share of menthol cigarettes has remained stable at 26% since the late 1980's, and 97% of cigarettes sold in 1992 were filtered.                                             Tobacco Control, Fall 1994, p. 289

11. Discount cigarette brands such as Misty, Doral, and Cambridge in 1993 had a 40% market share of the US market, up from 15% in 1989. Profit margins on these brands are 30 to 50% lower than on "premium" brands. Discount brands were first introduced in 1980, and in 1982 controlled only 2% of the US market.
                                                                   American Journal of Public Health, September 1993, p. 1212

12. Prior to the April 1993 price cuts, Philip Morris made a profit of about 55 cents a pack on Marlboro sales, but only 5 cents a pack on its discount brands. Thus, even with a 40 cent a pack price reduction, the company will make three times the profit on Marlboro compared to its discount brands.
                                                                                   Tobacco Free Youth Reporter, Spring 1993

13. In 1930, 75% of the tobacco grown in the United States was used for products other than cigarettes. By 1990, less than 15% was used for products other than cigarettes.

    Nicotine Dependence Conference, American Society of Addition Medicine, Atlanta, November 1993

14. Tobacco, the raw ingredient in cigarettes, accounts for only 9% of the price of a pack of cigarettes.

    *Nicotine Addiction*, p. 49

15. In 1993 the United States produced 1614 million pounds of tobacco. The leading states were North Carolina (606 million pounds produced), Kentucky (455), Tennessee (139), South Carolina (111), Virginia (100), and Georgia (96). Other states with small crops were Pennsylvania, Ohio, Florida, Indiana, Maryland, Wisconsin, Missouri, West Virginia, Connecticut, and Massachusetts.

    USA Today, May 18, 1994

16. Three insurance companies owned by the tobacco industry charge smokers nearly double for life insurance, because at any age, a smoker is about twice as likely to die as a nonsmoker.

    NEJM, April 7, 1994, p. 975 and Hospital Practice, August 15, 1994, p. 11

17. Smokers pay almost twice as much for term life insurance as nonsmoker "preferred" rates in a plan sponsored by the American Medical Association. A 30-year-old male nonsmoker pays $136 a year for a $100,000 policy; the rate increases to $225 for a smoker the same age. For a 50-year-old male, the rates are $361 and $679, respectively, for the same coverage, or 88% more for the smoker.

    AMA Life Insurance plan brochure, 1994

18. In a March 1997 advertisement for term life insurance, the United Services Life Insurance Company charged twice as much for smokers as nonsmokers for forty year olds, and two and a half times as much for 50-year-old smokers.

    US News and World Report, March 10, 1997

19. Term life insurance monthly rates for $100,000 of insurance are greatly increased for smokers. As an example, advertised monthly rates in 2003 for this coverage for a 40-year-old male was $11.90 for a nonsmoker and $22.49 for a smoker. For a 50-year-old male, the rates were $19.95 for a nonsmoker and $46.73 for a smoker; for a 60-year-old male, $42.61 a month for a nonsmoker compared to $106.14 for a smoker. Advertisement in U.S.

    News and World Report, March 2003

20. Nearly 25% of large insurance companies in 1997 charged smokers higher premiums for health insurance, up from less than 10% in 1992. Insurance claims for smokers average 18% more. USA Today, July 28, 1997, p. 1

21. Smokers who lie about their habit on life insurance applications may end up with no coverage at all. A federal appeals court allowed the New York Life company to avoid paying a claim in such a case, even though the policy holder died of a cause not related to his smoking.

    *Reducing the Health Consequences of Smoking*, p. 545

22. Health insurance policies in the US generally require nonsmokers to subsidize smokers by charging most the same rate.

    ASH Review, November-December 1994, p. 6

23. In 1991, only 25% of private health insurers in California had premium differentials based on smoking status, and fewer than 5% sold policies that covered smoking cessation services.

    Tobacco Control, Summer 1994, p. 124

24. In a 1987 study from a major city hospital emergency room, tobacco related illness accounted for 7% of total visits and 12% of total billings. Extrapolation to total national emergency visits of 81 million results in about 5.7 million visits and $1.2 billion in ER expenses for tobacco-related illness.

    American Journal of Emergency Medicine, March 1989, p. 187

25. A study from Dow Chemical found that smokers average 5.5 more days of work absence and 8 more days of disability leave each year than nonsmoking workers.

    Time, October 12, 1992, p. 76 (Andrew Tobias)

26. There are 77 to 80 million work days lost because of smoking each year in the U.S. Smokers' disability rates are 15% higher than those of nonsmokers, and the rate of absenteeism from work is 50% higher in smokers.

*Southern Medical Journal, January 1990, p. 13*

27. Cigarette smokers are absent from work about 6.5 days more per year than nonsmokers, and make about six visits more to health care facilities per year.

*NEJM, April 7, 1994, p. 975*

28. Smokers have a 33% to 45% higher absentee rate from work than nonsmokers. The average one-pack-plus-per-day smoker, over a lifetime, will cost an employer $624 per year. Lung cancer costs US private industry an estimated $785 million annually.

*Tobacco, p. 7*

29. US employees pay out an average of $960 extra per year in lost work time and health expenses for every smoker on their payroll.

*World Watch magazine, July-August 1997, p. 25*

30. Smokers are absent from work 50% more often than nonsmokers, and they are also 50% more likely to be hospitalized than workers who do not smoke. They also have 45% more sick days taken, and 15% higher disability rates.

*Passionate Nonsmoker's Bill of Rights*, p. 145, and Southern Medical Journal, January 1990, p. 13

31. The average smoker costs his or her employer more than $4500 each year in absenteeism, higher insurance and medical costs, lost productivity, and increased cleaning and maintenance costs.

*American Medical News, August 24, 1990*

32. Dr. William Weis published a study in the May 1981 edition of Personnel Administrator entitled "Can you afford to hire smokers?" The study assumed that the employer also allowed smoking in the workplace in addition to hiring smokers. The total cost per smoker per year (in 1981 dollars) was estimated at $4611, including $1820 for on the job time lost and the other factors of excess medical care, absenteeism, and morbidity and early mortality.

33. Smokers are admitted to hospitals twice as often as nonsmokers and utilize the health care system 50% more. Smokers are also absent from work 50% more, and have twice as many on-the-job accidents and 50% more traffic accidents than nonsmokers.

*Washington Post National Weekly Edition, September 26, 1994,
Hospital Practice, June 15, 1993, p. 8, Newsweek, January 13, 1986, p. 9,
and JAMA, October 16, 1987, p. 2085*

34. On the average, an employee who smokes wastes 6 percent of his working hours with the smoking ritual, takes 50 percent more sick leave, and uses the health care system at least 50 percent more.

*American Medical Association Fact Sheet on Smoking*

35. Employees who take four 10 minutes work breaks a day to smoke actually work one month less per year than workers who don't take breaks, and this lost productivity costs companies $29 billion a year.

*ASH Review, March-April 1994, p. 7*

36. About one third of all US hospital beds are devoted to tobacco-caused disease.

*Time, October 12, 1992 (Andrew Tobias)*

37. Smokers are admitted to hospitals twice as often as nonsmokers.

*Hospital Practice, June 15, 1993, p. 8*

38. As contrasted with smokers who successfully quit, continued smokers (average age 44 years) over 5 years of follow-up have a 7 to 15% increase in outpatient visits, a 30 to 45% increase in hospital admissions, and a 75 to 100% increase in hospital days.

*Archives of Internal Medicine, September 11, 1995, p. 1789*

39. In a study of 2500 postal employees, the absentee rate for smokers was 33% higher than for nonsmokers (5.43% compared to 4.06%).

*American Journal of Public Health, January 1992, p. 29*

40. The actual cost of tobacco contributes only about six cents to the price of a pack of cigarettes. Advertising and promotion contribute more than twenty cents to the price of each pack.

*Tobacco Use: An American Crisis*, p. 87

41. The Tobacco Institute claims that 2.3 million jobs in America depend on tobacco, and that more than 3500 of them would be lost for every penny increase in the cigarette tax. However, Arthur Andersen Economic Consulting called these figures "grossly inflated," noting that only 11% of the 2.3 million jobs, or 259,600, were actually in the tobacco growing, manufacturing, and wholesaling industry.

American Medical News, November 14, 1994, p. 16

42. The tobacco industry is trying to scare the public into believing that hundreds of thousands of jobs will be lost if excise taxes are increased. Their figures are based on the mistaken idea that money not spent on cigarettes will simply disappear from the economy, instead of being spent on other goods and creating new jobs in the process.

INFACT Newsletter, Summer 1994

43. A 1994 study refuted the economic argument by the tobacco industry that lower consumption would cost jobs and revenue. This would be true only in tobacco-producing states, since about half of the dollars that consumers spend on tobacco are "exported" to the tobacco states. The industry's estimates greatly exaggerate tobacco's economic importance.

JAMA, March 9, 1994, p. 771

44. Kenneth Warner, a health economist from the University of Michigan, published a review "The Economics of Tobacco: Myths and Realities" in the spring 2000 issue of Tobacco Control (pp. 78-89). He made the following points. Although the economies of the six state "tobacco bloc" in the southeastern United States are perceived to be heavily economically reliant on tobacco growing and manufacturing, only 1.6% of jobs in these six states are associated with the core tobacco sector of the economy.

Dr. Warner next disputes the notion that tobacco imposes an enormous financial burden on a country from lowered productivity and increased health care costs. In fact, studies indicate that net costs of smoking – the costs of treating smoking-related illness minus the additional expenditures on non-smokers because they live longer–are small or nonexistent. The magnitude of any fiscal concern pales in comparison with the enormity of the burden that smoking exacts from the public's health.

The tobacco industry argues that a large tax increase is undesirable because it will lead to lower sales and hence lower government revenue. However, there are no documented cases of tax revenues declining when taxes were increased.

45. "Even if smokers reduce the net costs imposed on others by dying young, it would be misleading to suggest that society is better off because of these premature deaths. To do so would be to accept the logic that says society is better off without its older adults."

*Curbing the Epidemic*, p. 36

46. It is common for the tobacco industry to claim that smoke-free ordinances create severe economic problems for restaurants and bars. A study by Glantz et al "debunks the tobacco industry allegation that smoke-free restaurant laws adversely affect tourism, including international tourism. Quite the contrary, implementation of these laws is often associated with an increase in the rate of growth of tourism revenues."

JAMA, May 26, 1999, pp. 1911-1918

47. The economic benefits associated with tobacco would not disappear if the industry did not exist; money now spent on tobacco products would instead be spent on other goods and services. Much of the revenue from tobacco spending in a non-tobacco state goes to tobacco-producing states and to tobacco company stockholders. Therefore, tobacco produces a net drain on the economy of non-tobacco states.

*Nicotine Addiction*, p. 51

48. The tobacco industry provides 800,000 jobs. There are more than 400,000 tobacco-caused deaths each year. "This means that one person must die each year to sustain two jobs. Put another way, at least 22 people must die to support the 44-year career of a Philip Morris employee. Surely, no one would argue that this is an acceptable trade-off. It is absurd for the tobacco industry to use lost jobs as a rationale for not saving lives."

*Tobacco Use: An American Crisis*, p. 86

49. The Tobacco Institute estimates that if tobacco were banned, 662,000 jobs and $15 billion to the economy would be lost. But University of Michigan health economist Kenneth Warner disagrees. "The tobacco industry implies that if there were a prohibition, tobacco money would disappear. What everyone fails to mention is that the money would be spent on other things...I'd bet my bottom dollar that if tobacco consumption declines, it will actually increase employment in at least 40 of the 50 states." If spending were reallocated from tobacco to other consumer items, most states would actually gain jobs because tobacco dollars would remain within the local state economy.                    Los Angeles Times magazine, August 10, 1997, p. 10

50. "Contrary to the tobacco industry's claims, reductions in spending on tobacco products will boost employment in every one of the 8 non-tobacco regions and will not diminish employment in the Southeast Tobacco region by as much as the industry estimates. The primary concern about tobacco should be the enormity of its toll on health and not its impact on employment." JAMA, April 24, 1996, p. 1241 (health economist Kenneth Warner)

51.     Nationally, tobacco accounts for only 0.002 of the gross domestic product, or one-fifth of one percent. North Carolina now produces more poultry and pork than tobacco.
Q. If tobacco is such a small part of the economy, how can the tobacco industry say that millions of jobs depend on it?
A. The tobacco industry seeks to perpetuate the myth that any action to reduce the US smoking rates would result in economic devastation of tobacco-growing regions. According to Arthur Andersen Economic Consulting, the tobacco industry's estimate that there are 2.3 million jobs dependent on tobacco relies on "a technique that cannot be used to determine whether a job is dependent on tobacco." In fact, the most recent tobacco industry data show only 259,616 jobs involved in the entire tobacco industry, including farming, manufacturing, warehousing and wholesaling. Even among those jobs directly related to tobacco, relatively few would be lost if US smoking rates declined. Reasons for this include:
    More than half of all tobacco grown in the US and more than 30 percent of all cigarettes are exported. That means that many of the 259,616 tobacco industry jobs would exist even if no one in the US smoked.
    When people stop smoking, the money they would have spent on cigarettes does not disappear from the economy, as the tobacco industry assumes. It is redirected to other goods and services, creating new jobs in other sectors. Economic studies have confirmed that in non-tobacco states, reduced smoking actually increases the number of jobs available.     Quote: Supporting FDA: Fact Sheet #5, August 7, 1995 (Advocacy Institute)

52. Q. Haven't the economies of tobacco-growing states already been hit hard by health restriction?
A. No. Due to rising cigarette exports, 25 billion more cigarettes were made in the US in 1992 than in 1982. Tobacco company profits grew by 300 percent over the same period. Health restrictions have not caused a reduction in tobacco growing or manufacturing.
Q. But haven't tobacco farmers and manufacturing employees lost tens of thousands of jobs over the past decade?
A. Yes. More than 40,000 tobacco farms disappeared over the past decade, and cigarette manufacturing jobs have fallen by more than 30 percent. Tobacco companies have caused these job losses by tripling the amount of foreign tobacco they import into the US since 1974, using more additives and less tobacco in each cigarette, and displacing workers through automation of manufacturing operations. As a result of tobacco companies' increased reliance on foreign tobacco, the tobacco farmer's share of the retail tobacco dollar fell from 7 percent to 3 percent between 1980 and 1991. The manufacturer's share increased from 37 percent to 50 percent over the same period. Tobacco companies have convinced many Americans, including tobacco industry workers, that health restrictions are responsible for job losses actually caused by the tobacco industry itself.
            Quote from Supporting FDA: Fact Sheet #5, August 7, 1995 (Advocacy Institute)

53. North Carolina produces three quarters of the nation's cigarettes. But the 18,600 factory jobs involved (down 30% since 1972) account for only 2% of the state's manufacturing employment and less than 1% of its total job base. Tobacco's $12 billion value is only about 8% of the state's $149 billion economy, and poultry now represents 29% of farm income, compared with 19% for tobacco.
                    American Medical News, November 14, 1994, p. 16

54. 25% of the nation's health care costs are directly related to smoking.
                    American Medical News, September 21, 1992, p. 22

55. Health care for smoking-related illnesses cost at least $50 billion in 1993, equal to $2.06 for each of the 24 billion packs of cigarettes sold. The federal government and state governments pay for 43% of all these smoking-attributed medical expenditures, and more than 60% for those over the age of 65. These figures are very minimum estimates, and likely to be lower than the actual costs. They do not include burns from fires caused by cigarettes, and low birth weight and other infant health problems caused by maternal smoking. If lost productivity and premature death were also included, it would at the least double the $50 billion figure for the total economic burden attributable to smoking. *New York Times*, July 8, 1994, p. A12

56. Cigarette smoking accounted for about 11.8% of total U.S. medical expenditures in 1993, totaling $72.7 billion. This is a much higher total cost than the estimated $50 billion projected by an earlier research study. *Public Health Reports*, September-October 1998, pp. 447-458

57. Most studies find the annual medical costs of smoking to constitute about 6 to 8% of American personal health expenditures. *Tobacco Control*, Autumn 1999, pp. 290-300

58. In high income developed countries, smoking-related illness accounts for between 6 and 15% of total health care expenditures. Despite their shorter lives, smokers' lifetime health costs are somewhat higher than nonsmokers'. *Curbing the Epidemic*, p. 4

59. In 1993, the estimated proportion of total medical expenditures attributable to smoking for the United States as a whole was 11.8%. Total U.S. medical expenditures attributable to smoking amounted to an estimated $72.7 billion in 1993. *Public Health Reports*, September-October 1998, p. 447

60. Smoking cost the Medicare system $20.5 billion in 1997, and the total Medicare bill that the U.S. government pays could be over $600 billion in the last three decades. *Reuters*, September 30, 1999

61. New York taxpayers spend $1.8 billion a year in Medicaid costs alone to treat smoking-related diseases. *New York Times*, June 5, 1999, p. A24

62. Smoking-related diseases account for 19% of the total medical costs among men, and 12% among women. *NEJM*, October 9, 1997, p. 1054

63. Smoking, drinking, and drug abuse cost the federal treasury $77.6 billion each year in health and benefit payments. This amounts to about 20% of the total $430 billion in 1995 taxpayer dollars spent on Medicare, Medicaid, Social Security disability insurance, and veterans health programs. *Reuters*, February 14, 1995, and *ASH Review*, March-April 1995

64. An estimated $16 billion of the $87 billion yearly inpatient medical expenses for Medicare patients are attributable to tobacco-induced disease. *ABC Radio*, February 9, 1995 (Dean Edell, M.D.)

65. Smoking will cost the economy more than $500 billion (in 1990 dollars) in excess lifetime health care costs for current smokers. This is an average of $7888 per male and $4143 per female smoker. That number grows by $9-10 billion annually due to the additional excess lifetime health care costs of the one million teenagers who take up smoking each year. *Milbank Quarterly*, Vol. 70, 1992, pp. 81-125

66. A male between the ages of 35 and 44 who smokes more than two packs a day will incur cigarette-related medical bills and lost work time adding up to a lifetime average cost of $58,987. *American Medical Association Fact Sheet on Smoking*

67. "Each year, more than one million youths become regular smokers. They're taking an average of 15 years off their lives, and committing our health care system to at least $8.2 billion in extra medical costs over their lifetimes." Dr. Paul Torrens, Professor of Health Services Administration at USC (*Denver Post*, September 14, 1994, p. 5A)

68. The estimated average lifetime medical costs for a smoker exceed those for a nonsmoker by more than $6000. The costs for smoking in terms of health care expenditures and lost productivity exceed $100 billion per year in the US.
NEJM, April 7, 1994, p. 975

69. Taxpayers subsidize cigarettes by about $1 a pack to pay the Medicare and Medicaid bills resulting from tobacco-related illnesses. Private insurance and other sources pay another $1 per pack because of the damage caused by cigarettes. These findings from the Centers for Disease Control do not include losses in productivity because of illness. Nor do they include the cost of premature death, burn injuries from fires caused by cigarettes, or prenatal damage or illness resulting from second-hand smoke.
San Francisco, Chronicle, July 18, 1994, p. A18

70. The shortened life span and premature death of just those smokers born in the single year 1920 will end up saving the Social Security System $14.5 billion. All told, smoking will reduce the obligations of the system by hundreds of billions of dollars.
New Yorker, June 13, 1994, p. 8

71. Each current smoker in the United States will save the government a total of about $35,000 in Social Security payments because of reduced life span. This amount multiplied by the current number of adult smokers, 46.3 million, equals $1.62 trillion ($1,620,000,000,000) in eventual Social Security payouts "saved" or reduced because smokers die earlier. If all smokers quit tomorrow, it would cost Social Security an extra $50 billion a year to start, and much more later on because of increased life expectancy.
*Lung Cancer Chronicles*, John Meyer, 1990, p. 155 and Medical Economics, October 19, 1992

72. Another study estimates that because of shorter life expectancy, the average male smoker receives $20,000 less in Social Security benefits than he contributes, and females, $10,000 less. Nonsmokers receive $3400 more than they pay in. This large differential results in a substantial net transfer of benefits from smokers to nonsmokers, and smokers subsidize Social Security income for nonsmokers. JAMA, October 16, 1987, p. 2085

73. "Stanford University tobacco researcher John Shoven, now dean of humanities and sciences, estimates that male smokers lose about $40,000 and female smokers $30,000 in future Social Security benefits."
Los Angeles Times magazine, August 10, 1997, p. 11

74. Some economists believe that smokers "pay their own way" despite their much higher medical costs. "Smokers…die young, so they don't recoup as much as nonsmokers in Social Security, Medicare and other programs for the elderly, even though they pay as much into those programs during their working years."
San Francisco Chronicle, August 29, 1994 (J. Marshall)

75. Some economists including W. Kip Viscusi of Duke University feel that because smokers die before collecting their full share of health and retirement benefits, they cover their own costs. This is the so-called "death benefit" argument. Viscusi estimated the costs and benefits to American society in 1993 per pack of cigarettes smoked. The costs are $1.37 per pack, including 55 cents for total medical care, 40 cents from lost taxes on earnings, 25 cents for secondhand smoke, 14 cents for group life insurance, two cents for fires caused, and a penny per pack for excess sick leave. The total benefit to society amounts to $1.95 per pack smoked, including 53 cents in excise taxes paid and the "early death benefits" of 23 cents in nursing home savings and $1.19 per pack in pension and Social Security outlays saved.
New York Times, May 5, 1996, p. E1

76. Companies and the government save $30 billion a year because of contributions that smokers pay into pension plans but never collect because they die younger.
CBS Evening News, June 23, 1997 (W. Kip Viscusi)

77. In 1990, cigarettes killed 33,404 New Yorkers, and health care related to smoking cost New York $2.6 billion in 1992. When lost productivity was added, the total cost was about $6 billion.
American Medical News, February 22, 1993

78. Smoking costs Floridians nearly $4.4 billion a year, a per capita cost of $616 a year for each resident over 34.
US News and World Report, March 6, 1995, p. 18

79. Tobacco manufacturers spend about $1.75 per pound for tobacco; there are 5 ½ ounces of tobacco in each carton of cigarettes. Of each dollar that the consumer spends on cigarettes, only 3 cents goes to the tobacco farmer. 16 cents is spent on advertising and promotion, and 25 cents on packaging and shipping. It costs just 11 cents of each dollar to actually manufacture the cigarettes.                60 Minutes, July 18, 1993 (Andy Rooney)

80. For each dollar spent on cigarettes, only 3 cents in 1991 went to the tobacco grower, down from 13 cents in 1950. The manufacturer's share in the same time interval increased from 21 cents to 50 cents.
                                                                American Medical News, November 14, 1994, p. 17

81. Most developing countries are net importers of tobacco, for which they spend scarce foreign exchange. In countries producing tobacco, land cultivated for this purpose denies rich farmland for food production, and food often has to be imported. Tobacco growing also depletes soil nutrients at a much faster rate than many other crops, thus decreasing the life of the soil.
            Panos Briefing, September 1994 (9th World Conference on Tobacco or Health, Paris, 1994)

82. In the United Kingdom, if 40% of smokers stopped their habit by the year 2000, the extra spending power could create up to 150,000 new jobs. Each year the UK has about 120,000 deaths from tobacco. There are 12,000 employees in tobacco manufacturing, which equals 10 deaths per employee per year.
                                                                            The Lancet, May 27, 1995, p. 1360

83. Even though smokers die younger than the average American, over the course of their lives current and former smokers generate an estimated $501 billion in excess health care costs. Smoking is the largest single drain on the Medicare trust fund, poised to take $800 billion over the next 20 years. On average, every pack of cigarettes smoked is directly responsible for more than $3.90 in health care costs and lost productivity. The tobacco industry argues that the total economic impact on society is less than would be expected because of the money saved when a smoker dies before collecting Social Security or a pension. Based on the tobacco industry's logic, all efforts to combat cancer, heart disease, and other diseases should cease because letting people die earlier saves money.                                        From "Saving Lives and Rising Revenue,"
                                                                Coalition on Smoking or Health, February 1995

84.     "The tobacco industry is using its enormous public relations and lobbying resources to try to convince Congress and the American public that a health tax on tobacco would do such a good job of reducing smoking that tobacco farmers would be devastated. This implies that Americans must keep smoking and dying in vast numbers to preserve tobacco industry jobs and the economic health of tobacco-producing states. This argument is both immoral and factually wrong.
        "Even if the debate were about industry jobs vs. human lives, only the tobacco processors would support the sacrifice of hundreds of thousands of lives to protect a much smaller number of jobs.
        "But the debate is not about jobs vs. lives. The tobacco industry has distorted the facts about jobs, just as it has manipulated the government and the tobacco farmers for so many years. One recent industry publication projected that the tax would cost 270,000 jobs even though there are only 256,616 jobs involved in the entire industry, including farming, warehousing, manufacturing and wholesaling."
                                                            Washington Post, February 9, 1994, p. A23 (Jimmy Carter)

85. In 1995, Medicare will pay more than $25 billion to treat tobacco-related medical conditions, and Social Security disability insurance will pay $4.6 billion to beneficiaries disabled by tobacco-related disease.
                                                                            NEJM, November 2, 1995, p. 1214

86. The total cost of smoking in California is estimated to be $10 billion per year, amounting to $2,014 per smoker and $314 per Californian. These are conservative health-sector costs. There are 4.3 million Californians who smoke, and if they were to pay for the cost of their extra health care related to smoking, it would add $1.82 to the price of each pack of cigarettes. If productivity were also included, the extra cost of each pack would rise to $5.06.                                                            Tobacco Control, Summer 1995, p. 545

87. "On average, at any given age, smokers incur higher medical costs than nonsmokers. However, nonsmokers live longer and therefore continue to incur medical costs over more years... The most recent research is the incidence-based study by Hodgson (Milbank Quarterly, Vol 70, 1992, pp. 81-125) who found that lifetime

medical costs for male smokers were 32 percent higher than for male neversmokers and lifetime medical costs for female smokers were 24 percent higher than for female neversmokers. Hodgson determined that the present value of the lifetime excess costs were about $9,400 in 1990 dollars... Adjusting by the consumer price index (CPI) for medical care raises the present value of Hodgson's excess medical cost per new smoker to $10,590 in 1994 dollars. Thus, those 1,000,000 young people under the age of 18 who currently become new smokers each year are responsible for excess lifetime medical costs measured at a present value of $10.6 billion (1,000,000 x $10,590). Since FDA projects that the proposed regulation would prevent 250,000 of these individuals from smoking as adults, the medical cost saving attributable to the proposed regulation is estimated at $2.6 billion per year." Federal Register, August 11, 1995, p. 41364

88. "Seattle University economist William L. Weis reported in 1983 that smokers devoted 6 percent of their workday to the ritual, took 50 percent more sick days, and made 50 percent greater use of the health-care system than non-smokers. If they hired only the latter instead, Weis added, employers would shave their personnel

89. costs by 20 percent, their insurance premiums by 30 percent, their office maintenance by 50 percent, and their disability outlays by 70 percent, for a claimed total savings of as much as $4,600 per worker per year."
*Ashes to Ashes*, p. 553

93. Tobacco use is the largest single drain on the Medicare trust fund. Over the next 20 years, Medicare will spend an estimated $800 billion caring for people with smoking-related illnesses.
Washington Post National Weekly Edition, June 9, 1997, p. 27

94. At any given age, health care costs for smokers are as much as 40% higher than for nonsmokers.
Associated Press, October 9, 1997

95. Smoking cost the United States $97.2 billion in health care costs and lost productivity in 1993. This included $50 billion to care for people with smoking related disease. In 1987, the most recent year data were collected, 43.3% of all medical care expenditures attributable to smoking were paid for by Medicare, Medicaid, and other federal and state sources of public funding.
American Lung Association Fact Sheet--Smoking Policies in the Workplace (August 1997 Update)

96. A. Robert Wood Johnson Foundation study estimated that the total economic cost of smoking, drinking, and drug abuse was $238 billion in 1990. This included $99 billion in alcohol-related costs, $72 billion from smoking, and $67 billion from drug abuse. San Francisco Examiner, October 18, 1993

97. "It has been known for a long time that smoking imposes a heavy cost on societies as a whole, in the form of medical expenses. An article in the September 13, 1908 edition of the Detroit Free Press, for instance, observed that smoking was costing the United States an estimated $385 million per year—at the time, a sum large enough to build the Panama Canal, run the Army and Navy, and make the interest payments on the national debt. Today, the United States spends $50 billion in medical expenses directly attributable to smoking—or $2.06 for every pack of cigarettes sold in the country. That figure doesn't include the indirect costs, such as the economic value of years of life lost to premature deaths, or lost productivity."
World Watch magazine, July-August 1997, p. 25 (Anne Platt McGinn)

98. The illness, lost productivity, and death caused by tobacco accounts for about one quarter of all public health expenditures in the countries of Canada and Australia. World Watch magazine, July-August 1997, p. 25

99. In all age groups, smokers incur higher health care costs than nonsmokers. The difference varies with the age group, but among 65 to 74 year olds, the costs are as much as 40% more for men and 25% more for women compared to nonsmokers the same age. However, these higher annual costs do not take into account the substantial lower longevity in smokers; the difference is 69.7 compared to 77.0 years life expectancy for men, and 75.6 versus 81.6 years for women. The lower yearly medical costs for nonsmokers are outweighed by their greater life spans; lifetime medical costs for smokers are an estimated $72,700 for men and $94,799 for women, compared to $83,400 and $111,000, respectively, for nonsmoking men and women. This amounts to lifetime costs for nonsmokers that are 15% higher for men and 18% higher for women. Therefore, although

smokers incur higher yearly medical costs, these are balanced by smokers' shorter life spans, and hence lower use of nursing homes, pensions, and Social Security payouts. NEJM, October 9, 1997, pp. 1052-57

100. In the United States, tobacco-induced disease is responsible for 6% of all medical care expenditures. As an offset to this gross cost, however, premature death from tobacco reduces the number of years that people consume medical care, so the net cost is somewhat less. In the elderly, 6 to 7% of state Medicaid expenses are for treating disease caused by tobacco.
10th World Conference on Tobacco or Health, Beijing, 1997 (Kenneth Warner and Richard Daynard)

101. Tobacco consumption results in an estimated net annual global loss of nearly $200 billion, about a third of which occurs in developing countries. The health care budgets of all developing countries combined are less than $100 billion. British Medical Journal, June 22, 1996, p. 1576

102. In the 1980's, about 6% of all employers refused to hire smokers, citing increased health care costs and a higher rate of absenteeism, with one study estimating increased costs of $5000 per employee. 28 states and the District of Columbia now have smokers' rights laws that prohibit this practice, and companies in these states (such as Pratt and Whitney in Connecticut) often charge smokers more for health insurance, usually an extra $250 to $500 per year. In Georgia, one of the states without smokers' rights laws, Turner Broadcasting System and Lockheed Martin do not hire smokers. New York Times, December 29, 1996, p. F13

103. Many small businesses in the United Kingdom are introducing two-tier pay for their employees, with lower pay for smokers because of their increased absenteeism and lower productivity. Smoking-related illness accounts for 50 million lost working days in the country each year. Other companies are docking pay for cigarette breaks. The London Sunday Times, December 28, 1997

104. If every American smoker smoked one less cigarette per day, it would cost the tobacco industry $750,000,000 in profits each year. Advocacy Institute, May 11, 1990

105. The president of RJR in 1978 said about antismoking measures, "If they caused every smoker to smoke just one less cigarette a day, our company would stand to lose $92 million in sales annually. I assure you that we don't intend to let that happen without a fight." International Journal of Health Services 1990; 20:424

106. Worldwide sales of cigarettes in 1996 were $295.8 billion (US dollars).
American Lung Association Fact Sheet

107.  In 1995, American smokers spent $45.8 billion to consume 24.35 billion packs of cigarettes. Of the $45.8 billion spent on cigarettes approximately $13.0 billion went toward payment of excise taxes levied by federal, state and local governments; $12.7 billion went to retailers and wholesalers; and $20.1 billion in manufacturers' receipts and estimated $7.6 billion was reported as operating profit, whereas the remaining $12.5 billion went for cigarette production and marketing including the costs of tobacco leaf.
 Thus, in 1995, Americans paid an average of $1.88 for each pack of cigarettes, of which 53 cents went to excise taxes; 52 cents went to retailers and wholesalers; and 83 cents went to cigarette manufacturers. Of the 83 cents per pack received by manufacturers, about 31 cents were reported as operating profit.
Quote from Tobacco Control, Winter 1996, p. 292 (Jeffrey Harris)

108. Total United States tobacco sales were $49 billion in 1993. $3 billion of this amount went for the raw material to the nation's 124,000 tobacco farms. The other $46 billion went to tobacco companies, retailers, wholesalers, vending machine operators, advertising agencies, and in taxes ($13 billion) to federal and state governments.
Washington Post National Weekly Edition, September 23-29, 1996, p. 29

109. For every dollar spent on tobacco in 1993, farmers received less than three cents (compared to 16 cents in 1957). Tobacco manufacturers and wholesalers received more than 63 cents, and the rest went to excise taxes (29 cents) and to retailers (5 cents). Tobacco Control, Autumn 1996, p. 193

110. The average U.S. retail price for a pack of cigarettes increased sharply to $2.88 in 1999 from $2.20 in 1998, as total cigarette sales in the United States dropped by 8.6% from the previous year.
*Associated Press, November 20, 1999*

111. With 1999 new taxes and price increases, a two pack a day smoker in California will now be paying $2800 a year for cigarettes. *San Francisco Examiner, February 7, 1999*

112. 70% of smokers earn less than $40,000 a year. *The Economist, February 13, 1999, p. 29*

113. 487 billion cigarettes were smoked in 1996 in the United States, and U.S. per capita consumption for the year was 2415 (population age 16 and older.) *American Lung Association Fact Sheet*

114. In 1996, U.S. consumer spending on tobacco products totaled $46.6 billion, or $185.30 per capita. The average price per pack was $1.91, and $13.1 billion (in 1996) was collected in federal, state, and local excise taxes. The world's highest annual spending on tobacco is in Denmark, $407.80 per capita.
*Wall Street Journal, June 1997*

115. The National Association of Convenience Stores estimates that cigarettes account for a quarter of the merchandise sales at the nation's 95,000 convenience stores. A new chain of stores, Cigarettes Cheaper!, was first opened in October 1994, and now has 393 branches in 8 states, with $250 million a year in sales.
*Los Angeles Times magazine, August 10, 1997, p. 10*

116. A two pack a day smoker who bought cigarettes at $1.75 a pack for 50 years would have $338,650 if the money were saved instead (assuming a constant price per pack and an annual interest rate of 5.5%).
*USA Today, February 20, 1997*

117. "There have been many estimates of the costs, direct and indirect, of smoking. Here's our take on just the out-of-pocket costs to the smoker. Say you're young and start smoking today and continue for 50 years, assuming it doesn't kill you first. A pack a day at $2.50 would add up to more than $900 a year, or $45,000 over 50 years. Put that money in the bank each year at 5 percent interest, and the total would quadruple. Add in extra life insurance costs (say an extra $20,000 over 20 years) and extra cleaning expenses of clothes, home and teeth, say $15,000 over the five decades). Now the total is more than $400,000. And that doesn't count the smoking-related medical expenses you'll have to face if one's health insurance doesn't cover everything."
*University of California Wellness Letter, September 1997*

118. How much does a smoker pay for cigarettes over a lifetime? "Let's make two assumptions: 1) A pack of cigarettes costs $2 and the price will rise 5% a year, a modest assumption given that cigarette companies usually raise prices twice a year and state and federal excise taxes are skyrocketing. 2) An average smoker buys a pack of cigarettes per day... If, instead of buying a pack of cigarettes, a 16-year-old smoker invested the same amount of money and earned 7% a year," the investment fund would be worth almost $26,000 at age 30, $260,000 at age 51, and $1,861,000 at age 66. For a two pack a day smoker, the above earnings would be doubled. *Smoke Free Air, Winter 1997-98 (Smoke Free Educational Services)*

119. In many developing countries, households with just one smoker commonly spend more on cigarettes than they do on all of their health care. *World Watch, July-August 1997, p. 25*

120. Nine of the 15 largest U.S. mutual funds list tobacco companies as one of their top 10 holdings.
*San Francisco Chronicle, November 18, 1996, p. B1*

121. The *Smoking Cessation: Clinical Practice Guideline* published in 1996 identifies efficacious interventions for primary care clinicians and smoking cessation specialty providers. The cost in 1995 dollars was determined per life-year or quality-adjusted life-year (QALY) saved. The guideline would cost $6.3 billion to implement in its first year. As a result, society could expect to gain 1.7 new quitters at an average cost of $3,779 per quitter, $2,587 per life-year saved, and $1,915 for every QALY saved. This is extremely cost effective compared with other preventive interventions, such as $61,744 for each life saved for annual mammography for women aged

122. Anti-smoking campaigns targeted at children cost between $20 and $40 per year of life gained, compared to $18,000 per year of life gained for lung cancer treatment. "Such campaigns are probably second only to childhood immunization programs as a cost-effective means of improving public health."

World Watch, July-August 1997, p. 27

123. Money spent on tobacco control is as cost-effective as is money spent for vaccination and immunization.

10th World Conference on Tobacco or Health, Beijing, 1997 (David Sweanor)

124. In a cohort of patients treated for nicotine dependence at the Mayo Clinic Nicotine Dependence Center, the cost of treatment was $6828 per net year of life gained. In comparison with the cost effectiveness of other medical services and interventions, treatment of nicotine dependence is relatively inexpensive.

Mayo Clinic Proceedings, October 1997, pp. 917-924

125. By way of comparison, screening mammograms for women between ages 40 and 50 cost $100,000 for each life saved from breast cancer. In women ages 50 to 70, the cost is $20,000 per life saved.

Dean Edell, M.D., ABC radio, December 24, 1997

126. A University of California San Francisco study by Stanton Glantz and James Lightwood published in Circulation in August 1997 showed that a seven year stop smoking program that reduced the smoking prevalence by one percent each year would result in 63,840 fewer hospitalizations for heart attack and 34,261 fewer hospitalizations for stroke, saving $3.2 billion in direct medical costs alone. In addition, such a program would prevent 13,100 deaths from heart attack that occur before victims can reach the hospital.

UCSF Medsounds, August 19, 1997

127. "The availability of discount/generic cigarettes has made smoking more affordable, which most likely has helped the cigarette industry retain customers sensitive to price, who might have otherwise reduced consumption or stopped smoking altogether." The reported use of discount/generic cigarettes increased from 6.2% in 1988 to 23.4% in 1993.

Tobacco Control, Winter 1997, p. S25

128. "It is no coincidence that in 1993 – the year that saw a sharp increase in the number of teenagers who started smoking – the tobacco companies lowered the price by 40 cents on the three brands that young people predominately smoke."

British Medical Journal, August 23, 1997, p. 448

129. In California, where Medicaid is called Medi-Cal, smoking-related costs account for 16% of the program's medical bills, or $1.7 billion in 1993.

San Francisco Chronicle, March 10, 1998, p. A1

130. Men who smoke are one third more likely to be hospitalized than nonsmokers, and people who quit smoking are no more likely to be hospitalized than people who never smoked. If men aged 45 to 64 years stopped smoking, hospital admissions in this group would decline by as much as 12.5%, therefore saving about $5.4 billion each year in the United States.

JAMA, April 15, 1998, p. 1153

131. During 1995-1999, the average annual mortality-related productivity loses attributable to smoking for adults were $81.9 billion. In 1998, smoking-attributable personal health-care medical expenditures were $75.5 billion, a total of $157.4 billion per year in lost productivity and health costs. For each of the approximately 46.5 million adult smokers in 1999, these costs represent $1,760 in lost productivity and $1,623 in excess medical expenditures, total economic costs of almost $3,400 per smoker per year. Productivity loses did not include the value of lost work time from smoking-related disability, absenteeism, excess work breaks, and secondhand smoke-related disease morbidity and mortality.

JAMA, May 8, 2002, p. 2356

132. For each of the approximately 22 billion cigarette packs sold in the U.S. in 1999, $3.45 was spent on medical care attributable to smoking and $3.73 in productivity losses were incurred, for a total cost of $7.18 per pack.

JAMA, May 8, 2002, p. 2356

133. In a study at Xerox Corp. in Rochester, New York, the yearly workers' compensation costs for smokers averaged $2,189, compared to only $176 for nonsmokers.　　　　　Reuters, August 11, 2001
　　　　　　　　　　　　　(from July 2001 Journal of Occupational and Environmental Medicine)

134. In 1998 among adults, the medical costs of smoking represented about 8% of personal health care expenditures.　　　　　JAMA, May 8, 2002, p. 2356

135. Smoking-attributable neonatal expenditures were $366 million in 1996, or $704 per maternal smoker. Maternal smoking accounted for 2.3% of total neonatal medical expenditures in 1996. The neonatal medical costs of maternal smoking understate the probable true costs of smoking-attributable conditions among children because the future medical costs for infants affected by maternal smoking and the current costs of treating newly diagnosed secondhand smoke-related conditions among children aged 1-4 years were not included.
　　　　　Quote from JAMA, May 8, 2002, p. 2356

136. Philip Morris manufactures about 80% of the cigarettes smoked in the Czech Republic, and in 2001 circulated a report claiming that the premature death of smokers saved the Czech government between $23.8 million and $30.1 million in health care, pensions, and housing for the elderly in 1999. Weighing all the costs and benefits, the report concluded that in 1999, the government had a net gain of $147 million from smoking.
　　　　　2002 AMA Annual Tobacco Report

137. A study sponsored by Philip Morris said that the Czech Republic saves $1,227 on health care, pensions, and housing every time a smoker dies.
　　　　　American Legacy foundation-sponsored poster of a tag on the toe of a cadaver, Newsweek, August 13, 2001

138. Philip Morris has apologized for a company-financed study in the Czech Republic that stated that the early deaths of smokers is one of the "positive effects" of smoking.　　　　　Associated Press, July 27, 2001

139. The cost of workplace smoking in Eurodollars in 2000: a company has 10,000 employees of which 3,000 smoke. Each smoker smokes 6 cigarettes per day at work. A cigarette break lasts 5 minutes. Each smoker wastes 30 minutes every working day. An employee on $8.64 per hour costs the company $1,037 per annum. The 3,000 smokers cost the company $3.1 million per annum.　　　　　The Tobacco Atlas, p. 75

140. The tobacco industry uses economic arguments to persuade governments, the media and the general population that smoking benefits the economy. It claims that if tobacco control measures are introduced, tax revenues will fall, jobs will be lost and there will be great hardship to the economy.

　　But the industry greatly exaggerates the economic losses, if any, which tobacco control measures will cause and they never mention the economic costs which tobacco inflicts upon every country.

　　Tobacco's cost to governments, to employers and to the environment includes social, welfare, and health care spending, loss of foreign exchange in importing cigarettes; loss of land that could grow food; costs of fires and damage to buildings caused by careless smoking; environmental costs ranging from deforestation to collection of smokers' litter, absenteeism, decreased productivity, higher numbers of accidents and higher insurance premiums.　　　　　quote from The Tobacco Atlas, p. 40

141. In a study of employees at Xerox, one of the most costly individual health risks was smoking. The workers' compensation cost for a smoker averaged $2,189, compared to $176 for a nonsmoker.
　　Journal of Occupational and Environmental Medicine, July 2001, reported in 2002 AMA Annual Tobacco Report

142. The average number of sick days off per year in 2001 in the United States was 3.86 for never smokers, 4.53 for former smokers, and 6.16 for current smokers.　　　　　The Tobacco Atlas, p. 40

143. In a study of 300 booking clerks at a U.S. airline, current smokers were absent from work for sickness for 6.16 days on average, compared with 4.53 days for former smokers and 3.86 days among never smokers. Employee productivity was also tracked, and current smoker production was 4.0% below never smokers and 8.3% below the former smoker group.　　　　　Tobacco Control, reported by The Age (Australia), September 5, 2001

144. In a young healthy active duty U.S. Army population, substantial fractions of hospitalizations (7.5% for men and 5.0% for women) and lost workdays (14.1% for men and 3.0% for women) were attributable to cigarette smoking.
                                                                          Tobacco Control 2000; 9:389-396

145. Taxpayers paid nearly $1.9 billion in benefits in 1994 alone to children whose parents had died from smoking-related diseases. This included 220,000 fatherless and 85,000 motherless children younger than 18 in the United States.
                                                                          Associated Press, May 6, 2000

146. For every dollar spent on tobacco in the United States, on average, 4 cents is for the tobacco itself, 7 cents is for non-tobacco materials, 43 cents is for manufacturing, 21 cents is for wholesale, retail and transport, 11 cents is for federal tax, and 15 cents is for state and local taxes.
                                                                          *The Tobacco Atlas*, p. 48

147. A $3.15 pack of Marlboros reaps $1.40 in revenues for Philip Morris, a 44% operating margin.
                                                                          Time, July 2, 2001, p. 38

148. "All told, more than 662,000 workers in the United States alone owe their livelihood – an estimated $15.2 billion in annual wages – to the business of growing, distributing, and selling tobacco products. The spiraling smoke of the cigarette business wafts through the economy as those workers pick up their paychecks and spend the money on more goods and services, creating another 1.15 million jobs worth another $39 billion in pay. Add up those direct and indirect jobs and salaries and you have $54.2 billion in U.S. wages – nearly 2% of the country's gross domestic product." In the United States, smokers spend $53 billion a year on cigarettes; worldwide, cigarette sales are $300 billion a year.
                                                                          *Cigarettes* (Parker-Pope), p. 22

149. Americans smoked 422 billion cigarettes in 2001, down 2% from 2000, and U.S. cigarette production fell to 580 billion in 2001 from 595 billion the previous year.
                                                                          U.S. Department of Agriculture

150. Domestic cigarette sales increased from 411.3 billion in 1999 to 413.5 billion cigarettes sold in 2000.
                                                                          Federal Trade Commission report, May 2002

151. California is saving $8 in health care costs for every dollar it spends to reduce smoking.
                                                                          U.S. News and World Report, December 17, 2001, p. 48

152. Most health insurance companies charge the same premiums for smokers and nonsmokers, thereby forcing the nonsmokers to subsidize the excess health costs for the smoking group. Smokers who learn that they may have to pay hundreds of dollars a year more in health insurance premiums would have a strong financial incentive to quit.
                                                                          ASH Smoking and Health Review, May-June 2002

153. CalPERS of the state of California, the largest pension fund in the U.S., in 2001 announced a complete divestment of all tobacco stocks, dumping $560 million in tobacco holdings, including $285 million in Philip Morris.
                                                                          INFACT Newsletter, Winter 2001

154. In West Virginia, the Public Employees Insurance Agency is adding a 30% surcharge to life insurance premiums for users of any form of tobacco, and a 10% discount for non-users.
                                                                          Charleston Daily Mail, October 5, 2002

155. "The typical poor smoker could easily add over 500 calories to the diet of one or two children with his or her daily tobacco expenditures. An estimated 10.5 million people currently malnourished could have an adequate diet if money spent on tobacco were spent on food instead. The lives of 350 children could be saved each day."
                                                      From an analysis of the economic impact of tobacco use on the poor in Bangladesh,
                                                                          Tobacco Control, June 2002, p. 160

156. Smoking costs in California are nearly $16 billion a year, or $3,331 per smoker per year for the 4.7 million smokers in the state (4.5 million adults and 207,000 adolescents). California deaths from smoking are 43,000 each year.
                                     UCSF Newsbreak, February 14, 2003, reporting data from the Tobacco Control Section
                                                                          of the California Department of Health Services

157. Smoking costs California $16 billion per year, or $475 per Californian, about $8.6 billion in health care costs, and the rest in lost productivity and premature death.             San Francisco Chronicle, January 19, 2003

158. A study from Johns Hopkins University estimates that "more than half of the annual medical costs of managing lung cancer...and 13% of the cost of managing coronary heart disease, stroke, and other smoking related cancers are attributable directly to smoking."          Reported in British Medical Journal, January 11,2003, p. 69

159. In 1997-1998 in England, 364,000 hospital admissions were attributable to smoking related illness.
British Medical Association (www.tobaccofactfile.org)

160. Between 1998 and 2000, U.S. cigarette sales declined by 9%, while wholesale prices increased by 58%.
Associated Press, June 7, 2000

# CHAPTER 38
# TAXATION

1. "Sugar, rum and tobacco, are commodities which are no where necessaries of life, which are become objects of almost universal consumption, and which are therefore extremely proper subjects of taxation."
Adam Smith, *An Inquiry into the Nature and Causes of the Wealth of Nations*, 1776

2. "This vice bring in one hundred million francs in taxes every year. I will certainly forbid it at once--as soon as you can name a virtue that brings in as much revenue."
Napoleon III (1808-1873) (from *Tobacco in History*, p. 191)

3. The first federal excise tax was imposed in 1862 to finance the Civil War, and tobacco taxes were the chief source of government revenue until the income tax.          American Medical News, November 14, 1994, p. 16

4. In 1880, tobacco taxes accounted for 31% of all federal tax revenues.
*The Story of Tobacco in America*, Joseph Robert, 1949

5. From the middle of the nineteenth century to the introduction of the income tax in 1913, taxes from tobacco accounted for 10 to 20% of all federal revenue. By 1981, tobacco taxes amounted to less than one percent of the total.                                  *Ashes to Ashes*, p. 10

6. In 1896, the South Carolina legislature passed a bill imposing a tax of 25 cents on each package of ten cigarettes sold. The current tax is 7 cents per pack of 20.          Tobacco Control, Autumn 1996, p. 250

7. In 1921, Iowa became one of the first states to tax cigarettes, charging two cents a pack on top of the six cent federal tax of the time.                                  *Ashes to Ashes*, p. 69

8. The US federal cigarette tax in 1998 was 24 cents per pack, the lowest of any industrialized country. In Canada in the early 1990's, taxes averaged $3.80 per pack (ranging up to $5.60 in the province of New Brunswick), and in Norway the average pack of cigarettes costs $8.74.

9. For teenagers, the "price elasticity of demand" for cigarettes is three times higher than the estimate for adults. For each 10% increase in the price of cigarettes, the demand falls by 14.4%, with most of this being 12% fewer teens making the decision not to begin to smoke at all. In Canada between 1979 and 1991, largely because of tax increases, the percentage of teenagers ages 15 to 17 who smoke dropped from 47% to 16%.
*Preventing Tobacco Use Among Young People*, 1994 Surgeon General report, p. 271, and Canadian Medical Association Journal, June 15, 1992, p. 2231

10. "This talk of $2 a pack is scaring us to death, and that's putting it mildly." Congressman Charlie Rose (D-NC). "Tobacco Country is Quaking over Cigarette Tax Proposal" (New York Times, March 22, 1993, p. A14). But the Wall Street Journal reported on March 12, 1993 that 70% of Americans believe that a $2-per-pack tobacco tax increase is an acceptable way to help pay for health care reform (SCARC, March 3, 1993). And Jimmy Carter wrote: "Our children are the most important reason for a major tobacco tax increase"
(New York Times, March 3, 1993, p. 16)

11. Conclusions from the Canadian experience are that while public education can result in moderate declines in tobacco consumption, major declines can be achieved from advertising bans and increased taxation.
American Journal of Public Health, July 1991, p. 902

12. North Carolina, where 56% of America's cigarettes are made, recently raised the per-pack tax from 2 to 5 cents. The number of tobacco farms there has fallen from 100,000 to 40,000 in the last decade, and poultry is now a bigger state business.                                  George Will column, February 10, 1992

13. An ABC/Washington Post Poll in May 1993 revealed that 65% of the American public supports raising the tobacco tax to $2 per pack.

14. Massachusetts voters approved a 25-cent a pack increase in the state cigarette tax in 1992. The most extreme tactic used by the tobacco industry was a last-minute effort to convince the state's anti-abortion voters that the tax revenue generated would be used by the state to fund abortion referrals and to distribute condoms.

    *Advocacy Institute, November 8, 1992*

15. Despite severe budgetary problems, the state of Virginia in 1991 rejected a bill to tax cigarettes at 20 cents a pack. Virginia's state tax has been 2 ½ cents since 1966, when it was reduced from 3 cents, and is the lowest of any state. The tobacco industry convinced the state legislature that Philip Morris, Richmond's biggest employer, might leave the state if the tax went through.

    *Tobacco Free Youth Reporter, Spring 1993*

16. "...the fiscal sense of using taxes to shape public behavior. When people smoke, they pass on costs to society - financial and physical strain on public health care, sick leave, disability benefits, and lost productivity. By including those otherwise-unpaid costs in the price of a pack of cigarettes, governments ensure that private decisions about smoking take into account the full impact that smoking has on society."

    *World Watch magazine, September-October 1992 (Hal Kane)*

17. Each penny of the federal cigarette excise tax generates almost $300 million in revenue.

    *Tobacco Use: An American Crisis, p. 69*

18. Major health organizations estimate that a $2 increase in the federal cigarette tax, and indexed to inflation, would raise an additional $35 billion in annual revenue and result in 7 million fewer American smokers. Eventually, almost 2 million premature smoking-related deaths would be avoided as a result. Current revenue from all local, state, and federal tobacco taxes is $11.3 billion. A 50-cent tax increase would mean 2.5 million fewer smokers, 600,000 lives saved, and $11 billion in increased revenue.

    *American Journal of Public Health, September 1993, and ASH Review, September-October 1993*

19. If cigarette prices were increased by 50%, 3.5 million current smokers (12.5% of the total) would give up smoking. A Centers for Disease Control study found that the effect of price increases varied greatly by race; the above tax increase would cut smoking rates by 7% among whites, 16% among blacks and up to 95% among Hispanics.

    *Morbidity and Mortality Weekly Report, July 31, 1998*

20. US tobacco taxes in 1991 amounted to $13 billion. By comparison, Canada, with one-tenth the population of the United States, raised $7.2 billion, and the United Kingdom, with less than a quarter of the US population, raised $10 billion in tobacco taxes.

    *Tobacco Use: An American Crisis, p. 60*

21. Premature death is not usually considered to be cost-effective. However, the assumption that early death saves future Social Security and Medicare expenses is essential to the tobacco industry's (incorrect) assertion that cigarette excise taxes "pay their own way" and cover the extra cost to government of diseases caused by smoking.

    *JAMA, March 2, 1994, p. 644*

22. More than $325,000 worth of tax-free cigarettes were sold in the Capitol and House office buildings in 1993. Senate figures are unavailable.

    *San Francisco Chronicle, July 19, 1994*

23. The US federal government taxes smokeless tobacco products at about one-tenth the rate of cigarettes, or 2.7 cents per tin of moist snuff and 2.3 cents per pouch of chewing tobacco.

    *Tobacco Control, Winter 1994, p. 299*

24. In terms of taxes levied to help pay for health coverage for the uninsured, the public expresses its greatest support for sin taxes on alcohol, cigarettes, and guns and ammunition. Seven of 10 Americans support an increase in federal taxes on alcohol (71%) and cigarettes (69%), while 65% favor a new tax on guns and ammunition. The least public support is for an increase in the federal income tax (22%) or a new national sales tax (23%).

    *JAMA, May 18, 1994, p. 1541*

25. "Senators and Congressmen should be happy to find a tax that is actually popular. Polls show that almost 80% of Americans...support a large cigarette tax. So those members of congress elected on a 'no new taxes' pledge can go along with this one. *Cigarette taxes are indeed different.*"

C. Everett Koop, M.D., Washington Post, September 21, 1993

26. If lost productivity is included, the Rand Corporation estimates that it would take a $5-per pack tax to pay for the health costs of tobacco use.

Hospital Practice, June 15, 1993, p. 8

27. In 1990, 16 states had no excise taxes on smokeless tobacco, while all states had excise taxes on cigarettes.

*Spit Tobacco and Youth*, p. 11

28. When the United Kingdom cut cigarette taxes 15% between 1987 and 1990, smoking rates rose 2% overall, but by 25% among children and adolescents age 17 and younger, the most "price-sensitive" group.

World Watch, September-October 1992, p. 9

29. In Canada from 1981 to 1992, taxes per pack increased from an average of 96 cents per pack to $3.58. Cigarettes sold in this time frame dropped by 44%, a decline from 71.3 billion in 1981 to 40.1 billion in 1992.

Washington Post, September 15, 1993, p. D1

30. The prevalence of smoking among young people in Canada declined by 52% between 1980 and 1989 as the price of cigarettes doubled.

American Journal of Public Health, September 1997, p. 1520

31. The average price of cigarettes per pack is $3.27 to $5.32 in the US, depending on the state tax, $2.76 in France, $6.33 in the UK, $4.02 in Australia, , and $7.56 in Norway.

ASH Smoking and Health Review, July-August 2002

32. In 2002, cigarette taxes per pack were $3.77 in Denmark, $5.03 in the UK, $2.89 in New Zealand, $2.77 in Australia, $2.08 in France, and $5.99 in Norway.

ASH Smoking and Health Review, July-August 2002

33. Eight of the 10 states with the lowest cigarette taxes - Virginia, Kentucky, North Carolina, South Carolina, Wyoming, Tennessee, Indiana and West Virginia - have higher than average rates of adult smoking. Similarly, seven of the 10 places with the highest excise taxes on cigarettes - Washington State, the District of Columbia, Hawaii, Arizona, Massachusetts, Connecticut and Minnesota - have lower than average smoking rates.

US News and World Report, February 5, 1996, p. 16

34. For every 25 cents of a federal tobacco tax increase, about one million Americans alive today would be discouraged from smoking, and between 200,000 and 300,000 premature deaths would be prevented.

Saving Lives and Raising Revenues, Coalition on Smoking or Health, February 1995

35. In 1983, total tobacco taxes amounted to $8 billion in the United Kingdom and $7 in Germany compared to $9.4 billion tax revenue for the United States. In Haiti in 1983, tobacco taxes accounted for 41% of all central government tax revenue, and in Argentina, 23%.

*Tobacco in History*, p. 11

36. Every 25-cent increase in excise taxes, indexed to keep pace with inflation, would discourage a million people from smoking, and save between 200,000 and 300,000 from premature death.

The Washington Monthly, May 1996, p. 20

37. Increasing cigarette prices by $1.10 a pack over five years would decrease teen smoking by 42% and prevent nearly one million premature deaths.

Associated Press, March 23, 1998

38. A cigarette tax increase of $2 per pack (supported by 66% of all voters, including a third of those who smoke) would result in $25 billion in new tax revenue, 7.6 million fewer smokers, and the prevention of 1.9 million future smoking-related deaths.

Newsweek, March 28, 1994, p. 27

39. Cigarette taxes in Japan are $24 billion a year, accounting for 8.3% of total tax revenue. U.S. taxes are $12.7 billion, 1.5% of total revenue.                    World Watch, July-August 1997, p. 24

40. The tobacco companies argue that excise tax increases will discourage smoking and thereby reduce government revenues. However, the fact is that "raising tobacco taxes, no matter how large the increase, has never once led to a decrease in cigarette tax revenues."
                    UICC Tobacco Control Fact Sheet 5, International Union Against Cancer, 1996

41. A frequently quoted 1981 study by Michael Grossman and Frank Chaloupka found that a 10% increase in the price of cigarettes would reduce the total number of youth smokers by 12%. A 1996 study by the same authors found that a 10% price increase would reduce the number of youthful smokers by 7%, a somewhat smaller effect than the earlier 12% projected. Cigarette consumption by all smokers, however, would decline by 6%, or three times larger than the decline of 2% projected in the 1981 study.Public Health Reports, July/August 1997, p. 295

42. A $2 a pack tax increase would reduce teen smoking by 70%, according to an estimate by the National Bureau of Economic Research. "Anything short of a sharp increase in price holds hollow promise of cutting teen smoking."                    Washington Post, September 7, 1997, p. C7 (Joseph Califano)

43. Tobacco companies are allowed to deduct the cost of advertising and promotion from their taxes as a business expense. This saves them in excess of $1 billion a year in taxes.
                    American Lung Association Fact Sheet, Cigarette Advertising and Promotion (August 1997 Update)

44. Republican Senator Orrin Hatch joined forces with liberal Edward Kennedy to introduce a bill to raise the federal cigarette tax by 43 cents (to 67 cents total) in order to provide health insurance for half of the nation's 10 million uninsured children. Senate majority leader Trent Lott was furious and publicly derided the proposal, saying that it would never become law on his watch. (It didn't.)                    Time, April 21, 1997, p. 78

45. If the proposed 43-cent increase cigarette tax in the Hatch-Kennedy bill had been enacted, the number of teenage smokers would have fallen by about 16%, and the number of cigarettes consumed by this group would have declined by 14%. This would translate into more than 2.6 million fewer smokers and more than 850,000 fewer smoking-related premature deaths in the current cohort of 0 to 17 year-olds.
                    Public Health Reports, July/August 1997, p. 291

46. The Senate in May 1997 defeated a plan sponsored by Senators Orrin Hatch (R-Utah) and Edward Kennedy (D-Mass) to raise the federal tobacco tax by 43 cents a pack in order to provide medical insurance for 5 million low income children who did not qualify for Medicaid. The Republican Policy Committee argued successfully that the bill should not be passed because it would create a hardship by depriving states of an estimated $6.5 billion in tax revenue over five years because of reduced cigarette sales. Senator Kennedy responded, "If fewer people smoke, states will save far more in lower health costs than they will lose in revenues from the cigarette tax," and Senator Hatch called the policy committee statement "absolutely preposterous."
                    New York Times, May 21, 1997, p. A20, and USA Today, May 23, 1997, p. 12A

47. An unsuccessful 1998 bill introduced by Senator Kent Conrad, Democrat from Montana, would have boosted cigarette prices by $1.50 a pack over three years, and raised $82 billion over five years, $10 billion of this going to tobacco farmers, and $13 billion for antismoking programs.
                    Wall Street Journal, February 12, 1998, p. A23 (Al Hunt)

48. A tax loophole allows tobacco products to be sold tax-free (of state taxes) on Indian reservations.
                    Roll Call, March 9, 1998, p. 29

49. "With regard to taxation, it is clear that in the US, and in most countries in which we operate, tax is becoming a major threat to our existence." "Of all the concerns, there is one--taxation--that alarms us the most. While marketing restrictions and public and passive smoking (restrictions) do depress volume, in our experience taxation depresses it much more severely. Our concern for taxation is, therefore, central to our thinking..."
                    From a 1985 Philip Morris International document "Smoking and Health Initiatives"
                    released by the Minnesota Attorney General's office in 1998

50. Two years after a 1997 Oregon cigarette tax increase from 38 to 68 cents a pack, per capita cigarette consumption in the state had declined by 11.3%, or the equivalent of 200 cigarettes (10 packs) per capita.
*Morbidity and Mortality Weekly Report*, February 26, 1999, p. 41

51. A 50% price increase could cause a 12.5% reduction in the total U.S. cigarette consumption, or about 60 billion fewer cigarettes smoked per year.
*JAMA*, December 16, 1998, p. 1979

52. On average, a 10% increase in cigarette prices reduces smoking by 4% overall in developed countries and 8% in poorer countries. A worldwide 10% increase would prompt 40 million people to quit and discourage others from starting.
*Wall Street Journal*, May 18, 1999, p. A28

53. A 10% cigarette price increase would reduce demand by about 4% in high-income countries (more in children and adolescents, who are more responsive to price increases), and by about 8% in low and middle-income countries. A 10% price increase worldwide would cause a minimum of 40 million smokers to quit, and would prevent at least 10 million tobacco-related deaths.
*Curbing the Epidemic*, p. 6

54. Domestic cigarette consumption has fallen 6 to 7% in 1998-1999, double the 3% average annual decline of the last decade. Analysts attribute the decline to a nationwide 25% per pack increase in the last year. In some states with high taxes such as California, Massachusetts, and Alaska, consumption declines from the previous year could be greater than 15%.
*Christian Science Monitor*, February 25, 1999, p. 1

55. The federal tax on large cigars is a maximum of 3 cents per cigar.
*NEJM*, June 10, 1999, p. 1830

56. 4 million teens spend $2 billion on a billion packs of cigarettes that they consume each year, paying $222 million in federal and $300 million in state tobacco taxes.
*ABC evening news*, June 30, 1999

57. The tobacco industry spent $29.8 million in an unsuccessful attempt to defeat California's Proposition 10, which raised the state cigarette tax by 50 cents a pack in 1999. Proponents of the tax spent $9 million, including director Rob Reiner's $1 million. The tobacco industry's position against the tax was supported by TV ads featuring Wilson Riles, a highly respected former state school superintendent, whom the industry paid $90,000. The tax passed by only 80,000 votes out 8 million cast.
*San Francisco Chronicle*, February 4, 1999, p. A1

58. "Will higher taxes keep young people from smoking?   Studies…find little or no relationship between higher prices and teen smoking."
Senator (new Attorney General) John Ashcroft in a letter
to Joel Moskowitz, June 17, 1998, responding to his Op-Ed
piece in the San Francisco Chronicle, March 20, 1998

59. The tobacco industry recognizes that increased taxes on tobacco products represent one of the greatest threats to the viability of the industry.
*Campaign for Tobacco-Free Kids*

60. The federal cigarette tax went from 32 cents to 37 cents a pack in January 2002.
*New York Times*, January 25, 2002, p. A21

61. The United States collects $15.5 billion a year in tobacco taxes.
*Cigarettes* (Parker-Pope), p. 39

62. In the United States, between 20% and 40% (depending upon the state) of the cost of cigarettes is taxes. In Canada, between 57% and 75% of the cost is taxes, depending upon the province. This compares to 86% of the total price being taxes in the United Kingdom, 82% in Denmark, and between 70% and 76% in France, Italy, Austria, Greece, Germany, the Netherlands, Sweden, Belgium, and Spain. *JAMA*, September 20, 2002, p. 1369

63. According to the World Bank, a price increase of 10% can reduce demand for tobacco products by about 4% in high-income countries and by about 8% in low-and middle-income countries. The Bank estimates that tax increases that would raise the real priced of cigarettes by 10% worldwide would cause about 42 million smokers to quit and prevent a minimum of 10 million tobacco-related deaths. The tobacco industry realizes the implications that higher taxes would have on their sales volume. It is not surprising that the tobacco industry

vehemently opposes increases in tobacco taxes and does everything it can to prevent governments from increasing taxes. Secret industry documents obtained in US litigation, from Philip Morris and British American Tobacco, express the industry's concerns: "Of all the concerns, there is one--taxation--that alarms us the most. While marketing restrictions and public and passive smoking do depress volume, in our experience taxation depresses it much more severely. Our concern for taxation is, therefore, central to our thinking about smoking and health," reveals one Philip Morris International's document. "Increases in taxation, which reduce consumption, may mean the destruction of the vitality of the tobacco industry," said BAT in a 1992 internal document. WHO calls on governments not to be deflected from their primary mission to protect public health and to resist industry pressure in taxation and other measures that will help save lives.

2002 AMA Annual Tobacco Report

64. In 1998, the Centers for Disease Control concluded that more lower income smokers quit than do higher income ones when the cigarette price increases, an effect that is more dramatic among young blacks and Hispanics. It is estimated that about one quarter of 18 to 24 year old Hispanic smokers and 10% of black smokers in this age group would quit smoking completely in response to a 10% price increase, whereas only about 1% of young white smokers would quit.                      The New Yorker, September 9, 2002, p. 78

65. According to the World Bank, taxation that increased cigarette prices by 10% worldwide would cause 40 million smokers to quit and prevent 10 million tobacco-related deaths.

Washington Post National Weekly Edition, January 21-27, 2002, p. 26

66. About 1.5 million of the country's 48 million cigarette smokers roll their own cigarettes to avoid taxes.

New York Times, October 18, 2002

67. When Dwight Watson sells a 700-pound bale of tobacco; he clears about $150 after expenses. That bale makes about 16,000 packs of cigarettes. If those packs are sold in New York City, the federal, state and local governments will have pocketed $58.000 in taxes on Watson's bale of tobacco. Each year, the tobacco industry generates about $13 billion in taxes.                      Quote from San Francisco Chronicle,
December 1, 2002, p. D4 (Joan Ryan column)

68. Some of the benefits of increasing tobacco taxes are intuitive and obvious--the more cigarettes cost, the less they will be smoked. Across the board, every 10% increase in the price of cigarettes reduces consumption by 4%. More recent research has established an even greater reduction for those who are more price-sensitive, less addicted, and more motivated to quit. The same 10% increase in the price of cigarettes reduces smoking among young people and pregnant women--key populations in reducing future prevalence and immediate health care costs--by 7%.                      Smokeless States National Tobacco Policy Initiative
(American Medical Association) 2nd quarter, 2002, p. 1

69. In June 2002, the New York City cigarette tax was increased by Mayor Bloomberg from 8 cents to $1.50 a pack, on top of the $1.50 New York state tax, raising the price of a pack of cigarettes in the city to about $7.50, the highest in the country.`                      The New Yorker, September 9, 2002, p. 77

70. The New York City cigarette tax increased to $1.50 a pack in July 2002. This is in addition to the New York state tax of $1.50 a pack, the highest state tax in the country. The two taxes increase the price of some brands to more than $7 a pack, nearly double the national average.                      New York Times, July 1, 2002, p. A15

71. A bill to raise the smoking age from 18 to 21 in California was not passed because the state would miss out on an estimated $25.7 million a year in tobacco tax revenue if it raised the minimum age. The state had a 2002 budget shortfall of $24 billion.                      San Francisco Chronicle, August 31, 2002, p. A17

72. In 1997, China collected 90 billion yuan (US $10.87 billion) in cigarette taxes, about 1% of all central government revenue. By introducing an additional 10% increase in cigarette tax, the tax revenue would twice exceed total losses in industry and tobacco farmers' income, and several million lives would be saved. China has 320 million smokers, 63% of men age 15 and over, and 3.8% of women (1996 data).

Tobacco Control, June 2002, p. 105

73. A $397 billion federal spending bill approved by Congress in 2003 includes $360,000 for research into alternative uses for tobacco as well as other projects derided as "pork" by John McCain and other senators. One example is $90,000 for the Cowgirl Museum and Hall of Fame in Fort Worth, Texas.

Associated Press, February 2003

74. 75% of Texans support an increase in the tobacco tax to balance the state's budget, compared to only 13% who are in favor of increasing the gasoline tax. (The figure includes 84% of nonsmokers and 46% of tobacco users in favor of the tobacco tax.)     From Bill Godshall at smokescreen.org, February 17, 2003

75. Kentucky is considering a 44-cent increase in its cigarette tax per pack, which is currently only three cents and has not increased since 1970.     Richmond, Virginia Times Dispatch, March 9, 2003

76. Raising tobacco taxes by 10% worldwide could save 16 million lives.

British Medical Association (www.tobaccofactfile.org)

77. In February 2003, the Interagency Committee on Smoking and Health, a 28-member panel of government and academic scientists chaired by Surgeon General Richard Carmona, unanimously endorsed raising the federal cigarette tax from 39 cents to $2.39 a pack. However, Health and Human Services Secretary Tommy Thompson testified to the House Budget Committee that raising the tobacco tax was not an option. "We are not contemplating it…This administration does not raise taxes." The proposed tax would generate an estimated $28 billion a year.     Washington Post, February 27, 2003, p. A25

78. The major tobacco producing states are Kentucky, Virginia, North Carolina, South Carolina, Georgia and Tennessee. As of early 2003, the average tax in these states is 8.3 cents per pack, compared to an average of 70 cents a pack in the other states.     Campaign for Tobacco-Free Kids flier

JAMA is Journal of the American Medical Association
NEJM is New England Journal of Medicine

State cigarette excise tax rates from lowest to highest, spring 2003 (Campaign for Tobacco-Free Kids brochure)

1. Virginia 2.5 cents
2. Kentucky 3 cents28.
3. North Carolina 5 cents
4. South Carolina 7 cents
5. Wyoming 12 cents
6. Georgia 12 cents
7. Alabama 16.5 cents
8. Missouri 17 cents
9. Montana 18 cents
10. Mississippi 18 cents
11. Colorado 20 cents
12. Tennessee 20 cents
13. New Mexico 21 cents
14. Oklahoma 23 cents
15. Delaware 24 cents
16. Idaho 28 cents
17. South Dakota 33 cents
18. Florida 33.9 cents
19. Arkansas 34 cents
20. Nevada 35 cents
21. Iowa 36 cents
22. Louisiana 36 cents
23. Texas 41 cents
24. North Dakota 44 cents
25. Minnesota 48 cents
26. New Hampshire 52 cents
27. Ohio 55 cents
28. West Virginia 55 cents
29. Indiana 55.5 cents
30. Nebraska 64 cents
31. Utah 69.5 cents
32. Wisconsin 77 cents
33. Kansas 79 cents
34. California 87 cents
35. Illinois 98 cents
36. Pennsylvania $1.00
37. Washington, D.C. $1.00
38. Maine $1.00
39. Maryland $1.00
40. Alaska $1.00
41. Connecticut $1.11
42. Arizona $1.18
43. Vermont $1.19
44. Puerto Rico $1.23
45. Michigan $1.25
46. Oregon $1.28
47. Hawaii $1.30
48. Washington $1.42
49. New Jersey $1.50
50. New York $1.50
51. Rhode Island $1.50
52. Massachusetts $1.51

# CHAPTER 39
# WORKPLACE, RESTAURANT and AIRLINE SMOKING RESTRICTIONS

## General

1. By 1991, 85% of American companies restricted smoking in the workplace, including 30% with outright bans. In 1985, only 27% of U.S. companies restricted or prohibited smoking.

    Michael Eriksen, 1993 Nicotine Dependence Conference,
    Atlanta, and Washington Post National Weekly Edition, September 26-October 2, 1994

2. 6000 companies in the United States, including CNN and Alaska Airlines, each with 6000 employees, refuse to hire smokers. Alaska Airlines was unsuccessfully sued to reverse its policy by a so-called "smokers rights" group organized and paid for by the tobacco industry.  Wall Street Journal, June 25, 1990

3. Seattle-based Pacific Northwest Bell telephone company with 15,000 employees banned all smoking in company facilities in 1985, the first large company to do so. Boeing followed the next year.

    New England Journal of Medicine, September 4, 1986, p. 647, and April 17, 1986, p. 1063

4. All indoor smoking was banned in Colonial Williamsburg, Virginia, in 1993.

    San Francisco Chronicle, January 15, 1993

5. In 1991, the Oakland Coliseum (home of baseball's Athletics) became the nation's first open-air stadium to ban smoking. By 1994, smoking was banned in 20 of 28 major league ballparks, 16 of them outdoors. And 20 ballparks in 1994 do not allow signs and billboards that advertise tobacco products. The Rose Bowl is also now nonsmoking.  American Medical News, June 20, 1994, p. 8, Sports Illustrated,
    June 3, 1991, p. 91, and New York Times March 20, 1994, p. E16

6. In a study from California, prevalence of regular smokers was significantly lower in smoke-free workplaces than in those with no restrictions (13.7% vs. 20.6%). In addition, continued regular smokers in smoke-free workplaces smoked significantly fewer cigarettes than in workplaces with no restrictions (296 vs. 341 packs per year). Consumption is 21% below that estimated if there were no smoking restrictions in California workplaces. If all workplaces were smoke-free, employee cigarette consumption would be 41% below the consumption expected if there were no workplace smoking restrictions. [A complete workplace ban did begin in California in 1995.]  Archives of Internal Medicine, June 28, 1993, p. 1485

7. In workplaces that ban smoking, 25% of smokers decide to quit, and the others reduced smoking by an average of 25%.  San Francisco Chronicle, January 7, 1994, p. A25

8. In another study, smokers with a mandatory worksite smoking ban reduce their total smoking on average by one pack a week, or 15%.  American Journal of Public Health, May 1994, p. 773

9. Smoking is prohibited in coal mines primarily because of the presence of methane, a highly flammable but odorless and colorless gas. Despite this, there have been 30 mine deaths secondary to smoking in the last 20 years, including eight in a coal mine explosion near Norton, Virginia, in December 1992.

    New York Times, September 9, 1994, p. 8

10. Two-thirds of Americans (including 39% of smokers) favor a ban on smoking in all public places.

    San Francisco Examiner, May 1, 1994, p. A7

11. The University of Wisconsin was the first "big ten" university to adopt a totally smoke-free policy for all university buildings. [The UW chancellor, Donna Shalala, became Secretary of Health and Human Services in the Clinton administration and is now president of the University of Miami.--editor]

    ANR Update, Summer 1991

12. Efforts by the Manville Corporation, a Texas asbestos manufacturer, to hire only nonsmokers and to ban workplace smoking have been stymied by litigation instigated by the International Machinists Union.

*Strategies to Control Tobacco Use*, p. 248

13. By early 1994, 3600 of the nation's 9100 McDonald's restaurants were smoke-free. The nation's largest fast-food chain banned smoking in all of its company-owned restaurants, and recommended that franchise restaurants follow the policy also. Jack-in-the-Box and Taco Bell also have smoking bans. The 3000 Dunkin Donuts restaurants went smoke-free in 1995.

New York Times, February 24, 1994, p. A13, and San Francisco Chronicle, February 24, 1994, p. A1

14. By 1996, 71% of all businesses were smoke-free, despite the absence of national regulations about smoking in the workplace. "The U.S. Occupational Safety and Health Administration has dallied since 1994 over a workplace smoking ban, trying to accommodate smoking interests. It's time it saved some lives instead."

USA Today editorial, May 22, 1997, p. 12A

15. Smoking was prohibited in 70% of buildings in the United States in 1995, up from 42% in 1991.

ASH Review, March-April 1995

16. In Australia, 79% of the public support workplace smoking bans, and 73% are in favor of smoking bans in restaurants.

Tobacco Control, Spring 1995, p. 30

17. The state of Nevada in 1995 had no nonsmoking casinos.

STAT conference, June 23, 1995, San Jose

18. In 1985, Telluride, Colorado, became the first U.S. city to ban smoking in restaurants. In 1990, Sacramento, California, became the first city to ban smoking in both restaurants and workplaces.

American Medical News, August 9, 1993, p. 14

19. San Francisco in 1983 became the first major city to enact restrictions against smoking in the workplace.

*Ashes to Ashes*, p. 554

20. The Supreme Court has let stand a Florida ruling that a city can require job applicants to swear they have not smoked or used tobacco products for the past year. The justices declined to review a Florida Supreme Court ruling that upheld North Miami's regulation requiring an affidavit denying tobacco use as a condition for being considered for a job.

Reuters, January 9, 1996

21. "...the control of smoking in the workplace may be the most significant step that can now be taken to further enhance the growing social unacceptability of smoking."

Tobacco Control, Spring 1996, p. 44

22. Costs of ventilation are much higher in buildings in which smoking is widely permitted. A 30% prevalence rate for smoking at a pack and a half a day would increase the ventilation rate requirement at least 2.5-fold, and smoking also increases the costs of cleaning, maintenance, and fire insurance.

Annual Review of Public Health 1991; 12:213

23. In 1977, asbestos manufacturer Johns-Manville banned workplace smoking, and smokers were no longer hired.

Annual Review of Public Health 1991; 12:209

24. Six months after institution of a workplace smoking ban in Australia, there was a reduction in consumption of 5.2 cigarettes per day on average for smokers. Over a two-year period, the estimated net effect of the ban was to reduce consumption by about 3.5 cigarettes per day.

Tobacco Control, Summer 1997, p. 131

25. A study from Australia found that in workplaces with smoking bans (either total or applied only to the usual work station), workday cigarette consumption was reduced by an average of five cigarettes per day compared with leisure-day consumption. This would decrease the yearly intake of the average smoker by 1150 cigarettes per year. Workplace smoking bans would result in a major loss in retail sales and revenue for tobacco companies, which is why they are aggressively fighting proposed workplace restrictions and smoking bans.

Journal of Occupational Medicine, July 1992, p. 693

26. Workplace smoking bans reduce consumption in smokers by an average of 4 to 5 cigarettes per day.
10th World Conference on Tobacco or Health, Beijing, 1997 (Nigel Gray)

27. Smoke-free worksite policies help employees to reduce or discontinue use of tobacco. In a study of 8,300 smokers in 22 cities in the United States and Canada, employees who worked in a smoke-free worksite were over 25% more likely to make a serious quit attempt, and over 25% more likely to achieve cessation than those who worked where smoking was permitted. Among continuing smokers, employees in smoke-free worksites consumed an average of three fewer cigarettes per day compared with those who worked in areas with non-restrictive smoking policies.
Tobacco Control, Winter 1997, p. S44

28. When people cannot smoke at work, their daily consumption falls by up to 25%, a level unprecedented by any other intervention, and smoking cessation is also prompted by workplace bans.
British Medical Journal, July 13, 1996, p. 98

29. The main public health impact of restrictions or bans on smoking in the workplace, reductions in smoking among smokers, should lead to reductions in tobacco-induced disease in smokers to a far greater degree than any health benefits for nonsmokers. In a survey of one nonsmoking workplace, the average smoker reduced consumption by 5.18 cigarettes a day. Light smokers did not change consumption, while moderate smokers reduced by an average of 5.8 cigarettes per day, and heavy smokers by 7.9 cigarettes.
International Journal of Health Services 1990; 20:417-427

30. In a 1997 study of 100,000 U.S. workers, only 46% reported completely smoke-free workplaces. Only 21% of food service workers had coverage by smoke-free policies, the lowest rate among different occupations; this group also has the highest rate of lung cancer among nonsmokers.
Tobacco Control, Autumn 1997, p. 164

31. The United States Occupational Health and Safety Administration, which regulates workplace and worker safety, regards a mortality risk on the job of greater than one per thousand as "very hazardous". This assessment is shared by the EPA (Environmental Protection Agency) and FDA (Food and Drug Administration). A study by the Direction de la Sante Publique de la Monteregie in Quebec reported on the health risks for nonsmoking restaurant workers exposed to environmental tobacco smoke in the workplace. The conclusion was that this smoke exposure creates a lifetime risk of 1% of dying from lung cancer for the average worker, and a 10% risk of dying from heart disease, over and above the likelihood of dying from these diseases for the general population.

32. Smoke-free workplaces in the United States reduced the number of cigarettes smoked by nearly 10 billion from 1988 to 1994. If all workplaces were smoke-free, U.S. cigarette consumption would be reduced by 20.9 billion cigarettes each year.
Reuters, July 1, 1999
(from July 1999 American Journal of Public Health, Dr. Simon Chapman)

33. Having 100% smoke-free workplaces reduced smoking prevalence by 6 percentage points and average daily consumption among smokers by 14% relative to workers subject to minimal or no restrictions. The authors from the Center for Economics Research in Research Triangle Park, North Carolina, concluded that requiring all workplaces to be smoke-free would reduce smoking prevalence by 10%.
Tobacco Control, Autumn 1999, pp. 272-277

34. A universal workplace smoking ban would result in 178,000 additional quitters in the Untied States each year.
Journal of the National Cancer Institute, March 17, 1999, p. 504

35. In Winston-Salem, North Carolina, the largest mall in the region has banned smoking, as have other malls in Greensboro and High Point, North Carolina.
NBC evening news, January 30, 1999

36. The establishment of smoke-free workplaces is important in contributing to the recent national declines in cigarette consumption in Australia and the United States. An estimated 22.3% of the decline in total cigarette consumption in Australia between 1988 and 1995 was attributable to the establishment of smoke-free workplaces, as was 12.7% of the decline in consumption in the United States between 1988 and 1994. These data "underscore the significance of the SFWs in a comprehensive approach to reducing tobacco consumption

in communities,. These estimates reinforce some of our earlier suggestions about why the tobacco industry devotes so much of its lobbying efforts to discrediting the scientific basis of restrictions on indoor smoking, funding "independent' scientific reports that concluded that the health risks posed by ETS are trivial, and undertaking expensive legal challenges to oppose government reports on ETS. Significantly, a 1991 tobacco industry memo stated, 'Of course ETS is the BIG ONE…Bans and restrictions are matters which will interest the marketing people in particular because these will affect the bottom line if they are effective' (emphasis in original)."                    American Journal of Public Health, July 1999, pp. 1018-1023

37. In a 1998 nationwide survey, 72% of white-collar workplaces, 52% of service-oriented workplaces, and 46% of blue-collar workplaces were covered by a smoke-free policy.     Washington Post, November 15, 1998, p. H4

38. In a study from Berkeley, California, more than 26% of smokers who were prohibited from smoking at work had quit in the preceding 6 months, compared with about 19% of smokers in communities with no antismoking ordinance.                        American Journal of Public Health, May 2000, p. 757

39. A study of workplace smoking restrictions published in the August 2001 issue of the *Journal of Occupational and Environmental Medicine* found that while over 80% of workers in states such as Maryland and Utah reported that their workplace is smoke-free, workers in most states report far lower rates of workplace protection.
Some key findings:
   - Nationally, 68.6%of all indoor workers reported working under a smoke-free policy in 1999 compared to 46% in 1993.
   - The five states with the highest rates of smoke-free workplace coverage in 1999 were: Utah--83.9%; Maryland--81.2%; California--76%; Massachusetts--76.8%; and Vermont--76.6%.
   - The five lowest ranked states were: Nevada--48.7%; Kentucky--55.9%; Indiana--58.1%; South Dakota--59.7%; and Michigan--60.7%.
   - In 1993, only two states, Washington and Utah, had 60% of its workforce reporting a smoke-free policy; 47 states and the District have now reached this level of coverage.
   - Major tobacco producing states have also seen significant progress. Only 31% of workers in North Carolina reported a smoke-free policy in 1993, by 1999, 61% were smoke-free. Other tobacco producing states and the percent of workers that were smoke-free in 1999 are:  Virginia--70.0%; Georgia--66.5%; South Carolina--64.1%; and Kentucky--55.9%.   2002 AMA Annual Tobacco Report

40. A Canadian study provides some of the most compelling scientific evidence yet for a total ban on workplace smoking, including bars and restaurants. The research, published in the *International Journal of Cancer* in July 2001, found that a non-smoking woman who lives with a smoker has a 21% higher risk of developing lung cancer over her adult lifetime. But if the woman lived with a smoking parent as a child, her risk jumps 63% above that of someone who has always lived in a smoke-free home. A woman who has always lived in a smoke-free home but works where smoking is permitted sees her risk of developing lung cancer jump by 27 per cent. That risk climbs steadily over time, and increases based on the number of smokers in the workplace. The new research found that when the number of "occupational smoker years" (the number of smokers in the workplace multiplied by the worker's years of service) reaches 26, the risk of lung cancer has doubled. That could mean two smoking co-workers over 13 years or five smoking co-workers over five years. It could also mean 26 customers daily for a year in a bar. When researchers looked at the upper third of workers--those exposed to the most second-hand smoke--they found the lung cancer risk was more than tripled. AMA Annual Tobacco Report

41. The effects of workplace passive smoke exposure on lung function was examined in a Scottish study, published in the journal *Occupational and Environmental Medicine* (2001; 58:563-568). Three hundred one never smokers were the subject of pulmonary function testing, correlated with exposure to ETS at work and home. Compared with unexposed subjects, those with the highest work exposures had a 254 ml reduction in FEV-1, and a 273 ml reduction in FVC after adjustment for confounders. Case-control analysis also showed a significant exposure-relation between ETS exposure at work and lung function. This nearly 10% drop in pulmonary function was statistically significant ($p<.05$) and is yet another clear indication for smoke-free workplace policies.                        2002 AMA Annual Tobacco Report

42. Smoke-free workplaces cut cigarette consumption per smoker and also lower the prevalence of smoking. A totally smoke-free policy (as opposed to one allowing smoking in designated areas) was associated with a 3.8% drop in smoking prevalence and, in addition, the number of cigarettes consumed per day per smoker decreased by 3.1. Policies that allowed smoking in some areas were about half as effective in reducing prevalence and consumption as those that prohibited smoking.                  British Medical Journal 2002; 325:188-194

43. Utah has the highest percentage of workers in smoke-free workplaces, 84%, and Nevada the lowest, 49%. The 1999 average nationwide was 70%.                  Associated Press, August 11, 2001

44. Finland adopted national smoke-free workplace legislation in 1995, and was successful in both reducing exposure to ETS in the workplace, as well as decreasing daily smoking prevalence among workers.
                  American Journal of Public Health, September 2001, p. 1416

45. A new study conducted by researchers at the University of California, San Francisco, demonstrates that smoke-free policies not only protect nonsmokers from the dangers of secondhand smoke but also encourage smokers to quit or reduce consumption. Twenty-six studies on workplaces in the United States, Australia, Canada, and Germany were subjected to a process of systematic review and meta-analysis. Entirely smoke-free workplaces were associated with a 3.8% reduction in smoking prevalence. Of those employees who continued to smoke, there was an average reduction in consumption of 3.1 cigarettes per day. The combined effects of increased cessation and decreased consumption corresponded to a 29% relative reduction in tobacco use among all employees.                  Quote from ANR (Americans for Nonsmokers' Rights) Update, Fall 2002

46. Philip Morris' own research shows that prohibiting smoking in the workplace not only reduces consumption, but also increases quitting rates. A 1992 memo summarizing these findings states: "Total prohibition of smoking in the workplace strongly affects industry volume. Smokers facing these restrictions consume 11%-15% less than average and quit at a rate that is 84% higher than average." The memo goes on to state that, "If smoking were banned in all workplaces, the industry's average consumption would decline 8.75%-10% from 1991 levels and the quitting rate would increase by 74%."   Smokeless States National Tobacco Policy Initiative
                  (American Medical Association), 2nd quarter, 2002, p. 4

47. Smoking will be banned in the main press center and in the bleachers at all outdoor sports arenas (including beach volleyball) at the 2004 Athens Olympics. In Greece, smoking is not allowed on public transportation and indoor public areas.                  2003 AMA Annual Tobacco Report

48. After a citywide indoor smoking ban (including restaurants and bars) passed in Helena, Montana, the incidence of heart attacks dropped sharply.                  Associated Press, April 3, 2003

49. Bowdoin College in Brunswick, Maine, has banned smoking in all buildings, including dorms and student housing; outside smokers must be 50 feet from any building.                  New York Times, January 6, 2003

50. Smoking is not allowed in 70% of American homes, ranging from 78% in the West to 64% in the Midwest, where it is most tolerated.                  San Francisco Chronicle, November 29, 2000, p. A8

## Federal and State Workplace Regulations

1. In April 1994, the Pentagon banned smoking in the workplace, a move affecting 3.6 million civilian and military employees. One top medical officer suggested that in the future, consideration might be given to recruiting only nonsmokers.                  Associated Press, March 8, 1994
2. The White House became completely smoke-free in February 1993, and the White House smoking ban has been continued in the Bush administration.       Journal of the National Cancer Institute, March 17, 1993, p. 430

3. Beginning in 1997, President Bill Clinton, by executive order, banned smoking in federal buildings. This did not include offices outside the executive branch--congressional offices and federal court buildings.
                  Associated Press, August 10, 1991

4. The Postal Service prohibited smoking in all of its buildings in June 1993. *Associated Press, June 1993*

5. The first Bush administration declined three requests by Secretary of Health and Human Services, Dr. Louis Sullivan, to sign an executive order banning smoking in federal buildings. *Tobacco Use*, p. 50

6. Rep. Henry Waxman (D-Calif.) in 1994 sponsored a bill, H.R. 3434, to make virtually all buildings open to the public smoke free. And Secretary of Labor Robert Reich proposed OSHA regulations that could potentially make 6 million workplaces smoke-free. *ANR Update, Summer 1994, p. 1*

7. The Occupational Safety and Health Administration (OSHA) is considering a rule that would ban smoking in all U.S. workplaces. Philip Morris hired the Washington lobbying firm of Bonner and Associates to generate letters against the proposed regulation. Bonner earned at least $1.4 million for a campaign that produced only 7,300 letters, and, additionally, was paid more than $100 for each of 1,500 faxes to members to Congress. *ASH Review, November 1994, p. 3*

8. The Occupational Safety and Health Administration (OSHA) is considering a proposal to ban smoking in the workplace nationally, adding up to 92 million workers at 6 million workplaces. Pat Tyson, former acting head of OSHA during the Reagan administration, was hired by Philip Morris to testify against the proposed workplace ban. *Washington Post National Weekly Edition, September 26, 1994*

9. Philip Morris and RJR have each hired a former head of OSHA (the Labor Department's Occupational Safety and Health Administration) to try to stymie agency efforts to restrict smoking in the workplace. *Common Cause, Spring 1995, p. 22*

10. Philip Morris pulled out of 1994 federal hearings on proposed workplace smoking restrictions. After grilling witnesses, including the AMA, who favor the Labor Department measure, Philip Morris refused its own turn at being cross-examined on grounds that the hearings were biased against tobacco. *American Medical News, December 12, 1994, p. 2*

11. The benefits of banning smoking in all public places in the U.S., as proposed by Rep. Henry Waxman, would outweigh the costs by at least $39 billion a year. More than 1 million smokers might quit immediately if such a ban became law, 50,000 to 100,000 more teenagers would not take up the habit, and 11,000 to 20,000 deaths of nonsmokers a year would be averted because of reduced exposure to secondhand smoke. *New York Times, April 22, 1994, p. A9*

12. A nationwide smoking ban in all public buildings would prevent as many as 12,900 premature deaths each year and save $39 to $72 billion a year, the Environmental Protection Agency (EPA) estimates. *San Francisco Chronicle, April 22, 1994, p. A3, and New York Times, February 24, 1994, p. A13*

13. With all the attention to the FDA proposed rules, the OSHA (Occupational Safety and Health Administration) proposed workplace smoking ban introduced in 1994 has received very little press. This would eliminate smoke exposure in the workplace for 75 million Americans; however, the tobacco industry has been successful in indefinitely stalling this proposal, and OSHA has reduced the number of employees working on the smoking rule from 12 to one. *Washington Legal Times, November 20, 1995 and ASH Smoking and Health Review, March-April 1996 and September-October 1996*

14. "While the public health community has mobilized aggressively in support of the FDA's proposal, the Occupational Safety and Health Administration's (OSHA) proposal to make workplaces smoke-free has been ignored... Creation of a smoke-free workplace reduces smoking prevalence by around 25% and tobacco consumption among continuing smokers by about 20%." *American Journal of Public Health, February 1996, p. 157 (Stanton Glantz)*

15. While President Clinton has won praise for backing the Food and Drug Administration's drive against youth smoking, a sweeping anti-smoking initiative with less political appeal has languished in the federal bureaucracy, all but forgotten. The proposed ban on workplace smoking, announced two years ago by the Occupational Safety and Health Administration, is going nowhere. It is being stalled by fierce opposition from

tobacco and restaurant interests and fear of antagonizing congressional Republicans who have sought to cut OSHA's enforcement powers. The proposal has been down-graded to a list of OSHA "long-term" actions, and nearly all staff members involved with the rule have gone on to other projects...

If smoking bans prompted the country's 48 million smokers to cut down by just three cigarettes a day, retail tobacco sales would drop by about $5 billion a year. But the delay has been criticized by some health officials and anti-smoking groups, who also question why the Clinton administration has failed to act on a long-dormant proposal to ban smoking in federal buildings by executive order. Critics say the delays reflect a broader retreat on secondhand smoke...

OSHA estimates that about 700 cases of lung cancer a year and up to 13,000 deaths from heart disease are attributable to workplace exposure to secondhand smoke. The agency's proposed rule, announced in April 1994, would ban smoking at some 6 million jobsites, including restaurants and bars.

Quote from Contra Costa Times, September 29, 1996, p. 3D (Los Angeles Times--Myron Levin)

16. A new federal law mandates that schools ban all smoking inside buildings, with a penalty of $1000 fines and a withdrawal of federal funds. This clashes with a North Carolina law that requires the provision of designated smoking areas in the same buildings.  American Medical News, October 10, 1994, p. 17

17. A 1993 North Carolina preemption bill mandates that smoking be permitted in at least 20% of spaces in state-controlled buildings, with nonsmoking areas not required. Cities and counties may not adopt more restrictive regulations for any public or private buildings after 1993. Because of this, by the year 2000, 59% of private employees will not be guaranteed any protection from worksite environmental tobacco smoke.

JAMA, March 8, 1995, p. 805

18. In 1994, the states of Maryland, California, Washington, and Vermont passed bills that essentially banned workplace smoking.

New York Times, July 22, 1994, p. A8, and San Francisco Chronicle, March 5, 1995, p. A4

19. Utah and Vermont in 1997 required restaurants to be 100% smoke-free. California requires smoke-free workplaces and restaurants. Maryland and Washington ban smoking in all workplaces except restaurants.

USA Today, August 8, 1997, p. 14A

20. Vermont has a statewide smoking ban signed by Governor Howard Dean, M.D., which bars smoking in most workplaces other than restaurants, and motels, which came under the ban in 1995.

San Francisco Chronicle, July 12, 1993

21. The states of Maryland and Washington now ban smoking in almost all indoor workplaces. Several tobacco companies unsuccessfully sued to block the Washington ban.

Time, April 18, 1994, p. 58, and American Medical News, August 15, 1994, p. 18

22. Assembly Bill 13 in California effective in January 1995 effectively banned smoking in the workplace and in restaurants, with bars exempt until 1997. In 1994, the tobacco industry had mounted a massive $17 million ballot referendum campaign to overturn the bill before it took effect, but their effort was unsuccessful, getting only 29% of the vote.  San Francisco Chronicle, November 10, 1994

23. A 1987 state law in Massachusetts blocks the hiring of smokers for police or firefighter positions, and has been upheld by the Massachusetts Supreme Court.  USA Today, October 27, 1997, p. 5D

# Restaurants and Bars

1. In lobbying against laws mandating smoke-free restaurants, the tobacco industry ran full page newspaper ads reading: "What if they passed a law that took away 30% of your business?" However, this allegation was proved to be false in cities that banned smoking in restaurants, as business before and after was unchanged. The National Smokers Alliance has claimed that a nationwide restaurant smoking ban would cost the restaurant business $24.3 billion in revenues and 400,000 jobs.  American Journal of Public Health, July 1994, p. 1081

2. The battle to overturn a Los Angeles restaurant smoking ban, despite the appearance that restaurant owners led the opposition, was bankrolled by tobacco companies, who gave 98% of the $216,000 spent in the unsuccessful attempt to reverse the ban.                                                        Associated Press, December 18, 1993

3. San Francisco's first nonsmoking bar opened in 1992. When the owner advertised for bartenders to fill job openings, emphasizing that it would be a smoke-free environment, he had more than 600 applicants.
                                                        San Francisco Chronicle, July 1992

4. Sales tax revenues from California cities and counties that have banned smoking in bars suggest that the bans do not hurt business, contrary to what the tobacco industry says about keeping customers away.
                                                        Associated Press, November 3, 1997

5. In a follow-up to an earlier study, Stanton Glantz and Lisa Smith in the October 1997 issue of the American Journal of Public Health (pp. 1687-93) published an evaluation of the economic effects of ordinances requiring smoke-free restaurants and bars. The conclusion was the same as their 1994 study: these smoke-free ordinances do not adversely affect restaurant or bar sales or revenues. In a strongly worded editorial, Mervyn Susser, editor of the American Journal of Public Health, commented on the furor that Dr. Glantz has generated with the tobacco industry (pp. 1593-94). "The tobacco industry has launched a personal attack upon Dr. Glantz' credibility and integrity as a scientist. Plainly, the aim is to destroy his career. The industry has assailed him in press conferences and in letters to government representatives and has formed a public interest organization (Californians for Scientific Integrity) seemingly for the sole purpose of suing him and his employer (the University of California). Contrary to the tobacco industry's claims, Glantz' contributions to this Journal have been sound and valid and attest to an unceasing and imaginative effort to limit the tobacco epidemic... In a letter... to Richard Atkinson, President of the University of California, the National Smokers Alliance charged Glantz as a faculty member with scientific incompetence or fraud in respect to the same paper... All reviewers agreed that both the previous work and the new work are sound... Instead of a compelling critique, however, we find a melange of scientifically inadmissible manipulations of data to obtain a desired result."

6. "Sit in a smoky bar for two hours and you'll suck up as many carcinogens as if you had smoked four cigarettes, according to figures from the American Cancer Society." All 35,500 bars in California became nonsmoking in 1998; California was the first state in the nation to ban smoking in bars. There had been 850,000 bar and restaurant workers in California exposed to passive smoke.
                                                        San Francisco Examiner, December 28, 1997, p. A8

7. After establishment of smoke free bars in California in 1998, bartender exposure to ETS declined from a median of 28 to 2 hours weekly. There was a rapid reduction in respiratory symptoms as well as an improvement in forced vital capacity and to a lesser extent, forced expiratory volume in one second.
                                                        JAMA, December 9, 1998, pp. 1909-1914

8. 59% of bartenders reporting respiratory problems before a smoking ban in California bars no longer had them four to eight weeks after the ban took effect. More than three quarters of the bartenders with irritated eyes, noses or throats before the ban reported that these problems had resolved on their followup medical exams. The article concluded that establishment of smoke free bars in California was associated with a rapid improvement of respiratory health in workers.                     JAMA, December 9, 1998, pp. 1909-1914

9. A statewide ban on smoking in restaurants in Maine, affecting 40,000 restaurant workers, has been approved.
                                                        "Maine", USA Today, April 7, 1999

10. TobaccoScam is an educational program which combines monthly advertisements in the hospitality trade press with an extensive web site. It is designed to break the alliance between the tobacco and hospitality industry by educating restaurateurs about how and why the tobacco industry has duped them into thinking that smoke-free restaurants hurt business and that the solution is expensive and ineffective ventilation systems.
                                                        Quote from 2002 National Conference on Tobacco or Health, Abstract POLI-273

11. How does Big Tobacco manipulate the hospitality industry?
    - Falsely claims smoke-free measures will ruin restaurants and bars.
    - Hijacks national and state hospitality groups as propaganda vehicles.
    - Lures owners into buying expensive "accommodation" ventilation systems.
    - Uses groups and owners as fronts to fight cost-free smoke-free measures.
    - How does Big Tobacco fool restaurants and bar owners into thinking cost-free smoke-free measures are business poison?
    - It pays for biased surveys and distorts or ignores research counter to its own propaganda.
    - No properly conducted study shows a negative economic impact. Some even show that a smoke-free measure improves business. In the meantime, as evidence mounts about the dangers of secondhand smoke, so does the liability of employers including restaurants.

    from TobaccoScam brochure (www.TobaccoScam.ucsf.edu)

12. An article in Tobacco Control (June 2002, pp. 94-104) by Stanton Glantz, et al from the University of California, San Francisco, described "how the tobacco industry used the 'accommodation' message to mount an aggressive and effective worldwide campaign to recruit hospitality associations, such as restaurant associations, to serve as the tobacco industry's surrogate in fighting against smoke-free environments…The tobacco industry, led by Philip Morris, made financial contributions to existing hospitality associations or, when it did not find an association willing to work for tobacco interests, created its own 'association' in order to prevent the growth of smoke-free environments. The industry also used hospitality associations as a vehicle for programmes promoting 'accommodation' of smokers and non-smokers, which ignore the health risks of secondhand smoke for employees and patrons of hospitality venues.

    **Conclusion**: Through the myth of lost profits, the tobacco industry has fooled the hospitality industry into embracing expensive ventilation equipment, while in reality 100% smoke-free laws have been shown to have no effect on business revenues, or even to improve them. The tobacco industry has effectively turned the hospitality industry into its de facto lobbying arm on clean indoor air. Public health advocates need to understand that, with rare exceptions, when they talk to organised restaurant associations they are effectively talking to the tobacco industry and must act accordingly."

13. "TobaccoScam" ads were initially accepted and later rejected in two restaurant trade magazines. One shows New York restauranteur Michael O'Neal, who says, "Big Tobacco has been conning the restaurant business for years. Don't be a sucker. Go smoke-free."      New York Times, August 7, 2002, via tobacco.org

14. Economic impact studies in 100 sites around the world have shown that restaurant smoking bans have no effect, or a positive effect, on revenues.      Stanton Glantz lecture, San Francisco, November 19, 2002

15. The Honolulu City Council has banned smoking in all restaurants and most restaurant bars on the island of Oahu starting July 1, 2002. Smoking will be prohibited in the remainder of restaurant bars starting July 1, 2002. Stand-alone bars and nightclubs are exempt.      2002 AMA Annual Tobacco Report

16. As of early 2003, the Hawaiian islands of Oahu, Maui, and Kauai have smoke-free restaurants and a bill to establish the same policies on the island of Hawaii was being considered.
    Information from the Coalition for a Tobacco Free Hawaii, www.tobaccofreehawaii.org

17. In a survey from Minnesota, 72% of respondents said that they would select a smoke-free restaurant over one where smoking is permitted, and 70% said that they would prefer a smoke-free bar.
    Mayo Clinic Proceedings, February 2001, p. 134

18. In Florida, 71% of voters in 2002 approved a ban on smoking in most enclosed indoor workplaces, including restaurants and in-home child care. Stand-alone bars were exempted.
    American Medical News, November 25, 2002

19. "New York City will enact a sweeping ban on indoor smoking that will include nearly all bars and restaurants…and yesterday the Boston Public Health Commission voted to ban smoking in its 2300 bars and restaurants as well…"
    New York Times, December 12, 2002, p. A1

20. Former Chicago Bears coach now turned restaurant owner, Mike Ditka, is leading the charge against a proposed restaurant smoking ban in Chicago. In an interview, Ditka had a cigar in one hand and a drink in the other.

Chicago Sun-Times, January 10, 2003

21. Mayor Richard Daly and restaurant owner, Mike Ditka, have blocked efforts to pass a strong smoke-free ordinance in Chicago.

ANR Update, Spring 2003

22. In a survey from Hong Kong, in advance of a legislative proposal for smoke-free restaurants and tea bars, 69% of respondents said that they would support a totally smoke-free policy in restaurants.

Tobacco Control, September 2002, p. 195

23. "Five years after California banned smoking in bars, a new survey reveals widespread public support. Nearly 75% of bar owners and employee say they prefer to work in a smoke-free environment. That's up from 47% in 1998. And 87% of customers say they are more likely to visit bars or have not changed their bar-going habits as a result of the smoking ban. Three out of four patrons approve of the law." Support for the ban increased from 24% in 1998 to 45% in 2002 even among smokers.

Contra Costa (Calif.) Times, November 21, 2002, pp. A1 and A22

24. Two years after California's bars went smoke-free, 73% of bar patrons approved of the ban, including 44% of smokers surveyed who supported the law.

San Francisco Chronicle, October 17, 2000, p. A3

25. Norway in the spring of 2004 will be the first country in the world to outlaw smoking in restaurants and bars nationwide.

New York Times, April 10, 2003, p. A8

26. An article published in Tobacco Control 2003; 12:13-20, concluded that no-smoking policies in restaurants and bars do not harm business, despite concerted efforts by the tobacco industry to prove otherwise. Only one of 31 tobacco industry funded studies was published in a peer reviewed journal, and the papers claiming that restaurants and bars lose money when smoking bans are imposed, were biased and of poor quality, the Tobacco Control article showed. Of the 21 good quality studies reviewed, none reported a negative impact, and four reported a positive effect of a smoking ban on sales.

27. A smoking ban took effect in Dallas in March 2003 which bans smoking in restaurants, hotels except for designated rooms, bars that open into hotels or restaurants, bowling alleys, bingo parlors, and city-owned facilities.

Fort Worth Star-Telegram, January 22, 2003

# Airlines and Smoking

1. In 1971, United Airlines became the first major airline to institute separate smoking and non-smoking sections on its planes.

*Reducing Tobacco Use*, pp. 46-47

2. Aeroflot, one of the world's last major airlines to allow smoking, went smoke-free in April 2002.

San Francisco Chronicle, November 25, 2001, p. C2

3. Freedom Air, a charter airline between Los Angeles and Chicago catering to smokers in the smoke-free skies of scheduled airlines, was disbanded after three little-patronized flights in 1993. The promoter failed to recoup $175,000 of his $200,000 investment.

San Francisco Examiner, February 13, 1994, p. E7, and USA Today, November 16, 1993

4. Two businessmen, who like to smoke, in 1992 were seeking FAA certification for Smoker's Express Airlines to fly from the Space Coast airport in Titusville, Florida, to cities in the southern and eastern U.S. They hoped to finance some of the $3.5 million in startup costs by selling sponsorships to tobacco companies.

Forbes, February 15, 1993, p. 20

5. Airports in Australia have had total indoor smoking bans for several years.

Simon Chapman, PhD., editor, Tobacco Control, 1999

6. Thai Airways went 100% smoke-free in May 1999.    Action on Smoking and Health Foundation Thailand

7. All U.S. airline flights, both domestic and international, were smoke free by the end of 1998.
USA Today, December 15, 1998

8. Virgin Atlantic airlines is now handing out nicotine patches to its passengers who smoke.
Paul Harvey news, June 8, 1999

9. 18 of 59 major U.S. airports surveyed in 1995 completely banned smoking, up from five in 1993.
New York Times, November 5, 1995, Section 5, p. 3

10. Smoking is still allowed on many domestic airline flights in Africa.    New York Times, February 2, 2003, p. 3

## Hotels and Cruise Ships

1. The Carnival Cruise Lines' ship Paradise bans smoking anywhere on the ship; violators must disembark, forfeit their cruise fare, and return home at their own expense. There are also special seven-day Caribbean cruises, sponsored by the American Lung Association, for smokers trying to quit.
San Francisco Chronicle, October 20, 2002, p. C2

2. Carnival Cruise Lines' Paradise is the only completely smoke-free cruise ship. Passengers must sign a contract promising to abide by the no-smoking policy, and offenders are kicked off the ship at the next port and must pay their own way home. The Paradise was launched in 1998 and carries 2,040 passengers.
Los Angeles Times, December 17, 2000 and San Francisco Chronicle, August 2, 1991

3. Renaissance Cruises now bans smoking on all of its ten ships.    San Francisco Chronicle, April 22, 2001, p. T4

4. The Comfort Inn Midtown in New York, run by Apple Core Hotels, in 2001 became perhaps the country's first entirely no-smoking hotel.                2002 AMA Annual Tobacco Report

5. In North America in 1996, 97% of all hotels had designated nonsmoking rooms. The corresponding figures were 93% for Australia, 80% in Asia, 77% in Africa and the Middle East, and 69% for Europe.
Contra Costa Times, January 22, 1997, p. C1

6. In late 1997, LeMirador hotel in Switzerland became the first 5-star hotel in the world to go smoke-free.
reported by Smoke Free Educational Services, Inc.

## Hospitals

1. The Joint Commission on Accreditation of Health Care Organizations (JCAHO) adopted a standard in 1992 that required all accredited hospitals to adopt a hospital-wide no-smoking policy.    *Nicotine Addiction*, p. 173

2. A total smoking ban in a large urban teaching hospital resulted in a 40% reduction in tobacco consumption.
*Nicotine Addiction*, p. 398

3. In the year after a smoking ban was instituted at the Harvard School of Public Health, 27% of the smokers there quit. In smoke-free hospitals, 36% of employees who quit attribute their decision to the hospital's smoke-free policy.                Archives of Internal Medicine, January 1991, p. 32

4. The Mayo Clinic does not permit smoking anywhere on its hospital property, indoors or out.
JAMA, January 6, 1989, p. 95

5. After smoking was prohibited indoors at the Johns Hopkins Hospital in Baltimore, employee smoking prevalence decreased by a quarter, from 22% to 16%. In addition, the daily number of cigarettes smoked

decreased by 25% in employees who continued to smoke. JAMA, September 26, 1990, p. 1565

6. One year after the Ochsner Clinic in New Orleans implemented a no-smoking policy, employee smoking dropped from 22 to 14%, and of those who continued to smoke, 81% smoked less than eight cigarettes per day.
Chest, May 1990, p. 1198

7. After implementation of smoking restrictions at New England Deaconess Hospital in Boston, 26% of previous smokers quit, and a third of current smokers had reduced their cigarette consumption. Chest 1983; 84:206

8. In a survey of 51 academic medical centers, only 10 were truly "smoke-free." 30 allow smoking right outside hospital buildings, and 20 allow smoking inside as well. Skin and Allergy News, July 2001, p. 56

# Prisons and Jails

1. Before his execution, death row inmate Larry White was refused his last request, a cigarette, because of the non-smoking policy of the jail in Huntsville, Texas. News of the World, May 17, 1988

2. Nebraska prisons began a total ban on tobacco use in early 2002; inmates are offered nicotine patches during their "cold turkey" phase. 2002 AMA Annual Tobacco Report

3. "While smoking bans within the hospital and the workplace have become accepted public policy, smoking bans within prison facilities is controversial. Ten states have completely banned smoking within their state prisons and smoking is restricted in 90% of the state correctional facilities. More prisons are exploring the idea of banning smoking as a way to control medical costs. Medical costs in prisons currently account for 11% of the Department of Correction's budget and are expected to double in the next ten years, largely due to diseases related to smoking, HCV, and HIV."
Quote from 2002 National Conference on Tobacco Health, Abstract POLI-332

4. New York City jails will soon be nonsmoking, joining more than 600 penal facilities nationwide. Oregon, Texas, Utah, Maryland, and the District of Columbia forbid smoking in prisons; Vermont bans all smoking inside, and at least seven other states limit where inmates can smoke. Federal prisons have designated smoking areas. USA Today, August 27, 1996, p. 4A

5. Tobacco use is prohibited for 60% of the 15,000 inmates in jails in the state of Wisconsin. Nationwide, it is estimated that several million prisoners have smoking restrictions. JAMA, April 15, 1992, p. 2013

6. The nation's only complete ban on smoking in prisons was imposed in Vermont in 1992. It created so many problems that the state has been forced to ease it; black market cigarettes had been selling for $40 a pack.
Associated Press, November 25, 1992

7. The smoking ban at the McPherson, Kansas, county jail was applied to spinach as well, after the sheriff learned that inmates saved spinach from their meals, dried it, wrapped it in squares of toilet paper, and then lit up.
Associated Press, April 17, 1994

8. Since smoking was banned at the Portland, Maine county jail in 1992, smuggled cigarettes can fetch $5 each.
American Medical News, August 24, 1992

9. In a 1992 survey of U.S. prisons and jails, 70% to 90% of the inmates were addicted to tobacco.
Abstract OS 250, 10th World Conference on Tobacco or Health, Beijing, 1997

10. States are increasingly adopting smoke-free prison laws. Montana became the seventh state in the United States to adopt a prohibition on smoking in prisons, banning all smoking in the state prison in Deer Lodge, where 80% of the 1200 inmates and half the guards smoke or chew tobacco.
QuitNet News, Massachusetts Tobacco Control Program, January 28, 1998

11. Smoking will be banned inside New York state prisons in January 1, 2001. 10 states now have completely banned cigarettes in prisons, 36 have partial bans, and five allow unrestricted access to cigarettes.

Boston Globe, July 20, 1999

12. Colorado in 1999 banned all tobacco use in its 24 prisons.                  USA Today, March 2, 1999, p. A10

13. The Oklahoma State Penitentiary became smoke free in March 1999, a policy covering both inmates and employees.                         USA Today, February 26, 1999 p. A

14. The South Dakota State Penitentiary has gone smoke free, and inmates can no longer smoke. An exception was made for the use of ceremonial pipes for American Indian religious ceremonies.

USA Today, January 12, 1999, p. A11

15. The Supreme Court in June 1993 ruled that prisons had to provide separate but equal facilities for nonsmoking prisoners, just as restaurants do.                         New York Times, June 23, 1993, p. A12

16. The Supreme Court ruled that William McKinney, serving a life sentence for murder in Carson City, Nevada, should not be forced to share his cell with a five-pack-a-day smoker and that nonsmoking prisoners have a constitutional right to smoke-free cells. Dissenting from the ruling were Supreme Court justices Clarence Thomas and Antonin Scalia.                         New York Times, June 23, 1993, p. A12, and Reuters, June 1993

17. The Texas Board of Criminal Justice in 1995 authorized a complete ban on tobacco use both indoor and outside for the 100,000 inmates and 50,000 employees of the state's prisons.

Tobacco Free Youth Reporter, Spring 1995

NEJM is New England Journal of Medicine
JAMA is Journal of the American Medical Association

# CHAPTER 40
# MISCELLANEOUS

1. Because particulates in cigarette smoke can harm machinery and electronic equipment, Philip Morris prohibits smoking in its plants around the machines it uses to manufacture 900,000,000 cigarettes each day.

   *The Passionate Nonsmoker's Bill of Rights*, p. 144

2. Poison control centers report that there are 15,000 cases each year in the U.S. of children under age 6 who swallow cigarette butts or whole cigarettes. Many of these end up with nicotine poisoning.

   Dean Edell, MD, ABC TV, San Francisco, March 1, 1996

3. Smokers weigh about seven pounds less on average than nonsmokers.

   Archives of Internal Medicine, November 8, 1995, p. 2457

4. In a 1985 Harris poll, the general public ranked the most important things that one could do to protect one's health. Not smoking was ranked tenth in priority, behind such factors as "take adequate vitamins," "drink pure water," and "have a smoke detector in the house." Not smoking did rank number one with physicians.

   Circulation, February 1986, p. 388A and Clinics in Chest Medicine, December 1986, p. 561

5. Two new Chrysler cars introduced in 1994, Cirrus and Stratus, were the first American cars since the 1950's not to have ashtrays as standard equipment. Smokers may request models with the "ashtray option."

   New York Times, January 5, 1994

6. New cars are increasingly being manufactured without ashtrays and cigarette lighters. Models without standard ashtrays and lighters include all Dodge and Chrysler minivans, Saturn cars, the Cadillac Seville, the Infinity G20, and the Acura TL.          Journal of the National Cancer Institute, September 15, 1999, pp. 1538-1539

7. Charles Southwood, owner and founder of Death Tobacco Company, sold more than 75,000 cartons of Death Cigarettes in his first year of operation. He has 100 park benches in the Los Angeles area with his ads that say "Don't Smoke Death Cigarettes." The popular new brand is sold as a novelty item in Southern California for $3 a pack. They come in a black box with a large white skull and crossbones under the brand name DEATH. Southwood has also introduced a menthol brand packaged in a green box and called GREEN DEATH.

   Journal of the National Cancer Institute, May 20, 1992

8. An estimated 350,000 tons of paper is used each year for cigarette wrappers.

   Tobacco Control, Fall 1994, p. 191

9. Cigarettes make up 95% of all the tobacco products consumed in the US.          *Nicotine Addiction*, p. 7

10. The average smoker puffs 23 cigarettes each day. If a year's worth were placed end to end, they would be more than seven and a half football fields in length.          Ann Landers, April 18, 1993

11. A two pack a day smoker takes 400 puffs a day and inhales up to 1000 milligrams (one gram) of tar. This is 150,000 puffs and a quart of thick brown gooey carcinogenic tar into the lungs each year.

    AMA Fact Sheet on Smoking

12. The average pack-a-day smoker of 20 years has inhaled cigarette smoke over one million times.

    *Nicotine Addiction*, p. 64

13. The Bowman Gray School of Medicine, a cancer research center, is named for a former president of the RJ Reynolds Tobacco Co.          San Francisco Chronicle, April 28, 1994

14. Dr. Alan Blum reports a 22 year old pregnant woman, a high school graduate, who when questioned about smoking assured him that she and her friends would never smoke cigarettes with a warning label on the pack saying that cigarettes can harm the fetus--only the ones with the label saying that they contain carbon monoxide.

JAMA, January 6, 1989, p. 44

15. There are well over a million outlets for tobacco products in the US.   Adolescent Medicine, June 1993, p. 311

16. The tobacco industry uses most of the world's supply of licorice.                   *Nicotine Addiction*, p. 8

17. Smokers who lie about their habit on life insurance applications may end up with no coverage at all. A federal appeals court allowed the New York Life Insurance Company to avoid paying a claim in such a case, even though the policy holder died of a cause unrelated to his smoking.       Wall Street Journal, January 18, 1991

18. Glamour magazine in November 1993 ran a cover story "Health Payoffs: 20 little changes to make now." In order to avoid problems like heart disease and cancer, the magazine recommended measures including drinking pure water, wearing sunglasses, seeing a dentist, and devoting time to your feet. But avoiding smoking did not make the list.                               Tobacco Control, Summer 1994, p. 103

19. In the early 1990's, it was estimated that the Veterans Administration and Medicaid paid $210 million a year for home oxygen therapy, or 15% of the $1.4 billion annual cost. In a study of VA patients on supplemental home oxygen, 21.3% of the veterans who knew that they were coming to the hospital to re-certify for oxygen had recently smoked tobacco, as indicated by a carboxy-hemoglobin level of greater than 2.5%. The study authors posed two questions: "Is it cost-effective for the VA to continue to fund long-term supplemental oxygen for their patients who continue to smoke cigarettes? Would it be unreasonable to insist that hypoxemic patients who continue to smoke cigarettes and wish to use home oxygen assume the cost through private pay?"

Federal Practitioner, October 1997, pp. 62-63

20. Up to half of patients on home oxygen admit to smoking. In a study from Johns Hopkins, 21 patients on home oxygen suffered severe burns when their oxygen delivery system ignited while they smoked.

Burns 1998; 24:658

21. "Robert Auger, who has emphysema, blew up his home Saturday while trying to smoke a cigarette while breathing with the help of an oxygen tank." He was treated for minor injuries after the tank "went off like a bomb."                                                            USA Today, November 9, 1997

22. Home oxygen therapy is dangerous for patients who continue to smoke, and there have been several reports of house fires started from oxygen tubing and connections catching fire.        Chest, October 1996, p. 1130

23. Catecholamines, vasopressin, endorphin and cortisol are among hormones whose levels are increased by smoking. The consequences of these are far-reaching; they include adverse effects on blood pressure, pulse rate, metabolism and the body's reaction to physical stress.                              *Cigarettes*, p. 136

24. Cigarette smoke particles in the ambient air in Los Angeles accounted for 1.0 to 1.3% of the particulate air pollution and smog in a 1994 study. An earlier 1982 study had concluded that cigarette smoke accounted for about 2.7% of the organic aerosol emissions in the air in the Los Angeles basin.

Environmental Science and Technology 1994; 28:1375

25. Smokers have 50% more car accidents than nonsmokers; one reason is the distraction of lighting up and smoking while driving.                               New York State Journal of Medicine 1986; 68:459

26. Smokers are more likely to be involved in car crashes (one study estimated a 1.5-fold increased risk), and are also 1.4 to 2.5 times more likely to be injured at work.                              *Cigarettes*, pp. 164-165

27. In one experimental study, smokers deprived of cigarettes were involved in 67% more rear-end collisions than nonsmokers. But smokers who had just had a cigarette did even worse, being involved in three and a half times

more rear-end collisions than nonsmokers. Reader's Digest, March 1995, p. 130

28. An estimated 424,000 metric tons of tobacco are burned indoors annually in the US. *Nicotine Addiction*, p. 30

29. In the 1980's, the National Institute of Health (NIH) spent $500,000 in research on smoking by dogs.
World Watch, Spring 1990

30. Kimberly-Clark is the maker of Kleenex, Huggies and Kotex as well as surgical gowns, drapes and other hospital supplies. The company is also a major manufacturer of cigarette paper and filter material. In an ad in the 1995 Global Tobacco Industry guide, Kimberly-Clark boasted of being a company with "a rock solid commitment to the tobacco industry." JAMA, March 22, 1995, p. 907

31. Fifty-four nations of the world have issued anti-smoking stamps. The United States is not one of them.
Tobacco Control, Winter 1994, p. 305

32. Heart rates average 84 in smokers, compared to 72 in nonsmokers. Time, March 25, 1991, p. 55

33. Adults who spend four or more hours a day watching TV were more than twice as likely to be smokers and physically inactive as those who watch TV for an hour or less.
San Francisco Chronicle, March 19, 1994, p. A1

34. Clove cigarettes are imported from Southeast Asia, primarily Indonesia, and are composed of about a third shredded cloves and two-thirds tobacco, the latter delivering twice as much tar and nicotine as tobacco in US cigarettes. They also contain substantial amounts of eugenol, an anesthetic agent. Nearly 170 million were consumed in the US at the height of their popularity in 1984. Pediatrics, February 1991, p. 395

35. Flue-cured tobacco is acidic, a chemical property that makes the smoke from cigarettes relatively easy to inhale, while air-and-fire-cured tobacco smoke is alkaline. *Tobacco in History*, pp. 98-99

36. 8 billion cigarettes with defective filters were recalled by Philip Morris in June 1995 because they could cause coughing, wheezing, and eye and throat irritation. Albany, N.Y. smoker Chris Edwards ignored the recall, remarking, "I've never met a cigarette that didn't make me do that anyway. I thought that's what they were for."
US News and World Report, June 12, 1995, p. 25

37. If a young worker smoking two packs a day placed the same money in an 8 percent annuity, it would be worth more than $1 million at retirement. A patient who quits smoking at the birth of a child will have saved enough money over 18 years of abstinence to pay for the child's college education. *Tobacco and the Clinician*, p. 31

38. The dose of radiation needed for one chest x-ray has dropped from 20 rads in the 1920's to under 0.2 rads in 1995. Less than one cigarette produces a health risk equivalent to one x-ray.
US News and World Report, November 6, 1995, p. 16

39. Cigarette smokers have a high incidence of sleep disturbance; they are significantly more likely than nonsmokers to have difficulty going to sleep, staying asleep, daytime sleepiness, minor accidents, and depression. Archives of Internal Medicine, April 10, 1995, p. 734

40. Smokers have more trouble falling asleep and staying asleep, according to a survey of 3,500 adults. Women smokers complained of greater daytime drowsiness, while men reported a greater susceptibility to nightmares.
Time, September 5, 1994, p. 20

41. In a 1978 Gallup poll, a third of respondents were unaware that smoking caused heart disease, and 44% of smokers agreed with the statement that smoking can't really be all that dangerous; otherwise the government would ban cigarette advertising. In a 1980 Roper poll, a majority thought that air pollution caused more cases of lung cancer than did smoking; actually air pollution causes only one to two percent of lung cancer. Twice as many people ranked traffic deaths as higher than smoking deaths. Actually, eight times as many people die from

smoking.   *Selling Smoke: Cigarette Advertising and Public Health*, American Public Health Association, 1986

42. In a 1993 Gallup poll, 68% of smokers wanted to quit. 16% of this group were unaware that smoking causes lung cancer, 25% were unaware of the connection with heart disease, and 35% did not know of the link to strokes.
American Medical News, December 27, 1993, p. 8

43. Gallup and Roper polls were taken in 1978. "The combined findings were that many people in fact did not know just how dangerous smoking was and what specific diseases it was casually linked to:  20 percent did not know smoking caused lung cancer, more than 30 percent were unaware of its link to heart disease, 40 percent of smokers thought only heavy smoking was dangerous, half of those polled did not know smoking could be addictive, and 60 percent did not know it caused emphysema. Nearly half the college-educated subjects in the sampling did not believe the statement that in industrialized nations cigarette smoking was the greatest single cause of excess deaths (i.e., beyond normal actuarial probability); twice as many believed traffic accidents were a greater killer as those who knew the truth."
*Ashes to Ashes*, p. 445

44.     Cigarette packs are required to carry warning labels, but those warnings aren't nearly as extensive as on other products, the magazine Priorities points out. The spring publication of the American Council on Science and Health offers a comparison between the warning on Camel Lights and the warning on a Camel lighter.
    The cigarette pack says "Surgeon General's warning: Cigarette smoke contains carbon monoxide."
    The cigarette-package-shaped promotional lighter says: "Important. Read Carefully!  Failure to follow instructions may result in burn injury. Danger--lighter contains butane gas under pressure. Extremely flammable. Do not use near fire or flame. Do not puncture, incinerate or expose to temperature from sun or otherwise above 120° Fahrenheit. Do not attempt to refill. Keep out of reach of children. As with all lighters, hold away from face while igniting. Caution:  Be sure the flame is extinguished after use."
Quote from American Medical News, August 1992

45. "...it's ironic that as a society, we spend billions to keep people from breathing asbestos--the EPA estimates 17 non-occupational asbestos-related deaths a year--but billions more to promote smoking."
Time, October 12, 1992, p. 76 (Andrew Tobias)

46. "Every smoke is a tiny drop of old age, so small that for a long time it is unnoticed."
Elinor Glyn, an ally of Lucy  Gaston,
National Anti-Cigarette League, about 1910 (*They Satisfy*, p. 61)

47. Yale's endowment of $5.8 billion includes $16.9 million of tobacco company stock, less than a third of one percent of the total. Universities which have removed tobacco stocks entirely from their portfolios include Harvard, Tufts, Northwestern, and Johns Hopkins.
Yale alumni magazine, February 1998, p. 13

48. Mel Gibson has bought the film rights to Christopher Buckley's book *Thank You for Smoking*.
Tobacco Control, Spring 1996, p. 64

49. Author Christopher Buckley spoke of an interview with a Tobacco Institute spokesperson. "I was in awe of this woman's powers of rationalization. It was clear that in the kingdom of the morally blind, this woman could echo-locate like a bat."
Tobacco Control, Spring 1996, p. 65

50. As of 1991 in the United States, there were 18,000 physicians, 322,000 registered nurses, and 128,000 licensed practical nurses who still smoked. Between 1974 and 1991, smoking declined from 18.8% to 3.3% among physicians, from 31.7% to 18.3% among RNs, and from 37.1% to 27.2% among LPNs.
*Tobacco*, p. 183

51. By 1980 because of use of reconstituted tobacco, 523 cigarettes were made from each pound of tobacco, compared with 382 in the late 1960's.
*Ashes to Ashes*, p. 550

52. Of all the things that could be done to reduce illness or prevent premature death, 50 percent of the total benefit is related to lifestyle changes, including not smoking, proper diet and exercise, wearing seat belts, and limiting alcohol consumption. Another 20 percent can be achieved by creating a safe and healthy environment, and 20 percent is related to genetics and heredity. Preventive medical care represents only 10 percent of the total

benefit. The life expectancy of men has increased from 45 years in 1900 to 75 years now; only five of those years are attributable to improved medical care, while the other 25 years are due to better sanitation, nutrition and safety.                    Rear Admiral William R. Rowley, Commander, Naval Medical Center, Portsmouth, Virginia (U.S. Medicine, August 1996, p. 26)

53. Nitric oxide (NO), a gas produced by cells lining the respiratory tract, is decreased in the exhaled air of cigarette smokers; this reduction is reversible after smoking cessation. NO has been reported to inhibit replication of respiratory pathogens, and lower levels in smokers may contribute to the adverse effects of smoking such as an increased incidence of lower respiratory tract infection.          Chest, August 1997, pp. 313-317

54. Smokers have an increased metabolism of caffeine. When smoking cessation is successful, the amount of caffeine present after a standard cup of coffee is higher than before, and the result may be unaccustomed jitteriness.      *The Harvard Guide to Women's Health*, Karen Carlson, Harvard University Press, 1996, p. 584

55. Smoking increases the metabolism of caffeine, and smoking cessation increases caffeine levels by 50% to 60%.
                      American Journal of Psychiatry, October 1996 supplement, p. 9

56. Methyl bromide is a significant depleter of the ozone layer. One of its largest uses is as a soil fumigant on tobacco farms.          Abstract S10/1, 10th World Conference on Tobacco or Health, Beijing, 1997

57. Health food stores now carry chemical and "additive-free" cigarettes such as American Spirit, Born Free, and Pure. They tend to be high in tar and nicotine content, and command a premium price, about a dollar a pack higher than regular brands.                Wall Street Journal, April 14, 1997, p. A1

58. Non-health messages on warning labels may be very effective in reducing smoking. Several examples are:
    - Men prefer women who don't smoke.
    - Women prefer men who don't smoke.
    - Smoking leads to premature wrinkles.
    - Smoking reduces athletic performance.
    - Smoking increases the risk of impotence.          *Smoke and Mirrors*, p. 252

59. "Tobacco is a dirty weed. I like it.
    It satisfies no normal need. I like it.
    It makes you thin, it makes you lean.
    It's the worst darn stuff I've ever seen. I like it."          G.L. Hemminger (*Tobacco Advertising*, p. 263)

60. "How big tobacco supports religious activities and the rewards it receives for doing so...Despite allegations of concern about people's health and promoting commandments linking activities that undermine people's health and well being with sin, for all intents and purposes, the Judaeo-Christian religions have been remarkably silent on the morality of smoking."
          Abstract OS 368 (Michael Crosby), 10th World Conference on Tobacco or Health, Beijing, 1997

61. Adults who smoke are 53% more likely to have been divorced than nonsmokers. Smoking does not cause divorce, but "those who smoke have characteristics and life experiences that make them more divorce-prone than nonsmokers."          USA Today, December 28, 1998, p. D1

62. A discount cigarette store called "Cigarettes Cheaper!" has 430 stores in 13 states, and the owner boasts that he is opening six new stores every week.          Joel Moskowitz, Ph.D., July 29, 1999

63. An average of less than one research dollar is spent per nicotine-addicted patient, compared to $55 for each person with HIV infection.          Alameda County Nicotine-Free Network News, December 1998

64. Most smokers do not perceive themselves at increased risk for heart attack (71%) or cancer (60%).
                      JAMA 1999; 281:1019-1021

65. In a study from the Harvard School of Public Health, male smokers of more than 15 cigarettes a day had more than a fourfold increased risk of suicide compared to nonsmoking men. "Although inference about causality is not justified, our findings indicate that the smoking-suicide connection is not entirely due to the greater tendency among smokers to be unmarried, to be sedentary, to drink heavily, or to develop cancers."

American Journal of Public Health, May 2000, p. 768

66. Two studies by the Massachusetts Department of Public Health and the nonprofit American Legacy Foundation document that cigarette makers have increased their advertising in magazines with large readerships by teenagers since 1998, when they agreed in a court settlement not to target teens in their ads. In the first 9 months of 1999, the industry spent $119.9 million on cigarette ads in magazines with a significant percentage of teen readers such as Rolling Stone, Glamour, Motor Trend and Sports Illustrated.     Associated Press, May 18, 2000

67. Nitrous oxide, or laughing gas, may help smokers quit the habit when used as a first step in treatment.

Associated Press, May 18, 2000

68. RJR's reduced smoke brand Eclipse where the tobacco is heated rather than burned is marketed with the claims of lower health risk than regular cigarettes.                JAMA, May 17, 2000, p. 2507

69. In a study from Japan and Denmark, the male-to-female sex ratio at birth among children of heavy smokers was 0.82, significantly lower than the male-to-female ratio (1.21) among children of nonsmokers. The proportion of male children born to a nonsmoking mother and a father who smoked heavily (0.98) also was significantly lower. "Cigarette smoking seems to reduce the frequency of male babies," the researchers said. One possible explanation is that sperm cells carrying the Y chromosome are more sensitive to deleterious effects of toxins in cigarette smoke than X-chromosome-bearing sperm.

JAMA, May 8, 2002, p. 2353 (from The Lancet, April 20, 2002)

70. In a study from Japan, the offspring sex ratio (male to female) when either or both parents smoked more than 20 cigarettes per day, was compared with couples where neither parent smoked. The ratio was 0.823 (255 boys and 310 girls) in the group where both parents smoked more than a pack a day, compared to 1.214 (1975 boys and 1627 girls born) in the group with nonsmoking parents.                The Lancet, April 20, 2002, p. 1407-1408

71. Cigarette butts account for 20% of all the trash collected in the United States (1996).     *The Tobacco Atlas*, p. 40

72. Cigarette butts are the most littered item in the world.

2002 National Conference on Tobacco or Health Abstract PREV-193

73. The Center for Marine Conservation's volunteers found 775,438 cigarette butts during their annual nationwide beach cleanup, accounting for 17% of all the trash collected.     American Medical News, September 13, 1993

74. In a survey of U.S. beach and shoreline cleanups, cigarette butts comprised 34.7% of all debris items collected. Bags and food wrappers at 11.9% were second on the "top ten" list.

Coastal Connection newsletter (the Ocean Conservancy), Summer 2002

75. Cigarette butts take one to five years to break down, and accounted for almost 20% of all items collected in the International Coastal Cleanup Project.                British Medical Association

76. After the September 2001 terrorist attacks, the FAA proposed a list of items, including matches and butane cigarette lighters, to be banned henceforth from all airline flights. A source reported to Mississippi Attorney General Michael Moore, who launched the successful state lawsuits against the tobacco industry, that the industry lobbied the Bush administration to have the matches and lighters removed from the banned list. They were indeed removed, apparently to facilitate smokers being able to light up as soon as they leave the plane at the end of the flight. Stanton Glantz and Joe Cherner, who released this information in July 2002, asked sarcastically why smokers should be punished just so the skies can be safe.

# Bidis

1. Bidis imported from India are the latest smoking fad with teens. They have higher levels of tar, carbon monoxide, and nicotine than regular cigarettes, and pose greater risks for throat, mouth, and lung cancer. Because of their sweet aroma and low price, public health experts have begun calling them "cigarettes with training wheels." They come in flavors, including chocolate, vanilla, and strawberry. Bidi smoke has three times as much nicotine and carbon monoxide and five times as much tar as smoke from a regular cigarette. 70% of bidis sold in 1998 had no warning labels and a quarter of stores illegally sold them to minors.
   *USA Today, August 5, 1999, p. A1*

2. Bidis resemble marijuana joints and have flavors, including mango, strawberry, vanilla, chocolate, and cinnamon. Because they do not have filters and are wrapped in nonporous leaves, a smoker needs to inhale more often and more deeply to keep it lit. One bidi produces three times more carbon monoxide and nicotine, and five times more tar than a regular cigarette.
   *Journal of the National Cancer Institute, November 3, 1999, pp. 1806-1807*

3. "The trendiest smoke on college campuses these days emanates from Indian imports called beedies (from the Hindi bidi)." They have up to 8% nicotine compared to 1% to 2% in American cigarettes and are unfiltered. They are hand rolled in Indian ebony leaves (tendu), and popular brands include Kailasand Mangalore Ganesh. Though they may have cult status in the U.S., in India where 800 billion are smoked every year, they have little cachet and remain the "poor man's cigarette." *Time, October 28, 1996, p. 28*

4. The bidi is perhaps the cheapest tobacco smoking product in the world, costing about one-third of one cent in India, where they are 8 to 10 times more common than cigarettes. A bidi contains about a quarter of the tobacco of a cigarette, yet delivers a higher amount of tar and nicotine.
   *11th World Conference on Tobacco or Health, Chicago, 2000, Abstract CA 01*

5. Bidi cigarettes contain higher concentrations of nicotine than conventional cigarettes, findings that belie a popular belief among young smokers that bidis might be a safe alternative to standard cigarettes.
   *Tobacco Control, June 2001, p. 181*

6. A study in the December 2002 issue of Nicotine and Tobacco Research showed that bidis and additive-free cigarettes are no less toxic than conventional cigarettes.

# Filter Cigarettes

1. "The other important development of the 1950s was the introduction of the filter cigarette--not, the companies were keen to point out, that there was anything wrong with the unfiltered kind. It was just that modern smokers seemed to be demanding less tar and nicotine. Even so, the acceptance of filters was by no means instantaneous. One of the functions of the Marlboro Man was to undermine the commonly-held belief that they were for sissies, and in 1960, Pall Mall (selling point: 'You can light either end') overtook the equally unfiltered Camel as America's best-selling cigarette." *Faber Book of Smoking, p. 106*

2. "Filtered cigarettes, however, were comparatively flavourless. It seemed that the public were prepared to sacrifice taste for the perception of safety. RJR gambled against the trend toward tasteless cigarettes, opting to load their new filter tip with tar and nicotine, so that even after the filter had done its work, some taste and tar would remain intact, In deference, however, to the modern smoker's less discriminating palates, they decided that quality of taste could be compromised, and that their new filter brand might make use of the 30 percent or so of tobacco wasted in processing in the manufacture of normal cigarettes. After rigorous experiments with a coffee grinder and a pulp press, RJR came up with RST--Reconstituted Sheet Tobacco--which used all the stems, leaf ribs, tobacco scraps, and dust which had hitherto been thrown away. 'Winston', their new filtered wonder, made extensive use of RST. It was offered to the public with the promise 'Winston brings flavor back into cigarette smoking!' and the guarantee 'Winston tastes good, like a cigarette should." *Tobacco (Gately), p. 275*

3. More than 90% of all cigarettes sold worldwide have filters.

2002 AMA Annual Tobacco Report

4. In the United States, cigarettes produced with filters increased from 0.6% in 1950 to 98% in 1998.

*Women and Smoking*, p. 47

# Menthol Cigarettes

1. "Mentholated cigarettes were impregnated with an extract of peppermint, that was also used by vets as a local anesthetic. The first menthol brand was the evocatively named 'Spud', which had been introduced in the 1930s. It was not alone for long. A second tier manufacturer named Brown & Williamson, sensing a future in healthier cigarettes, introduced its own menthol brand which it baptized 'Kool.' Kool's marketing promised smokers the opportunity to indulge without fear of laryngeal irritation: 'Give your throat a Kool vacation!' By the 1950s, there was a range of menthol brands and the category was an independent and profitable market."

*Tobacco* (Gately), p. 273

2. "Does winter make your head feel stuffy? Steam-heated rooms parch your throat? Heavy smoking 'brown' your taste? Then you've three extra reasons for changing to KOOLS. They're mildly mentholated. Light up and feel that instant refreshment. Smoke deep; the choice Turkish-Domestic tobacco flavor is all there. Smoke long; your throat and tongue stay cool and smooth, your mouth clean and fresh. Change to KOOLS. It's a change for the better."

"Give your throat a Kool vacation! Like a week by the sea, this mild menthol is a tonic to hot, tired throats."

1933 ad (*Clearing the Smoke*, p. 62)

77. Because menthol cigarettes provide a sensation of cooling when smoked, they may promote deeper and more prolonged inhalation.

*Growing up Tobacco Free*, p. 56

3. The tobacco industry once promoted the mentholated cigarette as a health benefit. Yet, African American smokers, who disproportionately smoke menthol cigarettes, have an increased risk for cancer and cardiovascular mortality. In 1925, the first mentholated cigarette hit the market; however, it was in the mid-1950s, when R.J. Reynolds introduced Salem to compete with Brown & Williamson's Kool, that mentholated cigarettes increased in popularity. Lorillard's Newport brand quickly followed. By the 1960s, menthol cigarettes had doubled their market share and tobacco companies were actively seeking control of this market, as several new mentholated variations of existing brands were introduced. By the early 1990s, Newport had become the brand of choice for 75% of African American teenage smokers…Indeed, Newport, the top U.S. menthol brand, is now second only to Marlboro in market share. Because of the association of menthol with medications, many consumers believe that menthol cigarettes are safer. Far from being innocuous, menthol in tobacco has been shown to increase carbon monoxide and nicotine levels, expand the bronchial passages to increase particulate permeation into the lungs, and may result in increased retention of smoke constituents in the lungs, all contributing to increased body burden of toxins.

2002 National Conference on Tobacco or Health, Abstracts D+D-30 and 181 (quote)

4. "Menthol increases salivary flow and acts as a bronchodilator. Although mentholated cigarettes were first sold to the public in the 1920s, menthol market share remained low until the 1960s and now accounts for about 25% of all cigarettes sold domestically in the USA." Tobacco Control, December 2002, p. 368

# Warning Labels

1. One of the new Canada warning labels, picturing a mother smoking in front of her daughter: "WARNING. CHILDREN SEE, CHILDREN DO. Your children are twice as likely to smoke if you do. Half of all premature deaths among life-long smokers result from tobacco use." Tobacco Control, September 2002, p. 186

2. In January 2001, new warning labels began on cigarettes sold in Canada. The 16 rotating labels cover half the front and back panels of the packs, one side in English and the other in French. Some labels have photos of a

gangrenous foot, a diseased heart, lung cancer, and a sick baby connected to hospital monitors. Another has a picture of a limp cigarette with the caption, "Tobacco Use Can Make You Impotent."

San Francisco Chronicle, January 3, 2001, p. A9

3. In 2001, Canada began to require large graphic health warnings on cigarette packs. One features a limp cigarette with the logo "Tobacco use can make you impotent," and another, a photo of rotting gums and the warning "Cigarettes cause mouth diseases." Others show a damaged brain with a warning about strokes, and two children with the large caption "Don't poison us."

Newsweek, March 25, 2002, p. 9

4. Within a year of the graphic health warnings appearing on cigarette packets in Canada, about 44% of smokers said they felt like quitting; 58% said they had become more concerned about their health; 27% smoked less at home, and 62% thought the pictures made it unpleasant to look at cigarette packs. The industry is threatening legal action. Philip Morris claimed graphic health warnings would impair the use of the company's valuable trademarks by obscuring the packet face. The graphic warnings, it said, would "unnecessarily" limit the company's right to communicate with its customers because existing text health warnings already covered one-third of the package.

2003 AMA Annual Tobacco Report

5. Thailand will be the third country in the world, following Canada and Brazil, to have graphic health warnings printed on cigarette packets. Several tobacco-related diseases will be depicted, including lung cancer, heart failure, chronic obstructive pulmonary disease, stroke, erectile dysfunction, premature aging, oral cancer and stained teeth. The graphic warnings will cover half of the front and back of cigarette packs.

2003 AMA Annual Tobacco Report

6. Israel, China, Vietnam, and Romania do not require health warnings on cigarette packs.

Earth Island Journal, Spring 2002, p. 17

7. "Since smoking might injure your health, let's be careful not to smoke too much."

Japan's cigarette warning label (Tobacco Control, September 2001, p. 293)

# Internet Tobacco Sales

1. "The ideal product to sell online would be easy to pack and ship, be much cheaper than what's charged at the retail counter, and be craved by tens of million of people. Cigarettes, the internet was made for you." Hundreds of cigarette websites have sprung up, selling cigarettes for about 30% less than local stores, and without ID checks or the surgeon general's warning….Some of the proprietors ambitiously estimating that the online world will eventually gain as much as 20% of the $50 billion U.S. tobacco business." However, the states are getting tough on tax-evading online sales.

Washington Post, September 3, 2000 (David Streitfeld)

2. "…the internet continues to provide ready access to cheap, untaxed cigarettes without proof of age." At the end of 2000, there were 68 U.S. websites selling cigarettes.

Tobacco Control, September 2002, p. 226

3. A story in the September 24, 2001, *Wall Street Journal* describes tobacco sales over the Internet. "Visitors to BarbisButts.com can order a carton of Marlboros for $28.75--abut a third less than in a bricks-and-mortar store in New York. Serious bargain hunters can buy cut-rate cigarettes with names such as Market and Niagara for as little as $10 a carton, or $1 a pack. The website, decorated with a silvery profile a buxom woman, says the company ships its wares from an Indian reservation near Salamanca in western New York State. Barbi's Butts promises that all information about customer orders will be kept 'strictly confidential'--which could make it easier for smokers to avoid paying state excise taxes on the cigarettes they buy."

A survey by the Massachusetts Health Department found that over 200 websites sell cigarettes and other tobacco products. Some, like Barbi's Butts, are based on Indian reservations. Others are small retailers based in the U.S. and overseas. "Collecting taxes on cigarettes sold online isn't easy. A federal law, the Jenkins Act, requires companies that ship cigarettes across state lines to report the names and addresses of buyers (other than licensed distributors) to state tax authorities. The law says companies must file those reports every month or risk being fined. "But state tax collectors say that the law is widely flouted. Many websites promise not to divulge the identity of purchasers and states generally haven't been aggressive about pursuing them."

Another survey identified 88 internet cigarette vendors. Nearly half, or 43 websites, were located in New York state and many were in tobacco producing states with low excise taxes. Indian reservations housed 49 of the 88 sites.

2002 AMA Annual Tobacco Report

4.   A federal appeals court has upheld a New York state law that bans sales of cigarettes over the internet and by mail order. Tobacco companies had argued that the law violated the U.S. Constitution.

Wall Street Journal Interactive Edition, February 14, 2003

5.   State tax-evading internet cigarette sales are expected to make up 14% of the U.S. cigarette market by 2005, with lost state tax revenue of $1.4 billion. An 18-wheel truck can haul 800,000 packs of cigarettes; a smuggled load from Virginia, where the tax is 2½ cents a pack, to New York City, where the tax is $3, can evade over $2 million in taxes in a single truckload.          U.S. News and World Report, November 4, 2002, pp. 46-47

6.   The ongoing increase in internet sales of tobacco products is a major challenge to public health efforts to reduce smoking and other tobacco use. By failing to do adequate age verification, the sharply growing number of websites selling tobacco products make it easier and cheaper for kids to buy cigarettes. They also offer smokers a way to avoid paying state tobacco and sales taxes, thereby keeping cigarette prices down and smoking levels up...Up from only a handful in the late 1990s, more than 200 websites in the U.S. and many more based overseas sell tobacco products. Internet tobacco sales are growing rapidly and will account for 14 percent of the total U.S. market by 2005, according to a recent Prudential securities report. One in five cigarette-selling websites do not even say that sales to minors are prohibited, and more than half require only that the buyers say they are of legal age, according to an upcoming study in the American Journal of Public Health.

Three-quarters of all internet tobacco sellers explicitly say that they will not report cigarette sales to tax collection officials, thus violating federal law, according to the U.S. General Accounting Office. States lose as much as $200 million annually in uncollected tobacco taxes through internet sales.

quote from Special Report: Internet Tobacco Sales, March 5, 2003, www.tobaccofreekids.org

# CHAPTER 41
# CIGARETTES AND FIRES

1. Cigarettes are the number one cause of fires in the home, and fires from smoking in bed and other cigarette mishaps account for almost half a billion dollars in property damage annually in the United States.

   *Cigarette Confidential*, p. 6

2. "A large proportion of fires in homes and hotels are caused by smoking. Insurance companies estimate that there were 2500 deaths due to accidental fires caused by smoking in 1980. Additionally, smoking contributes to many motor vehicle accidents by causing carbon monoxide intoxication and by distracting the driver. It is estimated that smoking caused about 1500 excess deaths from accidents other than fire during 1980, for a total of 4000 excess deaths from all kinds of accidents attributable to smoking."

   American Journal of Preventive Medicine, April 1985, p. 12

3. Smoking materials (especially cigarettes) are responsible for 28% of all household fire deaths. There were 163,000 fires from this cause in 1992, resulting in 1075 deaths, 3232 injuries, and $318 million in property damage.

   *Cigarettes*, p. 164

4. Fire deaths caused by unattended smoldering cigarettes in upholstery and bedding total 1500 per year, including 130 children.

   *Nicotine Addiction*, p. 16

5. A December 1992 coal mine explosion in Virginia which killed 8 was caused by smoking, which is illegal in mines because of danger of flammable methane gas.

   New York Times, December 22, 1992

6. In 1996 there were an estimated 417,000 total residential fires (including those unrelated to smoking) in the United States, resulting in 4035 deaths, almost 19,000 injuries, and nearly $5 billion in property loss.

   JAMA, May 27, 1998, p. 1633

7. In 1994 there were 134,100 cigarette-caused residential fires in the United States, causing $446 million in property damage, 909 deaths, and 3,000 serious injuries. 39% of those killed in these fires were not the smokers themselves. The tobacco industry gives millions of dollars each year to fire departments and fire safety organizations; the result has been that these organizations have not been aggressive in promoting fire-safe cigarettes.

   Contra Costa (California) Times, January 18, 1998, p. F9

8. Technology has existed for more than ten years for designing a fire-safe cigarette by using less tightly packed tobacco and less porous rolling paper. The resulting cigarette would burn at a lower temperature and be less likely to cause a fire.

   Contra Costa (California) Times, February 20, 1998, p. A8

9. Cigarettes are responsible for about 1,000 fire deaths each year in the United States, about a quarter of the national toll. Many scientists and fire officials say that small changes in cigarette design would make them less likely to start fires, and many bills have been introduced in state legislatures and the US Congress to require cigarettes to meet a fire safety or resistance standard. The tobacco industry, however, has spent millions of dollars to make an alliance with fire safety organizations, and some of these groups, grateful for the financial support, seem to have accepted the industry's argument that fire-safe cigarettes are not feasible.

   Contra Costa Times, January 2, 1998 (from Los Angeles Times, Myron Levin)

10. 25% of fatal residential fires begin when smokers fall asleep in bed with lighted cigarettes, or a lighted cigarette is dropped on a couch or chair. In 1997, about 900 people, including 140 children, were killed in the 136,900 fires caused by tobacco materials, and there were 2479 injuries and $436 million in property damage.

   New York Times, January 11, 2000, and San Francisco Chronicle, May 17, 2000

11. Every year, a million fires are started by children using cigarette lighters.

   *The Tobacco Atlas*, p. 41

12. "Fires caused by smoking cause more than $27 billion in damage every year worldwide and kill hundreds of thousands."

   San Francisco Chronicle, October 23, 2002, p. D3

13. From 1994 to 1998, smoking caused an average annual death toll of 966 from residential fires.

JAMA, May 8, 2002, p. 2355

14. Cigarette fires kill 1000 Americans a year, accounting for one in four fire deaths. Tobacco companies have repeatedly tried to defeat fire safety bills in the states. The bills are designed to reduce cigarette flammability.

Los Angeles Times, August 21, 2000

15. A cigarette tossed from a vehicle caused a 10,500-acre fire in Alpine, California, near San Diego, in January 2001.

Associated Press

16. Cigarettes are the leading cause of fire death in the USA, accounting for an estimated 30% of all fire deaths. Each year in the USA, approximately 1000 people die and billions of dollars are spent in property damages, health care, lost productivity, and fire and emergency services due to fires caused by cigarettes. The USA suffers on of the highest fire death rates in the industrialized world, although cigarette fires remain a worldwide problem with 10% of global fire deaths attributable to smoking.

   The tobacco industry has opposed fire safe cigarette legislation for the last 25 years. The industry has claimed, on an assortment of grounds, that it was not feasible to produce a fire safe cigarette. At various times, the industry stated that (1) fire safe cigarettes would be unacceptable to consumers; (2) that no testing method would accurately predict whether a cigarette was fire safe; (3) that fire safe cigarettes would increase toxicity; and (4) that cigarettes were not the primary problem of cigarette caused fires. Internal industry documents, however, contradict the industry's public claims. The industry has done research on this issue for more than 25 years, and has had numerous projects dedicated to creating a fire safe cigarette. A fire safe cigarette with demonstrated consumer acceptability was developed years ago, and the tobacco industry did not place it on the market.

Quote from Tobacco Control, December 2002, pp. 346 and 351

17. The world's worst cigarette-caused fire was caused by several forestry workers in northeastern China in 1987. It burned 3.1 million acres of forest and killed 300 people.

*Tobacco Control in the Third World*, p. 141 and *The Tobacco Atlas*, p. 41

18. In 2000, New York became the first state to pass legislation (effective in late 2003) requiring cigarettes companies to produce cigarettes modified so that they are fire-safe and burn out rather than keep burning when no one puffs on them. Philip Morris test marketed a fire-safe Marlboro in 1987, but shelved the research until "public pressure builds unduly." The tobacco industry has successfully blocked all other legislation similar to that passed in New York.          New York Times, February 20, 2003, and Newsday, August 14, 2002

19. A few years ago, New York State passed a law requiring all cigarettes sold in the state of New York to be "fire-safe" or "low-ignition." New York gave cigarette manufacturers two years (until July 2003) to comply. Fire-safe cigarettes automatically go out when they are not being smoked, so a cigarette left by a smoker who falls asleep in bed would go out, instead of causing a fire. Philip Morris hates this law because it reduces the number of cigarettes sold. Instead of burning to the end, fire-safe cigarettes go out and can be re-lit by the smoker. The smoker need not buy new cigarettes. He/she can simply re-light old ones.

   If Philip Morris sells fire-safe cigarettes in New York, it cannot justify selling other cigarettes in the rest of the country. If it does, people who die in cigarette-caused fires in other states will sue, and Philip Morris will have no excuse.

   Consequently, Philip Morris is lobbying hard to prevent New York from implementing its law.

quote from Smokescreen.org e-mail of February 11, 2003 (Joe Cherner and Bill Godshall)

20. In 2000, fires caused by smoking worldwide killed 300,000 people, or 10% of all fire deaths, and cost a total of U.S. $27 billion.

*The Tobacco Atlas*, p. 41

# CHAPTER 42
# TOBACCO AND THE MOVIES

1. Lois Lane never smoked in the comic strip, but in *Superman II* prominently smoked Marlboro Lights.
   Canadian Medical Association Journal, December 1, 1990, p. 1351

2. For a reported payment of $42,000, Philip Morris purchased 22 exposures of the Marlboro logo in the 1980 movie *Superman II*. Lois Lane, a newspaper reporter and role model for teenage girls, has a Marlboro pack on her desk and is shown puffing merrily away. At one point in the film, a character is tossed into a van with a large Marlboro sign on its side, and in the climactic scene the super-hero battles foes amid a maze of Marlboro billboards before zooming off in triumph, leaving in his wake a solitary taxi with a Marlboro sign on top.
   Quote from Mother Jones, May-June 1996, p. 48

3. Philip Morris placed tobacco products in children's movies like the *Muppet Movie* and *Who Framed Roger Rabbit*.
   ANR Update, Summer 1998

4. In a review of 50 G-rated animated films, 56% portrayed one or more incidences of tobacco use, including all seven films released in 1996 and 1997.
   JAMA, March 24/31, 1999, p. 1131

5. In the 1996 John Grisham movie *A Time to Kill*, Sandra Bullock plays a hotshot law student who smokes for much of her time on camera. The chance that a top law student in the 1990's would be a smoker is less than one in ten.

6. In a study of 40 movies produced in 1935, 30% of heroines smoked, compared to only 2.5% of villainesses. The comparable figures that year were 65% for heroes and 22.5% for male villains.
   New York State Journal of Medicine, July 1985, p. 337

7. "Films present a smoker who is typically white, male, and attractive, a movie hero who takes smoking for granted. As in tobacco advertising, smoking in the movies is associated with youthful vigor, good looks, and personal/professional acceptance....Films reinforce misleading images and overstate the normalcy of smoking, which may encourage children and teenagers, the major movie audience, to smoke."
   American Journal of Public Health, June 1994, p. 999

8. Liggett and Myers paid $30,000 for cigarette placement in the movie *Supergirl*.
   USA Today, January 3, 1997, p. 12A

9. Philip Morris paid $350,000 to get Lark cigarettes featured in the 1989 James Bond movie *Licence to Kill*.
   San Francisco Chronicle, June 20, 1994, p. A5

10. Movie heroes are three times more likely to smoke than their real-life role models in American society. Although only 19 percent of Americans of high socioeconomic status smoke, 57 percent of their movie counterparts do.
    American Journal of Public Health, June 1994, p. 998

11. Eight was the average number of times a film from the 1970's or 1980's showed someone smoking or made a reference to cigarettes. Twenty five was the average number in a film of the late 1990's.
    Health magazine, July-August 1998, p. 18

12. A study of top-grossing movies found that movie stars smoke at three times the rate of the audiences watching them. The most frequent users of tobacco were young white men in leading roles who tended to be the heroes. The study author, Stanton Glantz, said that movies appear to suggest that smoking is normal and even admirable behavior. "Films portrayed the smoker in the same way that tobacco advertising does."
    American Journal of Public Health, June 1994, p. 989

13. In a study, which examined five top films chosen randomly for each year from 1990 through 1996, 57% of leading characters smoked, compared with 14% of people of similar demographic backgrounds in the general

population. Fully 80% of male leads smoked. The study, published by Stanton Glantz in the winter 1998 issue of Tobacco Control, found that tobacco was used once every three to five minutes, an increase from once every 10 to 15 minutes in movies from the 1970's and 1980's. *American Medical News*, April 6, 1998

14. Sylvester Stallone was offered $500,000 to use Brown and Williamson cigarettes in the films *Rambo, Rocky IV, Godfather III*, and *Rhinestone Cowboy*. The company spent $1 million over a four-year period to put images of its cigarettes into the movies. *New York Times*, May 20, 1994, p. A8

15. In 1983, Sylvester Stallone guaranteed in writing to smoke Brown and Williamson cigarettes in five of his upcoming films for a payment of $500,000. B & W terminated the contract before all the films were made because of disappointment with the lack of prominent placement achieved. *The Cigarette Papers*, p. 365

16. In a March 1996 study, 77% of 133 current movies portrayed tobacco use. Walt Disney Pictures was rated the best, with an average of "only" six smoking situations per movie, followed by 20th Century Fox and Universal Pictures. At the bottom were Miramax Films and Castle Rock Entertainment, with 45 and 34 incidents, respectively. While only 3 percent of the American population smoke cigars, they were depicted in more than half of those movies with tobacco use. *San Francisco Chronicle*, September 15, 1996, Datebook, p. 56

17. The American Lung Association studied 133 movies released in 1994 and 1995, and found that 77% showed tobacco use. Of 18 films playing in theaters in October 1996, only one was smokeless. 10 of these films featured more than 15 smoking scenes, and all of the top ten films featured tobacco use. *USA Today*, November 7, 1996, p. 6D

18. In 1991, 3.5% of American men smoked cigars. In a 1994-95 movie survey, 52% of the 133 movies featured cigar smoking, and in a survey of 18 current films, 56% included cigar smoking. *USA Today*, November 7, 1996, p. 6D

19. A survey of 1996 movies showed an average of 36 instances of smoking in each movie. *NBC Evening News*, Tom Brokaw, March 21, 1997

20. Half of the top grossing films between 1990 and 1995 had scenes where a lead character smoked, up from 29% in films of the 1970's. *San Francisco Chronicle*, September 18, 1997, p. A13

21. In the summer of 1997 in one week, all five of the top five box office films featured smoking: *Men in Black, Face Off, Hercules, Batman and Robin*, and *My Best Friend's Wedding*. Characters played by Arnold Schwarzenegger, Bruce Willis, Brad Pitt, John Travolta, Meg Ryan, Sharon Stone, and Julia Roberts all smoked onscreen. John Travolta is a nonsmoker, but he has smoked on screen in *Get Shorty, Broken Arrow, Michael, Pulp Fiction* and *She's So Lovely*. Every film nominated for best picture at the 1997 Academy Awards had smoking featured.
*USA Today*, August 25, 1997, pp. D1-D2, and *New York Times*, August 24, 1997, p. 1 (section 2)

22. In *Beverly Hills Cop*, Eddie Murphy holds a pack of Lucky Strikes and says: "These cigarettes are very popular with the children." He then says that he personally prefers king-size Kents. In *Who Framed Roger Rabbit*, Betty Boop offers Camels to the detective, and Lucky Strike ads are also featured. *UICC Tobacco Control Fact Sheet 1*, International Union Against Cancer, 1996

23. In Hollywood, the health plans of the Screen Actors Guild and unions representing screenwriters and directors have sued the tobacco industry to seek to recover millions of dollars in smoking-related medical costs. *Associated Press*, November 27, 1997

24. Representatives of the Screen Actors Guild, Directors Guild, and Writers Guild, along with model Christy Turlington, met at the White House on December 3, 1997, and joined Vice President Al Gore to announce voluntary restraints to end the glamorization of cigarettes in television and movies. 77% of all movies released in 1996 showed tobacco use. *The Advocacy Institute*, December 4, 1997

25. "Leonardo DiCaprio smoking pensively on the Titanic deck is classic Marlboro Man. The swells in first class trading cigarettes are Dunhill. The rough-and-tumble crowd in steerage rolling their own could be taken as coded reference to the no-frills, no-additive, no-bull Winston, while Kate Winslet blowing smoke in her mother's face is very much 'You've come a long way, baby'--Virginia Slims... In *Titanic*, smoking is sexy and social and sophisticated and genuine and rebellious..." New Yorker, March 9, 1998, P. 31 (Malcolm Gladwell)

26. California anti-tobacco leaders and Rep. Vic Fazio have organized the "Hackademy Awards" reviewing smoking in movies. 100 teenagers reviewed 250 movies for 1997-98, and gave the thumbs-down award to *Titanic*, a Marlboro award to *Men in Black* (recommending it be renamed Men with Black Lungs), and the Stinkin' Stogie award to *Batman and Robin*, where Arnold Schwarzenegger would not stop lighting his cigars. The Best Anti-Tobacco Movie award went to *As Good As it Gets*, which called attention to asthma and the negative effects of smoking. *The Lost World* and *Tomorrow Never Dies* were recommended as movies with a minimal amount of smoking. The California Aggie (U.C. Davis newspaper), April 16, 1998

27. "he tobacco industry also received an unintentional assist from Hollywood. During the 1930s and 1940s, actors, directors, and writers discovered the cigarette as a prop. The 1933 film *Roberta* features one of the most famous smoking moments in Hollywood as wafts of smoke surround Irene Dunne while she sings, "When a lovely flame dies, smoke gets in your eyes." Marlene Dietrich, Carole Lombard, Jean Harlow, and Claudette Colbert smoked up the screens, while Lauren Bacall, in the 1944 film *To Have and Have Not*, oozed sex appeal when she asked the simple question, "Anybody got a match?" Smoking could convey sophistication (Audrey Hepburn as Holly Golightly puffed on a cigarette holder in *Breakfast at Tiffany's*); strength and isolation (Humphrey Bogart in *Casablanca*); and tawdriness (Diane Keaton as the good-girl teacher gone bad in *Looking for Mr. Goodbar*). Quote from *Cigarettes* (Parker-Pope), p. 94

28. "Davis smokes all through the movie. In a age when stars used cigarettes as props, she doesn't smoke as behavior, or to express her moods, but because she wants to. She inhales needfully. The smoking is invaluable in setting her apart from others, making her separate from their support and demands; she is often seen within a cloud of smoke, which seems like her charisma made visible."
Roger Ebert describing Bette Davis in the 1950 movie *All About Eve*
*The Great Movies*, Broadway Books, 2002, p. 31

29. In the 1942 movie *Now, Voyageur*, Paul Henreid several times lit two cigarettes in his mouth, and then handed one to Bette Davis.

30. Actor James Dean, star of the 1955 movie *Rebel Without a Cause*, smoked both in his movie roles and in real life. *Tobacco* (Gately), p. 271

31. In *Superman II* in 1980, Lois Lane smoked Marlboros throughout the film despite the fact that she never smoked in the comic book series. Philip Morris paid a reported product placement fee of $42,000; Marlboro appeared 22 times, including one battle scene with a backdrop of Marlboro billboards. *Tobacco* (Gately), pp. 331-332

32. Sissy Spacek chain-smokes Marlboros in the 2001 movie *In the Bedroom*, and Marlboros are mentioned by name twice in the movie. New York Time, January 21, 2002, p. A15
(from Smoke Free Movies organization ad)

33. The American Lung Association will give its Hackademy Award to Sissy Spacek and *In the Bedroom* for using Marlboros throughout the film. Dishonorable Mentions will go to *Charlie's Angels* and *Save the Last Dance*-- smoke-filled movies aimed at adolescents. "Teens imitate onscreen behavior," says Doran. "And it's not enough to make the good guy a non-smoker because bad guys are cool." Quote from Time, March 18, 2002, p. 79

34. If the movie industry made every movie with smoking R-rated, "the hue and cry about free speech would disappear overnight--99 percent of the smoking in movies would evaporate."
Los Angeles Times, March 17, 2002

35. One of the documents was a 1983 draft of a speech prepared for a Philip Morris executive that referred to the anti-smoking efforts at the time, stating, "Smoking is being positioned as an unfashionable, as well as

unhealthy, custom. We must use every creative means at our disposal to reverse this destructive trend. I do feel heartened at the increasing number of occasions when I go to a movie and see a pack of cigarettes in the hands of the leading lady." Depictions of smoking in movies have been steadily increasing, with nearly 85 percent of the top 25 highest-grossing movies released from 1988 to 1997 showing tobacco use, according to a released in 2001 by Dartmouth Medical School. The depictions of smoking in movies have a direct correlation with teenagers who start smoking, according to the report. Teenagers who don't smoke but see their favorite actors frequently smoke on screen are 16 times more likely to have positive attitudes toward smoking in the future.

Quote from San Francisco Chronicle, March 13, 2002, p. A2

36. An article by Stanton Glantz and C. McKemson in Tobacco Control (March 2002, supplement, pp. 81-91) described the relationship between the tobacco industry and the entertainment industry, and how tobacco companies hired aggressive product placement firms to arrange for showing cigarette brands in Hollywood movies and television programs. By 2000, the average amount of smoking in movies exceeded levels observed in the 1960's. One production company pointed out to RJR in a memo that "film is better than any commercial. Because the audience is totally unaware of any sponsor involvement...." A 1989 Philip Morris marketing plan stated: "We believe that most of the strong, positive images for cigarettes and smoking are created by cinema and television. We have seen the heroes smoking in Wall Street, Crocodile Dundee, and Roger Rabbit. Mickey Rourke, Mel Gibson and Goldie Hawn are forever seen, both on and off screen, with a lighted cigarette."

37. In a study of school children ages 9 to 15 years, there was a strong association between seeing tobacco use in movies and trying cigarettes; the more smoking that the group saw in movies, the more likely they were to smoke themselves. This finding supports the hypothesis that smoking in films has a role in the initiation of smoking in adolescents.
British Medical Journal, December 15, 2001, pp. 1394

38. ". . . nearly half of the G-rated animated feature films available on video cassette show alcohol and tobacco use as normative behavior and do not convey the long-term consequences of their use."
Pediatrics, June 2001, p. 1369

39. A study of 87 G-rated animated (cartoon) feature movies made between 1937 and 2000 found that nearly half showed characters using alcohol or tobacco.
Associated Press, June 5, 2001

40. 87% of the top 25 annual box office movies from 1988 to 1997 featured some use of tobacco.
San Francisco Chronicle, September 20, 2002, p. A26

41. "While sports is by far the best avenue to attract, sample and influence our core target smokers, it's not the only way. International movies and videos also have tremendous appeal to our young adult consumers in Asia."
Philip Morris (from 2001 publication "How do you sell death?"<br>from Campaign for Tobacco-Free Kids)

42. Two out of three tobacco scenes from the 50 highest-grossing movies released from the spring of 2000 to March 2001 were in movies rated G, PG, and PG13; the previous year, only 21% of the tobacco spots were in "kid-rated" films.
Smoke Free Movies Flier (www.smokefreemovies.ucsf.edu)

43. The 20 top-grossing films featured 50% more instances of smoking each hour in 2000 compared to 1960.
Smoke Free Movies ad, April 2002

44. "Smoking in movies may have a powerful influence on the decision of young people to smoke", and seeing smoking in movies may account for about one third of adolescent smoking.
Conference on Tobacco or Health Abstract PREV-117 and<br>James Sargent, M.D. lecture, San Francisco, November 14, 2002

45. "Worst offenders include Julia Roberts, sitting splay-legged with her pack of Marlboros in My Best Friend's Wedding; Bruce Willis in The Last Boy Scout, punching out a kidnaper over a pack of Marlboros; Al Pacino sucking on Winstons in Sea of Love, and the endless, leitmotif-like appearance of packages of Kool throughout There's Something About Mary."
Globe and Mail, February 13, 2001

46. Leading a smoke-filled best picture category, *Chicago* received the "Thumbs Down" Hackademy Award by the American Lung Association of Sacramento-Emigrant Trails for its multitudinous scenes of gratuitous tobacco use as the stars used cigarettes and cigars to depict toughness, sexiness, rebelliousness, wealth and power.

In *Chicago*, supporting actress nominee Catherine Zeta-Jones tries to look sexier and more glamorous by smoking in almost every scene, even while dancing; Richard Gere chomps on a cigar to display his power and wealth; and fellow supporting actress nominee Queen Latifah smokes to show a rougher edge.

This is the seventh Hackademy Awards, and the second in a row in which every Best Picture nominee included scenes of tobacco use. *Chicago and Gangs of New York* both have excessive tobacco use, but *Chicago* got the nod for the Hackademy Award because of its PG-13 rating, which allows teenagers entrance without being accompanied by an adult.

The Hackademy Awards were begun in 1996 as a fun way to bring to light a serious problem--how tobacco use by movie stars entices teenagers to pick up the habit. Recent Dartmouth University studies indicate that teens exposed to extensive smoking in films are three times more likely to try smoking than teens with limited exposure. Non-smoking teens whose favorite stars smoke on screen are 16 time more likely to have positive attitudes toward smoking in the future.

For their "Thumbs Up!" Hackademy Award, the teens honored the movie *Legally Blonde*.

Quote from zap2it.com, March 19, 2003

# CHAPTER 43
# PERSONALITIES, CELEBRITIES, AND "FAMOUS DEATHS"

A comprehensive list of celebrities who have died from smoking is found online at www.tobacco.org - click on heading "A Few of Our Losses..."

Celebrities who died from smoking, some with diagnosis and age at death

Gracie Allen, actress, 58, heart attack. She lived with her husband, George Burns, an inveterate cigar smoker, for 38 years.

Steven Ambrose, author and historian, 66, lung cancer

Louis Armstrong, musician, 74, heart attack

Desi Arnaz, actor and husband of Lucille Ball, 69, lung cancer

Lucille Ball, actress, 78, aortic aneurysm

Tallulah Bankhead, actress, 65, lung cancer or emphysema

William "Count" Basie, bandleader, 79, pancreatic cancer

Jack Benny, comedian, 80, pancreatic cancer

Leonard Bernstein, composer and conductor, 72, heart attack and emphysema

Amanda Blake, actress (Miss Kitty on Gunsmoke), 60, throat cancer

Bill Blass, fashion designer ("the urbane couturier who defined American style by marrying comfort with elegance" –Time Magazine, June 2002), 79, throat cancer

Humphrey Bogart, actor, 57, cancer of the esophagus

Yul Brynner, actor, 65, lung cancer

Jack Buck, Hall of Fame sports broadcaster, 77, lung cancer

Rory Calhoun, actor, 76, emphysema

Herb Coen, San Francisco Chronicle columnist, 80, lung cancer

John Candy, actor, 43, heart attack

President Grover Cleveland, 71, mouth cancer

Rosemary Clooney, singer, 74, lung cancer

Ty Cobb, baseball player, 74, cancer and heart disease

Nat "King" Cole, singer, 45, lung cancer

Chuck Connors, actor, 71, lung cancer

Noel Coward, playwright, 73, heart attack

Gary Cooper, actor, 60, lung cancer

Bette Davis, actress, 81, stroke

Sammy Davis, Jr., entertainer, 64, throat cancer

Colleen Dewhurst, actress, 67, lung cancer

Joe DiMaggio, baseball player, 84, lung cancer

Joe DiMaggio, Jr., 57, emphysema

Everett Dirksen, former Senate majority leader, 75, lung cancer

Walt Disney, 65, lung cancer

T.S. Eliot, author and poet, 76, emphysema

Duke Ellington, composer and bandleader, 75, lung cancer

George Fennemen, announcer for Groucho Marx, 77, emphysema

F. Scott Fitzgerald, writer, 44, heart attack

Ian Fleming, author and James Bond creator, 56, heart attack

Errol Flynn, actor, 50, heart attack

James Franciscus, actor, 57, emphysema

Sigmund Freud, 83, cancer of the jaw

Clark Gable, actor, 59, heart attack

Jerry Garcia, Grateful Dead musician, 53, heart attack

A. Bartlett Giamatti, baseball commissioner and Yale president, 53, heart attack

Arthur Godfrey, actor, 80, emphysema

Roberto Goizueta, Coca Cola CEO, 65, lung cancer

John Gotti, celebrity gangster and Cuban cigar smoker, 61, throat cancer

Betty Grable, actress, 56, lung cancer

Ulysses S. Grant, 18th president, 63, throat cancer

George Harrison, Beatle, 58, throat and lung cancer

Susan Hayward, actress, 55, lung cancer

Hubert Humphrey, politician, 66, bladder cancer

Chet Huntley, reporter, 62, lung cancer

John Huston, director, 81, emphysema

Burl Ives, actor, 85, mouth cancer

Dennis James, game show host, 79, lung cancer

David Janssen, actor, 49, heart attack

Boris Karloff, actor, 81, heart and lung disease

Stubby Kaye, actor, 79, lung cancer

Buster Keaton, actor, 70, emphysema

Brian Keith, actor, 75, lung cancer (actual death a suicide)

Alan King, comedian, 76, lung cancer

King Edward VII of England, Queen Victoria's son, 69, pneumonia, heart disease and emphysema

King Edward VIII of England, Prince of Wales after his abdication, 77, throat cancer

King George V of England, 70, chronic bronchitis and respiratory failure

King George VI of England, Queen Elizabeth's father, 56, lung cancer and heart attack

Caroline Knapp, author (*Drinking: a Love Study*), 42, lung cancer

Ernie Kovacs, TV personality, 43, from auto accident while he was trying to light up his trademark cigar

Michael Landon, actor, 54, pancreatic cancer

Alan Jay Lerner, lyricist, 67, lung cancer

Larry Linville, Frank Burns in MASH TV series, 60, lung cancer

Julie London, singer, 74, stroke

Paul Lynde, actor and comedian, 55, heart attack

Lloyd Mangrum, golfer, 59, heart attack

Roger Maris, baseball player, 51, lung cancer (this is disputed; he may have died from lymphoma)

Dean Martin, singer, 78, emphysema

Lee Marvin, actor, 63, emphysema and heart failure

Walter Matthau, actor, 79, heart attack

Doug McClure, actor, 56, lung cancer

Wayne McClaren, former Marlboro Man, 51, lung cancer

Kathleen McGrath, U.S. Navy captain and the first woman to command a Navy warship, 50, lung cancer
(I was unable to verify that she was a smoker - editor)

Audrey Meadows, actress, 71, lung cancer

Melina Mercouri, actress, 68, lung cancer

Robert Mitchum, actor, 79, lung cancer and emphysema

Gary Moore, game show host, 78, emphysema

Gary Morton, Lucille Ball's second husband, 74, lung cancer

Edward Mulhare, actor, 74, lung cancer

Edward R. Murrow, newscaster, 57, lung cancer

Pat Nixon, 81, lung cancer

Roy Orbison, singer, 52, heart attack

Jesse Owens, track star, 66, lung cancer

Bert Parks, actor and singer, 77, lung cancer

George Peppard, actor, 65, lung cancer

Vincent Price, actor, 84, lung cancer

Princess Margaret, 71, stroke

Johnny Paycheck, country singer, 64, emphysema

Dick Powell, actor, 59, lung cancer

Giacomo Puccini, opera composer, 65, throat cancer

Eddie Rabbit, singer, 56, lung cancer

Harry Reasoner, reporter, 68, lung cancer

Pee Wee Reese, baseball player, 81, lung cancer

Lee Remick, actress, 55, lung cancer

R.J. Reynolds, Sr., founder of the RJR Tobacco Company, 67, pancreatic cancer

R.J. Reynolds, Jr. 58, emphysema

R.J. Reynolds, III, 60, emphysema

Babe Ruth, 52, throat cancer

George C. Scott, actor, 71, ruptured abdominal aortic aneurysm

Rod Serling, "Twilight Zone", 51, heart attack

Ernest Shackleton, Antarctic explorer, 46, heart attack

Dmitri Shostakovich, composer, 69

Frank Sinatra, 82, heart attack

Alexander Spears, Chairman of Lorillard and ex-smoker, 68, lung cancer
   (one of the tobacco executives who testified before Congress in 1994 that nicotine was not addictive)

Barbara Stanwyck, actress, 82, heart failure

Ed Sullivan, TV host, 72, lung cancer

William Talman, lost all of his 251 TV court cases to Perry Mason, 53, lung cancer

Gene Tierney, actress and former JFK flame, 70, emphysema

Spencer Tracy, actor, 66, heart attack

Sarah Vaughan, singer, 66, lung cancer

John Wayne, actor, 72, lung cancer

Carl Wilson, Beach Boys lead guitarist, 51, lung cancer

Wolfman Jack, disc jockey, 57, heart attack

Dick York, actor, 61, emphysema

Coleman Young, Detroit mayor, 79, emphysema
                          (From Tobacco Control, Winter 1994, p. 301, ASH Review, March-April 1993
               "A Few of our Losses…" at www.tobacco.org, and other media sources, including www.google.com)

1.   The deaths of Presidents LBJ and FDR were related to smoking.          Tobacco Control, Winter 1994, p. 305

2.   Yul Brynner died from smoking. Alan Jay Lerner, who gave Yul Brynner's eulogy, died from smoking. And
     Leonard Bernstein, who gave Alan Jay Lerner's eulogy, died from smoking.          Joel Dunnington, MD

3.   Actor Kevin Spacey chain smoked while eating organic food during an interview with Us magazine.
                                                                  Tobacco Control, Summer 1997, p. 143

4.   Doris Duke, whom the media called "The Richest Girl in the World", died at age 80 in 1993. Her father,
     tobacco magnate "Buck" Duke, left her $300 million when he died in 1925, after giving $107 million to found
     Duke University. She gave away $1 billion during her lifetime and left an estate worth $1.2 billion, most willed
     to charity.          New York Times, November 2, 1993, p. A13 and Associated Press, October 29, 1993

5.   Jacqueline Kennedy Onassis was "a lifelong chain smoker away from the cameras who reportedly stopped only
     when she was given the cancer diagnosis."          Tobacco Free Youth Reporter, Summer 1994, p. 11

6.   RJ Reynolds Sr., founder of the tobacco company bearing his name, was a tobacco chewer and died of
     pancreatic cancer at age 67. RJR Jr. was a cigarette smoker and died of emphysema at age 58. RJR III smoked
     cigarettes and died of emphysema at age 60.          Tobacco Control, Spring 1995, p. 95

7. The Bowman Gray School of Medicine, a cancer research center, is named for a former president of the RJ Reynolds Tobacco Co. San Francisco Chronicle, April 28, 1994

8. Columnist Herb Caen of the San Francisco Chronicle died in 1997 of lung cancer at age 80, more than 30 years after he quit smoking.

9. Actor James Garner in 1997 at age 68 gave up cigarettes after smoking a pack a day for 55 years, after having had heart and vascular surgery. USA Today, February 14, 1997, p. 2D

10. In 1996 during his final interview, actor Robert Mitchum interrupted breathing oxygen with smoke breaks. He died at age 79 of emphysema and lung cancer Biography, Arts and Entertainment television

11. John Wayne, a heavy smoker, recovered from lung cancer diagnosed at age 57 when his left lung was removed. He died from stomach cancer at age 72. Biography, Arts and Entertainment television

12. Hubert Humphrey, who died of bladder cancer, smoked two packs a day for much of his life.
Associated Press, February 9, 1998

13. Jesse Owens promoted Chesterfields in TV ads in the late 1960's. Cancer Wars, PBS television, 1998

14. Frank Sinatra was buried with some of his favorite things, including a bottle of Jack Daniels whiskey and a pack of Camels. May 24, 1998 media report

15. Football icon Charlie Connerly of the New York Giants was the first Marlboro Man.
Frontline, PBS television, May 1998

16. Al Gore's sister, Nancy Gore Hunger, died of lung cancer in 1984 at age 46.
US News and World Report, August 21, 1995, p. 15

17. Al Gore was a one pack a day smoker from 1968 to 1973. Washington Post National Weekly Edition, January 2000

18. Roger Maris, a cigarette smoker, appeared in Camel ads in the 1960's, and died from lung cancer at age 51.
Buffalo News, August 30, 1998, p. B2

19. From USA Weekend magazine, February 7, 1999, about actor Mel Gibson: "He is fidgety. Wired. Kicking a 30-year habit, he finally stopped smoking four months ago with the help of the antidepressant Zyban."

20. In 1941, "Times Square was graced with a 30-foot-high Joe (DiMaggio), announcing that Camels never irritated his throat." Newsweek, March 22, 1999, p. 54

21. King Hussein of Jordan smoked Marlboro Lights. Newsweek, February 15, 1999, p. 39

22. In 1964, golfer Arnold Palmer quit smoking and gave up the $10,000 a year he was being paid to throw an L&M on the green and then pick it up and take a puff after putting. Within 6 months, he had gained 20 pounds and resumed smoking, not to quit for good until 1975. Reader's Digest, April 1992

23. In the 1960's, Jack Nicklaus was a pack a day smoker, but unlike Arnold Palmer, he did not smoke on the course. The Story of Golf, CBS sports, April 8, 2000

24. Nick Price, the world's top-ranked golfer at the time, appeared at a tournament in 1994 in South Africa wearing a shirt and carrying a golf bag both with the Camel cigarette logo. His endorsement fee was not disclosed.
Golf magazine, February 1995, p. 36

25. One of the few professional golfers who still smoke is former PGA and British Open champion John Daly.

26. "I've quit too much other stuff to worry about quitting smoking."

27. "This is the wrong tournament to be talking about quitting smoking."
28. Golfer John Daly at the European Tour event sponsored by Benson and Hedges (Golf World, May 17, 2002)

29. "I detest the fact that I endorsed cigarettes years ago; I didn't even smoke. Lucky Strikes, Chesterfields, Granger pipe tobacco – I endorsed them all. At the Greenbriar they had those ads on the walls as decoration. I made them take them all down."
            Sam Snead in an interview several months before he died at age 89 (Golf Digest, April 2002, p. 194)

30. "I stayed in shape because I didn't smoke or drink. I advertised Lucky Strikes, Chesterfields and Viceroys, but I never smoked them."            Sam Snead at age 88 Golf World, June 16, 2000

31. George Knudson, Canada's most famous golfer who won eight PGA events in the 1960's and 1970's, died of lung cancer at age 51.            Journal of the American Medical Association, May 28, 1997, p. 1652

32. Referring to David Duval and Tiger Woods, Golf World magazine commented (April 23, 1999, p. 14): "It is disappointing that our game's two top-ranked players are among the worst culprits of this new and ever more common expression: spitting." (Duval at the time was a smokeless tobacco user.)

33. Pierce Brosnan (who is a smoker) did not smoke on screen and drove a BMW with a sign "Please do not smoke" on the dashboard in the 1999 Bond movie *The World Is Not Enough.*
            San Francisco Chronicle, February 25, 1999, p. D10

34. Mark Twain smoked at least 22 cigars a day, perhaps as many as 40.            Cigar Aficionado, December 1999

35. Sigmund Freud smoked 20 cigars a day, and had 30 operations for throat cancer before he died.

36. At age 98, George Burns said: "If I had taken my doctor's advice and quit smoking when he advised me to, I wouldn't have lived to go to his funeral."            Cigar Aficionado, December 1999

37. A cigarette butt smoked by Greta Garbo once fetched $352 at a Hollywood auction.
            Washington Post National Weekly Edition, November 29, 1999, p. 25

38. Evarts Graham, the renowned thoracic surgeon from Washington University in St. Louis, who performed the first pneumonectomy for lung cancer in the 1930's, stopped smoking in 1953, but he died of lung cancer in 1957.

39. Actor Steve McQueen died of lung cancer at age 50 and was a smoker, but his cancer type was mesothelioma, normally associated with asbestos exposure, not smoking. Whether he ever smoked Kents with micronite asbestos filters when they were marketed in the 1950's is not clear.
            Information courtesy of Lonnie Bristow, M.D., past president, American Medical Association.

40. "Sammy Davis, Jr. smoked two packs of cigarettes a day, although this fact was omitted from People magazine's cover story when he died of throat cancer in 1990. Tobacco advertising is important to Time Warner, Inc., publisher of Time, Life, People, and Fortune. And if people who smoke have less time on earth to enjoy life – well that's their problem, because by accepting tobacco ads, Time makes a Fortune."
            From *Kids Say Don't Smoke*, Andrew Tobias

41. Jackie Gleason appears on one list of "tobacco deaths." However, his website (access via google.com) lists his death at age 71 as from liver and colon cancer, which would not be smoking-related.

42. Bing Crosby died of a heart attack age 73. Although he is on one list of "tobacco deaths" and was a Chesterfields spokesman in the late 1940's, I have not been able to determine whether he smoked – editor.
43. Groucho Marx had a heart attack and strokes in his 80's, and died of pneumonia at age 86 – whether his death was due to longtime cigar smoking is unclear.

44. "Oh the irony, Russell Crowe won wide acclaim in the film *The Insider* as a fired tobacco-company executive whose whistle-blowing interview with *60 Minutes* never aired on account of its incendiary content. Now the actor has got the Australian version of the news program in trouble by lighting up during an interview that did air – twice. Crowe chain-smoked on the show and at one point brandished a pack of Marlboros. The following week, during its 'Mailbag' segment, *60 Minutes* showed portions of the footage again after viewers wrote in to complain about Crowe's habit."                                                    Time, July 29, 2002, p. 68

45. National media reported in September 2002 that Johnny Carson, 76, and lifelong smoker, suffers from emphysema.

46. The world's oldest person as well as oldest smoker, Jeanne Calment, died in 1997 in France at the age of 122.
*Tobacco* (Gately), p. 358

47. "A customary and extremely important comfort in the life of the guerrilla fighter is a smoke."
Che Guevara, *Guerilla Warfare*, 1961

48. "I would rather die with a cigar in my mouth than boots on my feet."
Daryl F. Zanuck, head of production at Warner Brothers, 1925

49. Model Christy Turlington quit smoking in 1994 and has crusaded against smoking since her father died of lung cancer in 1997, and has announced that she has early stage emphysema.   Newsweek, December 11, 2000, p. 87

50. True or false? Jennifer Aniston and Brad Pitt have stopped smoking in order to have a baby. "False," says Aniston. "We do want to have a baby. We will eventually quit smoking."
Quote from Time, August 19, 2002, p. 59

51. Tennis star Pancho Gonzalez was one of the few regular smokers in his sport.
*You Cannot Be Serious*, John McEnroe, Putnam's Sons, 2002

52. Prominent public health and tobacco control advocate John Slade, M.D., died in early 2002 at age 52.
Tobacco Control, June 2002, p. 162

53. Alan Landers, a former model for Winston cigarettes and Tiparillo cigars, now devotes his time to speaking out against tobacco marketing to children. He is a survivor of smoking-induced lung cancer, open heart surgery, emphysema, and reconstructed vocal cords.
11th World Conference on Tobacco or Health, Chicago, 2000, Abstract EPC 12

54. My name is Patrick Reynolds. My grandfather, R.J. Reynolds founded the tobacco company that makes Camels, Winstons, and Salems. We've heard the tobacco industry say there are no ill effects caused by smoking. Well, they ought to look at the R.J. Reynolds Family. My grandfather chewed tobacco and died of cancer. My father, R.J. Reynolds, Jr., smoked heavily and died of emphysema. My mother smoked and had emphysema and heart disease. My two aunts, also heavy smokers, died of emphysema and cancer. Currently three of my older brothers who smoke have emphysema. I smoked for 10 years and have small-airways lung disease. Now tell me. Do you think the cigarette companies are being truthful when they say smoking isn't harmful?
Patrick Reynolds, in a public-service spot prepared by Tony Schwartz.Joel Dunnington, M.D.

55. From an interview with 70-year-old Academy Award winner Peter O'Toole: "O'Toole consumes innumerable unfiltered Gauloises, each carefully sleeved in a cigarette holder..."       Newsweek, March 24, 2003, p. 55

56. In August 2002, German Formula One race car driver Michael Schumacher, bedecked with Marlboro patches as always, won his record tenth race of the season. He also holds the record for most Grand Prix wins, 63.
San Francisco Chronicle

57. "Arnold Schwarzenegger resigned in 1993 as chairman of the President's Council on Physical Fitness and Sports. At the same time, this fitness icon appeared virtually everywhere with a cigar dangling from his mouth.

To millions of kids who look up to him as one of the finest specimens of virility, health, strength and sex appeal, Schwarzenegger is setting a dangerous double standard. Welcome to the STAT Hall of Shame, Arnold."

Tobacco Free Youth Reporter, Summer 1993

58. John McMorran, the oldest living American man and fourth-oldest person in the world, died in 2003 at age 113. His obituary mentioned that he quit smoking cigars at age 97. Wire services report, February 25, 2003

# CHAPTER 44
# HUMOR

1. In the 1920's Lucky Strikes were promoted by famous opera singers. Tenor Giovanni Martinelli was later challenged about an ad where he claimed that "Luckies" did not irritate his throat. "How could they?" he replied. "I have never smoked."
Reader's Digest, April 1992

2. An award-winning poster by a 10 year old New York girl showed a skeleton with a cowboy hat riding a horse through a cemetery with the slogan "Come to where the cancer is."
*Kids Say Don't Smoke*

3. "An Arab Tale: Smoking is good for you because:
   - If you smoke enough you will smell so bad that dogs won't bite you
   - If you smoke enough you will cough even in your sleep and this will deter bank robbers who will think you are awake."
*Smoking: Third World Alert*, Uma Nath, 1986

4. The Minnesota Department of Health has launched an ad campaign rapping the tobacco industry for using images of glamour and success. One shows two male ad executives admiring a billboard of a slim, sexy woman smoking a cigarette. One proclaims "Women will love it." The woman on the billboard comes to life and snuffs out her cigarette on his head. Another billboard shows three women smoking and the slogan: "Women are making the rush to rich flavor." As some of the panels peel off the billboard, the message changes to say: "Women are making us rich."
Associated Press, September 1992

5. "The young couple traveling in a crowded train from the seashore to London started out necking. But one thing led to another, and soon they were engaged in passionate lovemaking. Passengers were stunned by the display, but managed to keep stiff upper lips until the couple got around to the final act of their amorous liaison: lighting up in a nonsmoking compartment. That was going a bit too far. Outraged riders stormed the train porters with complaints, and police arrested the man and woman when they got off. A judge fined them $240 each for the smoking and the indecent conduct."
Reported in Life Magazine, October, 1992

6. On a recent trip to Scotland, I stayed with my 73-year-old cousin. One morning she said "Where's the newspaper? I want to see who quit smoking." Amazed at this, I asked "Do they publish the names of people who quit smoking in the Scottish newspapers?" "Aye", she said, "in the obituary column."
Letter published in Dear Abby, February 1993

7. "My neighbor stopped smoking yesterday. He is survived by a wife and child."
San Francisco Chronicle, April 24, 1994 (Herb Caen)

8. "Houston is famous for big deals, big domes, and individuals who make up their minds. You decide...Dakota or Marlboro."
Ad for Dakota, a new cigarette designed for young virile females who "do what their boyfriends tell them to do."

9. "Houston, home of the largest medical center in the world, asks you to make up your mind; Dakota tumors or Marlboro radiation treatments? You decide...is it going to be Dakota, DaCough, DaCancer or DaCoffin?"
Ad from DOC (Doctors Ought to Care) running simultaneously in 1988
Editor note: because of bad publicity, the brand was later withdrawn from the market.

10. A raunchy diatribe in one of Steve Martin's routines concerns flatulence. When a young woman asks: "Do you mind if I smoke?" his reply is "Not at all; do you mind if I fart?"
San Francisco Chronicle, June 25, 1993 (Art Hoppe)

11. Examples of DOC posters available are one of a macho man with his shirt unbuttoned and a cigarette protruding from his nose with the caption "I Smoke for Smell." Another mimics the Newport "Alive with Pleasure" theme with Newcorpse Dead with Cancer.

12. An American Cancer Society poster has a picture of a dog, a pig, a deer, and a duck each with a lighted cigarette dangling from its mouth and the logo "It looks just as stupid when you do it." Another counterad has a coffin containing cigarettes and the title "The Merit Crush-Proof Box."

13. Among themselves, Tobacco Institute staff refer to the Department of Health and Human Services (HHS) as Helpless, Hopeless, and Stupid. 　　　　　　　　　　　Tobacco Control, Spring 1996, p. 64 (Christopher Buckley)

14. Dr. Simon Chapman comments on the concept of "smokers' rights":
    ...a generally unspecified allusion to an inalienable assumption of rights said to apply to smokers. These alleged rights bear some reflection against the history of arguably comparable "rights" that have long since eroded.

    In Elizabethan England, the free exercise of flatulence even among company was considered normal and not proscribed by considerations of politeness or offensiveness. Similarly, public expectoration was commonplace across all social classes in Victorian and Edwardian England, and the practice remains widespread in many countries today without drawing any social or legal approbation. There are some pertinent similarities between flatulence, spitting, and smoking. Each behavior is essentially personal but being not involuntary, is each capable of being exercised in both private and in public settings. In view of these parallels, it is salutary to speculate on the likely reception that would be given to earnest talk about "farters' rights" or "spitters' rights." Clearly, such terms would be greeted with derision, while "smokers' rights" continues to maintain some currency as a serious concept. 　　　　　　　　　　　International Journal of Health Services 1990; 20:425

15. "Philip Morris has announced that because of corporate downsizing, it plans to lay off two U.S. Senators."
    　　　　　　　　　As told by Ronn Owens on his KGO radio talk show, San Francisco, March 24, 1997

16. Massachusetts tobacco control advocate Greg Connolly was served by the tobacco industry with a discovery motion asking for hundreds of documents, including records of his discussions with a Reverend George Trask. As it turned out, Trask was an abolitionist who also led a campaign against tobacco, and who died in 1875.
    　　　　　　　　　　　　　　　　　　　　　　　　　Tobacco Control, Winter 1997, p. 355

17. The following newspaper notice from GASP, United Kingdom, was reproduced in the December 2000 issue of Tobacco Control, p. 349.
    REPLACEMENT SMOKERS
    A breathtaking opportunity exists for at least 300 new smokers every day to replace the previous post holders who have been 'promoted'. The ideal candidates will be young, healthy and have money to burn. No previous experience needed. Immortality an advantage.
    Excellent benefits for us with profits in the UK of over 900 million pounds per annum. The successful candidates will be rewarded with a package that includes an expensive addiction, short and long term health problems and up to 25 years of life lost. A pension scheme is unnecessary but you do pay for ours.
    Applications are invited from all groups in society. We particularly welcome applications from young women, minority ethnic groups and those on low incomes.
    See packs for details. You could join us today.

18. On one occasion, when a woman told him she had twenty-two children because she loved her husband, Groucho Marx responded, "I like my cigar, too. But I take it out of my mouth once in a while."
    　　　　　　　　　　　　　　　　　　　　　　　　　　　　　*Tobacco* (Gately), p. 250

19. The Doonsbury cartoon of January 27, 2002, where Mr. Butts converses with Mr. Jay, the marijuana cigarette:
    Mr. Jay: Hey, tough guy, how's it going?
    Mr. Butts: Great! Just got the new number in! Turns out I'm still smokin' over 400,000 folks a year! So how about you? How many did you kill?
    Mr. Jay: Uh...none
    Mr. Butts: None?
    Mr. Jay: Zippo. The only thing that I caused was 735,000 arrests.

"Hopefully, not long after the beginning of the 21$^{st}$ century, the ashtray will be viewed in much the same light we now view the spittoon–as an item for antique collectors – inviting curiosity by those whose only knowledge of smoking comes from reading history books and seeing old movies."

Donald Shopland (Seminars in Oncology, August 1990, p. 411)

# CHAPTER 45
# TOBACCO CONTROL ORGANIZATION WEBSITES

| | | |
|---|---|---|
| 1. | The American Legacy Foundation | www.americanlegacy.org |
| 2. | ASH – Action on Smoking and Health | www.ash.org |
| 3. | ASH United Kingdom | www.ash.org.uk |
| 4. | American Cancer Society | www.cancer.org/tobacco |
| 5. | Office on Smoking and Health, Centers for Disease Control and Prevention | www.cdc.gov/tobacco |
| 6. | Center for Tobacco Cessation | www.ctcinfo.org |
| 7. | Globalink – International Union Against Cancer, Geneva | www.globalink.org |
| 8. | INFACT | www.infact.org |
| 9. | American Lung Association | www.lungusa.org/tobacco |
| 10. | Mayo Clinic Nicotine Dependence Center | www.mayoclinic.org/ndc-rst |
| 11. | National Cancer Institute | www.nci.nih.gov |
| 12. | Americans for Nonsmokers' Rights | www.no-smoke.org |
| 13. | National Spit Tobacco Education Program | www.nstep.org |
| 14. | The Philip Morris website | www.philipmorrisusa.com |
| 15. | Quit Net web-based cessation services | www.quitnet.com |
| 16. | The Robert Wood Johnson Foundation | www.rwjf.org |
| 17. | DOC | www.bcm.tmc.edu/doc |
| 18. | Smoke Free Movies and Details on Hollywood and Big Tobacco | www.smokefreemovies.ucsf.edu |
| 19. | Smokescreen Action Network | www.smokescreen.org |
| 20. | Tobacco Control Resource Center and the Tobacco Products Liability Project, Northwestern University Law School, Boston | www.tobacco.neu.edu |
| 21. | News about Tobacco and Tobacco Control | www.tobacco.org |
| 22. | Tobacco Control: an International Journal | www.tobaccocontrol.com |
| 23. | The Foundation for a Smoke-Free America | www.tobaccofree.org |
| 24. | The National Center for Tobacco-Free Kids | www.tobaccofreekids.org |
| 25. | The Truth about smoke free restaurants and bars | www.tobaccoscam.ucsf.edu |
| 26. | Coalition on Smoking or health | www.tobaccodocuments.org |

# BIBLIOGRPHY
## (Books listed in alphabetical order by title)

1. *Advertising, the Uneasy Persuasion,* Michael Schudson, Basic Books, 1984.

2. *Ashes to Ashes,* Richard Kluger, Knopf, 1996.

3. *Assuming the Risk: The Mavericks, The Lawyers, And The Whistle-Blowers Who Beat Big Tobacco,* Michael Orey. Little, Brown and Company, 1999

4. *Best Practices for Comprehensive Tobacco Control Programs.* Centers for Disease Control, August 1999

5. *Cancer Wars,* Robert N. Proctor, Basic Books, 1995.

6. *Changes in Cigarette-Related Disease Risks and Their Implication for Prevention and Control,* National Cancer Institute Monograph 9, 1997.

7. *The Cigar Connoisseur,* Nathaniel and Andrew Lande, Clarkson Potter, 1997.

8. *Cigarette Confidential,* John Fahs, Berkeley Books, 1996.

9. *The Cigarette Papers,* Stanton Glantz, University of California Press, 1996.

10. *Cigarettes,* Tara Parker-Pope, The New Press, 2001.

11. *Cigarettes: the Battle over Smoking,* Ronald J. Troyer and Gerald E. Markle, Rutgers University Press, 1983.

12. *Cigarettes: What the Warning Label Doesn't Tell You,* William London, Elizabeth Whelan, Andrea Case, editors, American Council on Science and Health, 1996 (references marked *Cigarettes* in text are from this source).

13. *Cigars: Health Effects and Trends,* National Cancer Institute Monograph, 1998.

14. *Clearing the Smoke: Assessing the Science Base for Tobacco Harm Reduction,* Institute of Medicine, National Academy Press, 2001.

15. *Comprehensive Framework and Analysis of Tobacco Industry Strategies and Tactics* (draft), The Advocacy Institute, November 1994 (referenced as *Tobacco Industry Strategies* in text).

16. *Cornered: Big Tobacco at the Bar of Justice,* Peter Pringle, Henry Holt, 1998.

17. *Curbing the Epidemic: Governments and the Economics of Tobacco Control.* Prabhat Jha, editor. The World Bank, 1999

18. *Deadly Choices: Coping with Health Risks in Everyday Life,* Jeffrey Harris, Basic Books, 1993.

19. *FDA Proposed Regulations on Cigarettes and Smokeless Tobacco,* Federal Register Vol. 60 No. 155, August 11, 1987, pp. 41314-41787.

20. *The Faber Book of Smoking,* James Walton, editor, Faber and Faber, London, 2000.

21. *The Fight for Public Health,* Simon Chapman, BMJ Publishing Group, 1994.

22. *Global Aggression,* INFACT Annual Report, Apex Press, 1998 – A review of the influence of Philip Morris and RJR Nabisco in trade policy, and international tobacco marketing

23. *Growing Up Tobacco Free: Preventing Nicotine Addiction in Children and Youths,* BS Lynch and RJ Bonnie, editors, National Academy Press, 1994.

24. *The Harvard Guide to Women's Health,* Karen Carlson, Harvard University Press, 1996.

25. *The Health Benefits of Smoking Cessation,* A report of the Surgeon General, Department of Health and Human Services, 1990.

26. *The Health Consequences of Involuntary Smoking,* A report of the Surgeon General, Department of Health and Human Services, 1986.

27. *The Health Consequences of Smoking: Nicotine Addiction,* A report of the Surgeon General, Department of Health and Human Services, 1988.

28. *Health Effects of Exopsure to Environmental Tobacco Smoke: the Report of the California Environmental Protection Agency,* Amy Dunn and Lauren Zeise, editors. National Cancer Institute Smoking and Tobacco Control Mongraph 10, 1999

29. *Healthy People 2000: Health Promotion and Disease Prevention Objectives,* US Public Health Service, 1991.

30. *Holy Smoke,* G. Cabrera Infante, Harper and Row, 1985.

31. *How to Help Your Kids Choose To Be Tobacco-Free,* Robert Schwebel, Newmarket Press, 1999

32. *Interventions for Smokers: an International Perspective,* Robyn Richmond, editor, Williams and Wilkins, 1994.

33. *Kids Say Don't Smoke,* Andrew Tobias, Workman, 1991.

34. *Koop,* C. Everett Koop, M.D., Random House, 1991.

35. *Kretek: the Culture and Heritage of Indonesia's Clove Cigarettes,* Mark Hanusc, Equinox Publishers, 2000.

36. *The Last Puff: Ex-smokers Share the Secrets of their Success,* John Farquher and Gene Spiller, W.W. Norton, 1990

37. *Legislative Action to Combat the World Tobacco Epidemic,* Ruth Roemer, World Health Organization, 1993.

38. *Licit and Illicit Drugs,* Edward M. Brecher, Little, Brown, 1972.

39. *Merchants of Death: the American Tobacco Industry,* Larry White, William Morrow and Co., 1988.

40. *Minorities and Cancer,* Lovell A. Jones, Springer-Verlag, 1989.

41. *Mortality from Smoking in Developed Countries 1950-2000,* Richard Peto, Alan Lopez et al, Oxford University Press, 1994.

42. *Nicotine: An Old-Fashioned Addiction,* Jack E. Henningfield, Chelsea House Publishers, 1985.

43. *Nicotine Addiction,* C. Tracy Orleans and John Slade, editors, Oxford University Press, 1993.

44. *Nicotine and Public Health,* Roberta Ferrence, John Slade, Robin Room, and Marilyn Pope, editors, American Public Health Association, 2000.

45. *Nicotine Safety and Toxicity,* Neil L. Benowitz, editor, Oxford University Press, 1998

46. *No Smoking: the Ethical Issues,* Robert E. Goodin, University of Chicago Press, 1989.

47. *No Stranger to Tears,* William G. Cahan, Random House, 1992.

48. *A Passion for Cigars,* Joel Sherman, Andrews and McNeal, 1996

49. *The Passionate Nonsmoker's Bill of Rights,* Steve Allen and Bill Adler, William Morrow & Co., 1989.

50. *The People Versus Big Tobacco,* Carrick Mollenkamp, Bloomberg Press, 1998.

51. *Preventing Tobacco Use Among Young People,* A report of the Surgeon General, Department of Health and Human Services, 1994.

52. *Proceedings of the 10th World Conference on Tobacco or Health,* Beijing, China, 24-28 August 1997.

53. *A Question of Intent: a Great American Battle with a Deadly Industry,* David Kessler, Public Affairs, 2001.

54. *Reducing the Health Consequences of Smoking: 25 Years of Progress,* A report of Surgeon General, Department of Health and Human Services, 1989.

55. *Reducing Tobacco Use,* A report of the Surgeon General, Department of Health and Human Services, 2000.

56. *Respiratory Health Effects of Passive Smoking,* Environmental Protection Agency, 1993.

57. *The Rise and Fall of the Cigarette: A Cultural History of Smoking in the United States,* Allen Brandt, Basic Books, This book was originally scheduled for publication in 1998, but now has been delayed to early 2004 according to the publisher.

58. *Smart Ways to Stay Young and Healthy,* Bradley Gascoigne MD, Ronin Publishing, 1992.

59. *Smoke and Mirrors: The Canadian Tobacco War,* Rob Cunningham, International Development Research Centre, 1996.

60. *Smoke in their Eyes: Lessons in Movement Leadership from the Tobacco Wars,* Michael Pertschuk, Vanderbilt University Press, 2001.

61. *Smoke Ring,* Peter Taylor, The Bodley Head, 1984.

62. *Smoked: Why Joe Camel is Still Smiling,* Mike Males, Common Courage Press, 1999

63. *Smokescreen,* Philip Hilts, Addison-Wesley, 1996.

64. *Smokeless Tobacco or Health,* Smoking and Tobacco Control Monograph 2, National Institutes of Health, 1992.

65. *Smoking: Making the Risky Decision,* W. Kip Viscusi, Oxford University Press, 1992.

66. *Smoking: Risk, Perception, and Policy,* Paul Slovic, editor, Sage Publications, 2001.

67. *Smoking: Third World Alert,* Uma Nath, Oxford University Press, 1986.

68. *Smoking Policy: Law, Politics, and Culture,* Robert L. Rabin and Stephen Sugarman, Oxford University Press, 1993.

69. *Smoking: The Artificial Passion,* David Krogh, W.H. Freeman and Co., 1991

70. *Sold American,* American Tobacco Company, 1954.

71. *Spit Tobacco and Youth,* Office of the Surgeon General, Department of Health and Human Services, 1992.

72. *State of Health Atlas,* Judith Mackay, Touchstone Press, 1993.

73. *State Tobacco Control Highlights 1996,* Centers for Disease Control, 1996.

74. *Stop the Sale, Prevent the Addiction,* Program Guide for Reducing Youth Access to Tobacco, Centers for Disease Control, 1995.

75. *The Story of Tobacco in America,* Joseph C. Robert, University of North Carolina Press, 1949.

76. *Strategies to Control Tobacco Use in the United States,* US Department of Health and Human Services, 1991.

77. *Taken at the Flood: the Story of Albert Lasker,* John Gunther, Harper and Brothers, 1960.

78. *Thank You for Smoking,* Christopher Buckley, Random House, 1994.

79. *They Satisfy: the Cigarette in American Life,* Robert Sobel, Anchor Books, 1978.

80. *Tobacco,* Mark S. Gold, Plenum Press, 1995.

81. *Tobacco: A Major International Health Hazard,* D. Zaridze, Oxford University Press, 1987.

82. *Tobacco Advertising: the Great Seduction,* Gerard Petrone, Schiffer Publishing, 1996.

83. *Tobacco and Americans,* Robert K. Heimann, McGraw Hill, 1960.

84. *The Tobacco Atlas,* Judith Mackay and Michael Eriksen, World Health Organization, 2002.

85. *Tobacco in Australia: Facts and Issues, 1995,* Quit Victoria, P.O. Box 888, Carlton South, Victoria 3053, Australia.

86. *Tobacco Biology and Politics,* Stanton Glantz, Ph.D., Health Edco, 1999 (second edition). The reference pages cited in the text are from the 1992 first edition.

87. *Tobacco and the Clinician,* Smoking and Tobacco Control Monograph 5, National Institutes of Health, 1994.

88. *Tobacco Control Country Profiles,* Corrao MA, Guindon GE, Sharma N., Shokoohi DF (editors), American Cancer Society, 2000

89. *Tobacco Control Policies in Developing Countries,* Prabhat Jha and Frank Chaloupka, editors, Oxford University Press, 1999

90. *Tobacco Control in the Third World,* Simon Chapman, International Organization of Consumers Unions, Penang, Malaysia, 1990.

91. *The Tobacco Epidemic,* C. T. Bolliger and Karl Fagerstrom, S. Karger, 1998.

92. *Tobacco: the Growing Epidemic,* Rushan Lu, Judith Mackay, Shiru Niu, and Richard Peto, Springer, 2000. (Proceedings of the Tenth World Conference on Tobacco or Health, August 1997, Beijing, China)

93.  *Tobacco and Health,* Karen Slama, editor, Plenum Press, 1995.

94.  *Tobacco or Health: a Global Status Report,* World Health Organization, 1997.

95.  *Tobacco in History,* Jordan Goodman, Routledge, 1993.

96.  *Tobacco Industry Strategies* (see reference No. 12)

97.  *Tobacco Tycoon* (James Buchanan Duke), John K. Winkler, Random House, 1942.

98.  *Tobacco Use Among U.S. Racial/Ethnic Minority Groups*, A Report of the Surgeon General, 1998

99.  *Tobacco Use: An American Crisis,* American Medical Association, 1993.

100. *Tobacco Use in California: A Focus on Preventing Uptake in Adolescents,* California Department of Health Services, 1992.

101. *Tobacco War: Inside the California Battles*, Stanton Glantz and Edith Balbach, Universty of Califorina Press, 2000

102. *Trust Us. We're the Tobacco Industry*, Ross Hammond and Andy Rowell, Campaign for Tobacco-Free Kids and Action on Smoking and Health – U.K., 2001

103. *Women and Smoking*, a report of the Surgeon General, Department of Health and Human Services, 2001.

104. *1992 Worldwide Survey of Substance Abuse and Health Behaviors among Military Personnel*, Robert Bray, Research Triangle Institute, December 1992.

105. *1995 Department of Defense Survey of Health Related Behaviors Among Military Personnel*, Robert Bray, Research Triangle Institute, December 1995.

## Pertinent U.S. Surgeon General's Reports

| | |
|---|---|
| 1964 | *Smoking and Health: Report of the Advisory Committee to the Surgeon General of the Public Health Service* |
| 1967 to 1979 | Yearly reports, *The Health Consequences of Smoking* |
| 1980 | *The Health Consequences of Smoking for Women* |
| 1981 | *The Health Consequences of Smoking, The Changing Cigarette* |
| 1982 | *The Health Consequences of Smoking - Cancer* |
| 1983 | *The Health Consequences of Smoking - Cardiovascular Disease* |
| 1984 | *The Health Consequences of Smoking – Chronic Obstructive Lung Disease* |
| 1985 | *The Health Consequences of Smoking – Cancer and Chronic Lung Disease in the Workplace* |
| 1986 | *The Health Consequences of Involuntary Smoking* |
| 1988 | *The Health Consequences of Smoking – Nicotine Addiction* |
| 1989 | *Reducing the Health Consequences of Smoking - 25 Years of Progress* |

| 1990 | *The Health Benefits of Smoking Cessation* |
| 1992 | *Smoking in the Americas* |
| 1994 | *Preventing Tobacco Use Among Young People* |
| 1998 | *Tobacco Use Among U.S. Racial/Ethnic Minority Groups* |
| 2000 | *Reducing Tobacco Use* |
| 2001 | *Women and Smoking* |
| 2004 | *The Health Consequnces of Smoking* |

# INDEX
### (Bold Indicates Chapter Headings)

carpal tunnel syndrome, 133
Carter, Grady, 325
Cartier, Jacques, 28, 34
Casey, Ben, 65, 66, 296

Cash, Pat, 302
Castano lawsuit, 402
Castro, Fidel, 181, 184, 252
cataracts, 121
cervical cancer, 102, 237
cessation, 102, 105, 111, 114, 115, 116, 117, 118, 122,
    123, 145, 146, 158, 161, 207, 208, 212, 214, 215,
    217, 218, 219, 220, 221, 222, 223, 224, 225, 226,
    229, 231, 252, 301, 312, 317, 368, 369, 377, 412,
    421, 436, 438, 451, 476
Chamberlain, Richard, 65
Chesterfield cigarettes, 52, 54, 55, 57, 58, 59, 61, 63,
    64, 158, 290, 291, 293, 294, 308, 403
chewing tobacco, 10, 13, 17, 27, 28, 37, 38, 40, 42, 43,
    45, 46, 47, 48, 50, 51, 54, 56, 58, 67, 111, 159, 167,
    169, 170, 171, 172, 173, 174, 175, 176, 201, 206,
    217, 244, 247, 271, 272, 390, 427, see also
    smokeless tobacco
children and smoking, 7, 8, 12, 14, 16, 20, 31, 35, 48,
    53, 68, 71, 72, 73, 74, 75, 76, 77, 78, 79, 82, 83, 87,
    88, 89, 90, 103, 125, 126, 127, 141, 142, 143, 145,
    146, 149, 150, **151-168**, 169, 170, 174, 190, 199,
    207, 222, 223, 229, 250, 254, 255, 256, 257, 260,
    268, 271, 272, 273, 275, 277, 278, 284, 287, 295,
    298, 299, 300, 303, 306, 307, 308, 309, 310, 311,
    313, 314, 325, 360, 362, 363, 364, 365, 366, 369,
    374, 378, 380, 382, 391, 396, 398, 409, 422, 423,
    424, 426, 428, 429, 430, 447, 450, 452, 454, 455,
    457, 459, 460, 462, 471, 474
Chile, 249, 252, 254, 334
Chilean grapes, 191
China, 10, 13, 14, 15, 51, 71, 72, 75, 95, 103, 105, 118,
    131, 213, 237, 248, 249, 250, 254, 263, 270, 277,
    278, 279, 280, 281, 282, 283, 287, 288, 327, 328,
    329, 332, 336, 339, 342, 344, 345, 346, 348, 352,
    354, 361, 411, 431, 455, 458, 479, 480
cholesterol, 9, 84, 108, 109, 113, 116, 153, 219, 372
chronic obstructive pulmonary disease, 15, 118, 119,
    120, 185, 186, 282
Churchill, Winston, 61, 62, 181, 365
cigarette butts, 199, 447, 452
Cigarette Labeling and Advertising Act, 66, 301, 370,
    379
cigars, 10, 13, 17, 21, 26, 31, 35, 37, 38, 40, 41, 42, 43,
    44, 45, 46, 47, 50, 51, 54, 56, 61, 62, 65, 67, 70,
    160, 174, 180, 181, 182, 183, 184, 185, 186, 187,
    195, 207, 218, 232, 367, 430, 460, 461, 463, 470,
    471, 472
Cipollone, Rose, 400
City University of New York, 373
Civil War, 253

cleft lip, 147
Cleveland, President Grover, 464
Clinton, Bill, 80, 183, 359, 362, 363, 364, 366, 369,
    374, 381, 383, 384, 385, 391, 392, 434, 438, 439
Clooney, Rosemary, 464
clove cigarettes, 189, 288
Cobb, Ty, 48, 290, 464
cocaine, 45, 48, 140, 148, 180, 197, 199, 200, 201,
    202, 203, 206, 207, 228, 229, 230, 333, 336, 351
coffee, 41, 56, 60, 196, 201, 204, 253, 288, 292, 319,
    334, 341, 344, 379, 405, 451, 453
Cole, Nat "King," 464
colic, 36, 132, 133, 140
colon cancer, 96, 105, 106, 470
Colorado, 77, 170, 174, 314, 336, 371, 394, 395, 433,
    435, 446
Colucci, Anthony, 330
Columbia, 7, 20, 37, 38, 75, 155, 167, 168, 218, 229,
    231, 238, 250, 251, 252, 253, 298, 355, 406, 420,
    428, 445
Columbus, Christopher, 26, 27, 194
congenital anomalies, 147
congress, 13, 48, 66, 90, 93, 178, 198, 199, 200, 201,
    204, 246, 275, 296, 297, 315, 317, 322, 327, 333,
    338, 342, 343, 344, 363, 364, 365, 366, 367, 368,
    370, 371, 375, 376, **379-400**, 401, 402, 403, 407,
    418, 432, 439, 457, 468
Connolly, Greg, 18, 248, 249, 263, 264, 350, 389, 401,
    406, 474
Connors, Chuck, 464
Conrad, Kent, 429
Consumer Product Safety Act, 380
Cooper, Gary, 465
COPD, see Chronic Obstructive Pulmonary Disease
Copenhagen smokeless tobacco, 170, 176, 177, 178,
    179, 379
coronary heart disease, 83, 84, 100, 108, 109, 110,
    112, 113, 114, 116, 185, 186, 225, 226, 235, 425
cotinine, 70, 73, 74, 75, 76, 77, 88, 127, 172, 192, 221,
    238
cough reflex, 134
Council for Tobacco Research, 165, 316, 319, 322,
    323, 324, 325, 371, 372, 407
counteradvertising, 66
Covington & Burling, 390
Coward, Noel, 464
Crawford, Victor, 381, 385, 393
Crimean War, 39
Crohn's disease, 75, 128, 132, 207
cruise ship smoking bans, 444
cryptococcus infection, 131
Cuba, 26, 27, 37, 40, 65, 180, 181, 184, 252, 253
Cuban cigars, 180, 181, 184, 186, 465
Cullman, Joseph, 66, 147, 335, 337, 372
cyanide, 130, 187, 188, 191, 193, 229
cystic fibrosis, 73

France, 29, 36, 37, 39, 55, 74, 88, 132, 150, 242, 256, 257, 259, 260, 261, 264, 290, 328, 353, 411, 428, 430, 471
Franciscus, James, 465
Frank, Stanley, 324
French, Lynn, 408, 410
Freud, Sigmund, 59, 180, 181, 195, 465, 470
fungal contamination of cigarettes, 121, 131

## G
Gable, Clark, 465
Gallup polls, 112, 196, 201, 210, 211, 216, 449, 450
Garcia, Jerry, 465
Garner, James, 221, 469
Gaston, Lucy Page, 48, 52, 53, 232
gay men, 19, 302
Gehrig, Lou, 60, 137, 292
Germany, 29, 37, 41, 47, 60, 61, 62, 63, 89, 90, 91, 96, 195, 256, 257, 258, 261, 313, 328, 336, 338, 339, 347, 353, 361, 411, 428, 430, 438
Giamatti, A. Bartlett, 465
Gibson, Mel, 450, 462, 469
Gingrich, Newt, 365, 367, 383, 385, 387, 388, 389
Glantz, Stanton, 14, 46, 70, 160, 188, 192, 228, 303, 319, 321, 322, 372, 387, 397, 399, 414, 422, 439, 441, 442, 452, 459, 460, 462, 477, 480, 481
Godfrey, Arthur, 64, 465
Goerlitz, David, 298, 299, 311
Goethe, Wolfgang von, 38
Goizueta, Roberto, 465
Goldstone, Steven, 204, 331, 405
Gore, Al, 366, 392, 460, 469
Gotti, John, 378, 465
Grable, Betty, 465
Grady, Carter, 325, 405, 410
Graham, Evarts, 59, 63, 92, 470
Grand Prix motor racing, 300, 306, 313, 335, 471
Grange, Red, 291
Grant, Ulysses, 42
Graves' disease, 125
Gray, Al, 245
Great American Smokeout, 216, 373
Great Britain, 23, 25, 30, 32, 33, 37, 44, 59, 67, 88, 111, 175, 248, 258, 259
Greece, 18, 74, 82, 85, 109, 249, 257, 261, 262, 263, 264, 353, 411, 430, 438
Greeley, Horace, 180
Gretzky, Wayne, 53, 183, 187
Group A carcinogen, 69, 78, 81
gum disease, 127

## H
Hagen, Donald, 247
Happy Days smokeless tobacco, 179
Harper, Charles, 318
Harrison, George, 465
Hart, Gary, 398

Harvard University, 7, 18, 37, 53, 54, 61, 84, 102, 106, 109, 122, 124, 125, 132, 149, 156, 159, 233, 236, 237, 272, 324, 325, 349, 366, 372, 373, 408, 444, 450, 451, 452, 478
Hatch, Orrin, 429
Hawaii, 17, 20, 22, 335, 428, 433, 442
Hayward, Susan, 465
Hazardous Substances Act, 380
health benefits of cessation, 213, 214, 224, 225, 376, 436
health care costs, 129, 144, 159, 244, 251, 367, 399, 403, 414, 415, 416, 418, 419, 420, 424, 425, 431
Health Nazis, 320, 384
hearing loss, 127, 131
heart bypass surgery, 111
heart disease, 8, 25, 44, 68, 69, 70, 81, 82, 83, 84, 101, **108-117**, 118, 120, 135, 171, 186, 196, 210, 225, 235, 237, 254, 273, 280, 282, 283, 299, 321, 322, 324, 336, 337, 371, 374, 375, 402, 418, 436, 440, 448, 449, 450, 464, 466, 471
Heiman, Robert, 317
Helms, Jesse, 216, 275, 289, 384, 385, 387, 390
Henley, Patricia, 407, 409
Henreid, Paul, 461
Heston, Charlton, 294, 295
Hill, Jon, 36, 37
hip fracture, 128, 129, 237
Hirayama, Takeshi, 81, 83, 128, 275
History of tobacco, **26-67**
Hitler, Adolf, 60, 292
HIV, 19, 25, 124, 131, 143, 219, 228, 445, 451
Ho Chi Minh, 289
Hong Kong, 136, 175, 234, 249, 250, 279, 281, 283, 284, 286, 287, 297, 339, 354, 388, 390, 411, 443
Hornung, Paul, 295
hepatitis C viris, 133
Horowitz, Milton, 406
Horrigan, Edward, 319, 373, 386
Horton, Nathan, 405, 406
hospital smoking bans, 40, 444, 445
hotel smoking bans, 20, 43, 182, 268, 271, 440, 443, 444, 457
Houston, Tom, 79, 165, 369
Huber, Gary, 27, 29, 32, 33, 49, 212, 325, 326, 400
humor, **473-475**
Humphrey, Hubert, 164
Humphrey, Hubert III, 164, 367
Hungary, 147, 249, 257, 263, 264, 265, 302
Hunt, Al, 160, 363, 390, 429
Huntley, Chet, 465
Hussein, Saddam, 186, 356
Huston, John, 466
hypertension, 9, 109, 110, 112, 114, 116, 135, 142

## I
illicit drugs, 8, 10, 11, 140, 201, **228-231**, 258, 261
immune function suppression, 133

Moss, Kate, 236

mouth cancer, see oral cancer

movies, 62, 163, 241, 276, 279, 296, 323, 340, 372, 374, 375, **459-463**

Mulhare, Edward, 467

multiple sclerosis, 132

Murrow, Edward, 467

myocardial infarction, 83, 85, 108, 110, 114, 226

## N

National Cancer Institute, 10, 13, 17, 70, 77, 78, 80, 82, 83, 95, 97, 98, 100, 101, 102, 103, 105, 106, 116, 121, 157, 160, 173, 175, 177, 182, 185, 186, 189, 190, 200, 207, 208, 213, 214, 215, 216, 237, 241, 258, 271, 277, 287, 291, 292, 298, 302, 304, 308, 321, 322, 323, 331, 335, 343, 345, 349, 364, 368, 377, 387, 389, 400, 436, 438, 447, 453, 476, 477, 478

National Smokers Alliance, 322, 371, 376, 440, 441

Native American smokers, 16, 20, 38, 141, 169, 174

Navy, 10, 47, 48, 61, 137, 242, 243, 244, 245, 246, 247, 251, 295, 419, 467

Nazi, 60, 62, 96, 97, 181, 292

neonatal intensive care, 10, 141, 146

Nepal, 137, 270, 273

Netanyahu, Binyamin, 186

Netherlands, 107, 126, 133, 134, 249, 256, 257, 258, 259, 261, 262, 264, 411, 430

Neuborne, Bert, 302

Nevada, 15, 17, 20, 22, 70, 433, 435, 437, 438, 446

New York City, 21, 63, 98, 134, 293, 296, 312, 339, 394, 431, 442, 445, 456

New Zealand, 22, 83, 84, 88, 124, 175, 255, 256, 304, 411, 428

Newport cigarettes, 67, 151, 152, 161, 163, 239, 240, 241, 299, 303, 306, 307, 309, 310, 312, 328, 329, 454, 473

NEXT cigarettes, 203

Nicklaus, Jack, 67, 469

Nicorette, 223, 224, 313, 317, 377

nicotine, 26, 29, 31, 42, 47, 48, 49, 59, 66, 69, 70, 73, 88, 95, 98, 99, 108, 111, 116, 123, 124, 126, 127, 130, 132, 133, 134, 139, 158, 161, 165, 171, 172, 173, 176, 177, 178, 179, 182, 183, 185, 186, 187, 188, 189, 190, 191, 192, **194-209**, 210, 211, 212, 213, 214, 216, 217, 218, 219, 220, 221, 222, 223, 224, 227, 230, 238, 239, 240, 241, 249, 254, 257, 271, 279, 286, 287, 288, 294, 297, 303, 310, 313, 315, 316, 317, 319, 322, 325, 327, 331, 333, 336, 337, 338, 339, 346, 350, 351, 362, 364, 365, 369, 370, 375, 377, 380, 382, 385, 386, 389, 390, 398, 401, 402, 403, 411, 422, 444, 445, 447, 449, 451, 453, 454, 468

nicotine patch, 126, 207, 221

nicotine poisoning, 133, 199

nicotine replacement therapy,

nitrosamine, 171

nitrosamines, 69, 95, 171, 187, 188, 190, 191, 214

nitrous oxide, 44, 223

Nixon, Pat, 467

Nixon, Richard, 67, 379

North Carolina, 17, 26, 29, 31, 42, 43, 49, 51, 57, 126, 127, 131, 133, 140, 165, 189, 216, 217, 275, 289, 312, 318, 319, 320, 321, 342, 343, 344, 345, 346, 352, 357, 362, 368, 372, 379, 385, 387, 404, 412, 415, 426, 428, 432, 433, 436, 437, 440, 480

Norway, 48, 54, 72, 85, 132, 140, 237, 250, 256, 258, 259, 262, 353, 411, 426, 428, 443

Novelli, William, 326, 338

Novotny, Tom, 360, 361

## O

obesity, 9, 10, 25, 133, 145, 224

occupational health and safety, 70, 436

Ochsner, Alton, 56, 92, 445

Oklahoma, 20, 22, 160, 170, 177, 393, 433, 446

Old Gold cigarettes, 58, 59, 61, 291, 292, 293, 294, 308

Oliver Twist smokeless tobacco, 179

Omni cigarettes, 214

oral cancer, 54, 103, 104, 106, 169, 171, 172, 178, 241, 390, 409, 455

oral contraceptives, 108, 114

Orbison, Roy, 467

OSHA, 81, 439, 440

Osteen, William, 362

osteoporosis, 121, 128, 129, 131, 234, 235, 237

Osler, William, 46

Owens, Jesse, 467

oxygen, 84, 113, 116, 119, 130, 133, 137, 138, 140, 142, 146, 181, 185, 226, 448, 469

ozone, 451

## P

Pakistan, 22, 90, 237, 248, 250, 270, 271, 272, 273, 347, 348

Palmer, Arnold, 67, 216, 295, 469

pancreatic cancer, 102, 187, 464, 466, 467, 468

panic attacks, 124

Parker Bowles, Camilla, 258

Parkinson's disease, 126

Parks, Bert, 467

passive smoking, 8, 38, 68, 69, 70, 74, 77, 78, 79, 80, 81, 82, 83, 84, 86, 88, 89, 95, 109, 112, 260, 273, 320, 360, 383, 407, 429, 431

Paycheck, Johnny, 467

Pearl, Raymond, 60

Peppard, George, 467

peptic ulcer, 128

perinatal deaths, 139, 141, 142, 144

periodontal disease, 127, 171

peripheral vascular disease, 108, 114

peritonsillar abscess, 130

Printed in the United States
51372LVS00001B/2